© 2003 Martin Dunitz, an imprint of the Taylor & Francis Group plc

First published in the United Kingdom in 2003 by Martin Dunitz,
an imprint of the Taylor and Francis Group plc,
11 New Fetter Lane, London EC4P 4EE

Tel.:   +44 (0) 20 7583 9855
Fax.:   +44 (0) 20 7842 2298
E-mail: info@dunitz.co.uk
Website: http://www.dunitz.co.uk

Although every effort has been made to ensure that all owners of
copyright material have been acknowledged in this publication,
we would be glad to acknowledge in subsequent reprints or editions
any omissions brought to our attention.

A CIP record for this book is available from the British Library.

ISBN 1 84184 001 7 (book)
      1 84184 337 7 (book and CD)

Distributed in the USA by
Fulfilment Center
Taylor & Francis
10650 Toebben Drive
Independence, KY 41051, USA
Toll Free Tel.: +1 800 634 7064
E-mail: taylorandfrancis@thomsonlearning.com

Distributed in Canada by
Taylor & Francis
74 Rolark Drive
Scarborough, Ontario M1R 4G2, Canada
Toll Free Tel.: +1 877 226 2237
E-mail: tal_fran@istar.ca

Distributed in the rest of the world by
Thomson Publishing Services
Cheriton House
North Way
Andover, Hampshire SP10 5BE, UK
Tel.: +44 (0)1264 332424
E-mail: salesorder.tandf@thomsonpublishingservices.co.uk

Composition by Scribe Design, Gillingham, Kent, UK
Printed and bound in Spain by Grafos SA, Arte Sobre Papel

Dedications

ABI

To my parents, Urs and Marianne, my wife, Susann, and our sons, Florian, Pascal and Dominik for their love, encouragement and accepting the lifestyle of an orthopaedic surgeon, and to my fellows for their support and questions.

JBT

In honor of my wife, Alyse, and our children, Sam and Anna, who maintained their love and tolerance during this project; and in memory of my father, Marvin, a man who continues to be deserving of my reverence.

FHF

To my wife, Hilda, our son, Gordon and our daughter, Joyce.

Contents

Contributors

Jeffrey S Abrams MD
Princeton Orthopaedic and Rehabilitation Associates
Princeton NJ
USA

Jens D Agneskirchner MD
Department of Orthopaedic Sports Medicine
Technical University of Munich
Munich, Germany

Erwin Aschauer MD
General Hospital Salzburg
Salzburg, Austria

Louis U Bigliani MD
The Shoulder Service
New York Presbyterian Hospital
Columbia-Presbyterian Medical Center Campus
New York NY, USA

Don Buford Jr MD
Sports Medicine Clinic of North Texas
Dallas TX, USA

Andreas Burkart MD
Assistant Professor
Department of Orthopaedic Sports Medicine
Technical University of Munich
Munich, Germany

Stephen S Burkhart MD
Clinical Associate Professor
Department of Orthopaedic Surgery
The University of Texas Health Science Center at San Antonio
And the San Antonio Orthopaedic Group, LLP
San Antonio TX, USA

Dann C Byck MD
Fellow, Mississippi Sports Medicine
and Orthopaedic Center
Jackson MS, USA

† Richard B Caspari MD

Louis W Catalano III MD
The Shoulder Service
New York Presbyterian Hospital
Columbia-Presbyterian Medical Center Campus
New York NY, USA

Brian S Cohen MD
Center for Advanced Orthopaedics and Sports Medicine
Adena Health System
Chillicothe OH, USA

William W Colman MD
Orthopaedic Associates of Duchess County
Lagrangeville NY, USA

Rami El Abiad MD
Department of Orthopaedic Surgery
Saint Joseph University
Beirut, Lebanon

Roger J Emery MD
Department of Trauma and Orthopaedics
St Mary's Hospital
London, UK

Guido Engel MD
Department of Orthopaedic Sports Medicine
Technical University of Munich
Munich, Germany

James C Esch MD
Tri-City Orthopaedics
Oceanside CA
and Assistant Clinical Professor
Department of Orthopaedics
University of California, San Diego, School of Medicine
San Diego CA, USA

Mark S Falworth MD
Department of Trauma and Orthopaedics
St Mary's Hospital
London, UK

Gary S Fanton MD
Sports Orthopaedic and Rehabilitation Group
Menlo Park CA, USA

Larry D Field MD
Co-Director, Upper Extremity Service
Mississippi Sports Medicine and Orthopaedic Center
Clinical Instructor, Department of Orthopaedic Surgery
University of Mississippi School of Medicine
Jackson MS, USA

Evan L Flatow MD
Lasker Professor of Orthopaedic Surgery
Chief of Shoulder Surgery
Mount Sinai Medical Center
New York NY, USA

Leesa M Galatz MD
Assistant Professor
Shoulder and Elbow Service
Washington University Department of Orthopaedics
Barnes-Jewish Hospital
St Louis MO, USA

Luis A Garcia MD
Department of Orthopaedic Surgery
San Ignacio University Hospital
University of Javeriana
Bogota, Colombia

Dominique F Gazielly MD
Shoulder Unit
Institut de la Main
Clinique Jouvenet
Paris, France

Ariane Gerber MD
Shoulder Fellow
Department of Orthopaedics
University of Zurich
Zurich, Switzerland

Christian Gerber MD
Professor and Chairman
Department of Orthopaedics
University of Zurich
Zurich, Switzerland

James N Gladstone MD
Assistant Professor
Knee and Shoulder Surgery, Sports Medicine
Department of Orthopaedic Surgery
The Mount Sinai Hospital
New York NY, USA

Karl Golser MD
Universitätsklinik für Unfallchirurgie
Innsbruck, Austria

Jeffrey L Halbrecht MD
Medical Director
The Institute of Arthroscopy and Sports Medicine
San Francisco CA, USA

Frank Hoffmann MD
Klinik für Orthopädie und Sportorthopädie Rosenheim
Rosenheim, Germany

Klaus Johann MD
Orthopaedic Department
St Elisabeth Clinic
Saarlouis, Germany

Amir M Khan MD
Sports Orthopaedic and Rehabilitation Group
Menlo Park CA, USA

Steven J Klepps MD
Shoulder and Elbow Service
Washington University Department of Orthopaedics
Barnes-Jewish Hospital
St Louis MO, USA

Uwe König MD
Department of Orthopaedic Sports Medicine
Technical University of Munich
Munich, Germany

Franz Kralinger MD
Universitätsklinik für Unfallchirurgie
Innsbruck, Austria

Michael Kunz MD
Head, Orthopaedic Department
St Elisabeth Clinic
Saarlouis, Germany

Laurent Lafosse MD
Clinique Générale
Annecy, France

Franz Landsiedl MD
Orthopädisches Spital Speising GmbH
Vienna, Austria

William N Levine MD
The Shoulder Service
New York Presbyterian Hospital
Columbia-Presbyterian Medical Center Campus
New York NY, USA

Eric R McMillan MD
President and CEO
Central California Orthopedic Medical Associates, Inc
Turlock CA, USA

Vladimir Martinek MD
Department of Orthopaedic Sports Medicine
Technical University of Munich
Munich, Germany

Leslie S Matthews MD
Department of Orthopaedic Surgery
Union Memorial Hospital
Baltimore MD, USA

Thomas Merl MD
Consultant Radiologist
Department of Neuroradiology
Munich, Germany

Suzanne L Miller MD
Senior Resident
Department of Orthopaedics
The Mount Sinai Hospital
New York NY, USA

Douglas S Musgrave MD
Clinical Instructor
Department of Orthopaedic Surgery
University of Pittsburgh
Pittsburgh PA, USA

Gregory P Nicholson MD
Midwest Orthopaedics
Chicago IL, USA

Laurent Nové-Josserand MD
Clinique Sainte Anne Lumière
Lyon, France

Peter M Parten MD
Former Shoulder Arthroscopy Fellow
The San Antonio Orthopaedic Group
Summit Orthopaedics
Maplewood MN, USA

William T Pennington MD
San Francisco CA, USA

Herbert Resch MD
General Hospital Salzburg
Salzburg, Austria

Mark W Rodosky MD
Department of Orthopaedic Surgery
University of Pittsburgh Medical Center
Pittsburgh PA, USA

Anthony A Romeo MD
Assistant Professor
Director, Shoulder Section
Associate Professor
Department of Orthopaedics
Rush University
Chicago IL, USA

Felix H Savoie III MD
Co-Director, Upper Extremity Service
Mississippi Sports Medicine and Orthopaedic Center
Clinical Associate Professor, Department of Orthopaedic
Surgery
University of Mississippi School of Medicine
Jackson MS, USA

Julious P Smith III MD
Fellow
Mississippi Sports Medicine and Orthopaedic Center
Jackson MS, USA

Stephen J Snyder MD
Southern California Orthopedic Institute
Van Nuys CA, USA

Gernot Sperner MD
University Hospital Innsbruck
Innsbruck, Austria

Michael P Staebler MD
Department of Orthopaedic Surgery
Union Memorial Hospital
Baltimore MD, USA

Joseph C Tauro MD
Assistant Clinical Professor of Orthopedic Surgery
New Jersey Medical School
Ocean County Sports Medicine Center
Toms River NJ, USA

Armin M Tehrany MD
Former Shoulder Arthroscopy Fellow
The San Antonio Orthopaedic Group
Staten Island NY, USA

Gilles Walch MD
Clinique Sainte Anne Lumière
Lyon, France

Ralph Wischatta MD
Universitätsklinik für Unfallchirurgie
Innsbruck, Austria

Eugene M Wolf MD
Medical Director,
Shoulder Arthroscopy Fellowship Program,
California Pacific Medical Center
San Francisco CA, USA

Ken Yamaguchi MD
Associate Professor
Program Director, Shoulder & Elbow Fellowship
Chief, Shoulder and Elbow Service
Washington University Department of Orthopaedics
Barnes-Jewish Hospital
St Louis MO, USA

Dean W Ziegler MD
Blount Orthopaedic Clinic
Milwaukee WI, USA

Preface

When we first conceived this textbook dedicated to shoulder arthroscopy, it was a mere three years after we started the initial, and now companion, textbook *An Atlas of Shoulder Surgery*. In that preface we remarked, 'Shoulder surgery has progressed most rapidly over the past 25 years.' It was clear to us that shoulder surgery, in particular arthroscopic surgical techniques, had progressed (and continue to do so!) at a very rapid pace. Arthroscopic techniques have been developed and successfully utilized to address myriad pathologies formerly treated primarily with open procedures. It is in this context and as a result of these changes in the surgical approach to treatment of many conditions affecting the shoulder that we devised this book.

In this title, we have followed a similar formula and format to that of its companion textbook. Our focus is on the reader and the desire to provide useful and applicable arthroscopic shoulder surgical techniques. *An Atlas of Shoulder Arthroscopy* includes all of the more common techniques currently employed in arthroscopy of the shoulder. In addition, we recognize that the pace of advancement in arthroscopic shoulder surgery may turn some of the more advanced techniques we present in this textbook into more commonly utilized procedures in the near future. Our goal is to present all of these techniques, as described by authorities in the field of arthroscopic shoulder surgery from Europe and the United States, in a straightforward manner that can be applied in clinical practice. Many sections within this textbook present two or more alternative techniques to address the same clinical condition, in an effort to provide greater perspective for the reader. Arthroscopic images, color photographs and drawings are used to highlight the steps of each procedure. However, we do not expect or desire that these techniques be considered the only methods that should be used to treat particular shoulder conditions. It would be a greater service to the field of shoulder surgery if these techniques served to stimulate other surgeons to develop modifications of these techniques or, even, develop new ways to simplify

a procedure or expand our indications for use of the arthroscope in the shoulder.

An Atlas of Shoulder Arthroscopy comprises 40 chapters and is divided into sections, beginning with an introduction which includes an historical perspective, basic science and diagnostic techniques. The therapeutic sections begin with an excellent review of the diagnostic arthroscopy and approaches to arthroscopic knot tying. Arthroscopic techniques are presented for the treatment of instability and labral pathology, impingement and posterosuperior rotator cuff pathology, subscapularis tears, acromioclavicular joint arthritis, calcific tendonitis, biceps pathology, frozen shoulder, ganglion cysts, osteoarthritis, inflammatory synovitis and tumors, and scapulothoracic conditions. In addition, we are particularly proud to offer an optional CD-ROM which contains video clips for many of the techniques described in the textbook. This will allow the reader to take another step closer to the successful application of techniques for arthroscopic shoulder surgery.

As we stated in the preface of our first atlas, 'We hope that this atlas will serve as an invaluable resource for both the novice and accomplished shoulder surgeon.' Indeed, this book offers both fundamental and advanced techniques for arthroscopic shoulder surgery. It is our aim to offer physicians who practice arthroscopic shoulder surgery, both on the early part of the learning curve or at a more advanced level, the necessary tools to achieve a successful surgical outcome. For the patient, we also recognize that an operation completed to perfection will only be successful if the indications, preparation and rehabilitation are performed correctly. We encourage readers to further develop their understanding of gross and arthroscopic shoulder anatomy, as well as basic science concepts, in the 'pursuit of knowledge in all aspects of the shoulder.'

Andreas B Imhoff MD
Jonathan B Ticker MD
Freddie H Fu MD DSci (Hon)

Acknowledgements

As with all endeavours of this magnitude, there are many people who worked on this atlas and the optional CD-ROM who are deserving of our thanks and appreciation:

To the numerous contributors, it is clear to us that we could not have produced such a high level of achievement with this atlas if we had not had such an accomplished group of arthroscopic shoulder surgeons who were willing to contribute their knowledge to these chapters. We shall all benefit from these efforts, and we extend our gratitude to each one of you.

To the production and editorial staff at Martin Dunitz, including Charlotte Mossop, Abigail Griffin and Dan Edwards, we thank you for providing the necessary links between the editors, the authors and the publisher to reach our goals. The hundreds of e-mail messages that provided us with an improved method of communication and distribution of material will attest to these efforts.

To our commissioning editor at Martin Dunitz Publishers, Robert Peden, who provided us with the necessary guidance to achieve our goals, after having the knowledge of working with us on the first book. Your fortitude and perseverance are admirable.

Especially to Jens Agneskirchner, MD – the video images on the optional CD-ROM could not have been completed without your collective knowledge and skills.

Finally, to our office staffs and residents who rose to the challenge once again by providing invaluable assistance.

We thank you all from the bottom of our hearts.

ABI
JBT
FHF

Section I – Introduction and imaging

1   History of shoulder arthroscopy

James C Esch

Introduction

In 1931, Burman (Figure 1.1) performed the first arthroscopy of the shoulder on a cadaver.[1] He examined 25 cadaveric shoulders in the first study of this joint. Over time, the procedure has gradually gained wide acceptance for use in diagnosing and correcting a variety of pathologic conditions of the shoulder. Its ease of use, good results, and shorter recovery times have made arthroscopic shoulder surgery increasingly popular and a viable alternative to open shoulder surgery. Time will determine whether the long-term results of instability and rotator cuff surgery equal or better the outcomes of traditional open surgery.

Johnson's description in 1974 of performing shoulder arthroscopy on a professional baseball pitcher with the patient under local anesthesia is probably the first case performed in vivo (LL Johnson, personal communication). A photograph (Figure 1.2) of this rotator cuff tear appears in his 1986 book.[2] The initial clinical reports[3–10] informed surgeons regarding the use of the arthroscope in the shoulder. Andrews and Carson provided the first look at the glenohumeral joint and other structures as seen from inside the shoulder.[9] Later reports include those of Detrisac and Johnson,[11] Ogilvie-Harris and Wiley,[12] Ellman,[13] Paulos and colleagues,[14,15] Esch et al,[16] and Snyder.[17] Johnson performed the first arthroscopic repair in the shoulder for instability on August 12, 1982, on a New York City orthopedic surgeon who had had 100 dislocations with associated degenerative changes.[18] Three staples were inserted: two in the joint and one lost within the joint. The staples were removed in 1994 (LL Johnson, personal communication).

In 1986, Johnson said 'I believe any operation on the shoulder joint itself, or on the tissues nearby should be preceded by or combined with an arthroscopic examination. Furthermore, the diagnostic accuracy prevents empirical surgical decisions, especially for "impingement

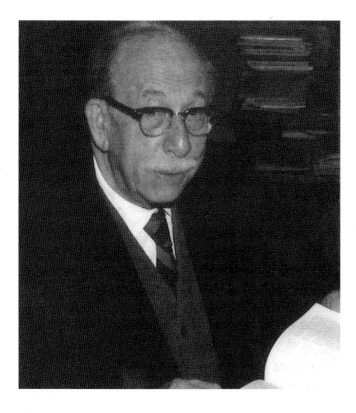

Figure 1.1

Burman performed the first shoulder arthroscopy in cadavers.

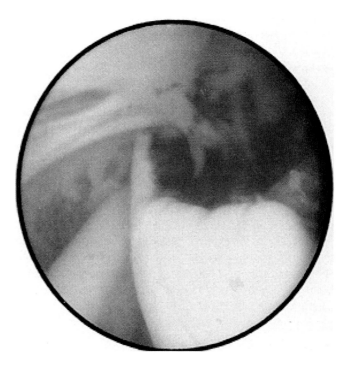

Figure 1.2

Rotator cuff tear in first shoulder arthroscopy by LL Johnson, MD. (Reproduced from Johnson[2] with permission, *Arthroscopic Surgery: Principles and Practices*, 1986).

syndrome" and replaces open surgical exploration.'[19] This quote was controversial at the time it was made, but remains true today. Rockwood expressed his concern regarding the early use of shoulder arthroscopy in an editorial for the *Journal of Bone and Joint Surgery*.[20] Rockwood acknowledged that shoulder arthroscopy provides excellent visualization, but was concerned that patients would gravitate to the arthroscopic surgeon and that socioeconomic considerations would lead to increased use of arthroscopy. His concern that the results of arthroscopic surgery for instability may be worse than the results of traditional open surgery is true today. Rockwood correctly challenged early zealots regarding the idea that arthroscopic subacromial decompression was a good treatment for patients with reparable rotator cuff tears. He stated 'It is unlikely that a middle aged patient who has a reparable cuff lesion would have a long term benefit from arthroscopic debridement of the cuff.'[20] He concluded his editorial by stating that the arthroscope is an adjunct tool for making the correct diagnosis in the shoulder and its use is still in the development stage.

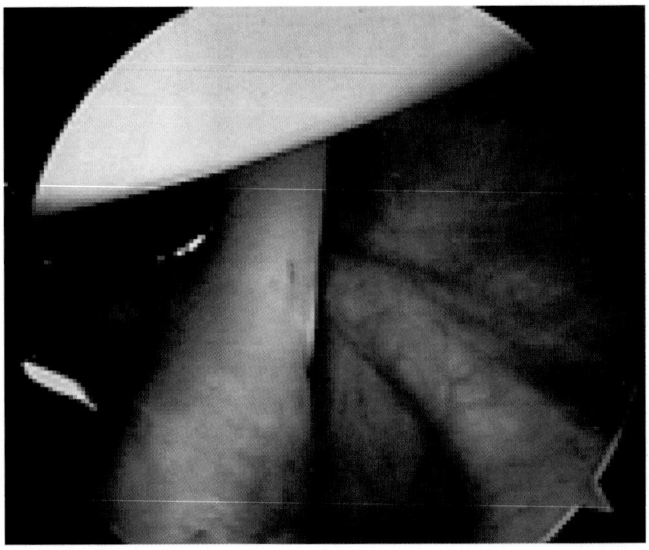

Figure 1.3

Rotator cuff 'ridge' anatomic variation.

Diagnostic arthroscopy

Diagnostic arthroscopy was the first application of this technique. Viewing is always done from the posterior portal with a secondary anterior portal. Early in the use of this procedure, surgeons struggled with determining the optimal placement of the anterior portal. The safety of creating the anterior portal from the outside to the inside of the glenohumeral joint was a major concern,[21,22] because a misplaced anterior portal could injure the brachial plexus.[23] Johnson described an inside-to-outside technique using a long metal rod that fits inside the metal arthroscopic cannula;[24] Wissinger had suggested this idea to Johnson during a visit to his operating room in 1982. The use of the Wissinger rod led to a safe, predictable method of creating an anterior portal.

Snyder emphasized a systematic approach for diagnostic arthroscopy and bursoscopy of the shoulder.[17] Distinguishing normal anatomy and its variants from pathologic anatomy was initially a dilemma. Rames et al described the normal range of variation in the glenohumeral ligaments.[25] A sublabral hole, a cord-like middle glenohumeral ligament, and Buford complex were some of the variations at the anterosuperior labrum.[26] A fibrous band within the rotator interval, later described as the rotator crescent (Figure 1.3) by Burkhart, is another variant. Snyder et al defined and classified the tear of the superior labrum from anterior to posterior, or the SLAP lesion.[27]

It was clearly important at this stage in the evolution of shoulder arthroscopy to define what was clinically significant pathology and what was normal variation. Detrisac and Johnson published their important anatomic study in 1986.[11] They had begun anatomic dissections of

210 shoulders in 1982 and their report included their findings in 310 shoulder arthroscopies between 1982 and 1985. They described the appearance and normal variations of the glenohumeral ligaments, labrum, biceps, rotator cuff, and bursa. This text provided a basis for understanding and differentiating normal anatomy from disease processes.

Surgeons noticed other anatomic differences in patients with shoulder instability. These findings included the classic Bankart lesion as previously seen at open surgery,[28,29] the absence of a Bankart lesion, and an anterior labral periosteal sleeve avulsion, which constitutes a Bankart lesion that has healed in an abnormal position.[30] Warren described a wide-open space known as the drive-through sign, which is indicative of capsular laxity (R Warren, personal communication). O'Brien et al,[31] Turkel et al,[32] Schwartz et al,[33] and others did anatomic and biomechanical studies of the inferior glenohumeral ligament and discussed its importance in shoulder stability.

Shoulder arthroscopy also helped define rotator cuff pathology. Findings included bursal side tears seen at traditional open surgery, articular side tears not seen at open surgery, and the concept of internal derangement. This led to ongoing studies of the relationship between glenohumeral joint stability and the rotator cuff.

Treatment of instability

The development of arthroscopy for shoulder instability is divided into four phases: glenoid fixation; transglenoid fixation; suture anchors; and capsular surgery.

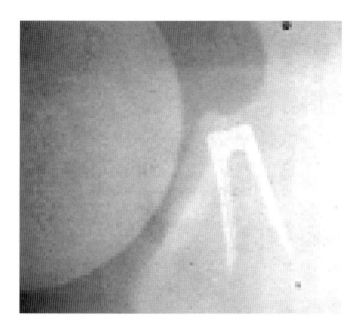

Figure 1.4

Radiologic view of staple.

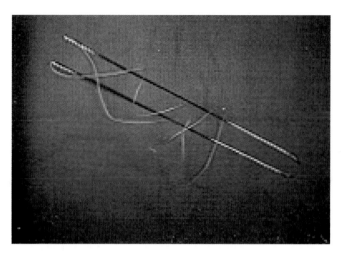

Figure 1.5

Needles designed by Morgan for arthroscopic instability repair.

Glenoid fixation

The first phase of arthroscopic surgery, glenoid fixation, began with the initial cases of arthroscopic stapling (Figure 1.4) by Johnson: two cases in 1982, and 18 cases in 1983. Other methods followed with the invention of various devices, including the removable rivet designed by Wiley in 1988[34] and the step staple designed by Gross in 1989.[35] At this time, some surgeons advocated abrading the glenoid and using a sling without internal fixation.[36] Because there was a question of the staple loosening, Wolf believed that more secure fixation was indicated, and a metal screw and washer were designed.[37] Warner et al published a technique using the first biodegradable fixation device in 1991.[38,39] Snyder developed the Biotac as part of a biodegradable research design (SJ Snyder, personal communication). Personal experience with a staple revealed that it allowed shifting of the tissues while achieving secure fixation. Two problems with this procedure were putting the staple on the glenoid neck rather than on the face of the glenoid and failing to grasp the tissue with the staple. The development of suture anchors that can be placed on the edge of the glenoid surface and allow tissue to be grasped independently of anchor insertion addressed these potential problems.

Transglenoid fixation

The second phase of arthroscopic surgery was transglenoid fixation. Morgan and Bodenstab initially

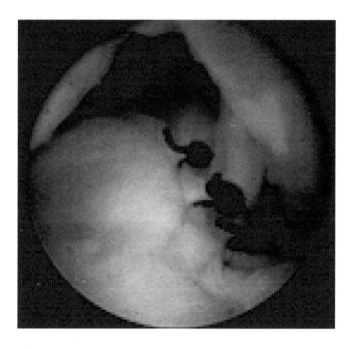

Figure 1.6

SLAP repair by Morgan using a sliding knot and PDS (Ethicon, Mitek, Norwood, MA, USA) suture.

described a suture technique using long needles (Figure 1.5) that were tied inside the joint onto the anterior labrum and capsule.[40,41] Rose introduced a guide for this procedure.[42] Morgan and Bodenstab[40] used the Duncan loop fishing knot (Figure 1.6). Shoulder arthroscopic surgeons have since rediscovered numerous other knots. Later, Maki described tying the knot over the bone posteriorly.[43] Caspari and colleagues modified this technique with a capsule–labrum tissue advancement.[44,45] They advanced the anterior capsulolabral tissue complex

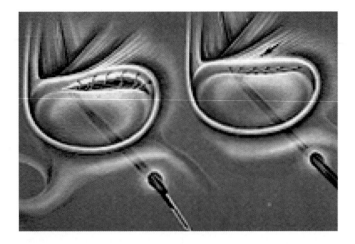

Figure 1.7

Caspari transglenoid technique.

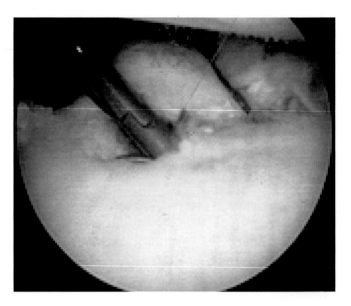

Figure 1.8

Suture anchor inserted into bone for labrum repair.

superiorly by grasping and passing sutures through the tissue with a suture punch. The sutures were passed through a hole drilled in the anterior glenoid from anterosuperior to posteroinferior (Figure 1.7). Torchia et al reported their long-term results.[46] The most common complication of this procedure is suprascapular nerve damage due to a misdirected drill hole through the glenoid. Caspari et al presented the use of fascial allograft substitution of the inferior glenohumeral ligament[44] and Lynch reported these results.[47] Today, this procedure is occasionally done for patients with absence of an anterior capsule and ligaments.

Suture anchors

Reports by Wolf[48] and Richmond et al[49] heralded the beginning of the suture anchor (Figure 1.8) phase of glenoid fixation in 1991. France had done strength studies of the initial anchor design.[50,51] This led to a host of other suture anchor devices in both push-in and screw-in forms. These devices were initially composed of metal and plastic, and biodegradable devices were later developed. Acceptance of this procedure required surgeons to learn and practise knots. Thal modified this technique by designing a knotless suture anchor in which the anchor catches a suture loop attached to the anchor, as an alternative to tying a knot.[52]

Capsular surgery

Capsular surgery to reduce excess volume is the most current phase of development for instability surgery. Using Caspari's transglenoid procedure, Savoie and Duncan reported on an arthroscopic capsular shift proce-

dure for the treatment of multidirectional instability.[53] Snyder et al,[54] using permanent sutures, and Wolf and Durkin,[55] using absorbable sutures, described capsular suturing to eliminate capsular redundancy. Arthroscopic closure of the rotator interval is now being performed.[56] Thermal modification of the collagen is currently in the developmental stages. Initial enthusiasm has been dampened by follow-up studies and anecdotal reports of failure, axillary nerve palsy, capsular holes, and frozen shoulders with excess capsular scarring.

One other area is arthroscopic repair following an acute first-time anterior dislocation. Diagnostic shoulder arthroscopy in young athletes with an acute shoulder dislocation demonstrates labrum tears, capsular tears, and bony lesions.[57,58] Early arthroscopic surgical repair of these lesions may reduce or possibly eliminate the high rate of recurrent anterior dislocation in this patient population.

My current practice for performing instability repair includes suture anchor reattachment of the labrum if torn, plication of the capsule, and suture closure of the rotator interval. Proper rehabilitation based on the strength of the repair is essential. The long-term redislocation rate following arthroscopic instability repair is 20% at 5 years. Surgeons doing this procedure also need to be aware of the fact that the 5-year dislocation rate is twice that of the 2-year rate.[46]

Rotator cuff

Ellman pioneered subacromial space surgery with arthroscopic subacromial decompression.[59–61] He taught this procedure to arthroscopic surgeons and was the bridge to introducing it to traditional shoulder surgeons. Interestingly, initially he did not look into the glenohumeral joint. Ellman demonstrated his belief in the future of shoulder arthroscopy by joining the Arthroscopy Association of North America (AANA) in 1989. Initial results with decompression were reported by Paulos et al,[62–64] Esch et al,[16,65] and Gartsman et al.[66]

Ellman taught the initial technique for arthroscopic subacromial decompression. One of the more popular variations is the cutting block technique in which the acromion is burred from posterior to anterior. This effectively removes the anterior and inferior bony prominence and is an excellent technique for both thin and thick acromions. Samson et al were the first to perform this technique.[67] Ellman tempered the zeal to perform an arthroscopic subacromial decompression on all patients with impingement syndrome by stating that some rotator cuffs require repair. Subacromial decompression is not indicated for all patients; good candidates include those with full-thickness rotator cuff tears, stiffness, significant partial-thickness rotator cuff tears, osteoarthritis, and massive rotator cuff tears.

The early stages in the arthroscopic approach to rotator cuff repair stressed diagnostic arthroscopy followed by repair of the tear through a small incision. The first arthroscopic cuff repairs were performed with a staple that was removed 4–12 weeks later, allowing a 'second-look' arthroscopic procedure that showed healing.

Snyder and colleagues classified tears into an 'ABC, 1234' system to differentiate among articular and bursal side partial tears and complete tears.[68,69] In this system the letters A, B, and C refer to the location of the tear (articular, bursal, or complete, respectively), and the numbers are used to designate the severity of a tear by depth. Burkhart brought mechanical engineering principles to the treatment of rotator cuff disease.[70] This included proper anchor insertion and margin convergence of large tears. Tippet presented cases of staged repairs.[71] Weber showed that the significant partial tear requires repair in addition to decompression.[72]

Today, arthroscopic repairs for partial and complete rotator cuff tears are most commonly performed with suture anchors. The reports of the short-term outcomes of arthroscopic rotator cuff repairs are equal to those treated with the traditional open repair.[73,74] The recovery time may be shorter with arthroscopic repair, and less deltoid muscle scarring may be produced.

SLAP lesions

Snyder et al called attention to the SLAP lesion and introduced a classification.[75] This was a lesion not recognized with open shoulder surgery. The relationship of this lesion to instability and rotator cuff problems have been proposed by Jobe,[76] Walch et al,[77] Burkhart and Morgan,[78] and Morgan et al.[79] Arthroscopic repair is the standard for treatment of SLAP lesions.

Frozen shoulder

Wiley,[80] Ogilvie-Harris and Wiley,[12] Haeri and Maitland,[7] Uitvlugt et al,[81] Detrisac and Johnson,[11] and Poehling[82] described and performed diagnostic arthroscopy of the frozen shoulder. Neviaser defined four stages of arthroscopic changes in adhesive capsulitis.[83] Poehling first called attention to an inflammation within the subacromial bursa.[82] Additionally, he noticed patchy vascular collections around the subscapularis and biceps associated with dense subscapular adhesions. Treatment of the frozen shoulder involves manipulation through arthroscopy. Esch and Baker described resecting the dense adhesions associated with this condition.[84] Arthroscopic release of adhesions and manipulation is the current standard of treatment for frozen shoulder.[85,86] Use of the arthroscope by researchers such as Rodeo et al[87] is leading to a better understanding of this disease. Mormino et al defined the postoperative 'captured shoulder' with scarring at the subacromial bursa and underneath the deltoid.[88]

Instrumentation

In the early days of arthroscopy, particular attention was paid to numerous tools, especially hand tools such as probes, graspers, knives, and elevators. Other instruments were designed to pass sutures; these include the suture punch, suture passers, suture grasper passers, and the cuff sew. Snyder designed the suture shuttle, which enables the surgeon to pass the suture from one portal to the other. Power shavers were introduced and progressed from a single to multiple shaver blades, with the addition of different burrs that can operate at different speeds.

Arthroscopic knot-tying presented early challenges. Initially, arthroscopic knot pushers were double-holed. Today, most surgeons find that the single-hole pusher affords better control of the suture and the knot. Knot nomenclature has become important and includes the knot post, loop, pass pointing, and knot security. Practicing knot-tying is essential for becoming familiar with the advanced arthroscopic repair techniques for instability, SLAP, and rotator cuff repairs. The development of cannulas has facilitated these techniques

Hemostasis and visualization

Early in the course of shoulder arthroscopy, the surgeon often struggled to control bleeding that obscured viewing through the arthroscope. High arthroscopic fluid flow and pressure helps to control bleeding by maintaining joint distension. This led to a design change in the arthroscopic cannula sheath that enables the inflow fluid to pass through the arthroscopic sheath. Higher pressures were maintained with infusion pumps and allowed better control of bleeding within the joint and subacromial space. Arthroscopic surgeons also became aware of the importance of maintaining the patient's systolic pressure at about 95 mmHg, which reduces the small vessel arterial pressure within the joint. Electrocautery devices are now essential for maintaining hemostasis and visualization. In addition, advances in camera technology have further contributed to our ability to see and operate arthroscopically.

Education

Arthroscopic shoulder procedures would not have advanced to the high level of today without a diligent effort to educate orthopedic surgeons. Shoulder arthroscopic techniques were initially taught at private courses given by Metcalf, Johnson, Esch, Nottage, Caspari, Myers, Whipple, Paulos, Snyder, and Curtis. The AANA pioneered cadaver surgery at its Fall course showing master surgeons performing various surgeries. This was initially done for the knee in 1985 in Colorado Springs, Colorado, and was followed the next year by a shoulder arthroscopic procedure. Sweeney pioneered the AANA Master's courses devoted to shoulder arthroscopy. The AANA was the impetus for a cooperative development with the American Academy of Orthopedic Surgeons: the Orthopaedic Learning Center in Rosemont, Illinois. Today, courses are offered in many countries by experienced surgeons to further advance arthroscopic shoulder surgery.

Numerous arthroscopic shoulder simulators have been valuable in training surgeons. These include devices as simple as blocks of wood for practice in tying sutures as well as a sophisticated shoulder simulator designed by Snyder called the Alex Shoulder Professor Design (Figure 1.9). Computer simulators such as the Swedish shoulder model are available to teach arthroscope rotation triangulation and feel.

Future

I have found that shoulder arthroscopy, just as any form of arthroscopic surgery, requires practice, dedication,

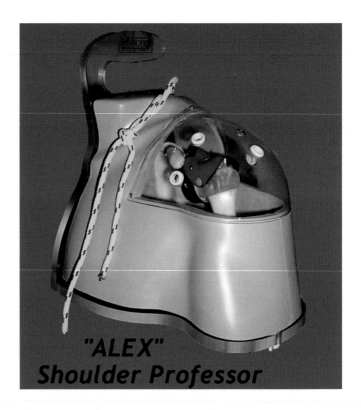

"ALEX" Shoulder Professor

Figure 1.9

Shoulder model 'Alex' can be used to practice arthroscopic procedures (Pacific Research Laboratories, Inc., Vashon, WA, USA).

enthusiasm, passion, and science. In the next decade, results will be better understood, indications for surgery will be refined, and anecdotal testimonials advocating one procedure or technique over another will be replaced with hard scientific evidence that supports the best technique for each condition and situation. Additionally, a better understanding of diseases that involve the shoulder, including frozen shoulder, instability, rotator cuff disease, and articular cartilage disorders, can be expected.

Acknowledgments

I would like to make a special tribute to Dr Steven Snyder, who has been an aggressive teacher of numerous shoulder surgeons; he also published his early results on arthroscopy of the shoulder and defined the SLAP lesion. Additionally, Dr Steve Burkhart, who has written extensively on the rotator cuff and brought engineering principles and science to the area of the rotator cuff treatment, also deserves special recognition.

References

1. Burman MS. Arthroscopy or the direct visualization of joints: an experimental cadaver study. *J Bone Joint Surg* 1931; **13**:669.
2. Johnson LL. *Arthroscopic Surgery: Principles and Practice.* St. Louis: CV Mosby, 1986; 1434.
3. Johnson LL. Arthroscopy of the shoulder. *Orthop Clin North Am* 1980; **11**:197–204.
4. Johnson LL. *Comprehensive Arthroscopic Examination of the Knee Joint.* St. Louis: CV Mosby, 1981.
5. Wiley AM, Older MW. Shoulder arthroscopy. Investigations with a fibrooptic instrument *Am J Sports Med* 1980; **8**:31–8.
6. Haeri GB. Ruptures of the rotator cuff. *Can Med Assoc J* 1980; **123**:620.
7. Haeri GB, Maitland A. Arthroscopic findings in the frozen shoulder. *J Rheumatol* 1981; **8**:149.
8. Caspari RB. Shoulder arthroscopy: a review of the present state of the art. *Contemp Orthop* 1982; **4**:523.
9. Andrews JR, Carson WG. Arthroscopy of the shoulder. *Orthopaedics* 1983; **6**:1157.
10. Cofield RH. Arthroscopy of the shoulder. *Mayo Clin Proc* 1983; **58**:501–8.
11. Detrisac DA, Johnson LL. *Arthroscopic Shoulder Anatomy: Pathological and Surgical Implications.* Thorofare, NJ: Stack, 1986.
12. Ogilvie-Harris DJ, Wiley AM. Arthroscopic surgery of the shoulder. A general appraisal. *J Bone Joint Surg [Br]* 1986; **68**:201–7.
13. Ellman H. Arthroscopic subacromial decompression: analysis of one- to three-year results. *Arthroscopy* 1987; **3**:173–81.
14. Paulos LE, Franklin JL. Arthroscopic shoulder decompression development and application. A five year experience. *Am J Sports Med* 1990; **18**:235–44.
15. Paulos LE, Grauer D, Smutz WP. Traumatic lesions of the biceps tendon, rotator cuff interval, and superior labrum [abstract]. *Orthop Trans* 1990; **15**:85.
16. Esch JC, Ozerkis LR, Helgager JA et al. Arthroscopic subacromial decompression: results according to the degree of rotator cuff tear. *Arthroscopy* 1988; **4**:241–9.
17. Snyder SJ. A complete system for arthroscopy and bursoscopy of the shoulder. *Surg Rounds Orthop* 1989. July
18. Johnson LL. *Diagnostic and Surgical Arthrosocpy of the Shoulder.* St. Louis: CV Mosby, 1993;318.
19. Johnson LL. *Arthrosopic Surgery: Principles and Practice.* St. Louis: CV Mosby 1986;1303.
20. Rockwood CA Jr. Shoulder arthroscopy. *J Bone Joint Surg* 1988; **70A**:639–40.
21. Wolf EM. Anterior portals in shoulder arthroscopy. *Arthroscopy* 1989; **5**:201–8.
22. Matthews LS, Terry G, Vetter WL. Shoulder anatomy for the arthroscopist. *Arthroscopy* 1985; **1**:83–91.
23. Matthews LS, Zarins B, Michael RH, Helfer DL. Anterior portal selection for shoulder arthroscopy. *Arthroscopy* 1985; **1**:33–9.
24. Johnson LL. *Diagnostic and Surgical Arthrosocpy of the Shoulder.* St. Louis: CV Mosby, 1993;83.
25. Rames RD, Morgan CD, Snyder SJ. Anatomical variations of the glenohumeral ligaments [abstract]. *Arthroscopy* 1991; **7**:328.
26. Snyder SJ, Buford D, Wuh HC. The Buford complex. Presented at the 59th Annual Meeting of the American Academy of Orthopaedic Surgeons, Washington, DC, February 1992.
27. Snyder SJ, Karzel RP, Del Pizzo W et al. SLAP lesions of the shoulder. *Arthroscopy* 1990; **6**:274–9.
28. Bankart ASB. Recurrent or habitual dislocation of the shoulder. *BMJ* 1923; **2**:1132.
29. Bankart ASB. The pathology and treatment of the recurrent dislocations of the shoulder joint. *Br J Surg* 1938; **26**:23.
30. Neviaser T. ALPSA lesion. Presented at the Annual Meeting of the Arthroscopy Association of North America, Boston, April 1992.
31. O'Brien SJ, Neves MC, Arnoczky SP et al. The anatomy and histology of the inferior glenohumeral ligament complex of the shoulder. *Am J Sports Med* 1990; **18**:449–56.
32. Turkel SJ, Panio MW, Marshall JL, Girgis FG. Stabilizing mechanisms preventing anterior dislocation of the glenohumeral joint. *J Bone Joint Surg* 1981; **63A**:1208–17.
33. Schwartz RE, O'Brien SJ, Warren RF, Torzilli PA. Capsular restraints to antero-posterior motion of the abducted shoulder: a biomechanical study. *Orthop Trans* 1988; **12**:727.
34. Wiley AM. Arthroscopy for shoulder instability and a technique for arthroscopic repair. *Arthroscopy* 1988; **4**:25–30.
35. Gross RM. Arthroscopic shoulder capsulorraphy: does it work? *Am J Sports Med* 1989; **17**:495–500.
36. Eisenberg JH, Redler MR, Hecht PJ. Arthroscopic stabilization of the chronic subluxating or dislocating shoulder without the use of internal fixation [abstract]. *Arthroscopy* 1991; **7**:315.
37. Wolf EM. Arthroscopic anterior shoulder capsulorrhaphy. *Tech Orthop* 1988; **3**:67.
38. Warner JJP, Warren RF. Arthroscopic Bankart repair using a cannulated absorbable fixation device. *Oper Tech Orthop* 1991; **1**:192.
39. Warner JJP, Pagnani M, Warren RF, et al. Arthroscopic Bankart repair utilizing a cannulated absorbable fixation device. *Orthop Trans* 1991; **15**:761.
40. Morgan CD, Bodenstab AB. Arthroscopic Bankart suture repair: technique and early results. *Arthroscopy* 1987; **3**:111–22.
41. Morgan CD. Arthroscopic transglenoid Bankart suture repair. *Oper Tech Orthop* 1991; **1**:171.
42. Rose DJ. Arthroscopic suture capsulorrahphy for anterior shoulder instability. *Orthop Trans* 1990; **14**:597.
43. Maki NJ. Arthroscopic stabilization: suture technique. *Oper Tech Orthop* 1991; **1**:180.
44. Caspari RB, Savoie FH, Meyers JF et al. Arthroscopic shoulder reconstruction. *Orthop Trans* 1989; **13**:559.
45. Caspari RB. Arthroscopic reconstruction for anterior shoulder capsulorrhaphy. *Tech Orthop* 1988; **3**:59.
46. Torchia ME, Caspari RB, Asselmeier MA et al. Arthroscopic transglenoid multiple suture repair: 2 to 8 year results in 150 shoulders. *Arthroscopy* 1997; **13**:609–19.
47. Lynch GJ. Arthroscopic substitution of the anterior inferior glenohumeral ligament [abstract]. *Arthroscopy* 1991:**7**:325.
48. Wolf EM. Arthroscopic Bankart repair using suture anchors. *Tech Orthop* 1991; **1**:184.
49. Richmond JC, Donaldson WR, Fu F. Modification of the Bankart reconstruction with a suture anchor: report of a new technique. *Am J Sports Med* 1991; **19**:343–6.
50. France EP. Technical report: fixation strength evaluation of Mitek suture anchors: applications in the shoulder. Salt Lake City: October 1989.
51. France EP. Fixation strength of double armed Mitek torpedo suture anchors: application in the shoulder. Salt Lake City: June 1990.
52. Thal R. A knotless suture anchor and method for arthroscopic Bankart repair [abstract]. Presented at the 18th Annual Meeting of the Arthroscopy Association of North America, Vancouver, British Columbia, Canada, 15–18 April, 1999.
53. Savoie B, Duncan R. Multidirectional instability: management by arthroscopic inferior capsular shift. A preliminary report [abstract]. *Arthroscopy* 1991; **7**:330.
54. Snyder SJ, Loren GJ, Karzel RP, Wichman MT. Extended success of arthroscopic capsular plication for glenohumeral instability in the absence of a Bankart lesion [abstract]. Presented at the 18th Annual Meeting of the Arthroscopy Association of North America, Vancouver, British Columbia, Canada, 15–18 April, 1999.
55. Wolf, EM, Durkin R. Arthroscopic capsular plication for multi-directional instability [abstract]. Presented at the 18th Annual Meeting of the Arthroscopy Association of North America, Vancouver, British Columbia, Canada, April 15–18, 1999.
56. Gartsman GM, Taverna E, Hammerman SM. Arthroscopic rotator

interval repair in glenohumeral instability: description of an operative technique. *Arthroscopy* 1999; **15**:330–2.

57. Wheeler JH, Ryan JB, Arciero RA, Molinari RN. Arthroscopic versus nonoperative treatment of acute shoulder dislocations in young athletes. *Arthroscopy* 1989; **5**:213.

58. Baker CL, Uribe JW, Whitman C. Arthroscopic evaluation of acute initial anterior shoulder dislocations. *Am J Sports Med* 1990; **18**:25–8.

59. Ellman H. Arthroscopic subacromial decompression. *Arthroscopy* 1987; **3**:173–81.

60. Ellman H. Diagnosis and treatment of incomplete rotator cuff tears. *Clin Orthop* 1990; **254**:64–74.

61. Ellman H. Arthroscopic treatment of impingement of the shoulder. *Instr Course Lect* 1989; **38**:177–85.

62. Paulos LE, Harner CD, Parker RD. Arthroscopic subacromial decompression for impingement syndrome of the shoulder. *Tech Orthop* 1988; **3**:33.

63. Paulos LE, Franklin JL, Harner CD. Arthroscopic subacromial decompression for impingement syndrome of the shoulder: a five-year experience. In: Paulos LE, Tibone JE, eds. *Operative Techniques in Shoulder Surgery.* Gaithersburg, MD: Aspen, 1991; 31.

64. Paulos LE, Franklin JL. Arthroscopic shoulder decompression development and application. A five-year experience. *Am J Sports Med* 1990; **18**:235–44.

65. Esch JC. Arthroscopy update #4. Arthroscopic subacromial decompression. Surgical technique. *Orthop Rev* 1989; **18**:733–5, 738–42.

66. Gartsman GM, Blair ME Jr, Noble PC et al. Arthroscopic subacromial decompression: an anatomical study. *Am J Sports Med* 1988; **16**:48–50.

67. Sampson TG, Nisbet JK, Glick JM. Precision acromioplasty in arthroscopic subacromial decompression. *Arthroscopy* 1991; **7**:301–7.

68. Snyder SJ, Pattee GA. Shoulder arthroscopy in the evaluation and treatment of rotator cuff lesions. In: Paulos LE, Tibone JE, eds. *Operative Techniques in Shoulder Surgery.* Gaithersburg, MD: Aspen, 1991; 45.

69. Snyder SJ, Pachelli AF, Del Pizzo WD et al. Partial thickness rotator cuff tears: results of arthroscopic treatment. *Arthroscopy* 1991; **7**:1–7.

70. Burkhart SS. Arthroscopic treatment of massive rotator cuff tears: clinical results and biomechanical rational. *Clin Orthop* 1991; **267**:45–56.

71. Tippett JW. Partial repair of rotator cuff tears greater than five centimeters [abstract]. Presented at the 17th Annual Meeting of the Arthroscopy Association of North America, Orlando, 30 April–3 May, 1998.

72. Weber SC. Arthroscopic debridement and acromioplasty versus mini-open repair in the treatment of significant partial-thickness rotator cuff tears. *Arthroscopy* 1999; **15**:126–31.

73. Tauro JC. Arthroscopic rotator cuff repair: analysis of technique and results at 2- and 3-year follow-up. *Arthroscopy* 1998; **14**:45–51.

74. Gartsman GM, Khan M, Hammerman SM. Arthroscopic repair of full-thickness tears of the rotator cuff. *J Bone Joint Surg [Am]* 1998; **80**:832–40.

75. Snyder SJ, Karzel RP, Del Pizzo W et al. SLAP lesions of the shoulder. *Arthroscopy* 1990; **6**:274–9.

76. Jobe CM. Posterior superior glenoid impingement: expanded spectrum. *Arthroscopy* 1995; **11**:530–6.

77. Walch G, Boileau J, Noel E et al. Impingement of the deep surface of the supraspinatus tendon on the posterior superior glenoid rim: an arthroscopic study. *J Shoulder Elbow Surg* 1992; **1**:238.

78. Burkhart SS, Morgan CD. The peel-back mechanism: its role in producing and extending posterior type II SLAP lesions and its effect on SLAP repair rehabilitation. *Arthroscopy* 1998; **14**:637–40.

79. Morgan CD, Burkhart SS, Palmeri M, Gillespie M. Type II SLAP lesions: three subtypes and their relationships to superior instability and rotator cuff tears. *Arthroscopy* 1998; **14**:553–65.

80. Wiley AM. Arthroscopic appearance of frozen shoulder. *Arthroscopy* 1991; **7**:138–43.

81. Uitvlugt G, Detrisac DA, Johnson LL. The pathology of the frozen shoulder: an arthroscopic perspective [abstract]. *Arthroscopy* 1988; **4**:137.

82. Poehling GG. Frozen shoulder. Presented at the 8th Annual Meeting of Arthroscopy of the Shoulder, San Diego, July 1991.

83. Neviaser TJ. Arthroscopy of the shoulder. *Orthop Clin North Am* 1987; **18**:361–72.

84. Esch JC, Baker CL. *Arthroscopic Surgery: The Shoulder and Elbow.* Philadelphia: JB Lippincott, 1993;205.

85. Warner JJP, Allen AA, Marks PH, Wong P. Arthroscopic release for chronic, refractory adhesive capsulitis of the shoulder. *J Bone Joint Surg* 1996; **78A**:1808–16.

86. Harryman DT, Matsen FA, Sidles JA. Arthroscopic management of refractory shoulder stiffness. *Arthroscopy* 1997; **13**:133–47.

87. Rodeo SA, Hannafin JA, Tom J et al. Immunolocalization of cytokines and their receptors in adhesive capsulitis of the shoulder. *J Orthop Res* **15**:427–36.

88. Mormino MA, Gross RM, McCarthy JA. Captured shoulder: a complication of rotator cuff surgery. *Arthroscopy* 1996; **12**:457–61.

2 Anatomy and biomechanics of the shoulder

Andreas B Imhoff and Jonathan B Ticker

Anatomy and function of the glenohumeral joint

The shoulder consists of five articulations: the sternoclavicular joint, the acromioclavicular joint, the glenohumeral joint, the subacromial space, and the scapulothoracic gliding plane. All of these function in a precise, synchronous manner to achieve a large range of motion. Movement of the hand requires motion of the clavicle, scapula, and humerus and requires many complex mechanisms to maintain joint stability.[1,2]

The glenohumeral joint has the greatest range of motion of all the joints in the human body. This functional situation is permitted by an anatomic arrangement where articular surface conformity offers little inherent stability;[3] therefore, joint stability is thought to be primarily achieved through static and dynamic soft-tissue restraints.[4-13] The static stabilizers, including osteoarticular geometry and the capsuloligamentous structures, as well as the effect of adhesion/cohesion and negative intra-articular pressure, must work together with a large number of muscles as the dynamic stabilizers to provide stability. Although the joint capsule and glenohumeral ligaments have been shown to limit excessive translation of the humeral head on the glenoid, most experimental studies have only provided indirect information about the tension or laxity in these structures during glenohumeral motion.[10-12,14-20] The rotator cuff and long head of the biceps brachii have been shown to contribute to joint stability through joint compression and steering effects that are dependent on arm position,[4,6,21,22] Disruption of one or more of these soft-tissue restraint mechanisms can lead to abnormal glenohumeral kinematics and can result in shoulder instability.[23-25]

The normal amount of anterior, posterior and inferior glenohumeral translation varies widely among individuals.[6] These translations associated with joint laxity should not be confused with glenohumeral instability. In this chapter, laxity is defined as the ability of the humeral head to translate passively on the glenoid, whereas instability is defined as a clinical condition in which excessive and undesired translation of the humeral head occurs and affects the function of the shoulder.

Static constraints

Articular components (humerus/glenoid)

The articular surfaces of the head of the humerus and the glenoid fossa of the scapula, although reciprocally curved, are oval and are not sections of true spheres. As the head of the humerus is larger than the glenoid fossa, only part of the humeral head can be in articulation with glenoid fossa in any position of the joint. The glenoid face offers a nearly pear-shaped surface, being narrow superiorly and wider inferiorly, with average anteroposterior and superoinferior dimensions of 25 mm and 35 mm, respectively. In contrast, the respective humeral head dimensions are 45 mm and 48 mm. Bigliani et al measured the humeral head and of the glenoid fossa using stereophotogrammetry: the radius of the humeral head was 25.23 ± 1.62 mm and that of the glenoid fossa was 27.03 ± 1.68 mm.[26] In any position only 25–30% of the humeral head is in contact with the glenoid surface.[27,28] The glenohumeral index, a ratio of maximum glenoid diameter to maximum humeral head diameter, has been determined to be approximately 0.6 in the transverse plane and 0.75 in the sagittal plane.[10,29,30] Examinations of the congruency of the articular surface at this joint have revealed the radii of curvature of the humeral head and the glenoid to be 23 mm and 24.5 mm, respectively.[31] The use of stereophotogrammetry by Soslowsky et al showed the true relationship between the two articular surfaces and determined that the glenoid cartilage was thicker peripherally than centrally, whereas the humeral cartilage was thicker centrally than peripherally. Consequently, the articular surfaces are closely congruent and nearly spherical.[31]

The humeral head and neck make an angle of 130–150° with the shaft, and are retroverted about 20–30° in relation to the transverse axis of the elbow. In 75% of subjects the glenoid is retrotilted by an average of 7.4° in relation to the plane of the scapula,[3,7,29,32] but in these studies, a wide range of normal values was established, including 25% of subjects possessing 2–10° of anteversion.[29] It has been suggested that this relationship is important in maintaining horizontal stability of the joint and counteracting any tendency toward anterior displacement of the humeral head.[29,33] Excessive retroversion of the glenoid cavity could be a cause of non-traumatic[32] or recurrent[34,35] posterior instability of the shoulder. However, this concept has not been supported by subsequent studies.[36]

In addition the glenoid is superiorly tilted by approximately 5°. This could be a necessary component for inferior joint stability, though it remains controversial. Galinat and Howell found no correlation between glenoid version and anterior or posterior instability,[5] while recent work of Itoi et al has implicated the importance of scapular inclination in the maintenance of inferior glenohumeral stability.[21]

Glenoid labrum

The labrum consists of fibrocartilage and fibrous tissue. However, it is not like the fibrocartilaginous meniscus and cannot withstand the type of meniscal stresses seen in the knee.[1,37] The labrum differs from the meniscus in lacking the microscopic architecture to disperse the hoop stresses that are important in meniscal biomechanics. The inner surface of the labrum is covered with synovium; the outer surface attaches to the capsule and is continuous with the periosteum of the scapular neck.

The function of the labrum is controversial. The role of the labrum both in increasing glenoid articular surface area and in load distribution has been suggested by the experimental work of several authors.[1,4,31] Galinat and Howell showed that the glenoid and labrum combine to form a socket with a depth up to 9 mm in the supero-inferior direction and 5 mm in the anteroposterior direction. Without the labrum the average anteroposterior depth was only 2.5 mm. They described a chock–block function to the labrum in preventing anterior translation.[5] The main function of the labrum may be to serve as an attachment for the glenohumeral ligaments, especially for the important inferior glenohumeral ligament complex, which is the primary ligamentous stabilizer.[20,38] Detachment of the labrum represents a Bankart lesion, in which the capsulolabral complex is torn from the glenoid rim.[39] However, every labral pathology is always accompanied by glenohumeral instability.[40,41]

Coracohumeral ligament

The coracohumeral ligament (CHL) is an important ligamentous structure in the shoulder complex. The ligament originates as a broad band from the base and lateral border of the coracoid process[42] or, rarely, as a continuation of the pectoralis minor tendon.[43,44] Neer et al[45] found that the origin at the base of the coracoid process extended along the lateral border of the coracoid for an average of 18 mm, while Ferrari measured this base as 25 mm.[46] The CHL passes obliquely downwards and laterally to the humerus, draping the interval – the so-called rotator interval – between the anterior margin of the supraspinatus tendon and the superior margin of the subscapularis tendon. Posteriorly the attachment to the supraspinatus blends with the fascia of the muscle along the length of the ligament. Anteriorly the ligament

blends with the insertion of the subscapularis tendon to the lesser tuberosity. Laterally the ligament separates into two major bands that insert into the greater and lesser tuberosities with a broad insertion over the anatomic neck of the humerus, creating a tunnel near the bicipital groove through which the biceps tendon passes (Figures 2.1 and 2.2). Inferiorly the CHL joins the superior glenohumeral ligament. This attachment occurs in the mid-portion on both the coracohumeral and the superior glenohumeral ligaments.

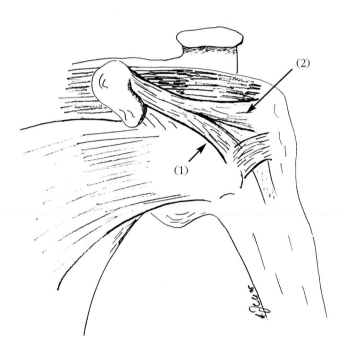

Figure 2.1

Schematic representation of CHL with anterior (1) and posterior (2) band (left shoulder).

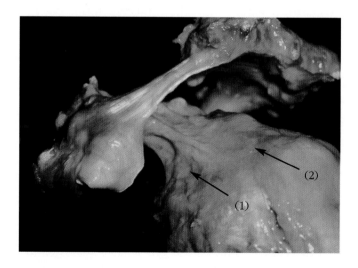

Figure 2.2

The CHL anterior (1) and posterior (2) bands showing intermingling of fibres with the antero-superior capsule, the supraspinatus, and the subscapularis (right shoulder).

Many investigators believe the CHL is the major structural ligamentous component in the anterosuperior region of the capsule.[5,45,47–49] Neer et al concluded from a study of 63 shoulder specimens (58 fixed and 5 fresh-frozen) that the CHL was well developed, and suggested it was important in preventing excessive external rotation. They went on to state that the CHL was found to be shortened in various pathologic states (e.g. frozen shoulder or adhesive capsulitis) and its release might be required to restore restricted external rotation.[45]

The structural interrelationships of the CHL, superior glenohumeral ligament (SGHL), and rotator cuff were described by Clark and Harryman,[50] who demonstrated that the rotator cuff and capsule are conjoined in this region. Harryman et al[16] described the interval as the region between the supraspinatus and subscapularis tendon. The CHL and the SGHL are considered to be the most constant structures of the fibrous joint capsule in the rotator interval, but each has separate origins and insertions. The transverse humeral ligament at the bicipital groove forms the apex of the interval. Edelson et al showed the CHL to be the main capsuloligamentous structure here.[47] Cooper et al in 1993[51] suggested that previous investigators might not have done a 'meticulous separation of the CHL and SGHL when examining the anatomy.' In addition, they suggested that because 'embalming increases the consistency of the tissue', previous studies using embalmed tissue may have led to the false belief that the CHL was a more significant structure than it actually is in vivo. A gross anatomy and histology study of the anterosuperior part of the capsule indicated that the SGHL was the major stabilizing component, while the CHL appeared to be no more than a thin fold of capsular tissue.[51] Strain gauge measurements by Terry et al[11] and O'Connell et al[52] have demonstrated that the CHL passively limits external rotation and inferior translation in the adducted glenohumeral joint.

Superior glenohumeral ligament

The SGHL represents the smallest of the three glenohumeral ligaments, although it is quite a consistent structure, being identifiable in up to 97% of shoulders.[43,53–55] The SGHL arises from the labrum and the anterosuperior edge of the glenoid near the origin of the tendon of the long head of the biceps. It passes the floor of the rotator interval and inserts on the top of the lesser tuberosity of the humerus with a portion of the CHL. Clark has defined the tissue layers at the glenohumeral joint in his anatomic studies and elucidated the structural interrelationships between the capsule, the rotator cuff tendons, the SGHL, and the CHL.[50]

Middle glenohumeral ligament

The middle glenohumeral ligament (MGHL) is not consistently present, but is significantly larger and also more variable in size than the SGHL, usually 1–2 cm wide and 4 mm thick.[42,43] It originates from the supraglenoid tubercle and the anterosuperior labrum below the SGHL on the superior glenoid, traverses the anterior capsule, and inserts anteriorly on the base of the lesser tuberosity of the humeral neck along with the posterior aspect of the subscapularis muscle. The ligament is intimately attached to the tendon of the subscapularis muscle. In younger patients the MGHL is better defined by the inferior subscapularis bursa, but it can still be visualized and palpated in older patients. After the age of 60 years the MGHL becomes very thin.

The MGHL prevents anterior translation of the humeral head in external rotation, but it is also an important anterior stabilizer in the lower to middle ranges of abduction (from 45° to 75°). Ferrari showed that the MGHL acts with the CHL to check external rotation from 0° to 60° of abduction.[46] At 60° the support of the CHL was lost. In the range 60–90° abduction and external rotation the MGHL has no function. Additionally, the MGHL is tightened over the anterior aspect of the humeral head in a position of extension and 45° of external rotation during abduction from 0° to 90°.

Inferior glenohumeral ligament complex

Composed of anterior and posterior bands and an axillary pouch, the inferior glenohumeral ligament complex (IGHLC) spans the anterior to posteroinferior capsule. Turkel et al described three parts of this ligament: the superior or anterior band, the anterior axillary pouch and the posterior axillary pouch or the posterior band.[56]

Posterior capsule

Finally, the thin posterior capsule alone occupies the posterosuperior quadrant, with no additional ligamentous thickening present. To understand the role the shoulder capsule plays in shoulder stability, it is often helpful to think of the capsule between the glenoid and humeral head as a circle. For dislocation to occur in one direction, there must be damage to both sides of the capsule. Therefore in cases of anterior instability there is also an increase in posterior laxity. Conversely, posterior dislocation cannot occur without anterior damage. The posterior capsule is secondary to the posterior band in conferring both anteroposterior and superoinferior stability.

Harryman et al have shown that a tight posterior capsule can cause anterosuperior translation with flexion,[6] resulting in anterior impingement. In contrast, Bigliani et al[26] showed, after tightening of the anterior capsule, that the head consistently translated posteriorly (0.63 ± 0.24 mm). However, there was no significant difference in medial–lateral and superior–inferior directions in neutral rotation or anterior tightening during the complete elevation. Articular contact patterns on the glenoid exhibited a corresponding posterior shift and a reduction in contact area in the tightened shoulders. In incongruent joints there was increased posterior translation (> 2.2 mm).

Dynamic factors

Rotator cuff

The rotator cuff is the musculotendinous complex formed by the attachment to the capsule of the tendon of the supraspinatus muscle superiorly, the subscapularis muscle anteriorly, and the teres minor and the infraspinatus muscle posteriorly.[57] These tendons blend intricately with the fibrous capsule. The four muscles of the rotator cuff and the long head of the biceps tendon contribute to the dynamic stability of the glenohumeral joint.[22]

The deltoid and the supraspinatus muscles are the primary movers of glenohumeral abduction. These muscles have been found to contribute equally to torque production in functional planes of motion. With the arm at the side, the directional force of the deltoid muscle is almost vertical: thus most of the deltoid force will cause an upward translation motion of the humeral head. The action lines of the infraspinatus, subscapularis and teres minor muscles are such that each tends to have a rotary component as well as a compressive force. Each also has a downward translation component that offsets the upward translation force of the deltoid. Infraspinatus, teres minor and subscapularis thus form a force couple with the deltoid and act to stabilize the humeral head on the glenoid fossa, allowing deltoid and supraspinatus to act as abductor of the humerus.

The rotator cuff has been thought to compress the humeral head into the glenoid, thus stabilizing the joint. Contraction of the cuff muscle would also influence the direction of joint force. For example, in abducting the arm, the contraction of the rotator cuff will assist the deltoid muscle in reducing the magnitude of the resultant joint force and the direction of the force relative to the glenoid surface.

Injuries to the rotator cuff such as those due to overload in an overhead athlete, may lead to diminished joint compression. As a result, increased translation in the anterior–posterior or superior–inferior direction may be possible. This excessive translation may cause overload of the capsuloligamentous structures and stretching or failure at their attachments, or stretching of the suprascapular nerve at the posterior capsule.[58–60] The increased translation may also cause shear forces on the glenoid and result in labral injuries.[2,61,62]

Biceps tendon

The biceps, the main flexor and supinator of the elbow, has the tendon of its long head across the glenohumeral joint. Theoretically, contraction of the biceps could provide a similar contribution to dynamic stabilization of the glenohumeral joint as the rotator cuff, preventing upward migration of the head of the humerus during powerful elbow flexion and forearm supination. Lesions of the long head of biceps therefore may produce instability and shoulder dysfunction.[22,61]

Soslowsky et al[63] demonstrated the contribution of the long head of the biceps on anterior shoulder stability through a range of translations. Tension in the long head of the biceps tendon demonstrated a large stabilization efficiency, even at low displacements. Due to its favorable line of action, the long head of the biceps directly absorbs subluxation energy, while the rotator cuff muscles provide stability by increased glenoid compression.[92]

An et al[64] have shown, in an experimental evaluation, that loading applied on the biceps causes displacement of the humeral head. In general, the head displaces superoanteriorly or posteriorly depending on arm abduction and axial rotational position. Loading of the biceps reduced the displacement of the humeral head under translational force with the arm in an abducted position.[22]

Negative intra-articular pressure

Negative intra-articular pressure is an effect of the vacuum created in the glenohumeral joint as a result of the joint capsule being a sealed structure with limited volume. This negative intra-articular pressure could limit glenohumeral translation. Warner and colleagues studied inferior translation in the intact and vented shoulder and found that negative intra-articular pressure had a role in the adducted shoulder, preventing inferior translation of the humeral head on the glenoid.[30,66] Kumar and Balasubramaniam observed that venting of the capsule in a cadaver resulted in significant inferior translation of the adducted shoulder.[66] With application of an inferior force Browne et al could measure an increase in the negative intra-articular pressure.[14] The average intra-articular pressure in the adducted shoulder of a cadaver was -42 cm H_2O and an inferior force increased this intra-articular pressure to -82 cm H_2O. This is most likely the result of the high osmotic pressure in interstitial tissue. This phenomenon is important in cases of capsular defects or increased joint volume, where the disrupted vacuum effect causes an increased tendency to excessive translation.

Adhesion and cohesion

The articular surfaces of the shoulder joint give additional stability through an adhesion–cohesion effect in the same way that the presence of water between two glass microscope slides prevents them from being pulled apart.

Biomechanics of the glenohumeral joint

First, some basic terms and testing techniques must be explained. The common experimental method used to study the mechanical behavior of ligaments and tendons is the tensile test. This test is used because the main physiologic function of the ligaments and tendons is to resist tensile loads. Such an experimental method can yield the structural properties of the bone–ligament–bone complex as well as the mechanical properties of the ligament substance.

Basic biomechanics

Structural properties are represented by a load–elongation curve. Typically, the curve is non-linear and concave upwards. Its initial region is referred to as the 'toe' region, representing low stiffness because the collagen fibres change from a crimped to an uncrimped alignment. As larger loads are applied, stiffness increases and the load–elongation curve becomes linear. Structural properties are represented by parameters such as stiffness, ultimate load, ultimate deformation, and energy absorbed at failure.

Mechanical properties of the ligament or tendon substance are determined from the stress–strain relationship. Stress is defined as load per unit of cross-sectional area; strain is the change in length per unit of original length. The stress–strain curve (or relationship), therefore, is independent of the specimen's size and shape. These properties reflect collagen fiber organization and orientation, as well as the microstructure of ligamentous tissue.[67] Mechanical properties of the ligament substance are represented by parameters such as the modulus, ultimate tensile strength, ultimate strain, and strain energy density. Failure of a bone–ligament–bone complex can occur through any of several mechanisms: fracture through a bone; avulsion, wherein the ligament pulls a small piece of bone free, leaving the insertion sites intact; insertion site failure, in which no bone is displaced; and mid-substance rupture of the ligament. Mechanical properties such as ultimate tensile strength and ultimate strain can be measured only if failure occurs within the substance of the tissue; therefore, it is important to report the failure mode of any tensile test.

Coracohumeral and superior glenohumeral ligaments

The stabilizing roles of the SGHL and the CHL have been appreciated only recently. Some have suggested that these structures act as restraints to inferior translation and external rotation of the adducted arm.[16,52,65] To further clarify the function of these two ligaments, their respective anatomic and structural properties were analysed in a recent study.[68,69]

Fresh-frozen cadaveric shoulders (donor age 55–76 years) were resected to allow fixation of the specimens in specially designed clamps. Specimens were deemed acceptable (no pathologic changes) based on an arthroscopic evaluation. In 10 specimens, the CHL was preserved, while in the other 10 specimens, the SGHL was preserved (Figure 2.3). This dissection left a bone–ligament–bone complex for tensile testing.

The cross-sectional area of each ligament was measured three times at the same location; repeatability was within 5%. In light of the obvious tapering of the SGHL from glenoid to humerus, its cross-sectional area was measured at three locations: at the proximal, middle, and distal thirds. The tapering of the cross-sectional area of the SGHL from origin to insertion was confirmed, the proximal area (20 mm²) being more than twice that of the distal area (9 mm²). In contrast, the CHL tended to fan out as it inserted on the humerus, merging with the rotator cuff tendons. The cross-sectional geometry of the two ligaments also differed. The cross-sectional area at

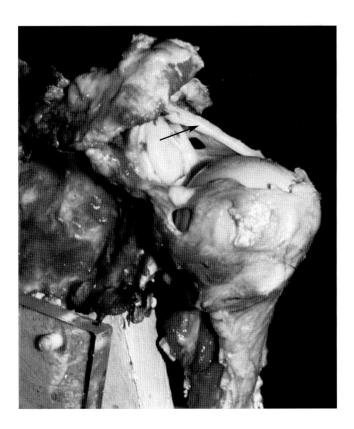

Figure 2.3

Posterior view of the left shoulder: The SGHL (arrow) arises from the labrum and the antero-superior edge of the glenoid near the origin of the tendon of the long head of the biceps.

the mid-portion of the CHL was found to be approximately 5 times that of the SGHL (54 mm^2 versus 11 mm^2).

Each specimen was then mounted in an Instron materials testing machine (Instron, Canton, MA, USA) using humeral and scapular clamps designed to allow proper longitudinal alignment and loading of ligament fibers. The stiffness, ultimate load, percentage elongation to failure, and energy absorbed to failure were derived from the load–elongation curve for each specimen. The stiffness, ultimate load, ultimate deformation, and energy absorbed to failure for the CHL were all significantly different from those of the SGHL. The CHL had twice the stiffness of the SGHL and 3 times the ability to withstand tensile loads compared with the SGHL. The CHL also absorbed 6 times the amount of energy to failure but only elongated 1.5 times as much as the SGHL during tensile testing. The values obtained for stiffness and ultimate load of the CHL were higher (150%) than those reported for the IGHLC components and the coracoacromial ligament (CAL)[70,72] but these values were much lower than those for the anterior cruciate ligament of the knee (15%).[67] All but one of the CHL specimens failed in the proximal ligament substance; the exception failed by bony avulsion at the coracoid process. In contrast, all of the SGHL specimens failed in the distal ligament substance near its insertion on the humerus.

The CHL is a discrete capsular thickening that behaves biomechanically like a ligament even if it lacks the typical histologic organization. As a significant capsuloligamentous structure it may function as a primary stabilizer in adduction and external rotation, maintaining glenohumeral stability by limiting inferior humeral translation and excessive external rotation.[13,30,52,54,65,72] Neer et al show that release of the CHL increased external rotation both with the arm at the side and with 90° of forward flexion.[46]

It is still controversial which ligamentous structure of the anterosuperior part of the glenohumeral capsule is most important in the prevention of inferior subluxation. The capsular cutting investigations performed by Oveson and Nielsen and later by Helmig et al confirmed this function of the superior capsule.[48,49,54,72,73] Work by Warner et al reconfirmed the importance of negative intra-articular pressure and the importance of the SGHL in limiting inferior humeral migration.[30] The SGHL becomes tight in adduction and is positioned to resist inferior and posterior translation. Posterior dislocation does not occur during selective cutting of the posterior part of the capsule until the anterosuperior structures have been released. In conclusion, the rotator interval is a primary restraint to inferior and posterior translation.

In summary, the CHL is much more robust than the SGHL and behaves biomechanically as a stiffer and stronger ligament. Because the SGHL tapers significantly toward its humeral insertion site, it failed in the distal portion when loaded in uniaxial tension. Conversely, the CHL, which fans out to merge with the rotator cuff tendons as it nears the humerus, failed proximally. Thus quantitative anatomic findings can be correlated with structural properties of the SGHL and CHL. Our data show that these two ligaments have significant structural properties.

Inferior glenohumeral ligament

Most studies have focused on the IGHLC[20,56,70] as the major static stabilizer of the abducted glenohumeral joint. Bigliani et al[70] examined the anatomic, geometric and mechanical properties of this complex. The superior or anterior band was found to be the thickest. Significant differences in total specimen strain at failure for the three IGHLC regions were observed for slow and fast strain rates. The anterior axillary pouch failed at a higher strain than either the anterior band or the posterior axillary pouch. Significant strain variations existed along the length of each region of the IGHLC. The strain was higher near the bony insertion side: 65% of the specimens failed at the insertion sites (40% at the glenoid and 25% at the humeral side), while 35% failed in the ligament mid-substance. In contrast, the failure stress in the anterior band and the anterior axillary pouch were significantly greater than in the posterior axillary pouch.

The geometric and biomechanical properties of the IGHLC appear to be well-suited to its role as a primary static anterior stabilizer of the glenohumeral joint. When the arm is abducted and externally rotated, a sudden traumatic event might overwhelm the dynamic stabilizers.[71]

The IGHLC is particularly important as it provides stability to the joint when the arm is in functional positions. The anterior band of the complex is the major stabilizer of the joint. It prevents anterior–inferior translation of the humeral head in abduction, external rotation and extension. In 90° abduction and external rotation the anterior band of the IGHLC wraps around the humeral head like a hammock to prevent anterior humeral migration (Figures 2.4–2.12). This suggests that the structure of the IGHLC provides stability during overhead motions, such as throwing, tennis serves, and freestyle swimming strokes.

Coracoacromial ligament and rotator cuff disease

Inflammation of the rotator cuff tendons and surrounding tissue is one of the most common causes of pain and disability in the upper extremity. Those who suffer range from the athlete and worker with repetitive overhead activities, to the elderly person with years of use. Despite the prevalence of this condition, its cause remains elusive.[74] It has been proposed that the supraspinatus tendon is damaged by compression under the coracoacromial arch.[18,46,75–80] The arch (consisting of the coracoid, acromion, and CAL (Figure 2.2)) is believed to cause pain, inflammation, and the ultimate rupture of the rotator cuff in association with abnormal joint kinematics.[58] In the absence of significant acromial abnormality, the CAL has been implicated in causing impingement at the joint. This conclusion was drawn from studies in which the CAL from pathologic specimens was noted to be qualitatively enlarged and stiffened with ultrastructural changes.[81,82] However, shoulder impingements are often situated much more anteriorly, between the coracoid process and the lesser tuberosity. The subacromial coracoclavicular space is divided into two compartments by the CHL. The normal space between the humeral head and the coracoid process in two functional positions of the arm was measured by Gerber and colleagues in 1985 using computerized tomography in adduction and flexion. The average distance was 8.7 ± 2.4 mm and decreased to 6.8 ± 2.9 mm in flexion.[83,84] Overuse in flexion and internal rotation may lead to displacement of the humeral head (for example in gymnastics, lance throwing or swimming). The coracohumeral space can be crowded by an isolated traumatic tear of the subscapularis usually associated with a dislocation of the long head of the biceps.[85] In addition to its role in impingement, the CAL supports the acromion and the coracoid as loads are transmitted to them through the surrounding musculature.

The CAL consists of two distinct bands: lateral and medial. These bands are similar in length and thickness, but the lateral band is consistently wider and has a much greater cross-sectional area. When shoulders with and without rotator cuff tears were compared, the lateral band was significantly shorter and the cross-sectional area was significantly larger in the group with rotator cuff tears. Because the lateral band is in the region where impingement of the rotator cuff can occur, it is reasonable to conclude that a shorter lateral band with a larger cross-sectional area could impinge on the underlying rotator cuff tendon. Whether such changes contribute to rotator cuff tears or occur as a result of cuff tears is not certain.[81]

With the growing awareness of the roles of the CAL, Soslowsky et al also compared the tensile properties of this ligament from shoulders with and without rotator cuff injuries. They found no statistically significant differences between normal and rotator cuff tear groups in structural properties (stiffness, ultimate load, and ultimate elongation) in the lateral band of the CAL. The medial band was not tested as it is relatively lax in this position. Assessment of the mechanical properties of the CAL showed a significant reduction in modulus and ultimate tensile strength in the shoulders with rotator cuff tears.[81,86] This finding corroborated previous work that the CAL in shoulders with rotator cuff tears have disorganized tissue and a loss of normal collagen fiber orientation.[56]

Glenohumeral joint capsule and age-related changes

Two types of tissue disruption in acute dislocation of the shoulder occur in humans: one is capsular rupture; the other is intracapsular dislocation in which the glenoid labrum or capsule is avulsed. These injuries differ in age distribution, capsular rupture predominating in the elderly and intracapsular dislocation being an injury of the young. This difference suggested that the relative strength of the components of the anterior retaining structures might alter with age.[87] Two studies examined the age-related properties of the glenohumeral joint capsule and capsular structures.

Kaltsas[88] studied the relationship between the age and the force required to rupture the capsule. Tensile testing performed on the entire joint capsule revealed that the strength of the capsule bears an inverse relationship to the age of the patient: that is, the capsule becomes weaker with increasing age. Studies have shown that the capsule weakens from the increase in calcification with age. Kaltsas also found that the anteroinferior part of capsule ruptured first, which suggests that this part of the capsule is the weakest and corresponds to clinical findings that anterior dislocation of the shoulder is most common.

Reeves[87] examined the age-related changes in the tensile properties of the subscapularis tendon and the anteroinferior part of the capsule. A total of 131 bone–ligament–bone or bone–tendon complexes were made, consisting of either the superior capsule, posterior capsule, or subscapularis tendon. The results from tensile testing showed that the strength of the subscapularis tendon varied with age and from specimen to specimen. This variation seems to be related to the cross-sectional area of the tendon and to the presence of ectopic areas of calcification in the tendon. Age-related calcification caused the tendon to rupture at a lower load per cross-sectional area than does normal tendon. Failure modes suggested that in the young, the weakest point in the anterior shoulder structures is the glenoid labral attachment, whereas in the elderly, the weakest point is the capsule and subscapularis tendon substance. These findings correspond to the age distributions for the two predominant shoulder dislocations as described above.

Comparison of ligaments of the shoulder and knee

Since the 1980s, there have been many well-controlled tensile tests on ligaments[68,89–93] most of which have focused on the anterior cruciate ligament (ACL) and the medial collateral ligament (MCL) of the knee. To put the biomechanical properties of ligaments from the shoulder in proper perspective, they should be compared with those of the knee.

The structural properties of the human femur–ACL–tibia complex (FATC) have been evaluated by Trent et al,[94] and by Noyes and Grood.[95] The structural properties of FATCs at 30° of knee flexion were compared among three age groups (*n* = 27 pairs).[67] The mean stiffness values for each group were 242 ± 28 N/mm (young, 22–35 years), 220 ± 24 N/mm (middle-aged, 40–50 years), and 180 ± 25 N/mm (old, 60–97 years). The ultimate load to failure of the young group (2160 ± 157 N) was approximately 50% higher than that of the middle-aged group (1503 ± 83 N) and more than three times higher than that of the oldest group (658 ± 129 N). The results for energy absorbed at failure were 11.6 ± 1.7 N.mm, 6.1 ± 0.5 N.mm, 1.8 ± 0.5 N.mm for the young, middle-ages, and old groups, respectively.

Woo et al also examined the mechanical properties of the rabbit MCL and ACL.[93] In the skeletally mature rabbit, the moduli for these two ligaments were 1120 ± 53 MPa and 516 ± 64 MPa. The tensile strength of the MCL and ACL substance was 35 ± 4 MPa, and 42 ± 5 MPa, respectively, while the strain at failure in the MCL was 4.1 ± 0.7% and in the ACL was 5.3 ± 0.5%.

Bigliani et al[70] studied the mechanical properties of the human IGHLC and reported that the modulus was greatest for the anterior band (62.6 ± 9.8 MPa) and least for the posterior band (39.9 ± 13.3 MPa). The tensile strength of the anterior and posterior bands and the axillary pouch ranged from 5.9 ± 1.7 MPa to 8.4 ± 2.2 MPa. The strain at failure was greatest for the anterior axillary pouch (10.8 ± 2.4%) and least for the posterior axillary pouch (7.8 ± 3.6%).

When the structural properties of the ACL were compared with those of the SGHL and the CHL in humans, significant differences were found in stiffness, the SGHL and CHL having approximately 10% the stiffness of the ACL. Ultimate load also differed significantly, with values for the SGHL being only 5%, and the CHL 15%, of the ACL value. The average modulus of the human IGHLC was only 10% of the modulus measured in rabbit MCL and the tensile strength of the IGHLC was only 15% that of the MCL. These differences suggest that the soft tissues at the shoulder do not function in the same capacity as those at the knee joint.

The stability of a joint can be described by the joint's stiffness, which for the shoulder, depends on the position of the arm. During the normal range of motion, the glenohumeral joint has a relatively low stiffness (laxity), which allows it to have a much greater range of motion than the knee joint. The minimal laxity of the knee accommodates its relatively limited range of motion (Table 2.1).

Discussion

Laxity or tension

This study evaluated tension and laxity (percentage elongation) in the glenohumeral ligaments during eight

Table 2.1		
	Length (L$_0$) *mean ± SD* *(mm)*	*Range widths* *mean ± SD* *(mm)*
SGHL	44.5 ± 3.6	38–53
MGHL	49.4 ± 8.1	34–60
AB-IGHLC	50.1 ± 4.9	43–59
PB-IGHLC	50.5 ± 7.8	45–76
AB-CHL	46.8 ± 12.6	33–67
PB-CHL	59.9 ± 11.1	48–76
CHL Origin	20.4 ± 3.1	
CHL Mid-portion	16.4 ± 4.4	
CHL Insertion	25.3 ± 4.7	
Humeral head radius	24.2 ± 1.4	21.5–25.02

AB, anterior band; CHL, coracohumeral ligament; IGHLC, inferior glenohumeral ligament complex; MGHL, middle glenohumeral ligament; PB, posterior band; SGHL, superior glenohumeral ligament.

motion paths of joint rotation. As no force was applied to displace the humerus out of the glenoid, no conclusions can be drawn as to the role of these ligaments in limiting excessive translations. Instead, information has been obtained that gives insight into the tension encountered by the ligaments during rotation of the normal shoulder joint. The physiologic amount of anterior, posterior, and inferior glenohumeral translation varies widely among individuals. These glenohumeral translations are associated with joint laxity but should not be confused with glenohumeral instability. The glenohumeral ligaments are discrete collagenous thickenings in the shoulder joint capsule with tensile properties that support their role in limiting excessive translations and rotations.[16,48,49,52,65,72,73] However, their role has been largely inferred indirectly from anatomic observations and ligament-cutting experiments.[12,20,38,51,52,56,70]

A few studies have attempted to give information about strain in these ligaments; however, the strain gauges used yielded information about only the small portion of the ligament in which they were placed.[11,52] Furthermore, most of these studies have been performed statically without any simulated rotator cuff muscle activity. A few studies have analysed the combined effect of static ligament restraint and dynamic rotator cuff and biceps muscle action on the anterior and posterior stability of the joint,[21,63] although these were ligament sectioning studies. Our laboratory previously demonstrated two-dimensional radiographic anatomy of these gleno-humeral ligaments in shoulders with simulated rotator cuff muscle activity;[12] however, the measurements were only semi-quantitative, being based on radiographs and did not account for the geometry of the ligament wrapping around the humeral head during rotation. The function of a ligamentous constraint depends on the tension and line of action of the force vector of the ligament. Stability in the glenohumeral joint is enhanced by the twisting or wrapping of the ligaments around the humeral head during joint rotation.

In the study described here we used the resting length (L_0) of the ligament as the reference value to determine if each ligament was lax or under tension. The degree of laxity or tension could be inferred from the percentage increase or decrease in the ligament's wrap-around length (L_w) relative to L_0. This allowed us to express glenohumeral anatomy with unprecedented precision. Moreover, muscle forces were applied in order to maintain the humeral head in the glenoid for concentric rotation. These muscle forces might also have affected the anatomy of the glenohumeral ligaments as the joint capsule and rotator cuff tendons have been shown to be anatomically conjoined in places.[50,68,69]

There was a high degree of variability in the reference length of each glenohumeral ligament, and this did not correlate with the humeral head size in each shoulder. This confirms the observations of DePalma[42] and others[20,33,46,51] that there is marked anatomic variability in the GHL and joint capsule anatomy (Figure 2.8). Moreover, these observations are consistent with those of Harryman and colleagues[6,16] and Warner et al[12] that the degree of laxity, or amount of translation of the humeral head on the glenoid, varies significantly in shoulders of normal individuals. Therefore, anatomically, the shoulder is not analogous to the knee, where the anterior and posterior cruciate ligaments are relatively constant structures. Instead, there is a wide range of length in the glenohumeral ligaments.

Coracohumeral ligament

Most reports on the CHL have failed to describe two distinct bands,[12,45,65,68,69,97] or only briefly mention that two bands exist.[97,98] In our study, we found that in all 10 fresh-frozen shoulders tested, the CHL was composed of two bands, the anterior and the posterior band, and that these bands were consistently present, well-developed, palpable anatomic structures. The posterior band was found to be longer than the anterior one, and the SGHL. The CHL as a whole (both bands together) resembled an hourglass in shape, with the mid-portion being the narrowest, and the insertion width the widest.

By separately quantifying percentage elongation (tension) and laxity in each band of the CHL through twelve different arcs of motion, our study clarified the function of these ligaments during rotations of normal glenohumeral joints. The reference length (L_0) of the ligament was used to determine if the CHL's two bands were lax or under tension during glenohumeral motion. The degree of laxity or tension could be determined by the percentage increase or decrease in the ligament's wrap-around length (L_w) relative to L_0. This comparison permitted a more quantitative anatomic description of the ligaments.

Trends were observed for both bands of the CHL during different shoulder motions. For the anterior band, initial elongation was greatest with the humerus in external rotation and the arm at the side, because of the greater humeral head wrap-around effect in this position. During abduction with the arm in neutral rotation, there was an initial increase in length L_w with a peak elongation around 35° abduction, and then subsequent shortening of L_w. With abduction and the humerus in internal rotation, L_w was shortened throughout the arc of motion. From these observations it appears that the anterior band-CHL acts as an important static restraint in abduction with the humerus in neutral and external rotation. The significant elongation of the initial L_w during adduction and humeral neutral and exteral rotation suggests that the anterior band plays a role in resisting early excessive adduction translation in these positions.

In both abduction and adduction the posterior band of the CHL underwent the greatest initial elongation with the humerus in internal rotation and was most shortened (or lax) with the humerus in external rotation. This suggests that this band is an important static restraint with the humerus in internal rotation with up to 50° abduction and 30° adduction. Additionally, because of their increased tension up to 40° abduction and 30° adduction, both bands of the CHL are likely to prevent excessive translation in these positions.

Our findings demonstrate that the two bands of the CHL apparently function in different ways, while the anterior band functions like the SGHL in normal shoulders during the glenohumeral motions tested.

Superior glenohumeral ligament

The SGHL has the smallest width and length of the three glenohumeral ligaments, although it is a consistent structure, being identifiable in up to 97% of shoulders.[20,42,51,65] The capsular cutting investigations performed by Ovesen and Nielsen[73] and later by Helmig et al[72] confirmed that the most important function of the SGHL was to prevent inferior subluxation of the humerus. In our study, the SGHL exhibited the greatest length at the neutral position. Values of L_w for five of ten shoulders were greater than L_0 which means that the SGHL is under tension in adduction and is positioned to resist inferior translation.[41] In addition, most of our specimens demonstrated their greatest lengths during the initial 50° of abduction. In one specimen L_w was 77% longer than L_0 in this position. As the humerus approached maximal abduction, L_w decreased steadily to L_0, the ligament therefore becoming lax. The radially-oriented fiber bundles wrapped and twisted around the humeral head, causing the length (L_w) of the SGHL to be larger than L_0, not only during horizontal adduction, but also during horizontal adduction and internal rotation (Figure 2.3).

Middle glenohumeral ligament

The MGHL is not consistently present and exhibits a large variation in length (Figure 2.4).[99,100] In younger patients the MGHL is better defined by the inferior subscapularis bursa, but it can still be visualized and palpated in older patients. After the age of 60 years the MGHL becomes very thin,[101] consistent with the findings of Woo et al, who examined the age-related changes of the rabbit medial collateral ligament.[89,90] Several studies identified the MGHL as a secondary restraint to both inferior and anterior instability, playing a greater role for anterior stability of the shoulder when its morphology is cord-like.[30,57] Our findings do not support Ferrari's[46] conclusions, which were that the MGHL and the CHL work together to limit external rotation from 0° to 60° of abduction and act as an important anterior stabilizer in the lower to middle ranges of abduction (from 45° to 75°). In our experiments, the MGHL L_w varied little during abduction (difference between L_0 and L_w small), with five of ten shoulders undergoing a 10% increase in elongation up to 45° (range 29–65°) and then reaching a plateau, and four shoulders remaining lax throughout the whole motion arc of abduction. In the range 60–90° of abduction and external rotation the MGHL tightened over the anterior aspect of the humeral head.

Inferior glenohumeral ligament complex

Composed of anterior and posterior bands and an axillary pouch, the IGHLC spans the anterior to the posteroinferior capsule. Turkel et al[56] described three parts of this ligament: the superior band, the anterior axillary pouch, and the posterior axillary pouch. Bigliani et al[70] and Ticker et al[71] examined the anatomic, geometric and mechanical properties of the IGHLC. The superior or anterior band was found to be the thickest. Significant differences in total specimen strain at failure for the three IGHLC regions were observed. The geometric and biomechanic properties of the IGHLC appear to be well suited for its role as a primary static anterior stabilizer of the glenohumeral joint. The complex is particularly important because it provides stability to the joint when the arm is in functional positions.

Anterior band

In our study, the IGHLC was divided into the anterior band (superior band), axillary pouch, and posterior band. We did not specifically study the axillary pouch. In these experiments the anterior band exhibited large differences between L_0 and L_w. Values of L_w steadily increased during the initial 40° of abduction, then remained at a plateau until maximal abduction. During abduction and extension, there was an increase of the ligament length above the reference length ($L_w > L_0$) in all shoulders, although three specimens were nonfunctional or lax during this motion. With maximal abduction and internal rotation seven shoulders demonstrated laxity of the anterior band ($L_w < L_0$). In 90° abduction and external rotation the anterior band of the IGHLC wrapped around the humeral head like a hammock to prevent anterior humeral translation (Figures 2.5–2.9). These observations support prior work that has inferred a stabilizing role for the ligament in abduction.

Posterior band

Similar tests on the posterior band of the IGHLC showed that during flexion L_w remained at a constant elongation until 30° of flexion motion path (range 25–50°); L_w then decreases approximately 10% over the remaining range of motion, L_w becoming smaller than L_0. The posterior

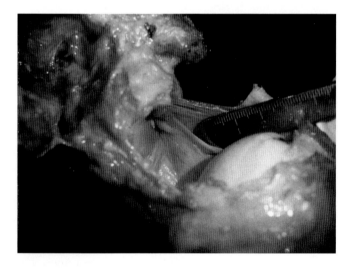

Figure 2.4

Posterior view of the left shoulder: The MGHL is variable in size and originates from the supraglenoid tubercle and the anterosuperior labrum below the SGHL and inserts anteriorly on the base of the lesser tuberosity of the humeral neck along with the posterior aspect of the subscapularis muscle. The MGHL is an important anterior stabilizer in the lower to middle ranges of abduction (from 45° to 75°).

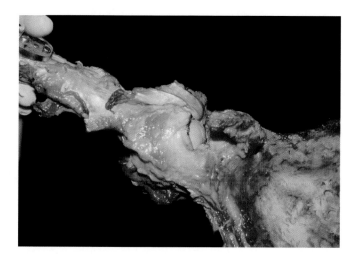

Figure 2.5

Anterior view of the right shoulder: anterior band of the IGHLC: abduction in the scapular plane with neutral rotation.

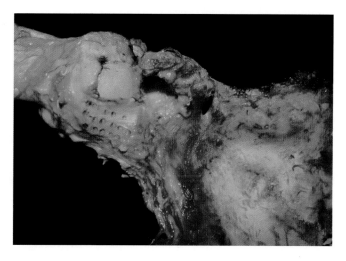

Figure 2.6

Anterior band of the IGHLC: internal rotation with the shoulder at 90° of scapularplane abduction.

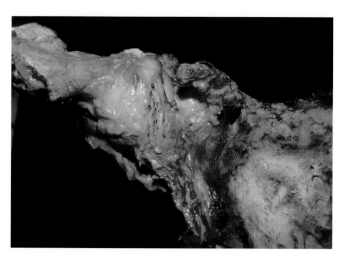

Figure 2.7

Anterior band of the IGHLC: external rotation with the shoulder at 90° of scapularplane abduction.

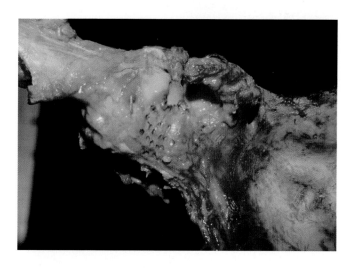

Figure 2.8

Anterior band of the IGHLC: flexion with the shoulder at 90° abduction.

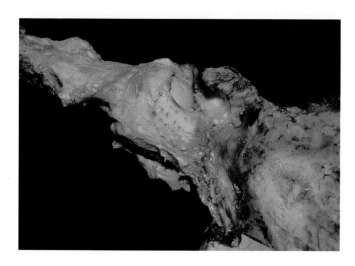

Figure 2.9

Anterior band of the IGHLC: extension with the shoulder at 90° abduction.

band therefore cannot prevent posterior dislocation.[10,13,35] With maximal abduction and external rotation, the posterior band in all shoulders was under tension, but the percent elongation of L_w was minimal.

In order to understand the role the joint capsule plays in shoulder stability, it is often helpful to consider the capsule between the glenoid and humeral head as a circle (Figures 2.10–2.12). For dislocation to occur in one direction, damage to both sides of the capsule must exist.[10,49] Therefore, an increase of posterior laxity must occur with anterior instability; conversely, posterior dislocation cannot occur without anterior capsular damage.

Conclusion

The circle concept includes the anterior and posterior bands of the glenohumeral ligaments and states that an injury must occur on both sides of the glenohumeral joint to produce instability (Figure 2.13). A reciprocal relationship exists between the portions of the capsule, each tightening and loosening during humeral rotation. Stability of the glenohumeral joint is enhanced by the twisting and wrapping of the glenohumeral ligaments around the humeral head. During abduction and external rotation the anterior band of the IGHLC is the most important stabilizer after 65°, while the posterior band is

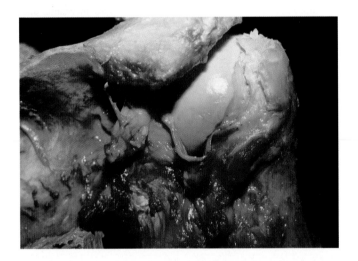

Figure 2.10
Posterior band of the IGHLC: adduction in the scapular plane with neutral rotation.

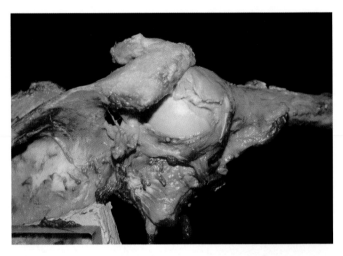

Figure 2.11
Posterior band of the IGHLC: abduction in the scapular plane with internal rotation.

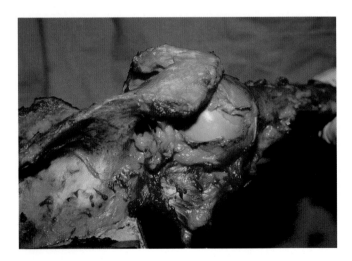

Figure 2.12
Posterior band of the IGHLC: flexion with the shoulder at 90° abduction.

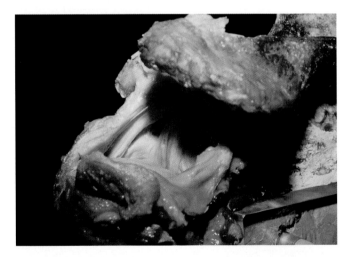

Figure 2.13
Posterior view of the left shoulder: anterior capsule with SGHL, MGHL, and anterior band of the IGHLC, axillary pouch of the IGHLC, posterior capsule with the posterior band of the IGHLC.

more important after 45° of abduction and internal rotation. Anterior stability is achieved not only by the anterior band of the IGHLC, but also by the posterior band and by the SGHL, and MGHL. The ligament length changes observed experimentally confirm the importance of the SGHL for stabilizing the glenohumeral joint during the first 30° of abduction, while in external rotation the IGHLC provides anterior stability. Posterior dislocation of the shoulder occurs clinically in flexion, adduction and internal rotation; this is the position where the posterior band is the primary restraint. In accordance with the circle concept, the anterior band has also been shown to increase stability in these positions.

References

1. Imhoff AB, König U (Hrsg.) *Schulterinstabilität – Rotatorenmanschette. Arthroskopische und offene Operationstechniken bei Schulterverletzungen des Sportlers; Endoprothetik.* Darmstadt: Steinkopff 1999; 335S.

2. Imhoff AB. A biomechanical approach for arthroscopic stabilisation procedures of the unstable shoulder (Suture anchor, Fastak, Laser assisted and elektrothermally assisted capsular shift). *Les annales d'arthroscopie, Societé francaise d'arthroscopie* 2000; S73–6.

3. Basmajian JV, Bazant FJ. Factors preventing downward dislocation of the adducted shoulder joint. *J Bone Joint Surg* 1959; **41A**: 1182–6.

4. Bowen MK, Deng XH, Warner JP et al. The effect of joint compression on stability of the glenohumeral joint. *Trans Orthop Res Soc* 1992; **17**: 289.

5. Galinat BJ, Howell SM. Excessive retroversion of the glenoid cavity. A cause of non-traumatic posterior instability of the shoulder. *J Bone Joint Surg* 1987; **69A**: 632–3.

6. Harryman DT, Sidles JA, Clark JM et al. Translation of the humeral head on the glenoid with passive glenohumeral motion. *J Bone Joint Surg* 1990; **72A**: 1334–43.

7. Inman VT, Saunders JB, Abbott LC. Observations on the functions of the shoulder joint. *J Bone Joint Surg* 1944; **26**: 1–30.

8. Lippitt SB, Vanderhooft JE, Harris SL et al. Glenohumeral stability from concavity-compression: A quantitative analysis. *J Shoulder Elbow Surg* 1993; **2**: 27–34.

9. Schai P, Imhoff A, Staubli AE, Morscher E. Differential diagnosis and therapy of communited humeral head fractures. An analysis of three clinical studies. *J Bone Joint Surg* 1993; **75B** Supp II: 195.

10. Schwartz RE, O'Brien SJ, Warren RF, Torzilli PA. Capsular restraints to anterior–posterior motion of the shoulder. *Trans Orthop Res Soc* 1988; **12**: 727.

11. Terry GC, Hammon D, France P, Norwood LA. The stabilizing function of passive shoulder restraints. *Am J Sports Med* 1991; **19**: 26–34.

12. Warner JJP, Caborn DNM, Berger R et al. Dynamic capsuloligamentous anatomy of the glenohumeral joint. *J Shoulder Elbow Surg* 1993; **2**: 115–33.

13. Warner JJP, Schulte KR, Imhoff AB. *Current Concepts in Shoulder Instability. Advances in Operative Orthopaedics.* Mosby Vol. 3, 1995; 217–48.

14. Browne AO, Hoffmeyer P, Tanaka S et al. Glenohumeral elevation studied in three dimensions. *J Bone Joint Surg* 1990; **72B**: 843–5.

15. Doody SG, Freedman L, Waterland JC. Shoulder movements during abduction in the scapular plane. *Arch Phys Med Rehab* 1970; **51**: 595–604.

16. Harryman DT, Sidles JA, Harris SL, Matsen FA. The role of the rotator interval capsule in passive motion and stability of the shoulder. *J Bone Joint Surg* 1992; **74A**: 53–66.

17. Imhoff A, Perrenoud A, Neidl K. MRI and instability of the shoulder – Correlations with CT-arthrography and arthroscopy [MRI bei Schulterinstabilität – Korrelation zum Arthro-CT und zur Arthroskopie der Schulter]. *Arthroskopie* 1992; **5**: 122–9.

18. Imhoff AB, Hodler J. Correlation of MR imaging, CT arthrography, and arthroscopy of the shoulder. *Bull Hosp Joint Dis New York* 1996; **54**: 146–52.

19. Matsen FA, Fu FH, Hawkins RJ, eds. *The Shoulder: A Balance of Mobility and Stability.* Rosemont, IL: American Academy of Orthopaedic Surgeons, 1993.

20. O'Brien SJ, Neves MC, Arnoczky SP et al. The anatomy and histology of the inferior glenohumeral ligament complex of the shoulder. *Am J Sports Med* 1990; **18**: 449–56.

21. Itoi E, Motzkin NE, Morrey BF, An KN. Scapular inclination and inferior stability of the shoulder. *J Shoulder Elbow Surg* 1992; **1**: 131–9.

22. Rodosky MW, Harner CD, Fu FH. The role of the long head of the biceps muscle and superior glenoid labrum in anterior stability of the shoulder. *Am J Sports Med* 1994; **22**: 121–30.

23. Blasier RB, Gulberg RE, Rothman ED. Anterior shoulder stability: contributions of rotator cuff forces and the capsular ligaments in a cadaver model. *J Shoulder Elbow Surg* 1992; **1**: 140–50.

24. Gerber C, Vinh TS, Hertel R, Hess CW. Latissimus dorsi transfer for the treatment of massive tears of the rotator cuff. A preliminary report. *Clin Orthop* 1988; **232**: 51–61.

25. Pettersson G. Rupture of the tendon aponeurosis of the shoulder joint in antero-inferior dislocation: a study on the origin and occurrence of the ruptures. *Acta Chir Scand Suppl* 1942; **77**: 1–187.

26. Bigliani LU, Flatow EL, Kelkar R et al. Effect of anterior tightening on shoulder kinematics and contact. *Proceedings of the Second World Congress of Biomechanics*, Amsterdam, The Netherlands, 10–15 July 1994: 304.

27. Bowen MK, Deng XH, Hannafin JA et al. An analysis of the patterns of glenohumeral joint contact and their relationship to the glenoid 'bare area'. *Trans Orthop Res Soc* 1992; **17**: 496.

28. Soslowsky LJ, Flatow EL, Bigliani LU et al. Quantitation of in situ contact areas at the glenohumeral joint: a biomechanical study. *J Orthop Res* 1992; **10**: 524–34.

29. Saha AK. Dynamic stability of the glenohumeral joint. *Acta Orthop Scand* 1971; **42**: 491–505.

30. Warner JJP, Deng X, Warren F. Superior inferior translation in the intact and vented glenohumeral joint. *Proceedings, Annual Meeting of the American Shoulder and Elbow Surgeons*, Anaheim 1991.

31. Soslowsky LJ, Flatow EL, Bigliani LU, Mow VC. Articular geometry of the glenohumeral joint. *Clin Orthop Rel Res* 1992; **285**: 181–90.

32. Brewer BJ, Wubben RC, Carrera GF. Excessive retroversion of the glenoid cavity. A cause of non-traumatic posterior instability of the shoulder. *J Bone Joint Surg* 1986; **68A**: 724–31.

33. Sarrafian SK. Gross and functional anatomy of the shoulder. *Clin Orthop Rel Res* 1983; **173**: 11–19.

34. Gerber C, Ganz R, Vinh TS. Glenoplasty for recurrent posterior shoulder instability. An anatomic reappraisal. *Clin Orthop* 1987; **216**: 70–9.

35. Perrenoud A, Imhoff A.B. Locked posterior dislocation of the shoulder. *Bull Hosp Joint Dis New York* 1985; **54**: 165–8.

36. Randelli M, Gambrioli PL. Glenohumeral osteometry by computed tomography in normal and unstable. *Clin Orthop Rel Res* 1986; **208**: 151–6.

37. Moseley HF, Overgaard B. The anterior capsular mechanism in recurrent anterior dislocation of the shoulder. *J Bone Joint Surg* 1962; **44B**: 913–27.

38. Cooper DE, Arnoczky SP, O'Brien SJ et al. Anatomy, histology and vascularity of the glenoid labrum. *J Bone Joint Surg* 1992; **74A**: 46–52.

39. Bankart AS. The pathology and treatment of recurrent dislocation of the shoulder joint. *Br J Surg* 1938; **26**: 23–9.

40. Bost FC, Inman VT. The pathological changes in recurrent dislocation of the shoulder: a report of Bankart's operative procedure. *J Bone Joint Surg* 1942; **24**: 595–613.

41. Lindblom K. On pathogenesis of ruptures of the tendon aponeurosis of the shoulder joint. *Acta Radiol* 1939; **20**: 563–77.

42. DePalma AF, ed. *Surgery of the Shoulder.* Philadelphia: JB Lippincott, 1983.

43. Imhoff A, Jacob HAC. *Biomechanics of instability of the shoulder* [Biomechanik der Schulterinstabilitaet]. Instructional Course. Deutscher Orthopaedenkongress (DGOT) 1994 Wiesbaden.

44. Jacob HAC, Imhoff AB, Franklin P, Wullschleger M. *In-vitro-Untersuchungen zur Biomechanik der Schulterinstabilität.* Instructional Course. Deutscher Orthopädenkongress (DGOT) 12–15 October 1994, Wiesbaden.

45. Neer CS, Satterlee CC, Dalsey RM, Flatow EL. The anatomy and potential effects of contracture of the coracohumeral ligament. *Clin Orthop* 1992; **280**: 182–5.

46. Ferrari DA. Capsular ligaments of the shoulder. Anatomical and functional study of the anterior superior capsule. *Am J Sports Med* 1990; **18**: 20–4.

47. Edelson JG, Taitz C, Grishkan A. The coracohumeral ligament. Anatomy of a substantial but neglected structure. *J Bone Joint Surg* 1991; **73B**: 150–3.

48. Helmig P. Sojbjerg JO, Sneppen O et al. Glenohumeral movement patterns after puncture of the joint capsule: An experimental study. *J Shoulder Elbow Surg* 1993; **2**: 209–15.

49. Ovesen J, Nielsen S. Anterior and posterior shoulder instability. A cadaver study. *Acta Orthop Scand* 1986; **57**: 324–7.

50. Clark JM, Harryman DT. Tendons, ligaments and capsule of the rotator cuff. *J Bone Joint Surg* 1992; **74A**: 713–25.

51. Cooper DE, O'Brien SJ, Arnoczky SP, Warren RF. The structure and function of the oracohumeral ligament: an anatomic and microscopic study. *J Shoulder Elbow Surg* 1993; **2**: 70–7.

52. O'Connell PW, Nuber GW, Mileski RA, Lautenschlager E. The contribution of the glenohumeral ligaments to anterior stability of the shoulder joint. *Am J Sports Med* 1990; **18**: 579–84.

53. DePalma AF, Callery G, Bennett GA. Variational anatomy and degenerative lesions of the shoulder joint. In: Blount WP, ed. American Academy of Orthopaedic Surgeons Instructional Course Lectures. Ann Arbor: JW Edwards, 1949; 225–81.

54. Ovesen J, Nielsen S. Stability of the shoulder joint. Cadaver study of stabilizing structures. *Acta Orthop Scand* 1985; **56**: 149–51.

55. Warner JJP, Micheli LJ, Arslanian LE et al. Scapulothoracic motion in normal shoulders and shoulders with glenohumeral instability and impingement syndrome. A study using Moir, topographic analysis. *Clin Orthop Rel Res* 1992; **285**: 191–9.

56. Turkel SJ, Panio MW, Marshall J, Girgis F. Stabilizing mechanisms preventing anterior dislocations of the glenohumeral joint. *J Bone Joint Surg* 1981; **63A**: 1208–17.

57. Codman EA. *The Shoulder. Rupture of the Supraspinatus Tendon and Other Lesions in or About the Subacromial Bursa.* Thomas Todd: Boston, 1934.

58. Demirhan M, Imhoff AB, Patel PR et al. Suprascapular nerve entrapment under the spinoglenoid ligament – an anatomic and morphologic study. *J Shoulder Elbow Surg* 1998; **7**: 238–43.

59. Imhoff A. Problems of the shoulder caused by neurologic syndromes [Schulterprobleme bei neurologischen Syndromen]. *Schweiz Rundschau Med (Praxis)* 1986; **75**: 571–6.

60. Warner JJP, Krushell RJ, Masquelet A, Gerber C. Anatomy and relationships of the suprascapular nerve: anatomical constraints to mobilization of the supraspinatus and infraspinatus muscles in the management of massive rotator-cuff tears. *J Bone Joint Surg* 1992; **74A**: 36–45.

61. Burkart A, Imhoff AB. Arthroskopische Fixierung der Typ II-SLAP-Läsion. *Arthroskopie* 2000; **13**: 226–8.

62. Imhoff AB, Agneskirchner JD, König U et al. Obere Labrumpathologie beim Sportler. *Orthopäde* 2000; **29**: 917–27.

63. Soslowsky LJ, Malicky DM, Blasier RB. Anterior glenohumeral stabilization factors: Relative and progressive effects in a biomechanical model. *Proceedings of the Second World Congress of Biomechanics*, Amsterdam, The Netherlands, 10–15 July 1994: 303.

64. An KN, Browne AO, Korinek S et al. Three-dimensional kinematics of glenohumeral elevation. *J Orthop Res* 1991; **9**: 143–9.

65. Warner JJP, Deng X, Warren F, Torzilli PA. Static capsuloligamentous restraints to superior–inferior translation of the glenohumeral joint. *Am J Sports Med* 1992; **20**: 675–85.

66. Kumar VP, Balasubramaniam P. The role of atmospheric pressure in stabilising the shoulder. An experimental study. *J Bone Joint Surg* 1985; **67B**: 719–21.

67. Woo SL, Gomez MA, Seguchi Y et al. Measurement of mechanical properties of ligament substance from a bone–ligament–bone preparation. *J Orthop Res* 1983; **1**: 22–9.

68. Boardman ND, Debski RE, Taskiran E et al. Structural and anatomic properties of the coracohumeral and superior glenohumeral ligaments. *Trans Orthop Res Soc* 1995; **20**.

69. Boardman ND, Debski RE, Warner JJP et al. Tensile properties of the superior glenohumeral and coracohumeral ligament. *J Shoulder Elbow Surg* 1996; **5**: 249–54.

70. Bigliani LU, Pollock RG, Soslowsky LJ et al. Tensile properties of the inferior glenohumeral ligament. *J Orthop Res* 1992; **10**: 187–97.

71. Ticker JB, Flatow EL, Pawluk RJ et al. The inferior glenohumeral ligament: a correlative biomechanical, biochemical and histological investigation. *Trans Orthop Res Soc* 1992; **18**: 313.

72. Helmig P, Sojbjerg JO, Kjaersgaard-Andersen P et al. Distal humeral migration as a component of multidirectional shoulder instability. An anatomical study in autopsy specimens. *Clin Orthop Rel Res* 1990; **252**: 139–43.

73. Ovesen J, Nielsen S. Experimental distal subluxation in the glenohumeral joint. *Arch Orthop Trauma Surg* 1985; **104**: 78–81.

74. Agneskirchner J, Fredrich H, Imhoff AB. Acromion reconstruction after total arthroscopic acromionectomy: salvage procedure using a bone graft. *Arthroscopy* 2001; **17/5**: E18:1–4.

75. De Simoni C, Ledermann Th, Imhoff A. Holmium YAG-Laser beim 'Outlet Impingment' der Schulter – Mittelfristige Ergebnisse. *Orthopäde* 1996; **25**: 84–90.

76. Imhoff A, ed. Schulterarthroskopie. Deutsche Ausgabe, Uebersetzung und Bearb. In: Bunker T, Wallace A, eds. *Shoulder Arthroscopy* unter Mitarbeit von S. Plaschy und mit einem Geleitwort von A. Schreiber. Thieme: Stuttgart, 1992, 190 pp.

77. Imhoff A. Arthroscopy of the shoulder and the bursa subacromialis – *Indications and complications* [Arthroskopie der Schulter und der Bursa subacromialis]. Instructional Course Deutscher Orthopaedenkongress (DGOT) 1992 Mannheim. In: Springorum HW, Katthagen BD, eds. *Current concepts of Orthopaedics* [Aktuelle Schwerpunkte der Orthopaedie] Vol. 5. Thieme: Stuttgart 1994; 103–12.

78. Imhoff A, Ledermann Th. Arthroscopic subacromial decompression with and without the Holmium:YAG-Laser – a prospective comparative study. *Arthroscopy* 1995; **11**: 549–56.

79. Imhoff A. The use of lasers in orthopaedic surgery. Controversial topics in sports medicine. *Operative Techniques in Orthopaedics.* 1995; **5**: 192–203.

80. Imhoff AB. The Ho:YAG-Laser in Shoulder Surgery. In: Gerber BE, Knight M, Siebert WE, eds. *Laser in the Muskuloskeletal System.* Berlin: Springer 2001; 173–6.

81. Soslowsky LJ, An CH, Johnston SP, Carpenter JE. Geometric and mechanical properties of the coracoacromial ligament and their relationship to rotator cuff disease. *Clin Orthop Rel Res* 1994; **304**: 10–17.

82. Uhthoff HK, Hammond DI, Sarkar K et al. The role of the coracoacromial ligament in the impingement syndrome: a clinical, radiological and histological study. *Int Orthop* 1988; **12**: 97–104.

83. Gerber C, Terrier F, Ganz R. The role of the coracoid process in the chronic impingement syndrome. *J Bone Joint Surg* 1985; **67B**: 703–8.

84. Gerber C, Terrier F, Zehnder R, Ganz R. The subcoracoid space. An anatomic study. *Clin Orthop* 1987; **215**: 132–8.

85. Gerber C, Krushell RJ. Isolated rupture of the tendon of the subscapularis muscle. Clinical features in 16 cases. *J Bone Joint Surg* 1991; **73B**: 389–94.

86. Soslowsky LJ, An CH, Johnston SP, Carpenter JE. Geometric and mechanical properties of the coracoacromial ligament and their relationship to rotator cuff disease. *Trans Orthop Res Soc* 1993; **18**: 139.

87. Reeves B. Experiments on the tensile strength of the anterior capsular structures of the shoulder in man. *J Bone Joint Surg* 1968; **50B**: 858–65.

88. Kaltsas DS. Comparative study of the properties of the shoulder joint capsule with those of other joint capsules. *Clin Orthop* 1983; **173**: 20–6.

89. Woo SL, Hollis JM, Adams DJ et al. Tensile properties of the human femur–anterior cruciate ligament–tibia complex. The effect of specimen age and orientation. *Am J Sports Med* 1991; **19**: 217–25.

90. Woo SL, Newton PO, MacKenna DA, Lyon RM. A comparative evaluation of the mechanical properties of the rabbit medial collateral and anterior cruciate ligaments. *J Biomech* 1992; **25**: 377–86.

91. Woo SL, Orlando CA, Gomez MA et al. Tensile properties of the medial collateral ligament as a function of age. *J Orthop Res* 1986; **4**: 133–41.

92. Woo SL, Debski RE, Patel PR et al. Biomechanics of the full upper extremity in simple abduction: application of the Pittsburgh dynamic shoulder testing apparatus. In Wu JJ, ed. *Proceedings of the First Academic Congress on Asian Shoulder Association*, 16–19 November 1994, Taipei, Taiwan. Mosby 1995. 23–28.

93. Woo SL, Debski RE, Imhoff AB et al. Soft tissue restraints around the glenohumeral joint. In Wu JJ, ed. *Proceedings of the First Academic Congress on Asian Shoulder Association*, 16–19 November 1994, Taipei, Taiwan. Mosby 1995. 29–34.

94. Trent PS, Walker PS, Wolf B. Ligament length patterns, strength and rotational axis of the knee joint. *Clin Orthop Rel Res* 1976; **117**: 263–70.

95. Noyes FR, Grood ES. The strength of the anterior cruciate ligament in humans and rhesus monkeys. Age-related and species-related chnages. *J Bone Joint Surg* 1976; **58A**: 1074–82.

96. Weber SC, Caspari RB. A biochemical evaluation of the restraints to posterior shoulder dislocation. *Arthroscopy* 1989; **5**: 115–21.

97. Clark J, Sidles JA, Matsen FA. The relationship of the glenohumeral joint capsule to the rotator cuff. *Clin Orthop Rel Res* 1990; **254**: 29–34.

98. Burkhart SS, Esch JC, Jolson RS. The rotator crescent and rotator cable: an anatomic description of the shoulder's 'suspension bridge'. *Arthroscopy* 1993; **9**: 611–16.

99. Debski RE, McMahon PJ, Thompson WO et al. A new dynamic testing apparatus to study glenohumeral motion. *J Biomech* 1995; **28**: 869–74.

100. Kohn D. The clinical relevance of glenoid labrum lesions. *Arthroscopy* 1987; **3**: 223–30.

101. Keyes EL. Anatomical observations on senile changes in the shoulder. *J Bone Joint Surg* 11935; **7A**: 953–60.

3 Physical examination of the shoulder

Andreas Burkart and Andreas B Imhoff

Introduction

With an appropriate history and careful physical examination one can reach a working diagnosis for patients with shoulder discomfort. The examiner should question the patient about the chief complaint and take into consideration the patient's occupation, dominant hand, sports activities and any history of trauma. Chronic shoulder problems most commonly present with pain and instability. Secondary symptoms are stiffness, weakness, loss of motion, functional disability, catching, and crepitus.

When questioning a patient with instability, it is necessary to ascertain the degree (subluxation versus dislocation), the onset (traumatic, atraumatic, or overuse), and direction (anterior, posterior, or multidirectional). Subluxation refers to subjective feeling that the shoulder partially slips out of the joint but quickly reduces spontaneously.

The most common cause for shoulder weakness is a rotator cuff tear. A torn cuff is often associated with a feeling of crunching or crepitation with shoulder movement. Complaints of catching or pseudolocking are often associated with labral tears, particularly in the throwing shoulder. Trauma can cause rotator cuff injury and should be considered in the differential diagnosis of patients, who are participating in contact sports, such as in younger patients. It is also important to determine the position of the arm at the time of injury.

Pain is the most common shoulder complaint for the majority of patients. The localization of the pain is often difficult. Radiation of pain down the shoulder into the deltoid is common for impingement symptoms. It is most commonly insidious in onset, often associated with overhead activity and associated with severe night pain. The patient should also be questioned about neck pain and any neurologic symptoms. Radiation of pain from the neck to the shoulder should be excluded and a clinical examination of the cervical spine should be performed. Axial loading in various positions of flexion, extension, or lateral bending of the neck may reproduce shoulder symptoms. The dead-arm syndrome usually presents as inability to lift the arm without neurologic deficits. Crepitus is a frequent finding and is often asymptomatic. It can be seen with degenerative arthritis, acromioclavicular joint pathology, fractures, and rotator cuff tear.

Inspection

Inspection of the shoulder and upper extremity involves the attitude, muscle features, deformities, swelling, skin manifestations, and color. Often there is a visible asymmetry of the shoulder in patients with a very painful shoulder, which stands higher than the opposite side.

The most important muscles about the shoulder to note for wasting are the deltoid, the supraspinatus and the infraspinatus. Wasting of the deltoid is best visualized from the anterior aspect as squaring off the shoulder. If the supraspinatus or infraspinatus are wasted, one can observe an excessive prominence of the scapular spine. To confirm atrophy of the supraspinatus is much more difficult than for the infraspinatus because the supraspinatus is deep to the trapezius in a fossa above the scapular spine. The most common cause for wasting of the supraspinatus or infraspinatus is a rotator cuff tear, but one must consider diagnoses such as C5 root compression, suprascapular nerve entrapment, or myopathy. Rupture of the long head of the biceps tendon manifests as a 'Popeye' appearance of the biceps muscle belly when the patient is asked to flex the elbow. A rupture of the pectoralis muscle may be detected with resisted adduction of the arm at 90° of forward flexion and neutral rotation. In acute ruptures, existence of a hematoma and a loss of contour of the anterior axillary fold can be clearly visualized.

A high-riding distal clavicle suggests pathology in the acromioclavicular joint, dislocation or fracture about the clavicle. Winging of the scapula can be illustrated by having the patient flex the shoulder forward by 90°, or for subtle cases, by having the patient do a 'push-up' against the wall. It may be due to weakness of the serratus anterior or the trapezius muscles. If one has a paralysis of the serratus anterior, the scapula tends to migrate proximally and its inferior angle moves medially. Serratus anterior weakness can be caused by a long thoracic nerve palsy. If the trapezius is paralysed, the scapula migrates downward while its inferior angle moves laterally. This can easily be seen when the patient is asked to flex the shoulder against resistance.

Palpation

The sternoclavicular joint should be identified and noted for swelling, tenderness, and displacement. Palpation continues along the clavicle to identify local deformities such as a displaced fracture. Palpation of the coracoid process is of little value because tenderness occurs even in the normal shoulder. The acromioclavicular joint is a common cause for shoulder pain and palpation of its superior surface may elicit tenderness. To palpate the greater tuberosity of the humerus and the insertion of the supraspinatus, the arm must be slightly extended and internally rotated. Just distal to the anterior edge of the acromion, the greater tuberosity can be palpated as a prominence. Palpation of the bicipital groove is possible directly anterior when the arm is in 10° of internal rotation. Tenderness in this area is indicative of biceps tendinitis.

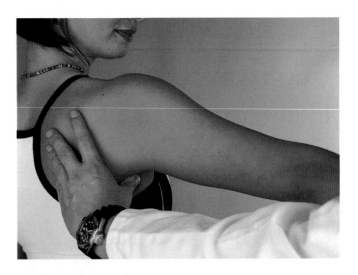

Figure 3.1
Testing glenohumeral abduction.

Range of motion

It is important to distinguish between scapulothoracic and glenohumeral movement. Movement at the glenohumeral joint can be quantified by observing the movement of the inferior angle of the scapula during abduction of the arm and by holding the scapula on rotation (Figure 3.1). Motion is mainly provided by the scapulothoracic articulation in diseases like osteoarthritis or adhesive capsulitis. Any asynchrony of motion should be observed. Asymmetry of the scapulohumeral rhythm may indicate compensation for pain. Patients with a painful, weak, or frozen shoulder may show a complex set of movements when elevating the shoulder in order to compensate for decreased glenohumeral motion. Labral pathology may cause catching pain and often has a 'click' phenomenon.

According to the American Academy of Orthopedic Surgeons all joint motions are measured from a defined reference point as the zero starting position. Thus, the degrees of joint motion are added in the direction that the joint moves from the zero position. For the shoulder the zero point refers to the position when the patient is standing with the arm at the side in neutral rotation, the palms facing the thighs. The injured side should be compared with the normal opposite side. If the opposite side is not normal one should compare the range with the average motion of an individual of similar age, sex, and physical build.

Motion is defined as active or passive. If possible, the extremity should be examined with the patient in a position of greatest comfort. According to the Society of American Shoulder and Elbow Surgeons the following arcs of motion should be documented:

1. Total elevation (or flexion) active and passive (Figure 3.2);
2. Total extension;

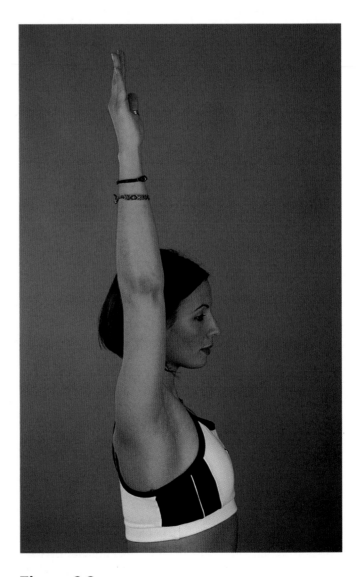

Figure 3.2
Total elevation/flexion.

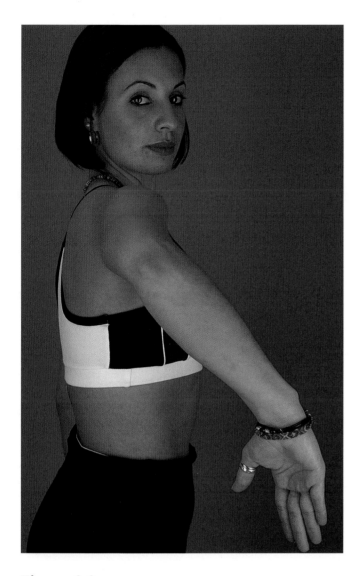

Figure 3.3

Internal rotation in 90° abduction.

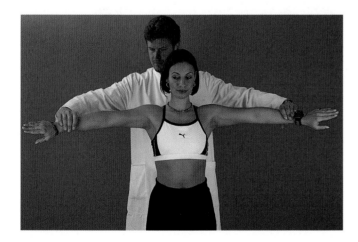

Figure 3.4

Testing the supraspinatus.

3. External rotation with the arm at the side (both actively and passively);
4. External rotation at the 90° of abduction;
5. Internal rotation;
6. Internal rotation at the 90° of abduction (Figure 3.3).

Internal rotation can be measured by a rule, starting from C7 down to the tip of the thumb. Common reference points that the thumb reaches are the greater trochanter, buttock, superior gluteal fold, and various spinous processes of the lumbar and thoracic vertebrae. Internal rotation can also be measured in the 90° abducted position.

Muscle testing

Testing of muscle strength evaluates the integrity of the musculotendinous unit and the neuromuscular elements. Muscle strength is rated by the following grading system:

0 = No palpable contraction;
1 = Muscle contracts, but part normally motorized does not move, even without gravity;
2 = Muscle moves the part but not against gravity;
3 = Muscle moves the part through a range against gravity;
4 = Muscle moves the part even against added resistance;
5 = Normal strength against full resistance.

Rotator cuff

Testing the supraspinatus

Loss of strength is not a reliable sign of rotator cuff tear, particularly in the young patient; resistance should be applied with the arm abducted 90°, maximally pronated, and flexed 30° forward (Figure 3.4).[1]

0 Grad abduction test

The arm is at the side of the body and the patient tries to abduct the arm against the resistance of the examiner. The starter function of the supraspinatus in initiating the first 30° of shoulder abduction is tested (Figures 3.5 and 3.6).

Testing the external rotators (infraspinatus/teres minor)

External rotation is mostly achieved through the action of the infraspinatus and teres minor. It can be tested with

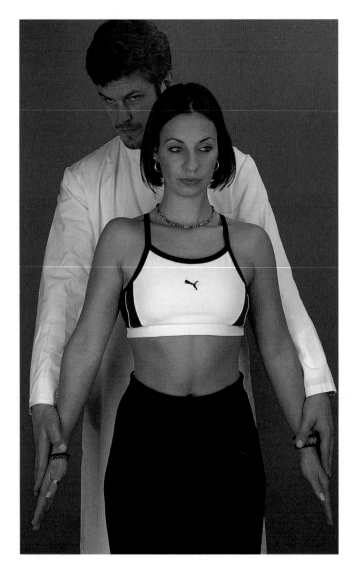

Figure 3.5
Abduction-test for supraspinatus.

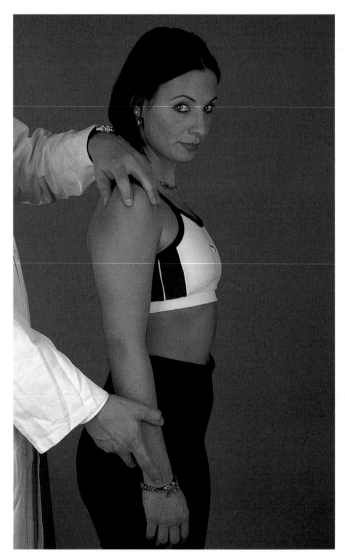

Figure 3.6
Abduction-test for supraspinatus (lateral view).

the arms starting at the side of the body in a neutral position. Resistance is then applied and compared with the opposite side. When the arm is abducted above 45° and externally rotated, the function of the teres minor is tested. It is also possible to test external rotation at 90° of abduction.

Hornblower's sign

According to Walch et al[2] the Hornblower's sign indicates an irreparable tear of infraspinatus and teres minor. The patient's arm is at 90° of abduction in the scapular plane and the elbow is flexed to 90°. The patient is asked to rotate the forearm externally against the resistance of the examiner's hand. A positive test occurs when the arm cannot be externally rotated. This

has a sensitivity of 100% and a specificity of 93% for the presence of fatty degeneration of the teres minor (Figure 3.7).

Dropping sign

According to Walch et al[2] a positive dropping sign indicates an irreparable tear of the infraspinatus. The examiner holds the patient's forearm at 45° of external rotation and 0° of abduction. The patient is instructed to maintain this position when the forearm is let go. The dropping sign is positive when the forearm drops back to 0° of external rotation, despite efforts to maintain the external rotation. This test has a sensitivity of 100% and specificity (100%) for the presence of fatty degeneration of infraspinatus (Figure 3.8).

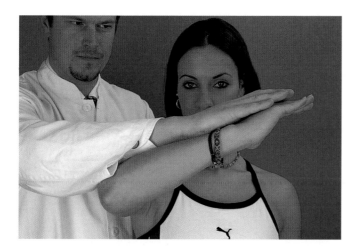

Figure 3.7
Hornblower's sign.

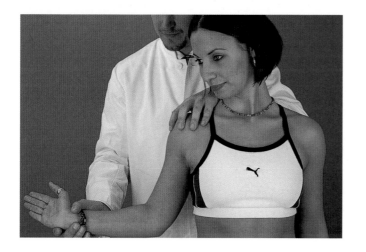

Figure 3.8
Dropping sign.

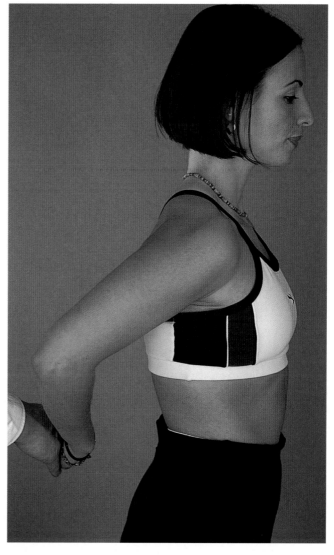

Figure 3.9
Lift-off test.

Testing the subscapularis

The so-called 'lift-off test' was first described by Gerber and Krushell.[3] This test is restricted by the lack of internal rotation. The patient must be able to internally rotate the arm sufficiently without too much pain. If the patient can lift the palm away from the small of the back, then the subscapularis is intact. The test can be refined by having the patient perform this test against resistance to estimate the sxrength of the subscapularis (Figure 3.9). If the patient is unable to internally rotate the arm, the elbow can be flexed to 90° and the palm is pressed against the abdomen. In our experience this test is very helpful and is called the 'Napoleon sign'.

Stability assessment

Glenohumeral translation (load and shift test)

At the beginning of the examination the humeral head must be reduced concentrically in the glenoid fossa. Patients with multidirectional laxity are especially prone to have an 'eccentric' resting position of the humeral head. The patient should be seated when the examiner applies a directional stress anterior and posterior, which means the humeral head is 'loaded'. The examiner places one hand over the shoulder and scapula to steady the limb girdle, while the opposite hand grasps the humeral head. Anterior and posterior stresses are applied. With increasing stress the humeral head may shift up or over the glenoid rim. Both shoulders should be tested by a grading system, as suggested by the Society of American Shoulder and Elbow Surgeons:[4]

0 = There is no translation;
1 = The humeral head moves slightly up face of glenoid (translation = 0–1 cm);
2 = The humeral head rides up glenoid face to but not over the rim (translation = 1–2 cm);
3 = The humeral head rides up and over the glenoid rim. This usually reduces, when the stress is removed, but can also remain dislocated (> 2 cm of translation).

Sulcus sign

The sulcus sign gives an impression of the amount of inferior glenohumeral translation. The elbow is grasped and inferior traction is applied. Dimpling of the skin below the acromion may be seen.[5] The space underneath the acromion is palpated for widening.

Anterior apprehension test

With certain positions of subluxation or dislocation subjective patient apprehension will be elicited. The apprehension test for anterior instability of a right shoulder is performed by abducting the arm 90° and externally rotating with the right hand. From behind, the examiner's hand is placed over the humeral head and the thumb pushes from posterior, anteriorly toward the fingers. The apprehension test is positive when the patient feels that the shoulder 'will come out' and the patient resists with muscular contraction. The test can be repeated in the supine position with the scapula supported by the edge of the examination table. If pain or apprehension is reproduced, the 'relocation test' is performed. If application of a posterior stress on the externally rotated humerus allows further external rotation, the relocation test is positive. The test can be quantified by measuring the change in external rotation (Figure 3.10).

Posterior instability

Posterior apprehension test

Physical examination may reveal pain with 90° of forward flexion and internal rotation. The shoulder may

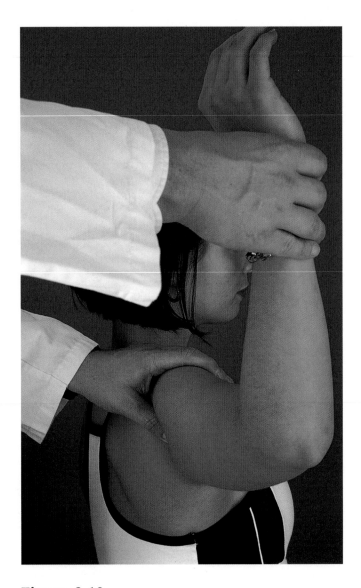

Figure 3.10
Apprehension test.

sublux posteriorly in this position. This can also be tested with the patient supine. The examiner may feel the humeral head sublux or dislocate when pressure is applied. The patient may also complain of apprehension during this maneuver.

Flexion pivot shift test for posterior instability

The supine patient is asked to flex the arm forward to 90° and adduct while posterior pressure is applied. The posterior subluxation or dislocation may not be palpated, but if the arm is slowly abducted to about 30–45°, the humeral head will reduce itself and a 'clunk' is heard.

Jerk test

To test posterior subluxation, the flexed arm is stressed posteriorly at 90° of flexion in neutral rotation. In this position the arm is in a subluxated position. One pushes towards the humeral head from a posterior direction during extension of the arm. Here, one can produce a clunk or obvious feeling of relocation of the subluxated humeral head.[6]

Relocation test

The supine patient is instructed to abduct and externally rotate the arm until pain is elicited. In this position the humeral head subluxes anteriorly. A posteriorly directed force will eliminate the pain.

Impingement tests

Impingement sign

The pronated arm is forcibly flexed. This maneuver often produces pain if the supraspinatus tendon is inflamed. With additional internal rotation, impingement of the supraspinatus tendon against the coracoacromial ligament may be achieved, also producing pain. A positive impingement sign may also occur in patients with an adhesive capsulitis, acromioclavicular or gleno-humeral joint arthritis, or calcific tendinitis (Figure 3.11).

Impingement test

One can distinguish shoulder pain from pain originating from other sources by an injection of lidocaine into the subacromial bursa.

Hawkins–Kennedy test

In this test the greater tuberosity is brought into contact with the lateral acromion. The arm is flexed forward to 90° and adducted. A forceful internal rotation of the arm against the fixed scapula produces anterior shoulder pain and indicates impingement (Figure 3.12).[7]

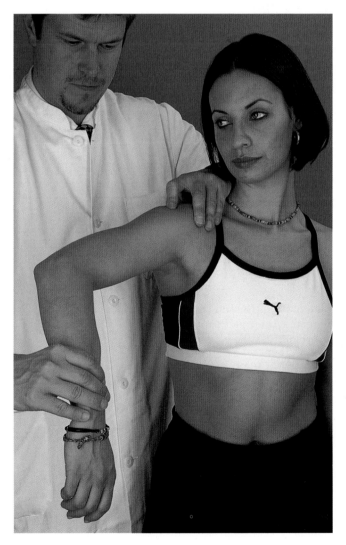

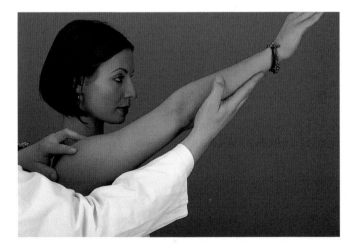

Figure 3.11
Impingement sign.

Figure 3.12
Hawkins–Kennedy test.

Painful arc

Another test for impingement is the traditional 'painful arc'. Pain is elicited when abduction occurs in the coronal plane between 60° and 100°. Increased pain can be observed by applying resistance to this abduction maneuver (Figure 3.13).

Acromioclavicular joint

Problems with the acromioclavicular joint can be found in conjunction with an impingement syndrome. Patients complain of pain at the acromioclavicular joint elicited by direct palpation. Pain can also be elicited by forcibly pushing the arm into the crossed-arm adduction at 90° of forward flexion. This test can also be painful in patients with a tight posterior capsule. Differentiation is possible by infiltration of local anesthesia into the acromioclavicular joint. It is a helpful test before resection of the acromioclavicular joint.

Biceps evaluation

Clinical complaints are pain, greater with overhead activity, and a painful 'catching' or 'popping' in the shoulder.[8] Superior labrum, anterior–posterior (SLAP) lesions may cause shoulder pain as a result of an interposition of the detached labrum between the humeral head and the glenoid. Most have marked deficits of internal rotation due to an acquired, tight posteroinferior capsule that is implicated as ultimately causing the SLAP lesions.[9]

Yergason's test[10]

The patient is asked to supinate the forearm from a pronated position while the elbow is flexed to 90°. Pain in the region of the bicipital groove may indicate pathology of the long head of the biceps (Figure 3.14).

Speed's test

This test is very similar to the Neer's impingement test. With an extended elbow and supinated forearm the patient is asked to flex the arm to approximately 60°. Resistance is provided by the examiner. The test is positive if the patient localizes pain in the area of the bicipital groove.[8]

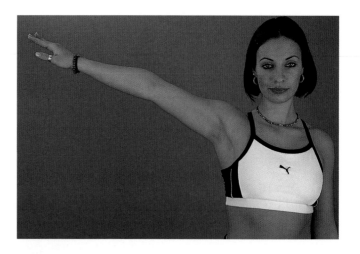

Figure 3.13
Painful arc.

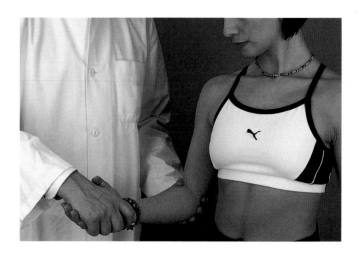

Figure 3.14
Yergason test.

O'Brien's test

O'Brien's cross-arm test is positive when the patient complains of shoulder pain with the arm adducted and flexed 90° across the chest with slight internal rotation (Figure 3.15).[9]

Biceps load test

The supine patient abducts the arm to 90°, flexes the elbow to 90°, and supinates the forearm. An anterior apprehension test is performed. If the patient experiences apprehension during that maneuver, external rotation is stopped. The patient is then asked to flex the

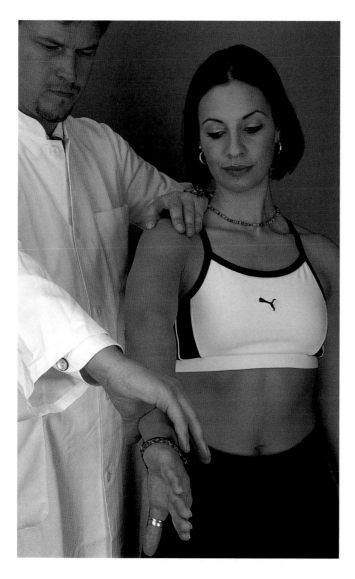

Figure 3.15

O'Brien test.

forearm pronation causes traction on the long head of the biceps tendon. Adduction entraps the unstable tendon and superior glenoid labrum between the glenoid fossa and humeral head. The test is repeated with the forearm supinated, which should diminish the pain by decreasing traction on the long head of the biceps tendon and reduction of the unstable labrum.

Crank test[13]

This test is considered to be positive when there is crepitus with the arm in an abducted, externally rotated position. It should be positive in labral pathology.

Jobe relocation test[14]

A positive Jobe relocation test occurs when shoulder pain and apprehension (produced by abduction and external rotation) is relieved by a posterior directed force applied to the humeral head.

elbow against the resistance of the examiner's hand. If the apprehension is lessened, the test is negative for SLAP lesions. This is because in shoulders with intact superior labra, the contraction of the biceps muscle reduces apprehension due to glenohumeral stability. The test is positive when the apprehension has not changed or pain increases.

Slapprehension test[12]

The arm is abducted to 90° and horizontally adducted, while the elbow is extended. Pronation of the forearm may result in pain in the bicipital groove, apprehension, and an audible or palpable click. Elbow extension and

References

1. Berg EE, Ciullo JV. A clinical test for superior glenoid labral or SLAP lesions. _Clin J Sport Med_ 1998; **8**:121–3.
2. Walch G, Boulahia A, Calderone S, Robinson AHN. The 'dropping' and 'hornblower's' sign in evaluation of rotator cuff tears. _J Bone Joint Surg_ 1998; **80B**:624–8.
3. Gerber C, Krushell RJ. Isolated rupture of the tendon of the subscapularis muscle. _J Bone Joint Surg_ 1991; **73B**:389–94.
4. King GJ, Richards RR, Zuckerman JD et al. A standardized method for assessment of elbow function. Research Committee, American Shoulder and Elbow Surgeons. _J Shoulder Elbow Surg_ 1999; **8**:351–4.
5. Neer CS, Foster CR. Inferior capsular shift for involuntary inferior and multidirectional instability of the shoulder. _J Bone Joint Surg_ 1980; **62A**:897–908.
6. Hawkins RT, Boker DJ. Clinical evaluation of shoulder problems. In: Rockwood CA, Matsen FA III. _The Shoulder_, Vol 1. Philadelphia: Saunders, 1990. 147–77.
7. Hawkins RJ, Kennedy JC. Impingement syndrome in athletes. _Am J Sports Med_ 1980; **8**:151–8.
8. Burkhart SS, Morgan CD, Kibler WB. Shoulder injuries in overhead athletes. The 'dead arm' revisited. _Clin Sports Med_ 2000; **19**:125–58.
9. O'Brien SJ, Pagnani MJ, McGlynn SR et al. The active compression test. _Am J Sports Med_ 1998; **26**:610–13.
10. Yergason RM. Supination sign. _J Bone Joint Surg_ 1931; **13**:160.
11. Berg EE, Ciullo JV. The SLAP prehension test. _J South Orthop Assoc_ 1995; **4**:237–8.
12. Liu SH, Henry MH, Nuccion SL. A prospective evaluation of a new physical examination in predicting glenoid labral tears. _Am J Sports Med_ 1996; **24**:721–5.
13. Jobe FW, Tibone JE, Jobe CM, Kvitne RS. The shoulder in sports. In: Rockwood CA, Matsen FA, _The Shoulder_, Vol 2. Philadelphia: Saunders, 1990. 961–90.

4 Imaging of the shoulder

Thomas Merl

Conventional radiography

High-quality radiographs in two orthogonal planes are the first step in imaging work-up of patients with diseases of the musculoskeletal system. Availability, costs, speed, and relative ease of interpretation make conventional radiography the first imaging choice and even magnetic resonance imaging (MRI) should never be performed or read without X-ray films.

Due to the complicated anatomy of the shoulder numerous projections for specific pathologies have been described although some of them have lost importance with the availability of computed tomography (CT) and MRI. Depending on clinical findings, tailored examinations should be performed, and routine X-ray examinations should include the lateral clavicle, glenohumeral joint, acromioclavicular joint and scapula.[1-4]

A trauma series for the shoulder should consist at least of a true anteroposterior view (including internal and external rotation) and (modified) axillary or scapular lateral view.

The 'true' anteroposterior view is angled 30–40° relative to the coronal plane in order to visualize the glenoid in profile, thus separating the glenoid from the humeral head (Figure 4.1). Although internal and external rotation anteroposterior views are highly informative, they do not adequately demonstrate the joint in a trauma patient as they do not represent two orthogonal planes

(Figure 4.2) They should (but in a trauma case, must) always be supplemented by a second view—orthogonal to the first. In most cases this is the axillary view (first described by Lawrence in 1915;[4] Figure 4.3). In patients who cannot abduct properly, modifications of the

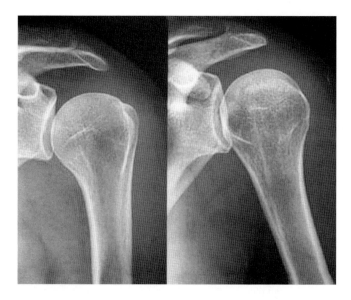

Figure 4.2

Internal and external rotation views allow assessment of greater and lesser tuberosity to assess fractures and calcifications.

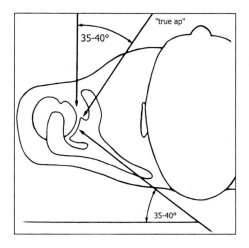

Figure 4.1

Schematic representation of positioning for 'true' anteroposterior projection. Only a 35–40° posterior oblique projection allows tangential depiction of the glenohumeral joint with only the coracoid process superimposed.

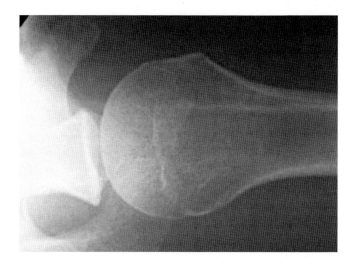

Figure 4.3

Axial views depict acromion and coracoid process, anterior and posterior humeral head contour and (sub-) luxations in the glenohumeral joint.

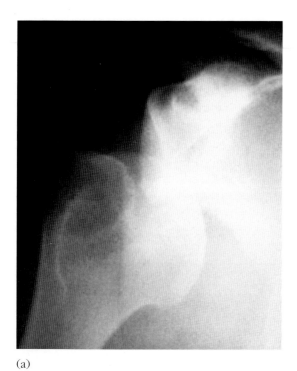

(a)

Figure 4.4

Anterior luxations. (a) Anterior luxation with impaction fracture.
(b) Anterior luxation with tuberosity fracture. In anterior
inferior luxation, impaction fractures of the posterolateral
humeral head and associated tuberosity fractures are usually
easily identified on plain anteroposterior radiographs.

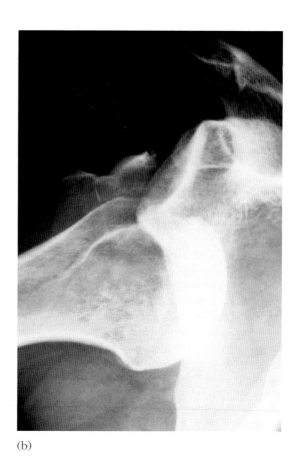

(b)

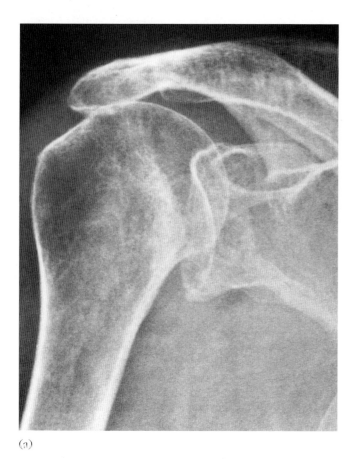

(a)

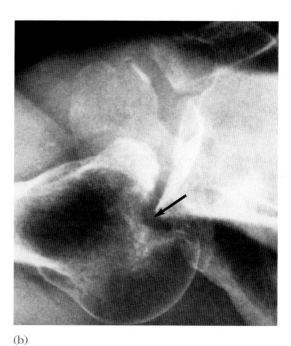

(b)

Figure 4.5

Posterior luxation. (a) Anteroposterior view; (b) axial view.
Posterior luxations are more difficult to assess on plain
anteroposterior films (a), sometimes the trough sign (arrow)
is not so obvious. Axial views (b) are extremely valuable in
determining extent of luxation and damage.

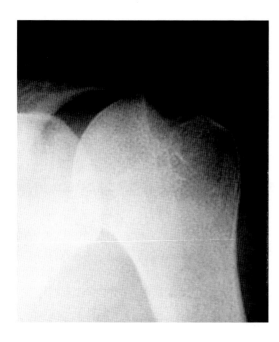

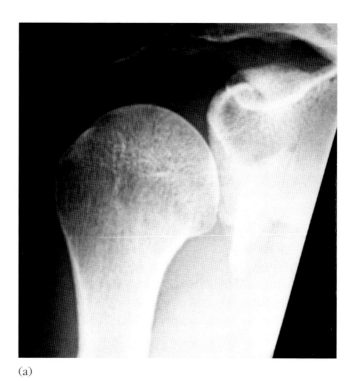

(a)

Figure 4.6

Hill–Sachs lesion. Large impaction fracture of the posterolateral humeral head ('Hill–Sachs') after anteroinferior luxation (anteroposterior view).

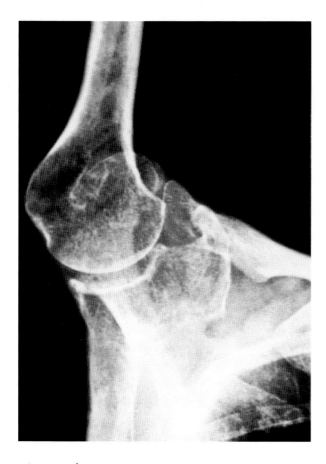

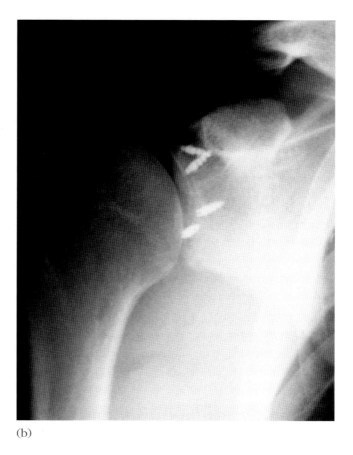

(b)

Figure 4.7

Stryker notch view. The Stryker notch view demonstrates defects in the posterolateral humeral head and is more sensitive than plain anteroposterior views.

Figure 4.8

Postoperative X-ray control. (a) Status 1 year after osseus stabilization procedure. (b) Status after refixation of the glenoid labrum with Fastak (Arthrex, Naples, FL, USA).

original axial projection have been described, the most popular of which are the West Point view and the apical oblique view. If these cannot be performed either, a true scapulolateral view (also known as the tangential lateral or 'Y' view) should be made.[4] These views are particularily helpful to rule out luxation.

Glenohumeral dislocations are easily detected with anteroposterior radiographs (Figure 4.4). For evaluation of patients with instability numerous projections have been described to depict the anterior and posterior margin of the glenoid rim and the humeral head: Hermodsson's tangential view, Stryker's notch view (see Figure 4.7), Didiee's view and the modified axial views, especially the so-called West Point view, are helpful (Figure 4.5).[4–6] While an anteroposterior view can reveal a large posterolateral humeral head impaction fracture (Figure 4.6), the Stryker notch view shows more subtle defects (Figure 4.7). However, as cross-sectional imaging modalities have evolved rapidly these special projections have also lost some of their importance.

In imaging of the rotator cuff conventional radiographs play a rather limited role. They are helpful in depicting anatomic predisposing factors to impingement, yet rotator cuff tears are not directly visible. Calcifications of the tendons and ligaments or subacromial spurs may be shown with an anteroposterior view with 20–30° caudal tilt or the outlet view with scapulolateral positioning and an additional 10° caudal tilt. The outlet view allows good assessment of acromial morphology (Bigliani types I–III and sloping). Unfortunately inter- and intraobserver agreement is comparatively poor in assessment of these pathologies and in many cases only fluoroscopy identifies spurs and calcification reliably.[7–14]

The acromioclavicular and sternoclavicular joints must be assessed for degenerative disease as well as for fractures, luxations, or ligamentous injuries. For the acromioclavicular joint this is usually accomplished with anteroposterior views with a 10–15° cephalic tilt, in the case of suspected ligament injury with weight stress.

The sternoclavicular joints are difficult to assess with standard radiography, even with special views. Hence, cross-sectional imaging should be the method of choice to rule out or quantify pathologies to these joints.[1,2,13–15]

In imaging of the postoperative patient radiographs are helpful in assessing metallic implants and extent of osseus morphology, yet the result of soft tissue reconstructions cannot be adequately demonstrated (Figure 4.8).

Computed tomography and CT arthrography

In addition to the information offered by conventional radiography, CT offers cross-sectional display of the complicated anatomy of the shoulder. Thus assessment of spatial relationships is made much easier and more

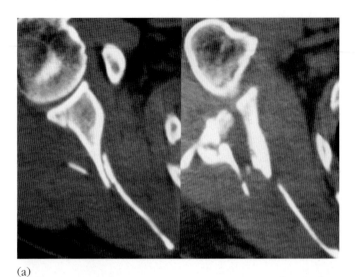

(a)

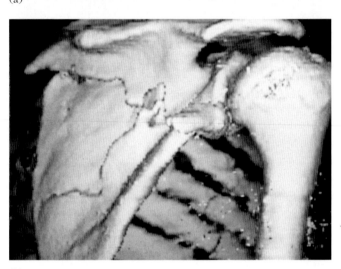

(b)

Figure 4.9

Complex scapular fracture in 2D axial slices and 3D rendering. (a) Reconstruction of complex scapular fractures using standard 2D axial planes and (b) 3D visualization technique facilitates assessment of the fracture.

reliable than with plain film imaging. Increased tissue contrast permits judgment of soft tissues, cortical and cancellous bone and, with modern thin slice spiral CT, the opportunity to reformat slices with remarkable quality. Hence CT has evolved as an excellent problem-solving tool in evaluation of the musculoskeletal system, especially the shoulder. Compared to MRI, CT still offers superior detection of calcification and gas, assessment of cortical disruption and is still faster than MRI. Many commercially available scanners offer 3D reconstruction possibilities that do not change radiologic diagnosis but make the enormous amount of source images easier to assess for the referring clinician, for example in complex fractures (Figure 4.9) or for computer-aided design (CAD) planning of protheses.

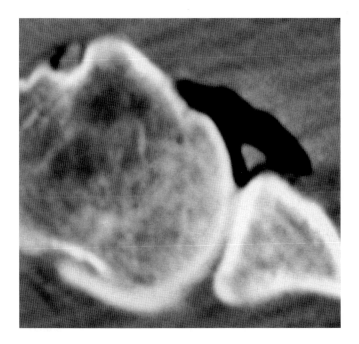

Figure 4.10

Bankart lesion in CT arthrography. Double contrast CT arthrography (after injection of 3 ml iodinated contrast and 10 ml of air) demonstrates detachment of the anterior labrum in a patient with instability.

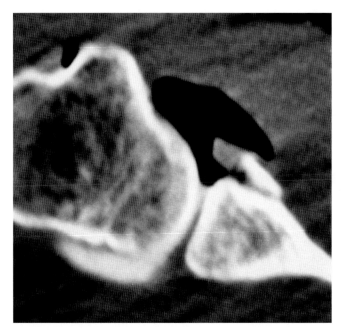

Figure 4.11

Bankart lesion in CT arthrography. Double contrast CT arthrography depicts a Bankart type lesion of the anteroinferior capsulolabral complex with a small osseus fragment.

CT arthrography was originally a development out of the combination of arthrography and conventional tomography, soon replacing them both essentially. In the hands of an experienced radiologist double-contrast arthrography is a safe and valuable tool to assess capsular integrity, full thickness or small articular partial thickness rotator cuff tears. When used in conjunction with CT as double-contrast CT arthrography this technique has, since its beginnings in the early 1980s, changed imaging strategies in shoulder disease (until MRI became available).[4,16–19]

CT arthrography is usually performed after (and usually in conjunction with) a conventional arthrography where 3–4 ml iodinated contrast medium and about 10 ml air are injected. Then, after short exercise, anteroposterior views in internal rotation and external rotation and magnified spot views of the area of suspected pathology are obtained. The patient is taken to the scanner without delay (to avoid extravasation of the contrast) and thin section imaging with the arm in neutral position is performed (Figures 4.10 and 4.11).

In evaluation of the rotator cuff, CT and CT arthrography are of rather limited value: CT can help in defining osseus predisposing factors to impingement, acromioclavicular joint degeneration or intra-articular loose bodies. The strength of CT arthrography lies in assessment of the glenohumeral ligaments, the glenoid labrum itself and only, with some limitations, the rotator cuff.

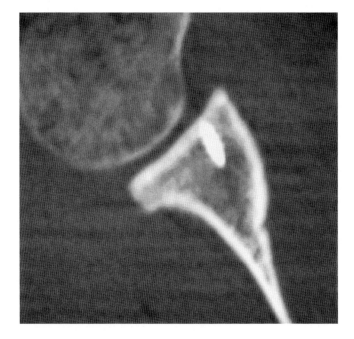

Figure 4.12

CT in postoperative monitoring. Suture anchor (Mitek, Westwood, MA, USA) in the glenoid of a patient with multidirectional instability. CT demonstrates localization of the implant and possible signs of loosening or infection. For metallic implants CT is superior to MRI.

Pathologies of the surface of the capsulolabral complex are detected with high accuracy (taking into account the enormous number of normal variants) yet lesions of the inner substance that do not communicate with the surface are difficult to assess.[3,5,6,16,20–23] Also, lesions of the rotator cuff are usually not adequately visualized with CT arthrography; however, with the advent of multislice CT scanners this may change again. These scanners allow simultaneus acqustion of multiple thin section slices and multiplanar reconstruction without step artifacts. In evaluation of the postoperative cuff this may become an alternative to MRI.

In the meantime MRI and MR arthrography have taken the place of CT arthrography in daily practice as they allow not only the assessment of superficial contours but also of intrasubstance and extra-articular pathologies with high accuracy. Only in cases where the smallest therapeutically relevant calcifications or osseous lesions not detectable with plain films are suspected are CT or CT arthrography still warranted (for example, postoperative monitoring; Figure 4.12).

Magnetic resonance imaging and magnetic resonance arthrography

MRI is the latest and most advanced of all imaging techniques. It has had tremendous impact in the diagnostic work-up of shoulder patients due to its ability to show not only bone but also soft tissues with high contrast and to assess in multiple planes internal changes in all joint-forming structures. Thus it has changed diagnostic and even therapeutic approaches to diseases of the shoulder joint. This section describes technical aspects of shoulder imaging, normal anatomy and common pathologic findings in MRI. Although MRI of the shoulder contributes to virtually every aspect of shoulder disease this section focuses on impingement-related disease, rotator cuff tears, and instability.

A detailed description of the physical background of MRI is beyond the scope of this chapter and the reader may find introductions in most standard textbooks of MRI.[6,18,24–29]

Technical considerations for MRI of the shoulder

Unique features of shoulder anatomy, such as the oblique orientation of key structures (often small with subtle pathologies), far lateral position in the body and the asymmetric external shape, make MRI of the shoulder technically demanding. In order to achieve high spatial resolution (necessary to identify, e.g. smallest labral tears) dedicated surface coils are required. The position of the shoulder in relation to the centre of the magnetic field (so called 'off-center imaging') requires an excellently maintained scanner with only minimal field inhomogeneities. Only then is homogenous and complete fat suppression possible, enabling the radiologist to pick up minute signal changes. Sophisticated magnet and coil design as well as powerful gradient systems are expensive yet mandatory.

Moreover, the complex anatomy and the abundance of normal variants make MRI of the shoulder demanding in terms of interpretation. Due to the rapid development of hardware and software the ideal examination protocol is still debated furiously; it depends on technical items such as scanner set-up and the software available as well as on patient history and the questions raised by the referring clinician.

Spin–echo (SE) sequences remain the mainstay of musculoskeletal imaging; fast SE (FSE) may replace conventional SE, although some caveats must be observed (for example, blurring and high fat signal). Frequency selective fat saturation (FS) has been shown to improve lesion conspicuity, for example in small rotator cuff tears although special care must be taken to ensure homogenous FS. Gradient echo sequences allow shorter acquisition times and 3D imaging but are more vulnerable to artifacts caused by metal or air and also to the magic angle effect. Unlike SE sequences, their image contrast depends, in a complex manner, on parameter settings, producing slightly different weighting, such as T2*, which basically resembles the SE T2 contrast, yet with somewhat more artifacts.

Short inversion time inversion recovery (STIR) technique is another FS method, not as vulnerable to field inhomogeneities as FS, but lengthy and with worse spatial resolution. It also suppresses gadolinium signal and so is not feasible with MR arthrographic techniques.

A typical examination routine (without intra-articular contrast) in a high-field scanner comprises a T2*-weighted axial gradient echo recalled sequence (GRE) sequence, T1 SE and T2 FSE (+FS) coronal and oblique sagittal T2 FS sequence; field of view not exceeding 18 cm, matrix 192 × 256 or better (preferably 256 × 512), and slices not thicker than 4 mm, with the gap between slices less than 20% slice thickness. Thus spatial in-plane resolution is in the vicinity of 1 mm and examination time overall should not exceed 40 minutes. Comfortable patient positioning, placement of the surface coil and choice of imaging planes and sequences are crucial to high quality images. The patient's arm is in neutral rotation, axial slices run parallel to the supraspinatus muscle, oblique coronal slices parallel to the long axis of the supraspinatus tendon and oblique sagittal slices run parallel to the glenoid fossa or perpendicular to the long axis of the supraspinatus muscle. Imaging in the ABER position (*ab*duction *e*xternal *r*otation) is helpful whenever pathology in the antero-inferior capsulolabral complex or small undersurface tears of the rotator cuff are suspected.[6,18,25,27–29]

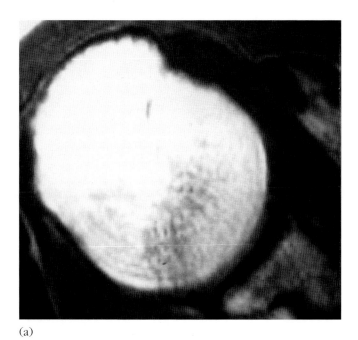

(a)

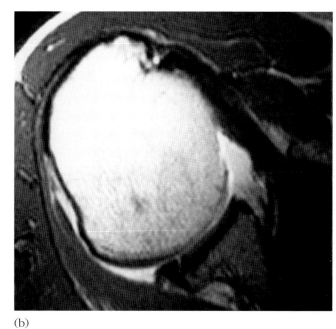

(b)

Figure 4.13

Imaging of the capsulolabral complex with MR arthrography. (a) Before intra-articular application of gadolinium, the extent of damage to the capsulolabral complex is almost impossible to assess exactly (coronal T1 SE). (b) After intra-articular application of gadolinium the extent of damage to the capsulolabral complex is perfectly visualized (axial T1 SE with ia gad).

Although open low-field scanners promise new insights in functional assessment of the shoulder joint, their physically inherent lower signal-to-noise ratio (and hence resulting lower spatial resolution) limit their application in high-end imaging. Most imaging centers use conventional whole-bore high-field scanners with field strengths from 1.0 or 1.5 Tesla and fast gradient systems (> 20 mT).

MR arthrography

MRI allows excellent visualization of muscles and tendons, but there is still some controversy about its ability to detect capsulolabral pathologies reliably. In particular, the injured or degenerated glenoid labrum, the glenohumeral ligaments, the rotator interval or the capsule itself, especially in patients with instability, are relatively difficult to assess in non-contrast-enhanced imaging. In the last couple of years several studies have shown significant diagnostic improvement when distending the joint before imaging. Intra-articular application of diluted gadolinium has meanwhile become the accepted standard: 12–15 ml 1/200 diluted gadolinium are injected (usually under fluoroscopic guidance) and triplanar T1-weighted sequences with FS are acquired. An additional oblique coronal T2 FS complements this routine. Many centers do a preinjection oblique coronal FSE T2 and axial T2* GRE. Alternatively, saline can be injected into the joint; scanning protocol would then mostly rely on

FSE T2 sequences. Another technique is 'indirect' MR arthrography: gadolinium is injected intravenously, the patient exercises for a couple of minutes and is scanned afterwards. Diffusion of gadolinium into the joint allows T1-weighted imaging of the joint fluid as it mixes with gadolinium. The advantage of a non-invasive technique (apart from IV injection of gadolinium) is in our opinion markedly reduced by the lack of joint distention (Figures 4.13 and 4.14).[19,30–38]

Normal anatomy in MRI of the shoulder

As macroscopic and arthroscopic anatomy is presented in detail in specific chapters of this book, only the cross-sectional anatomy relevant to MRI is reviewed. The shoulder joint is actually composed of four joints: the glenohumeral, acromioclavicular, sternoclavicular and scapulothoracic joint. All components of these joints can be evaluated using MRI. Matched pairs of axial slices in cross-sectional cryocuts and MRI slices run parallel to the supraspinatus muscle, oblique coronal slices run parallel to the long axis of the supraspinatus tendon and oblique sagittal slices run parallel to the glenoid fossa or perpendicular to the long axis of the supraspinatus muscle. They demonstrate the muscles of the rotator cuff, important osseus anatomical landmarks and the capsulolabral

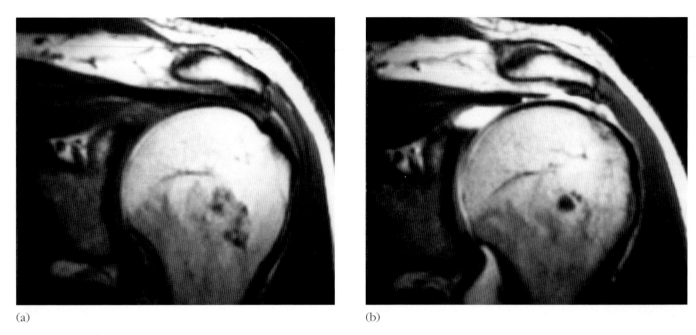

(a)   (b)

Figure 4.14

MRI imaging with direct MR arthrography. (a) Before intra-articular application of gadolinium a tear is suspected but difficult to assess (axial T1 SE). (b) After intra-articular application of gadolinium the rotator cuff tear is far better visualized, especially the extent of rupture and retraction (coronal T1 SE with intra-articular gadolinium (ia gad)).

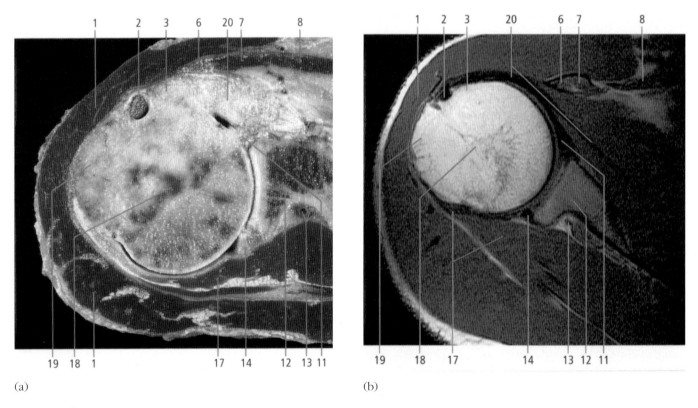

(a)   (b)

Figure 4.15

Normal anatomy. (a) Cryosection (axial). (b) MRI (T1 SE, axial). Reproduced from Burgkart et al[98] with permission.

1: Deltoid muscle	8: Pectoralis minor muscle	17: Infraspinatus muscle
2: Biceps tendon (long head)	11: Labrum, anterior	18: Humeral head
3: Lesser tuberosity	12: Angulus lateralis scapulae	19: Greater tuberosity
6: Biceps tendon (short head)	13: A, V, N suprascapularis	20: Subscapularis tendon
7: Coracobrachialis muscle	14: Labrum, posterior	

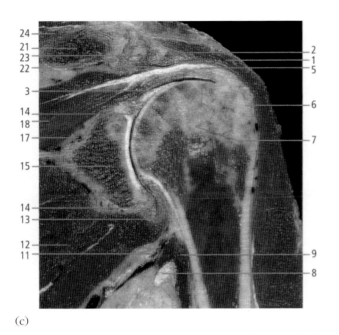

(c)

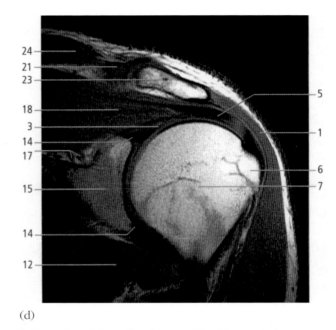

(d)

Normal anatomy. (c) Cryosection (coronal). (d) MRI (T1 SE, coronal). Reproduced from Burgkart et al[98] with permission.

1: Deltoid muscle
2: Coracoacromial ligament
3: Biceps tendon (long head)
5: Supraspinatus tendon
6: Greater tuberosity
7: Humeral head
8: Latissimus dorsi tendon

9: Teres maior muscle
11: A, V circumflex hum
12: Subscapularis muscle
13: Joint capsule and IGHL
14: Labrum, inferior and superior
15: Angulus latissimus scapulae

17: A, V suprascapularis
18: Supraspinatus muscle
21: Clavicle
22: Subacromial bursa
23: Acromion
24: Trapezius muscle

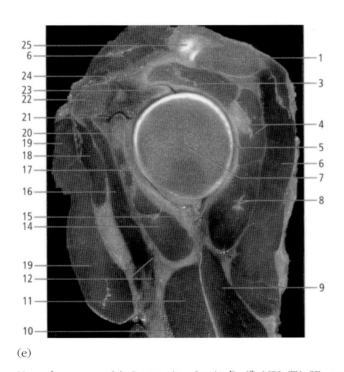

(e)

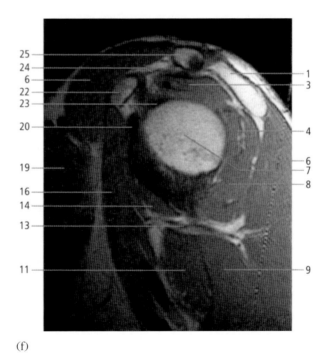

(f)

Normal anatomy. (e) Cryosection (sagittal). (f) MRI (T1 SE, sagittal). Reproduced from Burgkart et al[98] with permission.

1: Acromion
3: Supraspinatus muscle and tendon
4: Infraspinatus muscle and tendon
5: Joint capsule
6: Deltoid muscle
7: Humeral head
8: Teres minor muscle
9: Triceps muscle and tendon

10: Latissimus dorsi muscle and tendon
11: Teres major muscle
12: A, V, N brachialis
13: Circumflex artery
14: Subscapularis muscle
15: Joint capsule and IGH
16: Coracobrachialis muscle
17: Joint capsule and MGHL

18: Pectoralis minor muscle
19: Pectoralis major muscle
20: Subscapularis tendon
21: Bursa
22: Coracoid process
23: Biceps tendon (long head)
24: Coracoacromial ligament
25: Clavicle

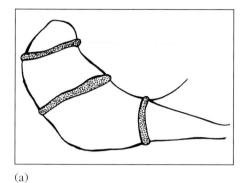

(a)

Figure 4.16

Os acromiale. (a) Schematic representation of variants of the os acromiale. (b) MRI of os acromiale (axial and sagittal T1 SE).

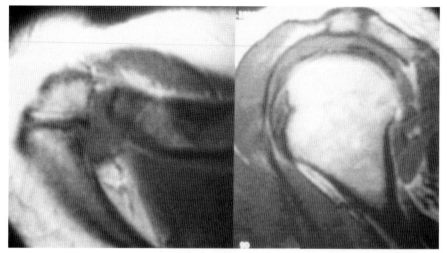

(b)

complex. The figures correlate representative MR images with cross-sectional specimen in axial, coronal and sagittal planes (Figure 4.15).

Problems and pitfalls in MRI of the shoulder

Most tendons demonstrate uniformly low signal on T1- and T2-weighted sequences and hence signal alterations are usually pathologic. The rotator cuff tendons however quite often show high signal on T1 or proton-density images, but these do not represent pathologic signal constellations in patients with no clinical findings related to the shoulder.[27,39]

These signal alterations are partially related to anatomic phenomena. If imaging is performed in internal rotation, the tendons of the infraspinatus and supraspinatus muscle overlap in coronal cross-sectional view, giving the tendons a 'stippled' appearance, even mimicking a tear. In addition, there are usually two main tendon bundles in the supraspinatus muscle, one of which courses 10–15° more anteriorly than the other and also contributes to high signal.[40]

The 'critical zone' of hypovascularity 1 cm central to the insertion of the supraspinatus tendon often is hyperintense on short TE or proton-density sequences. This is usually related to 'magic angle effect' (an artificial signal elevation when immobile hydrogen protons bound to a collagenous matrix are oriented 55° relative to the main magnetic field), but it may also represent physiological mucinous degeneration or partial tear. Only very careful examination of this critical area using different weightings allows correct diagnosis. Further medially, there is sometimes a high signal attributed to interdigitating fat or muscle fibers at the musculotendinous junction.[4,27,41,42]

Partial volume averaging also contributes to high signal intensity especially at the rim of the supraspina-

tus tendon where fat or fluid (in the biceps tendon sheath) is volume averaged; this is particularily puzzling when trying to assess rotator interval lesions.

Indirect signs of impingement such as a discontinous subacromial fat stripe, effusion in the subacromial–subdeltoid bursa, moderate thickening of the coracoacromial or coracohumeral ligaments, relative narrowing of the subacromial space or rotator cuff lesions are either non-specific, late-stage signs or sequelae of an impingement syndrome. As explained above, many are also found in patients without shoulder complaints.[40–53]

Rotator cuff

Rotator cuff pathologies may be attributed to a variety of conditions and the debate about the relative importance of the contributing factors is still ongoing.[7,18,54] Impingement—primary external and internal or instability-related secondary impingement—is a difficult challenge to the diagnostic radiologist. Impingement as a functional impairment is not directly visualized on static MR images with the patient in the magnet bore and the arm in neutral position. Nonetheless MRI is the only imaging modality able to assess the status of the rotator cuff (including early signs of degeneration and small tears) and to identify morphologic features predisposing to impingement.

MRI can reliably detect anatomic predisposing factors to impingement such as certain acromial shapes, subacromial spurs, acromioclavicular joint disease, or supraspinatus hypertrophy and in addition assess the rotator cuff itself.

Bigliani and Morrison's classification of acromial types based on plain films (and anatomical findings) found a higher incidence for rotator cuff lesions with 'hook' Type 3; surprisingly, subsequent studies using MRI to classify did not match the plain film classification well, mostly due to technical reasons (projection phenomena, site of

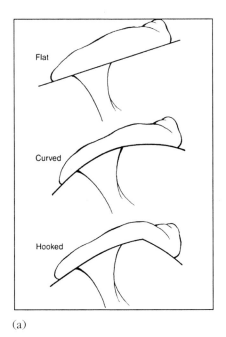

(a)

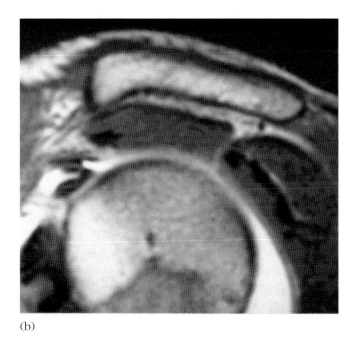

(b)

Figure 4.17

Acromial shapes. (a) Schematic drawing of acromial morphology (modified after Rockwood and Matsen 1998.[4]). (b) A Type 3 acromion with encroachment of the supraspinatus (oblique sagittal T1 SE).

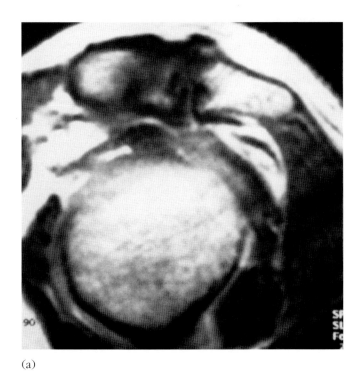

(a)

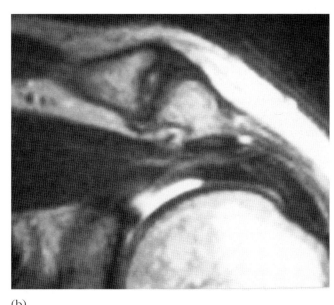

(b)

Figure 4.18

Degenerative acromioclavicular joint changes encroaching the rotator cuff. (a) Oblique sagittal T1 SE; (b) Coronal T1 SE.

assessment), so care should be taken when trying to compare acromial shape in plain films and MRI. The presence of an os acromiale, subacromial spurs or downward sloping of the acromion nevertheless seem to be important predisposing factors in the pathogenesis of external subacromial impingement (Figures 4.16–4.18). Degenerative disease of the acromioclavicular joint with hypertrophic osteophytes also functionally narrows the subacromial space. If the coaracoid process is longer or larger than average and thus the distance between the coracoid and the lesser tuberosity less than 11 mm in internal rotation, subcoracoid impingement of the subscapularis tendon can occur.

Apart from external encroachment of the rotator cuff, primary internal derangement was recognized as an important factor in rotator cuff disease. Most partial tears

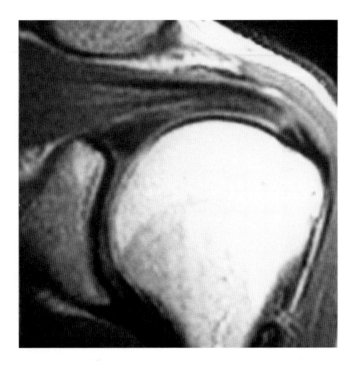

Figure 4.19

Signal intensity alteration due to tendinopathy at the Codman triangle (surgically proven intact rotator cuff) (coronal T1 SE).

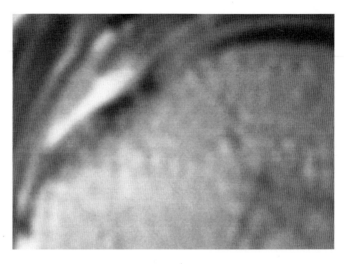

Figure 4.20

Small tear at the insertion of the supraspinatus at the greater tuberosity (T1 SE ia gad).

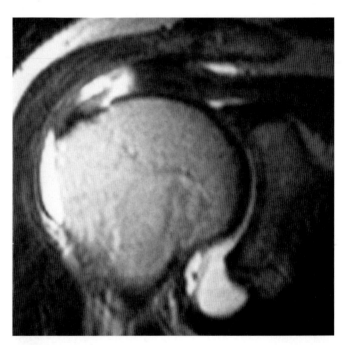

Figure 4.21

Full thickness rotator cuff tear (supraspinatus depicted in this slice) with retraction of the tendon to 12 o'clock position; wide axillary recess (T1 SE ia gad).

start at the articular side of the cuff, often at the critical hypovascular zone described by Codman.[4]

MRI is accurate in describing early signs of degeneration (some still clinically obscure) and also in describing subsequent stages of rotator cuff tears. Severe inflammatory tendinopathy, however, can be difficult to distinguish from subtle partial tears (Figure 4.19). Partial thickness rotator cuff tears actually represent a variety of different lesions from small surface fraying to degenerative tears that look like torn millefeuille pastry and hence are more difficult to assess than full thickness rotator cuff tears. Diagnosis of partial thickness rotator cuff tears was shown to be significantly improved with MR arthrography. Full thickness rotator cuff tears are reliably identified even on non-contrast-enhanced MR images with a fluid-filled gap as the hallmark lesion (Figures 4.20 and 4.21). It is very important to report not only the presence but also the exact location and size of a tear and the surrounding anatomy to facilitate surgical planning (arthroscopic versus mini-open versus open, portals, stabilizing procedures etc.). Hence, description of the rotator cuff must include size and location of a tear, quality and amount of retraction of the tendons, fatty degeneration of the rotator cuff muscles (a recently recognized important prognostic factor) (Figure 4.22), biceps tendon and rotator interval lesions, concomitant capsulolabral lesions and of course precise depiction of the predisposing factors (Figure 4.23). If a grading system is used at all to classify lesions, radiologist and surgeon should use the same system. Assessment is difficult in the patient with prior surgery where metal artifacts make diagnosis of subtle retears tricky, yet full thickness rotator cuff tears are detectable (Figure 4.24).[4,9,10,12,14,15,55–76]

MRI is an excellent tool to assess integrity of the rotator cuff and to define predisposing factors for impingement. Anatomic and technical pitfalls are numerous so that meticulous planning, scanning and interpre-

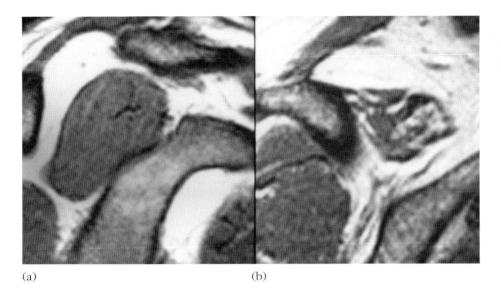

(a)   (b)

Figure 4.22

(a) Normal cross-sectional cut through supraspinatus. (b) Severe fatty degeneration of the supraspinatus.

tation are absolutely mandatory for consistently high diagnostic accuracy.

Instability

Whereas MRI has established a definite role in evaluation of the rotator cuff, indications for MRI in evaluating instability still differs tremendously from center to center.

This is largely due to the referring physician's personal preference as to how to diagnose and treat patients with instability. As new treatment options allow minimally invasive stabilization procedures and fewer patients now have to be hospitalized for open reconstruction, presurgical tests must provide information to the surgeon about which procedure is adequate. This is particularly true in high-level athletes, patients with prior and failed surgery or if clinical examination is equivocal.

In most cases history and physical examination by an experienced surgeon reveal type, cause, direction and acquisition of instability. MRI can help further define the type and can assess the extent of pathologies related to instability. As in assessment of the rotator cuff not only the primary determinants or sequelae of instability may

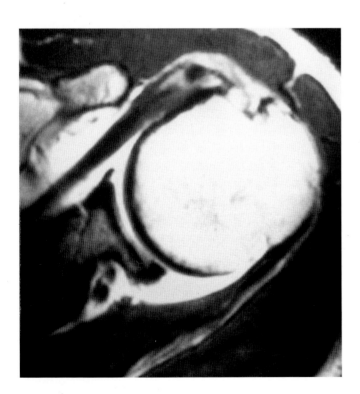

Figure 4.23

Subscapularis tear with luxation of the biceps tendon (axial T1 SE ia gad).

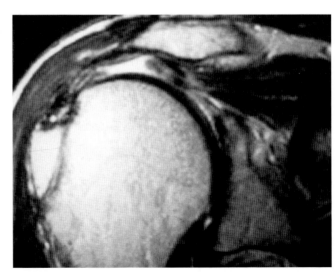

Figure 4.24

Retear after reconstruction of the rotator cuff (coronal T1 SE ia gad).

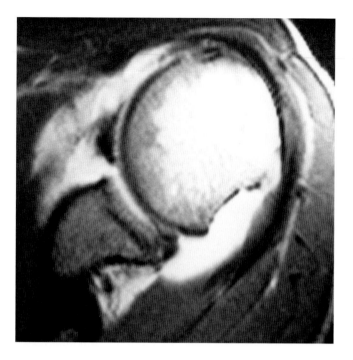

Figure 4.25

Hill–Sachs lesion in a patient with anterior instability (axial T1 SE ia gad).

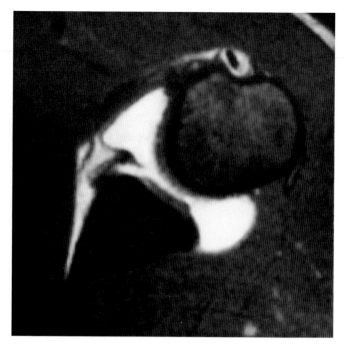

Figure 4.26

Lesion to the anterior inferior capsulolabral complex with detachment of the labrum and partial stripping of the periosteum (axial T1 SE ia gad).

be seen with MRI but also the rotator cuff and pathologies not readily detectable in clinical examination, for example notch cysts. Even though instability-related impingement is still difficult to diagnose as well clinically as with imaging, our growing understanding of pathophysiology and image patterns may enable us to define with more confidence those patients who should undergo subacromial decompression before stabilization and vice versa.

In MRI of patients with instability we rely almost solely on MR arthrography. Although some (even very experienced) musculoskeletal radiologists still advocate non-contrast examinations, in accordance with recent studies in the literature, we found accuracy markedly improved using intra-articular diluted gadolinium. This procedure is of course only justified in those patients willing to undergo therapy; as we provide imaging for a group of highly specialized orthopedic surgeons, almost all our patients (many of them high level professional athletes) opt for maximum diagnostic and therapeutic opportunities and a majority finally undergoes reconstructive surgery.[50,77]

The most common type of instability is anterior instability. It usually leads to an injury of the anteroinferior capsulolabral complex, typically a Bankart (or Bankart-like) lesion. When Bankart described the 'avulsed fibrous or fibrocartilaginous ligament (...from the glenoid margin)' in 1938 he did not state exactly whether this lesion was

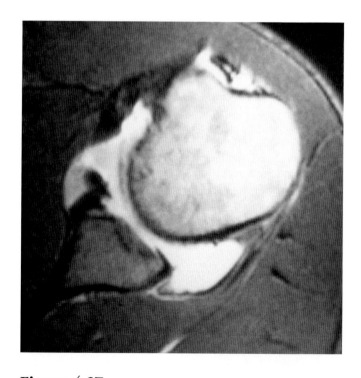

Figure 4.27

MR arthrogram in a patient with recurrent luxations revealing rotator cuff and biceps tendon tears as well as partially healed injuries to the anteroinferior capsulolabral complex (axial T1 SE ia gad).

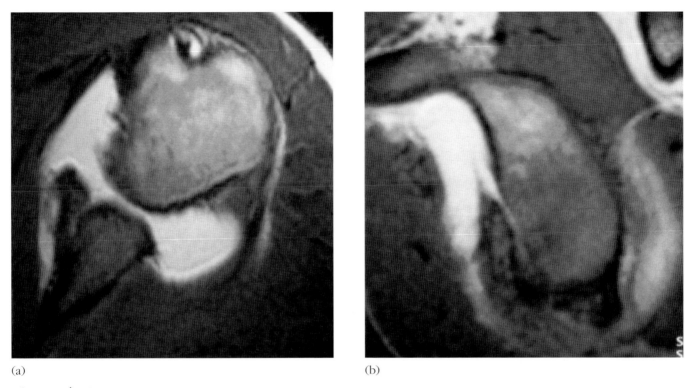

(a)

(b)

Figure 4.28

Bankart lesion with osseus defect. (a) Axial T1 SE ia gad; (b) sagittal T1 SE ia gad.

with or without osseus component (Figures 4.25–4.28).[4] Since then many different types of ligamentous, periosteal and osseus lesions related to instability have been described in the orthopedic and radiologic literature that are virtually pathognomonic on MR arthrography. Numerous acronyms have been coined to characterize these lesions: ALPSA, GLAD, HAGL and SLAP.[25,72,78–80]

ALPSA describes an anterior labroligamentous periosteal sleeve avulsion of the inferior glenohumeral ligament with an intact anterior scapular periosteum. Thus the avulsed labroligamentous complex can roll medially up the periosteum. GLAD stands for glenolabral articular disruption, an injury usually resulting from forced adduction out of abduction and external rotation. A superficial anteroinferior labral tear is associated with glenoid articular cartilage injury. HAGL stands for humeral avulsion of the glenohumeral ligament, a far less frequent injury than Bankart-type lesions. In Perthe's lesion the periosteum is intact but stripped away from the glenoid with the attached anteroinferior labroligamentous complex.

Posterior instability may cause similar damage to the posterior rim of the glenoid or the labroligamentous complex, resulting in a reverse Bankart. All these lesions can be identified on MR arthrography images with high accuracy. Precise documentation is crucial to successful planning of the arthroscopy portals and use of instrumentation.[81,82]

Assessment of the glenoid labrum itself is more difficult than one might expect, as normal variations and physiologic degeneration do not always readily allow differentiation between normal and abnormal. In particular, the anterosuperior quadrant of the glenoid labrum shows a wide variety of normal variants. Neumann and colleagues[23,83] found considerable range of normal variants in labral shape, DePalma[4] described in 1983 the normal variants in foramina and recesses in the anterosuperior quadrant of the capsulolabral complex. The labrum may be completely absent, sometimes coincide with a thick cord-like middle glenohumeral ligament (Buford complex) or the different labral configurations originally described by Detrisac and Johnson.[4] Several different biceps tendon insertions with different recesses and varying degrees of cartilage undercutting make confident diagnosis of a detachment of the labrum extremely difficult. In addition, longitudinal clinical and cadaveric studies showed an increasing degeneration in the signal in the substance of the glenoid labrum, fraying of the surface and physiologic detachment of the labrum beginning in the fifth decade.[4,22,23,50,82–96]

Snyder et al[80] described a complex lesion of the superior labrum, extending from anterior to posterior, in some cases even with extension into the biceps tendon, as the SLAP lesion. Although clinical diagnosis may be difficult, MRI findings are mostly straightforward, especially in types III and IV.[27,31,80,97] One must pay atten-

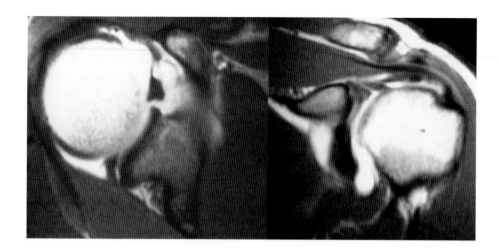

Figure 4.29

SLAP IV lesion. Axial and oblique coronal MR arthrogram (T1 SE) reveals a lesion to the superior labrum from anterior to posterior involving the biceps anchor (type IV Snyder).

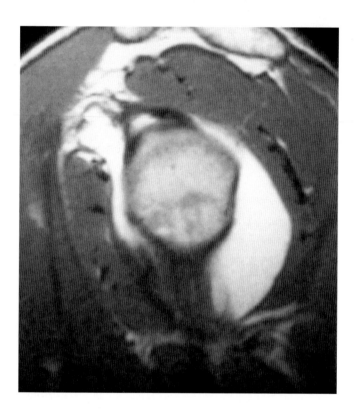

Figure 4.30

Rotator interval lesion of the unstable type involving parts of the SGHL and the CHL (surgically proven) (T1 SE ia gad).

tion, however, to the different normal variations in labral morphology and biceps tendon attachment to avoid overcalling (Figure 4.29). The rotator interval has attracted a lot of interest among shoulder surgeons recently, so far only MR arthrography can delineate pathology in the rotator interval (Figure 4.30).

MR arthrography is an excellent technique to assess intra-articular morphology and pathology of patients with instability. Like no other modality it is able to quantify intra- and extra-articular pathology of bone and soft tissues. Unfortunately the enormous spectrum of normal variants makes it diffcult for the radiologist (and the surgeon) to distinguish the normal from the abnormal and completely pathological.

References

1. Bernau A. *Orthopädische Röntgendiagnostik.* Munich: Urban & Schwarzenberg, 1995.
2. Lutz KC. *Einstelltechniken in der Traumatologie.* Stuttgart: Thieme, 1992.
3. Resnick D. Shoulder imaging. Perspective. *Magn Reson Imaging Clin N Am* 1997; **5**:661–5.
4. Rockwood CA, Jr, Matsen FA. *The Shoulder.* 2nd edn. Philadelphia: WB Saunders, 1998.
5. Iannotti JP, Williams GR. *Disorders of the Shoulder: Diagnosis and Management.* Philadelphia: Lippincott Williams & Wilkins, 1999.
6. Resnick D. *Diagnosis of Bone and Joint Disorders.* 3rd edn. Philadelphia: WB Saunders, 1995.
7. Bigliani LU, Morrison DS, April EW. The morphology of the acromion and its relationship to rotator cuff tears. *Orthop Trans* 1986; **10**:228.
8. Cone ROD, Resnick D, Danzig L. Shoulder impingement syndrome: radiographic evaluation. *Radiology* 1984; **150**:29–33.
9. Gold RH, Seeger LL, Yao L. Imaging shoulder impingement. *Skeletal Radiol* 1993; **22**:555–61.
10. Haygood TM, Langlotz CP, Kneeland JB et al. Categorization of acromial shape: interobserver variability with MR imaging and conventional radiography. *Am J Roentgenol* 1994; **162**:1377–82.
11. Kilcoyne RF, Reddy PK, Lyons F, Rockwood CA Jr. Optimal plain film imaging of the shoulder impingement syndrome. *Am J Roentgenol* 1989; **153**:795–7.
12. Newhouse KE, el-Khoury GY, Nepola JV, Montgomery WJ. The shoulder impingement view: a fluoroscopic technique for the detection of subacromial spura. *Am J Roentgenol* 1988; **151**:539–41.
13. Ogata S, Uhthoff HK. Acromial enthesopathy and rotator cuff tear. A radiologic and histologic postmortem investigation of the coracoacromial arch. *Clin Orthop* 1990; **254**:39–48.
14. Ozaki J, Fujimoto S, Nakagawa Y et al. Tears of the rotator cuff of the choulder associated with pathological changes in the

acromion. A study in cadavera. *J Bone Joint Surg* 1988; **70A**:1224–30.

15. Tuite MJ, Toivonen DA, Orwin JF, Wright DH. Acromial angle on radiographs of the shoulder: correlation with the impingement syndrome and rotator cuff tears. *Am J Roentgenol* 1995; **165**:609–13.

16. Rafii M, Firooznia H, Golimbu C et al. CT arthrography of capsular structures of the shoulder. *Am J Roengenol* 1986; **146**:361–7.

17. Rafii M, Firooznia H, Bonamo JJ et al. Athlete shoulder injuries: CT arthrographic findings. *Radiology* 1987; **162**:559–64.

18. Rafii M. Update on the shoulder. *Magn Reson Imaging Clin N Am* 1997; **5**:787–811.

19. Rafii M, Minkoff J. Advanced arthrography of the shoulder with CT and MR imaging. *Radiol Clin North Am* 1998; **36**:609–33.

20. Chandnani VP, Yeager TD, DeBerardino T et al. Glenoid labral tears: prospective evaluation with MRI imaging, MR arthrography, and CT arthrography. *Am J Roentgenol* 1993; **161**:1229–35.

21. Deutsch AL, Resnick D, Mink JH et al. Computed and conventional arthrotomography of the glenohumeral joint: normal anatomy and clinical experience. *Radiology* 1984; **153**:603–9.

22. Nelson MC, Leather GP, Nirschl RP et al. Evaluation of the painful shoulder. A prospective comparison of magnetic resonance imaging, computerized tomographic arthrography, ultrasonography, and operative findings. *J Bone Joint Surg* 1991; **73A**:707–16.

23. Neumann CH, Petersen SA, Jahnke AH Jr et al. MRI in the evaluation of patients with suspected instability of the shoulder joint including a comparison with CT-arthrography. *Am J Roentgenol* 1986; **146**:361–7.

24. Holt RG, Helms CA, Steinbach L et al. Magnetic resonance imaging of the shoulder: rationale and current applications. *Skeletal Radiol* 1990; **19**:5–14.

25. Resnick D, Kang HS. *Internal Derangement of Joints.* Philadelphia: WB Saunders, 1997.

26. Rodkey WG, Steadman JR, Ho CP. Role of MR imaging in sports medicine research. Basic science and clinical research studies. *Magn Reson Imaging Clin North Am* 1999; **7**:191–203.

27. Steinbach LS, et al. *Shoulder Magnetic Resonance Imaging.* Philadelphia: Lippincott-Raven, 1998.

28. Stoller D. *MRI in Orthopedics and Sports Medicine.* 2nd edn. Philadelphia: Lippincott-Raven, 1997.

29. Zlatkin MB. *MRI of the Shoulder.* New York: Raven Press, 1991.

30. Kopka L, Funke M, Fischer U et al. MR arthrography of the shoulder with gadopentetate dimeglumine: influence of concentration, iodinated contrast material, and time on signal intensity. *Am J Roentgenol* 1994; **163**:621–3.

31. Monu JU, Pope TL Jr, Chabon SJ, Vanarthos WJ. MR diagnosis of superior labral anterior posterior (SLAP) injuries of the glenoid labrum: value of routine imaging without intraarticular injection of contrast material. *Am J Roentgenol* 1994; **163**:1425–9.

32. Palmer WE, Caslowitz PL, Chew FS. MR arthrography of the shoulder: normal intraarticular structures and common abnormalities. *Am J Roentgenol* 1995; **164**:141–6.

33. Recht MP, Kramer J, Petersilge CA et al. Distribution of normal and abnormal fluid collections in the glenohumeral joint: implications for MR arthrography. *J Magn Reson Imaging* 1994; **4**:173–7.

34. Tirman PF, Stauffer AE, Crues JV III et al. Saline magnetic resonance arthrography in the evaluation of glenohumeral instability. *Arthroscopy* 1993; **9**:550–9.

35. Tirman PF, Bost FW, Steinbach LS et al. MR arthrographic depiction of tears of the rotator cuff: benefit of abduction and external rotation of the arm. *Radiology* 1994; **192**:851–6.

36. Tirman PF, Feller JF, Janzen DL et al. Association of glenoid labral cysts with labral tears and glenohumeral instability: radiologic findings and clinical significance. *Radiology* 1994; **190**:653–8.

37. Tirman PF, Bost FW, Garvin GJ et al. Posterosuperior glenoid impingement of the shoulder: findings at MR imaging and MR arthrography with arthroscopic correlation. *Radiology* 1994; **193**:431–6.

38. Vahlensieck M, Peterfy CG, Wischer T et al. Indirect MR arthrography: optimization and clinical applications. *Radiology* 1996; **200**:249–54.

39. Davis SJ, Teresi LM, Bradley WG et al. Effect of arm rotation on MR imaging of the rotator cuff. *Radiology* 1991; **181**:265–8.

40. Vahlensieck M, Pollack M, Lang P et al. Two segments of the supraspinatus muscle: cause of high signal intensity at MR imaging? *Radiology* 1993; **186**:449–54.

41. Kaplan PA, Bryans KC, Davick JP et al. MR imaging of the normal shoulder: variants and pitfalls. *Radiology* 1992; **184**:519–24.

42. Kjellin I, Ho CP, Cervilla V et al. Alterations in the supraspinatus tendon at MR imaging: correlation with histopathologic findings in cadavers. *Radiology* 1991; **181**:837–41.

43. Chandnani V, Ho C, Gerharter J et al. MR findings in asymptomatic shoulders: a blind analysis using symptomatic shoulders as controls. *Clin Imaging* 1992; **16**:25–30.

44. Davidson PA, Elattrache NS, Jobe CM, Jobe FW. Rotator cuff and posterior–superior glenoid labrum injury associated with increased glenohumeral motion: a new site of impingement. *J Shoulder Elbow Surg* 1995; **4**:384–90.

45. Epstein RE, Schweitzer ME, Frieman BG et al. Hooked acromion: prevalence on MR images of painful shoulders. *Radiology* 1993; **187**:479–81.

46. Erickson SJ, Cox IH, Hyde JS et al. Effect of tendon orientation on MR imaging signal intensity: a manifestation of the 'magic angle' phenomenon. *Radiology* 1991; **181**:389–92.

47. Kieft GJ, Bloem JL, Rozing PM, Obermann WR. Rotator cuff impingement syndrome: MR imaging. *Radiology* 1988; **166**:211–14.

48. Liou JT, Wilson AJ, Totty WG, Brown JJ. The normal shoulder: common variations that simulate pathologic conditions at MR imaging. *Radiology* 1993; **186**:435–41.

49. Middleton WD, Kneeland JB, Carrera GF et al. High-resolution MR imaging of the normal rotator cuff. *Am J Roentgenol* 1987; **148**:559–64.

50. Minkoff J, Stecker S, Cavaliere G. Glenohumeral instabilities and the role of MR imaging techniques. The orthopedic surgeon's perspective. *Magn Reson Imaging Clin N Am* 1997; **5**:767–85.

51. Mirowitz SA. Normal rotator cuff: MR imaging with conventional and fat-suppression techniques. *Radiology* 1991; **180**:735–40.

52. Monu JU, Pruett S, Vanarthos WJ, Pope TL Jr. Isolated subacromial bursal fluid on MRI of the shoulder in symptomatic patients: correlation with arthroscopic findings. *Skeletal Radiol* 1994; **23**:529–33.

53. Tsao LY, Mirowitz SA. MR imaging of the shoulder. Imaging techniques, diagnostic pitfalls, and normal variants. *Magn Reson Imaging Clin North Am* 1997; **5**:683–704.

54. Neer CSD, Impingement lesions. *Clin Orthop* 1983; **173**:70–7.

55. Farley TE, Neumann CH, Steinbach LS et al. Full-thickness tears of the rotator cuff of the shoulder: diagnosis with MR imaging. *Am J Roentgenol* 1992; **158**:347–51.

56. Gagey N, Ravaud E, Lassau JP. Anatomy of the acromial arch: correlation of anatomy and magnetic resonance imaging. *Surg Radiol Anat* 1993; **15**:63–70.

57. Goutallier D, Postel JM, Bernageau J et al. Fatty muscle degeneration in cuff ruptures. Pre- and postoperative evaluation by CT scan. *Clin Orthop* 1994; **304**:78–83.

58. Ho CP. MR imaging of rotator interval, long biceps, and associated injuries in the overhead-throwing athlete. *Magn Reson Imaging Clin N Am* 1999; **7**:23–37.

59. Hodler J, Kursunoglu-Brahme S, Snyder SJ et al. Rotator cuff disease: assessment with MR arthrography versus standard MR imaging in 36 patients with arthroscopic confirmation. *Radiology* 1992; **182**:431–6.

60. Iannotti JP, Zlatkin MB, Esterhai JL et al. Magnetic resonance imaging of the shoulder. Sensitivity, specificity and predictive value. *J Bone Joint Surg* 1991; **73A**:17–29.

61. Imhoff A, Hodler J. [Arthroscopy and MRI of the shoulder: a comparative retrospective analysis]. *Z Orthop Ihre Grenzgeb* 1992; **130**:188–96.

62. Imhoff AB, Hodler J, Perrenoud A. [Possibilities of shoulder arthroscopy in comparison with magnetic resonance tomography and arthro-computerized tomography]. *Z Unfallchir Versicherungsmed* 1993; **86**:4–17.

63. Jobe FW. Impingement problems in the athlete. *Instr Course Lect* 1989; **38**:205–69.

64. Jobe CM. Posterior superior glenoid impingement: expanded spectrum. *Arthroscopy* 1995; **11**:530–6.

65. Kaneko K, De Mouy EH, Brunet ME. MR evaluation of rotator cuff impingement: correlation with confirmed full-thickness rotator cuff tears. *J Comput Assist Tomogr* 1994; **18**:225–8.

66. Needell SD, Zlatkin MB, Sher JS et al. MR imaging of the rotator cuff: peritendinous and bone abnormalities in an asymptomatic population. *Am J Roentgenol* 1996; **166**:863–7.

67. Neumann CH, Holt RG, Steinbach LS et al. MR imaging of the shoulder: appearance of the supraspinatus tendon in asymptomatic volunteers. *Am J Roentgenol* 1992; **158**:1281–7.

68. Park JG, Lee JK, Phelps CT. Os acromiale associated with rotator cuff impingement: MR imaging of the shoulder. *Radiology* 1994; **193**:255–7.

69. Patten RM, Spear RP, Richardson ML. Diagnostic performance of magnetic resonance imaging for the diagnosis of rotator cuff tears using supplemental images in the oblique sagittal plane. *Invest Radiol* 1994; **29**:87–93.

70. Patten RM. Tears of the anterior portion of the rotator cuff (the subscapularis tendon): MR imaging findings. *Am J Roentgenol* 1994; **162**:351–4.

71. Rafii M, Firooznia H, Sherman O et al. Rotator cuff lesions: signal patterns at MR imaging. *Radiology* 1990; **177**:817–23.

72. Seeger LE, Gold RH, Bassett LW, Ellman H. Shoulder impingement syndrome: MR findings in 57 shoulders. *Am J Roengenol* 1988; **150**:343–7.

73. Thomazeau H, Rolland Y, Lucas C et al. Atrophy of the supraspinatus belly. Assessment by MRI in 55 patients with rotator cuff pathology. *Acta Orthop Scand* 1996; **67**:264–8.

74. Tuite MJ, Yandow DR, DeSmet AA et al. Diagnosis of partial and complete rotator cuff tears using combined gradient echo and spin echo imaging. *Skeletal Radiol* 1994; **23**:541–5.

75. Tuite MJ, Yandow DR, De Smet AA et al. Effect of field of view on MR diagnosis of rotator cuff tears. *Skeletal Radiol* 1995; **24**:495–8.

76. Williamson MP, Chandnani VP, Baird DE et al. Shoulder impingement syndrome: diagnostic accuracy of magnetic resonance imaging and radiographic signs. *Aust Radiol* 1994; **38**:265–71.

77. Kwak SM, Brown RR, Trudell D, Resnick D. Glenohumeral joint: comparison of shoulder positions at MR arthrography. *Radiology* 1998; **208**:375–80.

78. Neviaser TJ. The GLAD lesion: another cause of anterior shoulder pain. *Arthroscopy* 1993; **9**:22–3.

79. Neviaser TJ. The anterior labroligamentous periosteal sleeve avulsion lesion: a cause of anterior instability of the shoulder. *Arthroscopy* 1993; **9**:17–21.

80. Snyder SJ, Karzel RP, Del Pizzo W et al. SLAP lesions of the shoulder. *Arthroscopy* 1990; **6**:274–9.

81. Ferrari JD, Ferrari DA, Coumas J, Pappas AM. Posterior ossification of the shoulder: the Bennett lesion. Etiology, diagnosis, and treatment. *Am J Sports Med* 1994; **22**:171–5.

82. Garneau RA, Renfrew DL, Moore TE et al. Glenoid labrum: evaluation with MR imaging. *Radiology* 1991; **179**:519–22.

83. Neumann CH, Petersen SA, Jahnke AH. MR imaging of the labral–capsular complex: normal variations. *Am J Roentgenol* 1991; **157**:1015–21.

84. Green MR, Christensen KP. Magnetic resonance imaging of the glenoid labrum in anterior shoulder instability. *Am J Sports Med* 1994; **22**:493–8.

85. Gross ML, Seeger LL, Smith JB et al. Magnetic resonance imaging of the glenoid labrum. *Am J Sports Med* 1990; **18**:229–34.

86. Gusmer PB, Potter HG, Schatz JA et al. Labral injuries: accuracy of detection with unenhanced MR imaging of the shoulder. *Radiology* 1996; **200**:519–24.

87. Legan JM, Burkhard TK, Goff WB 2nd et al. Tears of the glenoid labrum: MR imaging of 88 arthroscopically confirmed cases. *Radiology* 1991; **179**:241–6.

88. Loredo R, Longo C, Salonen D et al. Glenoid labrum: MR imaging with histologic correlation. *Radiology* 1995; **196**:33–41.

89. McCauley TR, Pope CF, Jokl P. Normal and abnormal glenoid labrum: assessment with multiplanar gradient-echo MR imaging. *Radiology* 1992; **183**:35–7.

90. Palmer WE, Caslowitz PL. Anterior shoulder instability: diagnostic criteria determined from prospective analysis of 121 MR arthrograms. *Radiology* 1995; **197**:819–25.

91. Pappas AM, Goss TP, Kleinman PK. Symptomatic shoulder instability due to lesions of the glenoid labrum. *Am J Sports Med* 1983; **11**:279–88.

92. Rafii M, Firooznia H, Golimbu C. MR imaging of glenohumeral instability. *Magn Reson Imaging Clin N Am* 1997; **5**:787–809.

93. Tirman PF, Feller JF, Palmer WE et al. The Buford complex—a variation of normal shoulder anatomy: MR arthrographic imaging features. *Am J Roentgenol* 1996; **166**:869–73.

94. Tuite MJ, De Smet AA, Norris MA, Orwin JF. MR diagnosis of labral tears of the shoulder: value of T2*-weighted gradient-recalled echo images made in external rotation. *Am J Roentgenol* 1995; **164**:941–4.

95. Tuite MJ, Orwin JF. Anterosuperior labral variants of the shoulder: appearance on gradient-recalled-echo and fast spin-echo MR images. *Radiology* 1996; **199**:537–40.

96. Williams MM, Snyder SJ, Buford D, Jr. The Buford complex—the 'cord-like' middle glenohumeral ligament and absent anterosuperior labrum complex: a normal anatomic capsulolabral variant. *Arthroscopy* 1994; **10**:241–7.

97. Hodler J, Kursunoglu-Brahme S, Flannigan B et al. Injuries of the superior portion of the glenoid labrum involving the insertion of the biceps tendon: MR imaging findings in nine cases. *Am J Roentgenol* 1992; **159**:565–8.

98. Burgkart R, Merl T, Weinhart H et al. Schnittenanatomie des Schultergelenkes. *Sportorthopäde-Sporttraumatologie* 1996; **12**:222.

5 Ultrasound of the shoulder

Dean W Ziegler

Introduction

Shoulder disorders and dysfunction can be severely debilitating. While many shoulder problems respond readily to non-operative treatment, those that require more invasive management do best if the management plan can be implemented as efficiently and effectively as possible. Thorough history-taking and physical examination are mandatory in the evaluation of any shoulder complaint and can help in determining its severity. Plain radiographs are also essential and excellent for evaluating degenerative glenohumeral joint disease and advanced rotator cuff tear arthropathy. They can give hints at complete or partial-thickness tears of the rotator cuff as well as recurrent instability of the shoulder, but cannot diagnose these entities; a method is therefore needed to definitively evaluate the soft tissues of the shoulder, especially the rotator cuff. Arthrography was until recently the primary method of documenting tears of the rotator cuff.[1] Excellent results have been reported for complete tears, but deep surface partial-thickness tears are difficult to evaluate and superficial tears cannot be diagnosed arthrographically. Other disadvantages include the invasiveness of the technique, with the possibility of neurovascular injury, infection, allergic reaction to dye injection, and pain.[1,2]

Magnetic resonance imaging (MRI) is now commonly used to evaluate the soft tissues of the shoulder.[1] It is reported to give excellent results for diagnosing full-thickness tears of the rotator cuff and is potentially better than arthrography at evaluating partial-thickness tears, especially those involving the superficial surface. Although MRI is presented as being non-invasive, arthrogram or injection MRI scans are more commonly done; additionally, many patients find lying for extended periods in the scanner to be uncomfortable and for some intolerable. An MRI examination is also time-consuming, expensive and variable in quality, depending on the type of scanner and the skills of the technician.

Diagnostic ultrasonography can fulfil the required conditions for imaging the soft tissues of the shoulder, especially the rotator cuff. It is non-invasive, efficient in terms of both cost and time, and has virtually no side-effects. Most importantly, it permits dynamic and functional evaluation of the shoulder.

The brothers Pierre and Jacques Curie initiated the development of ultrasound in 1880 with the discovery of the piezoelectric effect, which when inverted produces ultrasound.[3] In 1949 Douglas Howry, a radiologist, and W R Bliss, an engineer, developed an impulse–echo system for medical application.[3] In 1951 they developed a compound technique that allowed the production of the first ultrasound images but had limited clinical success. The first real-time scanner was developed in 1967 and in 1972 the gray-scale method of imaging significantly improved screen resolution. By the late 1970s real-time gray-scale imaging combined with the use of digital computers significantly advanced the use of ultrasound, especially in orthopedics.[3]

The first publication on shoulder sonography was written by Mayer and presented in 1977 at the American Institute of Ultrasound and Medicine in Dallas, Texas.[3,4] In 1983 Farrar et al, at the American Academy of Orthopedic Surgeons Annual Meeting, described the use of dynamic sonography to evaluate the shoulder in 48 patients.[5] They found 91% sensitivity and 76% specificity for diagnosing complete rotator cuff tears. In 1984 Middleton and colleagues described the normal ultrasonic anatomy of the shoulder,[6] in 1985 the criteria for diagnosing tears of the rotator cuff,[7] and in 1986 the pitfalls of sonography that may lead to poor results.[8] In 1985 Mack et al described a technique for examination, stressing the use of dynamic sonographic evaluation of the shoulder.[9]

There have been many studies, with variable results (Table 5.1), of the usefulness of ultrasound in diagnosing rotator cuff tears as well as other shoulder disorders.[2,5,7,9–24] Regardless of the results, these reports and others stress the importance of the role of the operator.[25–29] The sonographer must be present during both static and dynamic imaging, have an excellent three-dimensional understanding of shoulder anatomy and function,[30] and be proficient with the imaging techniques of diagnostic ultrasound. If these criteria are met, ultrasonography provides an effective method for evaluating the soft tissues of the shoulder and allows efficient implementation of the management plan.

Principles

Ultrasound consists of electromechanical waves with frequencies above those audible to humans (> 20 000 Hz). Those used for medical diagnosis have frequencies of 1–12 MHz. The waves are generated by inversion of the piezoelectric effect, in which a mechanical deformation will generate a voltage at a crystal surface. The piezoelectric crystal therefore acts as both a transmitter and receiver.[3]

Table 5.1 Efficiency of ultrasonography in diagnosis of rotator cuff tears

Study	Year	No. of shoulders	Verification	Full-thickness tear		Partial-thickness tear	
				Sensitivity (%)	Specificity (%)	Sensitivity (%)	Specificity (%)
Farrar et al[3]	1983	48		91	76		
Mack et al[9]	1985	72	Arthrography	93	97		
Mack et al[9]	1985	47	Surgery	91	100		
Middleton et al[15]	1985	39	Arthrography	93	83		
Middleton et al[15]	1986	106	Arthrography	91	91		
Brandt et al[11]	1989	62	Arthrography	68	90		
Brandt et al[11]	1989	38	Surgery	57	76		
Soble et al[20]	1989	75	Arthrography	92	84		
Soble et al[20]	1989	30	Surgery	93	73		
Miller et al[18]	1989	57		58	93		
Burk et al[12]	1989	10	Surgery	63	50		
Vick and Bell[23]	1990	81	Arthrography 79, Surgery 2	67	93		
Drakeford et al[2]	1990	50	Arthrography	92	95		
Kurol et al[16]	1991	58	Surgery	67	74		
Hedtmann and Fett[15]	1995	1227	Surgery	97.3	94.6	91	94.6
van Holsbeeck et al[21]	1995	52	Surgery			93	94
van Moppes et al[22]	1995	41	Arthrography, Surgery	86	91		
Chiou et al[13]	1996	157	Arthrography	92	97.2		
Alasaarela et al[10]	1998	20	Surgery	83	57		
Read and Perko[19]	1998	42	Surgery	100	97	46	97
Fabis and Synder[14]	1999	74	Surgery	98.2	90	50	96.3

Ultrasound waves follow the laws of acoustics and therefore can be reflected, absorbed and scattered.[3] Reflection forms the basis of the pulse-echo imaging in which an image is created by the use of energy being reflected back to the source. Reflection of ultrasound waves occurs where there is a difference in the acoustic impedance between two tissues. The greater the difference in impedance, the more waves will be reflected at the tissue interface. Absorption leads to attenuation of the ultrasound waves and increases linearly with frequency. Higher frequency results in less penetration of the ultrasound waves. Scatter occurs if ultrasound waves do not travel in a direction perpendicular to an interface. Therefore the best images are formed when there is a large difference in acoustic impedance between two tissues, while using a transducer whose frequency has a focal region at the depth of the tissue of interest, and whose waves are directed perpendicularly to the structure being imaged.

Ultrasonic examination of the shoulder is performed using real-time scanning. High-resolution linear array transducers are essential to deliver an image free from distortion.[3] The ideal frequency for imaging the structures of the shoulder is 7.5 MHz. In larger patients in whom deeper penetration is required, a 5.0 MHz transducer may be useful. The introduction of broadband technology with improved electronic focusing has further improved spatial and contrast resolution. This has allowed 10 MHz and even 12 MHz transducers to become more common. Using the latest models of these high-resolution scanners combined with the proper examination technique allows for excellent ultrasound images of the shoulder.[3,31]

Examination technique

Ultrasonic examination of the shoulder is extremely operator-dependent, with results improved by dynamic imaging.[3,9,19,25–28,32,33] Therefore the individual issuing the report must examine the patient in order to view both static and dynamic images of the shoulder. Interpreting the static images alone decreases the effectiveness of the examination.

Prior to the sonographic examination, a thorough history should be obtained from the patient followed by physical examination of both shoulders and review of plain radiographs of the involved shoulder. Bilateral ultrasonic shoulder examinations should always be performed.[34] This usually does not take longer than 10 minutes. The asymptomatic shoulder is evaluated first in

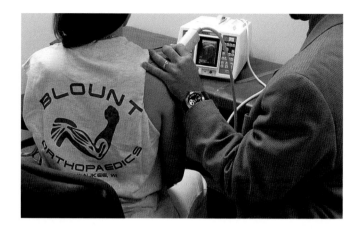

Figure 5.1

Position of patient and examiner during shoulder ultrasound examination.

order to define the normal anatomy of that patient's shoulder. This provides an opportunity to educate the patient about the shoulder, and also allows the patient to experience the examination of an asymptomatic shoulder in order to give a better indication of abnormal tenderness in the involved shoulder.

The examiner and patient should both be seated on rolling, rotating stools. A small back support may be helpful to encourage the patient to sit upright (Figure 5.1). The examiner and patient sit in an angled position that allows them both to see the screen on the monitor and gives the examiner access to the patient's shoulder. Positions may be switched when the opposite shoulder is examined.

A number of techniques have been presented regarding ultrasonic examination of the shoulder. Described here is a modification of the technique presented by Mack and colleagues,[9,33] who emphasized a dynamic examination of the shoulder in six planes, using active muscle contraction against resistance to accentuate rotator cuff defects. The sequence of shoulder imaging described here includes (in order of viewing):

- transverse view of the biceps tendon; longitudinal view of the subscapularis tendon; transverse view of the supraspinatus tendon;
- longitudinal view of the infraspinatus tendon, posterior glenoid and labrum;
- longitudinal view of the infraspinatus muscle;
- longitudinal view of the biceps tendon;
- transverse view of the subscapularis tendon attachment; longitudinal view of the supraspinatus tendon (both static and dynamic with elevation);
- longitudinal view of the supraspinatus muscle; longitudinal view of the supraspinatus tendon with the arm in internal rotation and extension, and transverse view of the supraspinatus tendon with the arm in internal rotation and extension.

This sequence has been effective when evaluating the shoulder and specifically the rotator cuff. However, any sequence may be used as long as all pertinent structures are properly evaluated.

Biceps tendon: transverse view

The transducer is initially placed over the anterior aspect of the shoulder, perpendicular to the intertubercular groove at the proximal humeral shaft (Figure 5.2). The intertubercular groove should be visualized along with the biceps tendon, which appears as a round, echogenic structure in the groove. If there is any difficulty in identifying the biceps tendon or the intertubercular groove, the humerus can be passively rotated while imaging the proximal humerus until the groove and tendon enter the field of view. The transducer can be moved superiorly to evaluate the intra-articular portion of the tendon and then distally to fully evaluate the tendon in the groove. In the face of an acute rupture of the biceps there may be an 'empty groove' sign. If there is no effusion in the glenohumeral joint, excessive fluid present around the biceps tendon in its sheath represents tenosynovitis of the biceps. Fluid present in the biceps tendon sheath must be differentiated from fluid in the subacromial bursa and the subdeltoid bursa. If fluid is present in both, it is an indication of a rotator cuff tear.

Subscapularis tendon: longitudinal view

From the biceps tendon position the transducer is moved in a slightly superior and medial direction while the shoulder is passively externally rotated. The insertion of the subscapularis to the lesser tuberosity is then visualized, as is the body of the tendon. The tendon appears as a convex cuff of tissue following the convex contour of the underlying humeral head. With passive internal and external rotation the movement of the tendon can be evaluated to assure that the tendon tissue moves with the humeral head. If the tissue overlying the humeral head does not move with rotation, it indicates a disruption of the subscapularis. Imaging the tendon during resisted internal rotation helps to further identify any defects in the tendon and allows assessment of the subscapularis muscle's contractility. Moving the transducer medially during passive and active rotation allows evaluation of the muscle–tendon unit as it moves under the coracoid process and the coracoacromial ligament. Any roughness at this interface can be evaluated. A static image of the tendon is obtained and the thickness of the tendon is measured and recorded.

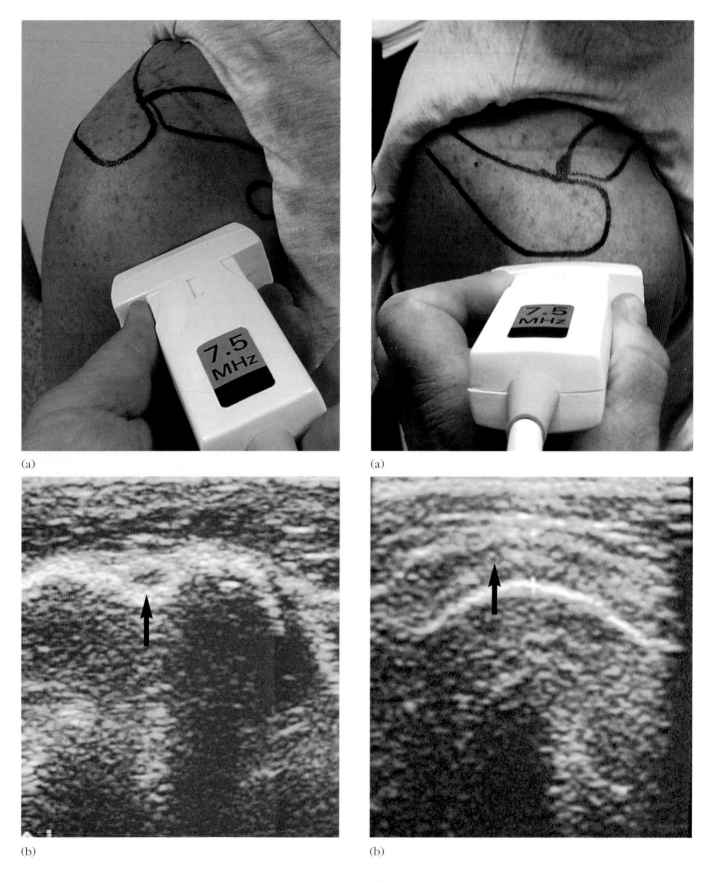

(a)

(a)

(b)

(b)

Figure 5.2

(a) Initial examining position evaluating the biceps tendon transversely. (b) Transverse ultrasonic image of the biceps tendon within the bicipital groove (arrow).

Figure 5.3

(a) Transducer position for transverse imaging of the supraspinatus tendon. (b) Transverse ultrasonic image of the supraspinatus tendon (arrow) including measurement of tendon thickness.

Supraspinatus tendon: transverse view

The transducer is then placed over the lateral edge of the acromion, moved distally, and directed toward the proximal humerus (Figure 5.3). The supraspinatus tendon is seen as a convex cuff of tissue with moderate echogenicity found between the weakly echogenic deltoid and the strongly echogenic humeral head. Portions of two concentric echogenic circles should be visualized: the outer circle is the reflection from the interface between the deltoid and the supraspinatus, and the inner circle is from the interface between the supraspinatus and the humeral head. While there may be slight thinning of the posterior supraspinatus, the tendon should be of uniform thickness. Any significant thinning of the anterior supraspinatus represents a tear of the tendon. A massive tear of the supraspinatus is evident if there is no tendon present and the undersurface of the deltoid abuts the greater tuberosity. The subacromial subdeltoid bursa is located superficial to the tendon and deep to the deltoid and should be less than 2 mm thick. If it measures more than 2 mm in thickness an effusion is present. A static image of the tendon is obtained and the thickness is measured and recorded. The transducer can be moved posteriorly to obtain a transverse view of the infraspinatus tendon.

Infraspinatus tendon: longitudinal view

The transducer is placed over the posterior acromion and the scapular spine and moved inferiorly, directed towards the posterior humeral head (Figure 5.4). The infraspinatus tendon is imaged at its attachment to the lesser tuberosity. The humerus is passively rotated and the attachment is evaluated. Moving the transducer distally permits evaluation of the inferior infraspinatus and the teres minor attachments. Moving the transducer medially allows evaluation of the posterior glenoid and labrum. Rotation of the humeral head demonstrates its congruence with the glenoid and labrum, and the tightening of the posterior capsule with internal rotation and laxity of the capsule with external rotation. The deeper fibers of the infraspinatus should be no more than 2 mm from the labrum – a greater distance represents an intra-articular effusion. The posterior humeral head can also be evaluated for abnormalities such as a Hill–Sachs lesion. A static image of the infraspinatus is obtained with the arm in internal rotation and the thickness of the infraspinatus tendon is measured and recorded.

Infraspinatus muscle: longitudinal view

The transducer is moved even further medially to image the infraspinatus muscle. The contractility of this muscle

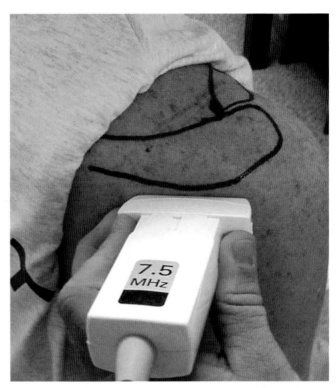

(a)

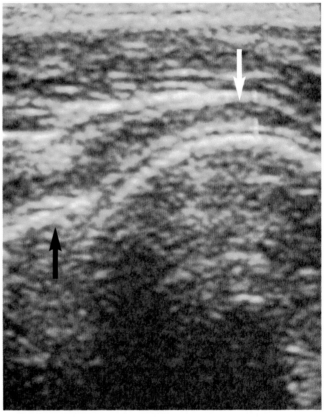

(b)

Figure 5.4

(a) Transducer position for longitudinal imaging of the infraspinatus tendon. (b) Longitudinal ultrasonic image of the infraspinatus tendon (black arrow) including the posterior humeral head, glenoid (white arrow) and labrum.

is evaluated during resisted external rotation of the shoulder, which also allows differentiation between the infraspinatus and the overlying deltoid. A static image is obtained and the width of the muscle at its thickest point is recorded. The muscle thickness can also be recorded during resisted external rotation in order to document its contractility. Asymmetric thinning of the infraspinatus muscle belly and decreased contractility of the muscle may accompany a massive rotator cuff tear or supra-scapular nerve dysfunction. The spinoglenoid notch can also be evaluated by orienting the probe slightly superior while moving it medially from the glenoid rim.

Biceps tendon: longitudinal view

The transducer is moved back to the anterior aspect of the shoulder and placed parallel to the intertubercular groove. If this is difficult to find, the groove can be imaged transversely and the transducer rotated 90°. The biceps is seen as a strong echogenic structure adjacent to the humeral head. It may be necessary to angle the transducer superiorly to visualize the tendon fully. The tendon has a fine, fibrous pattern; loss of this pattern implies an abnormality of the tendon.

Subscapularis tendon attachment: transverse view

The transducer is moved medially and superiorly while maintaining the same orientation. This allows visualization of the subscapularis where it attaches to the lesser tuberosity. Any abnormality in the insertion can be detected.

Supraspinatus tendon: longitudinal view

The transducer is placed over the anterolateral edge of the acromion and as it is advanced distally over the humeral head the supraspinatus attachment to the greater tuberosity is visualized (Figure 5.5). The acromion casts an ultrasonic shadow, limiting the ability to evaluate the tendon medially. However, the transducer can be moved anteriorly and posteriorly to image the entire supraspinatus attachment. Any loss in continuity of the tendon represents a tear at the attachment. Partial-thickness tears are evident when there is a mixed hyper-echoic and hypoechoic focus in the critical zone of the supraspinatus; patients will often complain of tenderness during imaging over such an abnormality in the tendon. The patient is then taken through passive elevation of the shoulder in the plane of the scapula. The clearance

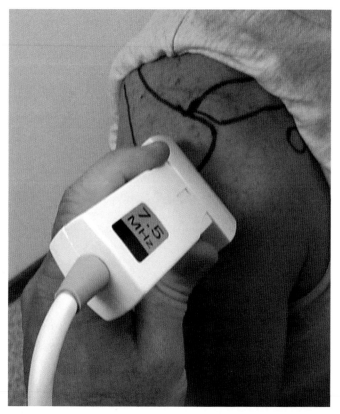

(a)

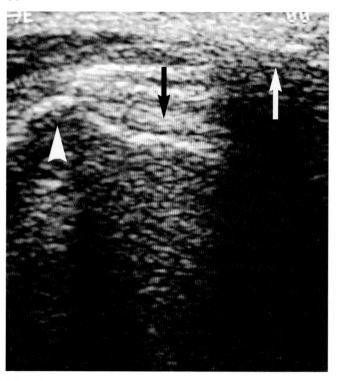

(b)

Figure 5.5

(a) Transducer position for static longitudinal imaging of the supraspinatus tendon with the arm at the side. (b) Longitudinal ultrasonic image of the supraspinatus tendon (black arrow) with the arm at the side, including the greater tuberosity (white arrow head) and anterior acromion (white arrow).

of the supraspinatus and greater tuberosity under the acromion are evaluated. A similar evaluation is made during active elevation. It should be determined whether the patient can smoothly clear the greater tuberosity under the acromion or if there is roughness, pain or abutment of the greater tuberosity onto the acromion and therefore an inability to elevate the humerus further. Elevation against resistance is imaged, which accentuates a defect of the supraspinatus attachment.

Supraspinatus muscle: longitudinal view

The transducer is moved medially, over the acromion and on top of the supraspinatus fossa. The supraspinatus muscle belly is visualized. Resisted abduction demonstrates the contractility of the muscle and differentiates it from the overlying trapezius muscle. A static image of the supraspinatus muscle belly is obtained and its thickness is recorded. The thickness of the supraspinatus during resisted abduction can also be recorded in order to document the contractility of the muscle. The probe can be orientated laterally and then posteriorly and anteriorly in this region in order to evaluate possible masses (e.g. ganglion cysts). However, the shadow cast by the acromion may limit the ability to visualize the superior glenoid and the arterior spinoglenoid notch.

Supraspinatus tendon

Internal rotation/extension longitudinal view

The patient's arm is placed behind the back, with the dorsum of the hand resting on the sacrum. This brings out a larger portion of the supraspinatus from underneath the acromion. The transducer is oriented obliquely over the prominence of the proximal humerus and a longitudinal image of the supraspinatus as it attaches to the greater tuberosity is obtained (Figure 5.6). The transducer is moved anteriorly and posteriorly to visualize the entire attachment of the supraspinatus. The position of the arm not only facilitates evaluation of the tendon but also accentuates any defects in the supraspinatus attachment. Again, it should be noted whether tenderness is felt when imaging over an abnormal portion of the supraspinatus attachment.

Internal rotation/extension transverse view

The transducer is rotated 90° to give a transverse image of the supraspinatus tendon. As with transverse imaging of the supraspinatus with the arm at the side, two concentric echogenic circles should be seen and the tendon should be a uniform thickness. Any significant thinning or

absence of the tendon is evidence of a tear. A static image is obtained and the thickness of the tendon is recorded.

Other approaches

The technique described above gives a thorough and extensive sonographic evaluation of the shoulder,

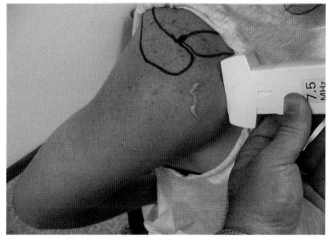

(a)

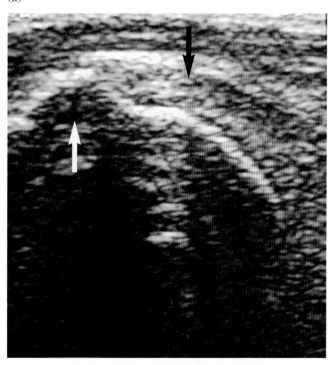

(b)

Figure 5.6

(a) Transducer position for longitudinal imaging of the supraspinatus tendon with the shoulder in internal rotation/extension. (b) Longitudinal ultrasonic image of the supraspinatus tendon (black arrow) with the shoulder in internal rotation/extension including the supraspinatus attachment to the greater tuberosity (white arrow).

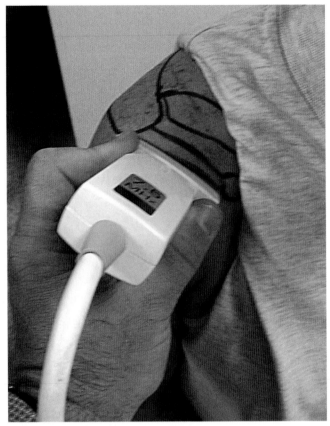

(a)

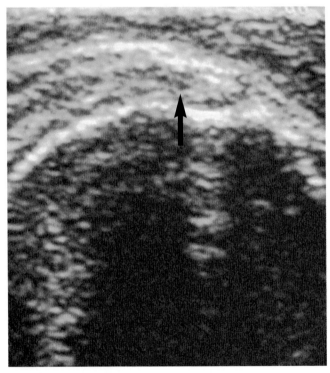

(b)

Figure 5.7

(a) Anterosuperior transducer position parallel and just lateral to the coracoacromial line. (b) Ultrasonic image from antero-superior transducer position showing the critical zone of the supraspinatus attachment. Arrow shows supraspinitus tendon.

allowing longitudinal and transverse views of all rotator cuff tendons and using passive and dynamic motion of the shoulder to evaluate the rotator cuff and the gleno-humeral joint. However, other possible techniques may be more efficient or emphasize other structures.

Hedtmann and Fett stress that an investigation to exclude or confirm rotator cuff tears can be economi-cally performed using only anterosuperior probe positions.[25] Their standard probe positions include one parallel and just lateral to the coracoacromial line (Figure 5.7), and another perpendicular to the first. This allows excellent visualization of the critical zone of the supraspinatus attachment. With internal rotation and extension of the shoulder the posterior portion of the rotator cuff is brought into the coracoacromial window. As long as there is no limit to internal rotation the entire infraspinatus can be imaged from this position. They also stress that dynamic investigation is integral, record-ing the sliding behavior of the subacromial/subdeltoid bursa and the underlying rotator cuff. Indentation of the rotator cuff or bursa during rotation implies a rotator cuff tear.

Other structures that can be evaluated with ultrasound include the anteroinferior labrum[35] and the acromioclav-icular and coracoclavicular intervals.[36,37] To evaluate the anteroinferior labrum the patient is placed in a supine position and both arms are abducted and externally rotated. The transducer is placed in the longitudinal direction, parallel to the border of the pectoral muscle, with a ventrocaudal tilt. The anteroinferior labrum and capsule are evaluated and compared with the opposite side. The acromioclavicular interval can be evaluated and the distance recorded from a superior and anterior position. From the anterior position the clavicle and coracoid process are imaged and the interval between the two is measured. These intervals are then compared with the normal shoulder. Along with these intervals, the integrity of the deltotrapezial fascia can be evaluated in high-grade acromioclavicular separations.

Criteria for diagnosing rotator cuff tears

Understanding the criteria needed to diagnose a tear of the rotator cuff is essential for maximal effectiveness of shoulder ultrasonography. Normal rotator cuff tendons have homogeneous echogeneity.[3,6,31] There may be some areas of abnormality in the signal, but in the normal tendon these abnormalities are usually mirrored in the opposite shoulder.

Disruption of the rotator cuff tendon may present itself in a variety of ways, and the criteria for diagnos-ing both partial and complete rotator cuff tears have been documented in many studies.[2,7,9,13,17,20,21,24,25] Findings in *complete tears* of the rotator cuff include focal thinning of the rotator cuff tendon; complete non-visualization of the rotator cuff tendon, which is similar to focal thinning but no normal tendon tissue is identified; focal discontinuity in the homogeneous echogenicity of the rotator cuff without focal thinning; inversion of the superficial bursal contour; and hyperechoic material in the location of the tendon that fails to move with the humeral head during real-time dynamic imaging. Findings in *partial tears* of the rotator cuff include a hypoechoic discontinuity in the rotator cuff tendon in which the lesion involves either the bursal or articular side of the tendon; or a mixed hyperechoic and hypoechoic region within the tendon which is thought to be due to a separation of the torn edge from the rest of the tendon, resulting in a new interface within the tendon. Often when imaging over an area of a partial tear (and at times over a complete tear) the patient will report tenderness as the transducer moves over the defect and pressure is applied to visualize the tear. This sensation should be compared with that experienced during imaging of the asymptomatic shoulder to ensure that the tenderness is not normal for that patient.

It is important to have an excellent understanding of the normal sonographic anatomy of the shoulder in general and in particular of the patient's 'normal' shoulder anatomy. Together with this, application of the above criteria has been documented to enhance the results of shoulder ultrasonography (Figures 5.8–5.17). Some authors have stressed the value of a two-criteria model,[25] in which a defect is only diagnosed if a criterion is reproducible either in different joint positions or in different transducer positions, or if a second criterion (e.g. a static along with a dynamic criterion) is present in different positions. Finally, it is important to understand that the 'formal' criteria of thinning, non-visualization, discontinuity of the tendon or disruption, or inversion of the superficial bursal contour are not prone to artifacts, in complete contrast to the criteria of echogenicity. Variations in tendon echogenicity should be recorded, but care is needed in making a diagnosis solely based on this criterion.

Images from a 55-year-old man following shoulder dislocation with difficulty on shoulder elevation and supraspinatus weakness

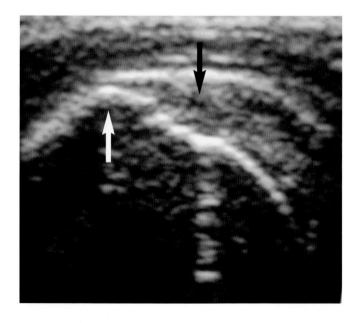

Figure 5.8

Longitudinal view of the supraspinatus tendon with the arm in internal rotation and extension demonstrating the intact attachment (black arrow) of the tendon to the greater tuberosity (white arrow) in the contralateral shoulder.

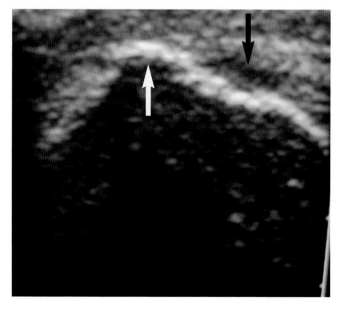

Figure 5.9

Longitudinal view of the supraspinatus tendon with the arm in internal rotation and extension demonstrating a focal discontinuity in the homogenous echogenicity of the tendon indicating a full thickness tear (black arrow).

Images from a 45-year-old man following a fall with significant supraspinatus weakness and an inability to actively elevate the arm

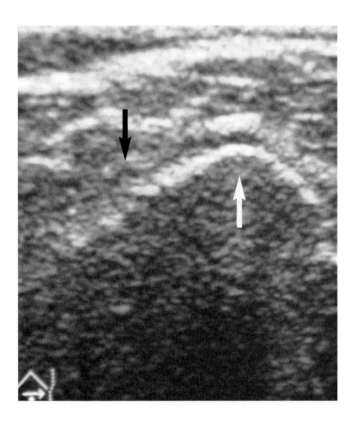

Figure 5.10

Longitudinal view of the supraspinatus tendon with the arm in internal rotation and extension demonstrating the greater tuberosity (white arrow) but complete non-visualization of the tendon, indicating a complete tear of the supraspinatus with retraction (back arrow).

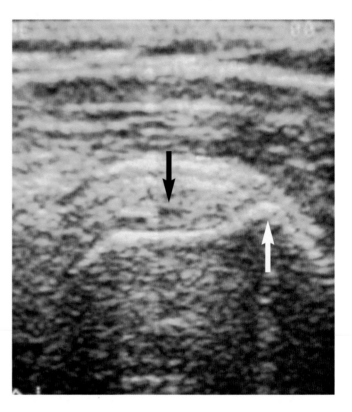

Figure 5.11

Longitudinal view of the supraspinatus tendon with the arm in internal rotation and extension demonstrating the intact attachment (black arrow) of the tendon to the greater tuberosity (white arrow) in the contralateral shoulder.

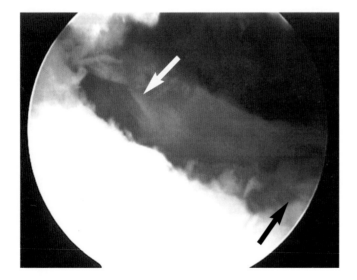

Figure 5.12

Arthroscopic view from the posterior portal confirming the complete tear of the supraspinatus tendon (white arrow) with retraction from the greater tuberosity (black arrow).

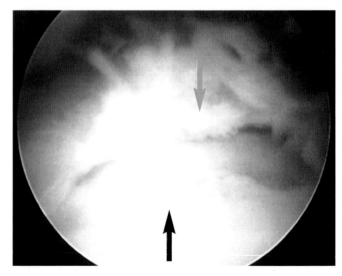

Figure 5.13

Arthroscopic view from the lateral portal confirming the complete tear of the supraspinatus tendon (tinted arrow) with retraction from the greater tuberosity (black arrow).

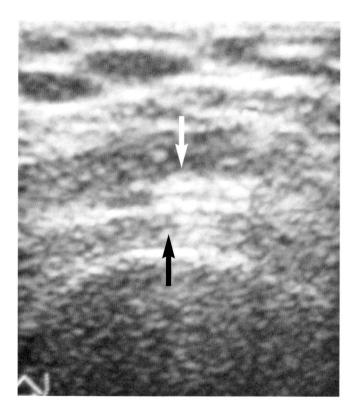

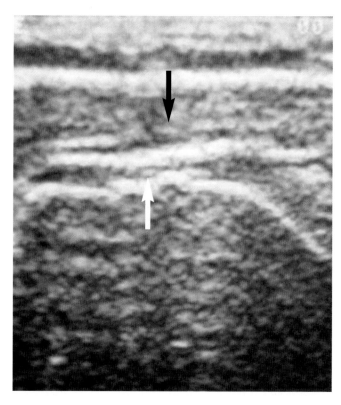

Figure 5.14

Transverse view of the supraspinatus tendon (black arrow) with the arm in internal rotation and extension in the intact shoulder demonstrating a uniform thickness of tendon tissue between superficial (white arrow) and two deep concentric echogenic circles in the contralateral shoulder.

Figure 5.15

Transverse view of the supraspinatus tendon with the arm in internal rotation and extension demonstrating inversion of the superficial bursal contour (black arrow) and complete non-visualization of the tendon (white arrow), indicating a complete tear of the supraspinatus with retraction.

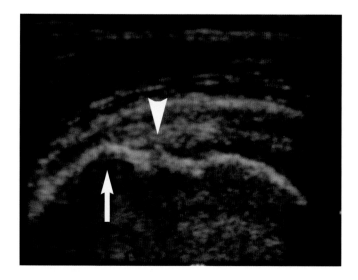

Figure 5.16

Longitudinal view of the supraspinatus tendon with the arm in internal rotation and extension demonstrating the intact attachment of the tendon to the greater tuberosity (white arrow) in the shoulder following rotator cuff repair (arrow head).

Image from patient with shoulder pain and shoulder effusion

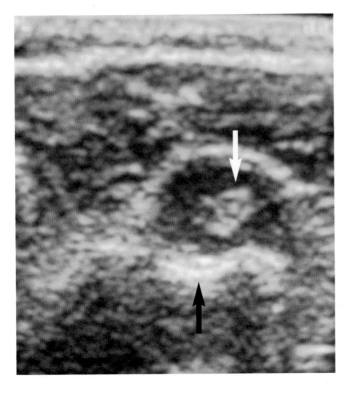

Figure 5.17

Transverse view of the bicipital groove (black arrow) and biceps tendon (white arrow) with an effusion surrounding the tendon in its sheath.

Pitfalls

When done properly, ultrasonography is an excellent technique for imaging the soft tissues of the shoulder and particularly the rotator cuff. However, numerous series report less than satisfactory results from ultrasound evaluation of shoulder disorders.[10–12,14,16,18,19,23] The technique is highly dependent on operator skills, but results can be markedly improved if a specific technique is followed and certain errors of interpretation are avoided.[8,25,31,34]

One of the most common errors in sonography of the shoulder is a misinterpretation of normal anatomy. This may occur when the echogenicity of the rotator cuff – specifically the supraspinatus – is similar to that of the overlying deltoid. This is uncommon, but does occur in older patients. Another problem area is the anterior supraspinatus near the biceps, where the hyperechoic biceps tendon or the hypoechoic area just posterior to the biceps may be misinterpreted as a partial thickness or small full thickness tear. Other misinterpretations of normal anatomy include thinning of the posterior supraspinatus and infraspinatus as seen on the transverse view, and mild variations in echogenicity of the rotator cuff tendons. All of these potential misinterpretations can be avoided by comparing the findings with the asymptomatic shoulder.

Other potential errors of shoulder sonography are due to soft tissue or bony abnormalities. A calcific nodule within the rotator cuff tendon (calcific tendinitis) is one such soft tissue abnormality, and a greater tuberosity fracture or inferior subluxation of the glenohumeral joint is an example of a bony abnormality. Errors due to abnormalities of bone or soft tissue can be avoided by evaluating radiographs of the shoulder prior to ultrasonography.

Technical limitations of ultrasound imaging can also lead to errors in interpretation. An example of such a limitation is the inability to image a portion of the supraspinatus tendon because of the overlying acromion. This can be corrected by positioning the arm in such a way that the supraspinatus is better exposed (e.g. internal rotation and extension).

There are many potential errors that might lead to the variable results reported when using ultrasound to image the shoulder. The technique requires an examiner who is proficient in using ultrasound and has an excellent three-dimensional understanding of the shoulder. Other pitfalls can be avoided by evaluating both shoulders and thus using the asymptomatic shoulder as a control, reviewing plain radiographs of the shoulder, positioning the shoulder to maximize visibility of the cuff tendons, and using passive and active motion of the shoulder during the imaging process.

Conclusion

Diagnostic ultrasonography provides a superb method for evaluating the rotator cuff and other soft tissues of the shoulder. It is non-invasive, cost- and time-efficient, and allows static, dynamic, and functional imaging of the shoulder. It is also an educational tool for patients, giving them an opportunity to participate in the evaluation and management of their shoulder disorder.

Many studies document excellent results when using ultrasound to diagnose tears of the rotator cuff. While there are studies in which the results are not as favorable, pitfalls that may cause these poor results have been presented. In order to maximize its effectiveness the ultrasonic investigation should be performed by an examiner dedicated to the technique, who is comfortable using ultrasound as an imaging tool, and who has an excellent three-dimensional understanding of shoulder anatomy. The patient's history, physical examination and plain radiographs should be reviewed and a bilateral ultrasonic examination of the shoulders should be performed, including static and dynamic imaging using both active and passive motion. Any perceived abnormalities found in the symptomatic shoulder must be compared with the asymptomatic side to verify that the findings are not 'normal' for that particular patient. By following these guidelines the pitfalls that lead to false positive and negative results can be avoided, maximizing the benefits of ultrasonic shoulder evaluation for both patients and physicians.

References

1. Matsen FA, Arntz CT, Lippitt SB. Rotator cuff. In: Rockwood CA, Matsen FA, eds. *The Shoulder*, 2nd edn. Philadelphia: WB Saunders, 1998; 789–91.

2. Drakeford MK, Quinn MJ, Simpson SL et al. A comparative study of ultrasonography and arthrography in evaluation of the rotator cuff. *Clin Orthop* 1990; **253**:118–22.

3. Katthagen BD. *Ultrasonography of the Shoulder*. New York: Thieme, 1990.

4. Mayer B. Ultrasonography of the rotator cuff. *J Ultrasound Med* 1985; **4**:607–8.

5. Farrar EL, Matsen FA, Rogers JV et al. Dynamic sonographic study of lesion of the rotator cuff [abstract]. Presented at the American Academy of Orthopedic Surgeons 50th Annual Meeting. 10–15 March 1983; 49.

6. Middleton WD, Edelstein G, Reinus WR et al. Ultrasonography of the rotator cuff: technique and normal anatomy. *J Ultrasound Med* 1984; **3**:549–51.

7. Middleton WD, Edelstein G, Reinus WR et al. Sonographic detection of rotator cuff tears. *Am J Roentgenol* 1985; **144**:349–53.

8. Middleton WD, Reinus WR, Melson CL et al. Pitfalls of rotator cuff sonography. *Am J Roentgenol* 1986; **146**:555–60.

9. Mack LA, Matsen FA, Kilcoyne RF et al. US evaluation of the rotator cuff. *Radiology* 1985; **157**:205–9.

10. Alasaarela E, Leppilahti J, Hakala M. Ultrasound and operative evaluation of arthritic shoulder joints. *Ann Rheum Dis* 1998; **57**:357–60.

11. Brandt TD, Cardone BW, Grant TH et al. Rotator cuff sonography: a reassessment. *Radiology* 1989; **173**:323–7.

12. Burk DL, Karasick D, Kurtz AB et al. Rotator cuff tears: prospective comparison of MR imaging with arthrography, sonography, and surgery. *Am J Roentgenol* 1989; **153**:87–92.

13. Chiou HJ, Hsu CC, Chou YH et al. Sonographic signs of complete rotator cuff tears. *Chung Hua I Hsueh Tsa Chih* (Taipei) 1996; **58**:428–34.

14. Fabis J, Synder M. The sensitivity and specificity of sonographic examination in detection of rotator cuff. *Chir Narzadow Ruchu Ortop Pol* 1999; **64**:19–23.

15. Hedtmann A, Fett H. Sonography of the shoulder in subacromial syndromes with diseases and injuries of the rotator cuff. *Orthopade* 1995; **24**:498–508.

16. Kurol M, Rahme H, Jilding S. Sonography for diagnosis of rotator cuff tear. *Acta Orthop Scand* 1991; **62**:465–7.

17. Middleton WD, Reinus WR, Totty WG et al. Ultrasonic evaluation of the rotator cuff and biceps tendon. *J Bone Joint Surg* 1986; **68A**: 440–50.

18. Miller CL, Karasick D, Kurtz AB et al. Limited sensitivity of ultrasound for the detection of rotator cuff tears. *Skeletal Radiol* 1989; **18**:179–83.

19. Read JW, Perko M. Shoulder ultrasound: diagnostic accuracy for impingement syndrome, rotator cuff tear, and biceps tendon pathology. *J Shoulder Elbow Surg* 1998; **7**:264–71.

20. Soble MG, Kaye AD, Guay RC. Rotator cuff tear: clinical experience with sonographic detection. *Radiology* 1989; **173**:319–21.

21. van Holsbeeck MT, Kolowich PA, Eyler WR et al. US depiction of partial-thickness tear of the rotator cuff. *Radiology* 1995; **197**:443–6.

22. van Moppes FI, Veldkamp O, Roorda J. Role of shoulder ultrasonography in the evaluation of the painful shoulder. *Eur J Radiol* 1995; **19**:142–6.

23. Vick CW, Bell SA. Rotator cuff tears: diagnosis with sonography. *Am J Roentgenol* 1990; **154**:121–3.

24. Wiener SN, Seitz WH. Sonography of the shoulder in patients with tears of the rotator cuff: accuracy and value for selecting surgical options. *Am J Roentgenol* 1993; **160**:103–7.

25. Hedtmann A, Fett H. Atlas und Lehrbuch der Schultersonografie, 2nd ed. Stuttgart: Enke, 1991.

26. Helweg G, Moriggl B, Sperner G et al. Ultrasound diagnosis of the shoulder. *Radiologe* 1996; **36**:971–80.

27. Mellerowicz H, Kefenbaum A, Stelling E. Soft tissue diagnosis of the shoulder joint using sonography, computerized tomography and magnetic resonance tomography (MRT). *Zentralbl Chir* 1989; **114**:209–21.

28. Sonnabend DH, Hughes JS, Giuffre BM et al. The clinical role of shoulder ultrasound. *Aust NZ J Surg* 1997; **67**:630–633.

29. Tallroth K. Shoulder imaging. A review. *Ann Chir Gynaecol* 1996; **85**:95–103.

30. Balogh B, Fruhwald F, Neuhold A et al. Sonoanatomy of the shoulder. *Acta Anat* (Basel) 1986; **126**:132–5.

31. Ptasznik R. Sonography of the shoulder. In: van Holsbeeck MT, Introcaso JH, eds. *Musculoskeletal Ultrasound*, 2nd edn. St Louis: Mosby, 2001; 463–516.

32. Lick-Schiffer W. Ultrasound examination of the shoulder joint. *Wien Med Wochenschr* 1996; **146**:121–3.

33. Mack LA, Nyberg DA, Matsen FA. Sonographic evaluation of the rotator cuff. *Radiol Clin North Am* 1988; **26**:161–77.

34. Casser HR, Sulimma H, Straub A, Paus R. Sources of error in sonographic diagnosis of the rotator cuff. *Ultraschall Med* 1991; **12**:256–62.

35. Wittner B, Holz U. Ultrasound imaging of the ventrocaudal labrum in ventral instability of the shoulder. *Unfallchirurg* 1996; **99**:38–42.

36. Kock HJ, Jurgens C, Hirche H et al. Standardized ultrasound examination for evaluation of instability of the acromioclavicular joint. *Arch Orthop Trauma Surg* 1996; **115**:136–40.

37. Sluming VA. Technical note: measuring the coracoclavicular distance with ultrasound – a new technique. *Br J Radiol* 1995; **68**:189–93.

Section II – Basic techniques

6   Diagnostic shoulder arthroscopy: The 23-point arthroscopic evaluation with normal anatomical variants and pathology

Don Buford Jr and Stephen J Snyder

Introduction

The past 20 years has seen a remarkable increase in the number of shoulder arthroscopies performed for both diagnosis and treatment of a wide range of shoulder conditions. With the ongoing development of arthroscopic techniques and equipment, many procedures can now be accomplished arthroscopically that used to be performed as open procedures. The arthroscopic surgeon's goal is to treat the pathology in a minimally invasive fashion. In order to accomplish this, the surgeon should have a standard arthroscopic diagnostic evaluation so that all pathology is identified.

Surgical principles

The initial decision that the shoulder arthroscopist must make is whether to use the beach chair or lateral decubitus position. Each position has its advantages and disadvantages. The beach chair position offers advantages of easy airway management and easy access for an arthrotomy if necessary. The beach chair position also provides an anatomic visualization of the intra-articular structures. Disadvantages of the beach chair position include difficulty in visualizing the anterior capsular structures and difficulty in maintaining joint distraction. The lateral decubitus position allows for good visualization of the intra-articular structures and the ability to position the arm with a constant distraction force. Hypotensive anesthesia, which is important for visualization during subacromial bursoscopy, is safer with the patient in the lateral decubitus position. Additionally, it is possible to perform a deltoid splitting rotator cuff repair or a biceps tenodesis or a subscapularis repair with the patient in the lateral decubitus position.

Surgical technique

At our institutions, diagnostic and operative shoulder arthroscopy is performed with the patient in the lateral

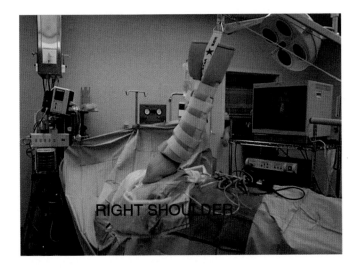

Figure 6.1
Operating room set-up showing lateral decubitus position.

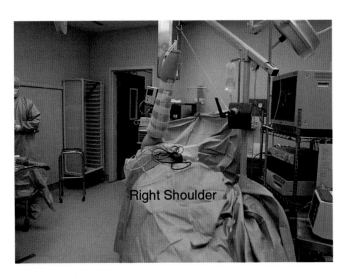

Figure 6.2
Operating room showing lateral decubitus position.

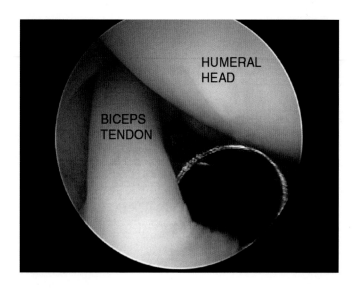

Figure 6.3

Point 1 of the arthroscopic shoulder evaluation.

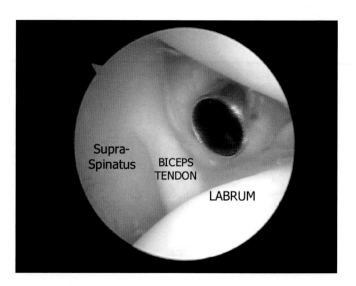

Figure 6.4

Biceps attaching into rotator cuff tendon.

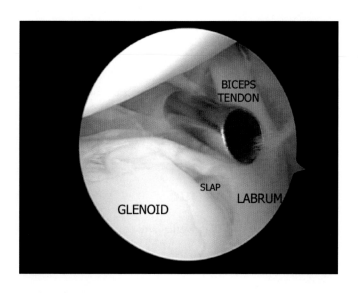

Figure 6.5

Type II SLAP lesion.

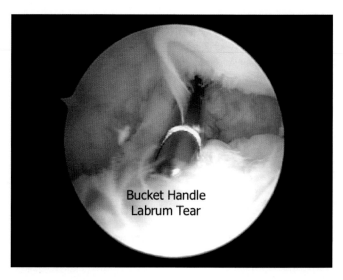

Figure 6.6

Type III SLAP lesion.

decubitus position. The patient is positioned so that the torso is rolled back approximately 20° in relation to the operating table. We always use an axillary roll and take care to pad all bony prominences. A beanbag is used to support the patient and a shoulder holder supports the upper extremity in approximately 70° of abduction and 15° of flexion (Figure 6.1). Ten pounds of traction weight is placed initially and small adjustments are made based on patient size. After positioning the patient in the lateral decubitus position, the surgical team can then rotate the bed approximately 45° to make more room at the head of the table (Figure 6.2). Pressure and flow controlled

pump are initially set at 40 mmHg and medium flow. Epinephrine is not routinely added to the arthroscopic fluid.

A thorough diagnostic shoulder arthroscopic exam was presented by Snyder in 1989.[1] Initial arthroscopic evaluation of the shoulder is done from a posterior portal made approximately 2-cm medial and 2-cm inferior to the posterolateral edge of the acromion. A blunt tipped obturator is used to insert the arthroscopic cannula into the glenohumeral joint. After inserting the arthroscope into the joint, the rotator interval is identified and a switching stick is used to make an anterior portal in the

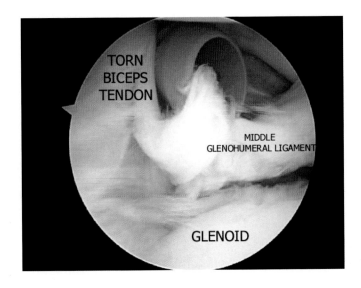

Figure 6.7
Type IV SLAP lesion.

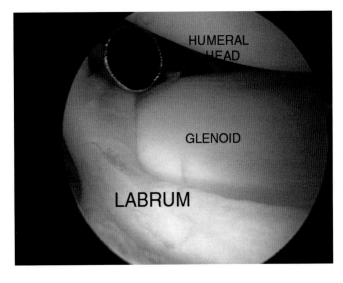

Figure 6.8
Point 2 of the arthroscopic evaluation.

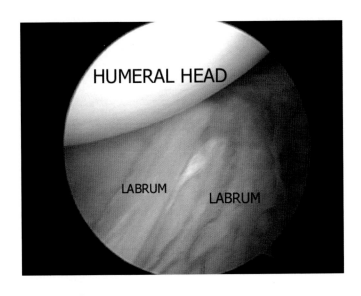

Figure 6.9
Posterior labral tear.

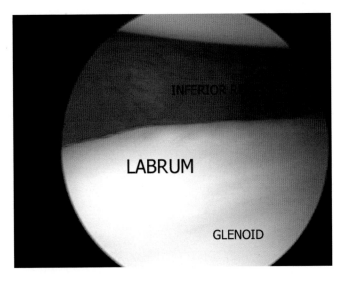

Figure 6.10
Point 3 of the arthroscopic evaluation.

rotator interval. A metal outflow cannula connected to gravity drainage is inserted over the switching stick into the rotator interval. After the outflow cannula is located in the rotator interval anteriorly, the diagnostic arthroscopy can then begin.

It is important to have a systematic method of assessing shoulder anatomy arthroscopically. The camera is rotated so that the glenoid is parallel to the floor and the humeral head is superior. Our comprehensive examination begins with an evaluation of the biceps tendon (point 1). The biceps tendon is visualized from its attachment at the supraglenoid tubercle and superior

labrum up to where it exits the shoulder through the rotator interval (Figure 6.3). The supraglenoid recess can also be inspected at this time. Tears of the biceps tendon can be easily visualized at this point. One interesting finding seen at this point is the biceps tendon blending into the undersurface of the rotator cuff tendon (Figure 6.4). We evaluate the stability of the biceps anchor and superior labrum at this time to see whether the patient has a SLAP lesion (biceps anchor—superior labrum detachment from anterior to posterior) (Figures 6.5–6.7).[2] We then rotate the camera to visualize the posterior labrum and the posterior joint capsule where

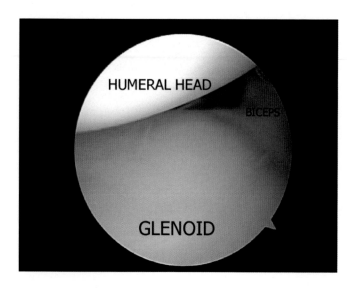

Figure 6.11

Point 4 of the arthroscopic evaluation.

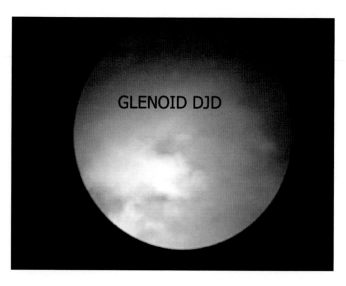

Figure 6.12

Glenoid osteoarthritis. DJD, degenerative joint disease.

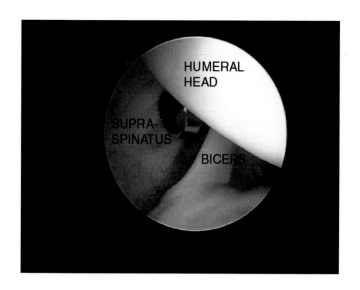

Figure 6.13

Point 5 of the arthroscopic evaluation.

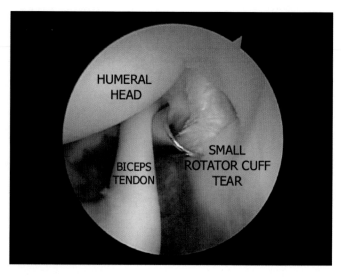

Figure 6.14

Small supraspinatus tendon tear.

it attaches to the glenoid (point 2) (Figure 6.8) At this point, posterior labral tears and posterior capsule pathology can be identified (Figure 6.9). The next point to evaluate is the inferior recess, where loose bodies may be present (point 3) (Figure 6.10). Then evaluate the articular surface of the glenoid by rotating the camera to view the anterior aspect of the joint (point 4) (Figure 6.11). Any glenoid chondrosis can be evaluated at this time (Figure 6.12). We then rotate the camera superiorly to view the supraspinatus tendon and its insertion into the humeral head (point 5) (Figure 6.13). Start anteriorly just posterior to the biceps tendon and slowly progress to view the entire attachment of the supraspinatus tendon. Tears in the rotator cuff tendon most commonly begin just posterior to the biceps tendon and can be visualized at this time (Figure 6.14). Large rotator cuff tears can sometimes be deceiving because the surgeon can look directly into the subacromial space. It is important to view these tears from posterior, anterior, and the lateral bursal positions to fully evaluate the tear size and shape (Figure 6.15). Continue by viewing the posterior insertion of the rotator cuff and eventually come to the posterior bare area of the humerus (point 6) (Figure 6.16). The articular

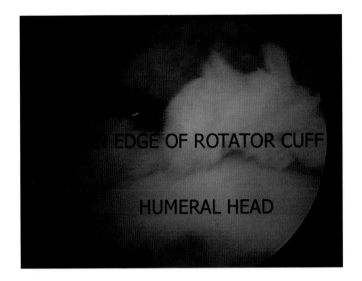

Figure 6.15

Large rotator cuff tear.

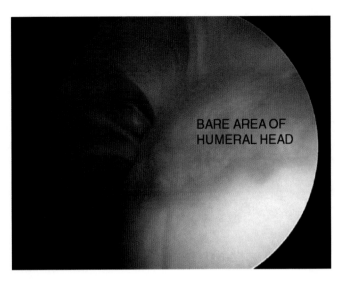

Figure 6.16

Point 6 of the arthroscopic evaluation. IGL, inferior glenohumeral ligament.

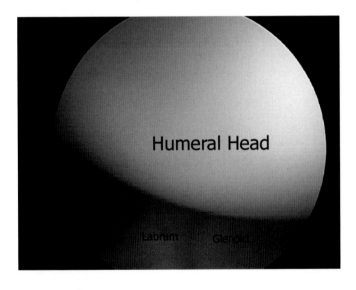

Figure 6.17

Point 7 of the arthroscopic evaluation.

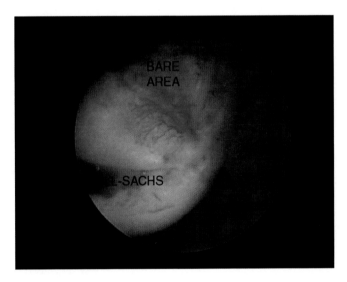

Figure 6.18

Hill–Sachs lesion.

surface of the humeral head is then visualized from posterior to anterior (point 7) (Figure 6.17). Hill–Sachs lesions can be assessed at this time (Figure 6.18). We then maneuver the arthroscope to the anterosuperior quadrant of the shoulder. The anatomical structures to be evaluated at this time include the subscapularis tendon and the middle glenohumeral ligament crossing the subscapularis tendon at a 45° angle (point 8) (Figure 6.19). The middle glenohumeral ligament can be difficult to identify, or it can be a very well defined cord-like ligament. The most common appearance of the middle glenohumeral ligament is as an easily identified

capsular fold that crosses the subscapularis tendon. The next point to evaluate is the middle glenohumeral ligament attachment and the anterosuperior labrum (point 9) (Figure 6.20). Once again, there are several anatomical variations that the arthroscopist must be able to identify. Some patients may have a sublabral foramen in this area or no labral tissue at all. The configuration of a cord-like middle glenohumeral ligament attaching at the biceps insertion with no anterosuperior labral tissue has been termed a 'Buford complex' (Figure 6.21).[3] The final point to evaluate from this position is the inferior glenohumeral ligament and the inferior

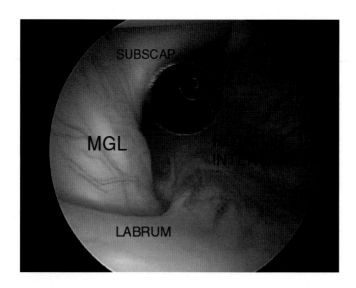

Figure 6.19

Point 8 of the arthroscopic evaluation.

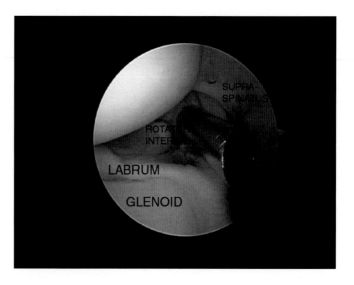

Figure 6.20

Point 9 of the arthroscopic evaluation.

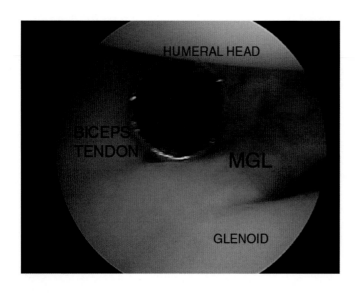

Figure 6.21

Buford complex: cord-like middle glenohumeral ligament inserting into biceps tendon anchor and absent superior labrum. MGL, middle glenohumeral ligament.

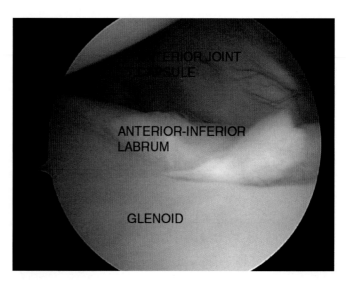

Figure 6.22

Point 10 of the arthroscopic evaluation.

labrum (point 10) (Figure 6.22) Bankart lesions can be identified at this time but are best evaluated with the arthroscope in the anterosuperior portal.

We then switch the arthroscope to the anterior portal and move the outflow cannula to the posterior portal. The first assessment from this position is the posterior labrum and posterior joint capsule (point 11) (Figure 6.23) The surgeon can then rotate the arthroscope superiorly to view the posterior aspect of the rotator cuff (point 12) (Figure 6.24). The rotator cuff insertion can be followed around anteriorly and viewed both anterior and posterior to the biceps tendon. The

camera is rotated to view the anterior glenoid, labrum, joint capsule, and glenohumeral ligaments (point 13) (Figure 6.25). Bankart lesions are best seen from this perspective (Figures 6.26 and 6.27). The next point is the subscapularis tendon and its recess (point 14) (Figure 6.28). Loose bodies may be found in the subscapularis recess. The final intra-articular assessment is of the subscapularis tendon attachment to the humeral head (point 15) (Figure 6.28). Also visualize the anterior humeral articular cartilage and the humeral insertion of anterior joint capsule and glenohumeral ligaments.

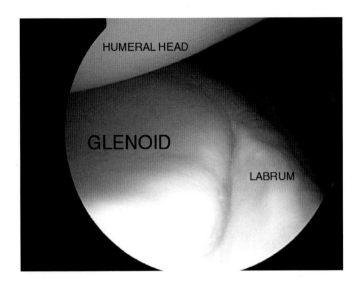

Figure 6.23

Point 11 of the arthroscopic evaluation.

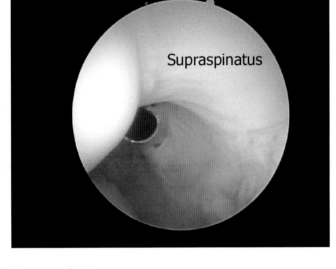

Figure 6.24

Point 12 of the arthroscopic evaluation.

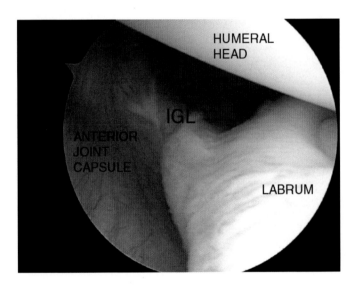

Figure 6.25

Point 13 of the arthroscopic evaluation.

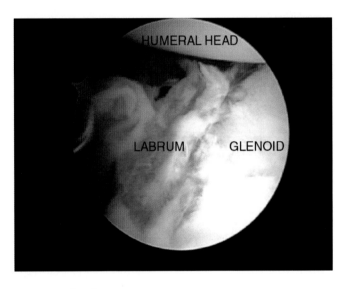

Figure 6.26

Bankart lesion.

Complete assessment of the shoulder requires an evaluation of the subacromial bursa. Change the direction of traction on the arm so that the arm is abducted 15–20° and traction is applied in line with the patient's body. We typically apply 15 pounds of weight with the arm in this position. The initial portal is the same posterosuperior portal used for the intra-articular arthroscopy. A metal cannula with a blunt tipped obturator can be used to palpate the posterior edge of the acromion and then slide underneath the acromion into the subacromial space. Then direct the cannula anteriorly until resistance is met. A Wissinger rod is passed through the cannula and directed to the anterior skin portal. An empty cannula is passed over the Wissinger rod anteriorly and into the bursal space. The anterior cannula is inserted to approximately one-third of its length and the posterior cannula is inserted to approximately three-quarters of its length so that it is past the posterior bursal curtain. The arthroscope is inserted into the posterior cannula and gravity outflow is attached to the anterior cannula. It is sometimes necessary to use a shaver to debride some bursal tissue for good visualization but this should be keep to a minimum initially. The camera is oriented so that the

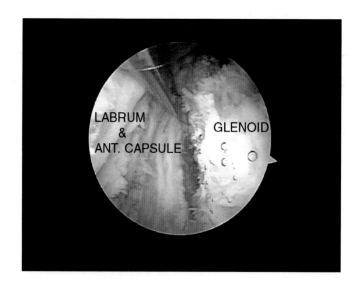

Figure 6.27

Preparation to repair a Bankart lesion.

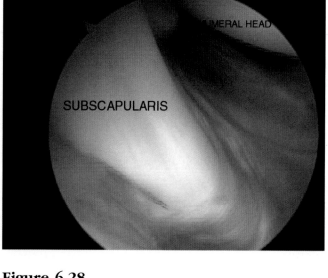

Figure 6.28

Points 14 and 15 of the arthroscopic evaluation. CA, coracoacromial

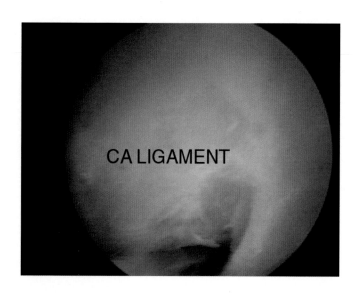

Figure 6.29

Point 16 of the arthroscopic evaluation.

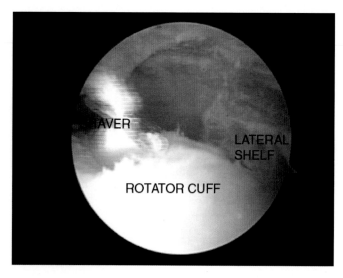

Figure 6.30

Point 17 of the arthroscopic evaluation.

acromion is above and the rotator cuff tendon is below. We first visualize the anterior inferior surface of the acromion and the coracoacromial ligament attachment (point 16) (Figure 6.29). By rotating the camera laterally, the lateral subdeltoid synovial shelf is assessed (point 17) (Figure 6.30). By further rotating the camera, the rotator cuff insertion into the humeral tuberosity can be identified (point 18) (Figure 6.31). By rotating the camera back medially, the rotator cuff tendon substance and the musculotendinous junction

is visualized (point 19) (Figure 6.32). Finally, look medially to assess the area of the acromioclavicular joint (point 20) (Figure 6.33). The best view of an anterior acromial bone spur is from the lateral portal (Figure 6.34).

Our next step is to switch the arthroscope to the anterior position and switch the outflow to the posterior portal. From this anterior portal we first visualize the posterior bursal curtain (point 21) (Figure 6.35). The surgeon can then see the posterior superior surface of

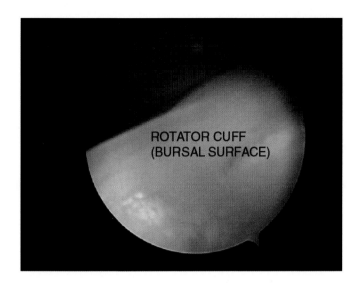

Figure 6.31

Point 18 of the arthroscopic evaluation.

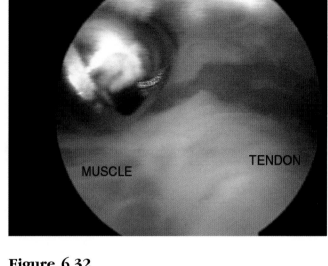

Figure 6.32

Point 19 of the arthroscopic evaluation.

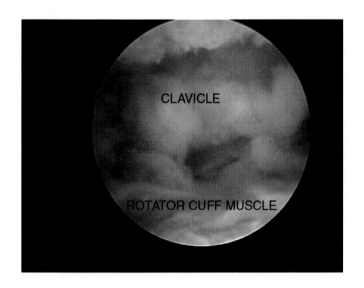

Figure 6.33

Point 20 of the arthroscopic evaluation.

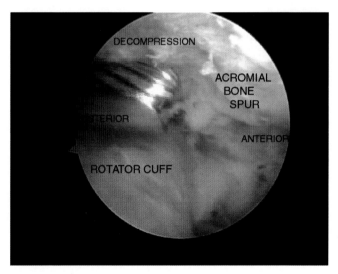

Figure 6.34

Anterior acromion bone spur.

the rotator cuff tendon (point 22) (Figure 6.36) The last area to assess is the rotator interval anteriorly and the superior border of the subscapularis tendon (point 23) (Figure 6.37).

At the end of our basic 23-point diagnostic shoulder arthroscopy, we have identified all pathology that can be visualized with the arthroscope. By having an easily reproducible and comprehensive examination, the surgeon can see all pathology from at least two vantage points.

Postoperative protocol

After arthroscopy, the portals are approximated with steri-strips. If a large cannula is used during the procedure then a single Vicryl suture is used subcutaneously to help approximate the portal. We place our patients in an arm sling that has a small pillow that maintains the shoulder in approximately 10° of abduction. The pillow also maintains the shoulder in a neutral rotation position. We also use a cooling pad on the shoulder

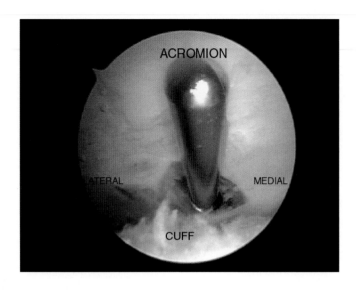

Figure 6.35

Point 21 of the arthroscopic evaluation.

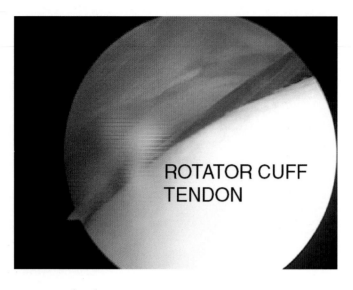

Figure 6.36

Point 22 of the arthroscopic evaluation. Middle glenohumeral ligament.

which decreases postoperative edema and helps to control postoperative pain. Specific postoperative protocols will depend on the surgical procedure performed.

References

1. Snyder SJ. A complete system for arthroscopy and bursoscopy of the shoulder. *Surgical Rounds for Orthopedics* 1989; **7**:57–65.
2. Snyder SJ, Karzel RP, Del Pizzo W et al. SLAP lesions of the shoulder. *Arthroscopy* 1990; **6**:274–9.
3. Buford DA, Williams MM, Snyder SJ. The Buford complex—the 'cord-like' middle glenohumeral ligament and absent anterosuperior labrum complex: a normal anatomic capsulolabral variant. *Arthroscopy* 1994; **10**:241–7.

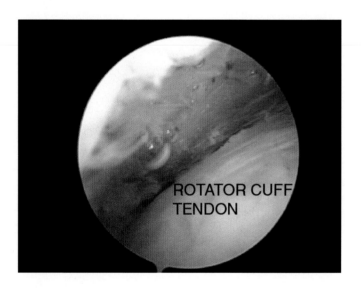

Figure 6.37

Point 23 of the arthroscopic evaluation.

7 Arthroscopic knot-tying techniques

Eric R McMillan and †Richard B Caspari

Introduction

One of the most important advances in the last two decades has been the development of devices that allow sutures to be passed and retrieved within joints. These devices have allowed arthroscopists to 'sew' within joints, and the need to tie knots arthroscopically has naturally followed.

Initially, knots used in open procedures such as the square knot were tried for arthroscopic applications. It became clear that these knots were not well suited to arthroscopic applications as it was very difficult to maintain tissue approximation tension when tying these knots arthroscopically. The search therefore began for knots that better lent themselves to arthroscopic techniques. Slip knots were found to be easily tied and to provide good tissue approximation tension, but they tended to loosen easily. Attention then turned to attempts to somehow 'lock' the slip knot so that it would not loosen so easily. Loutzenheiser et al[1] showed that the most effective way to secure a sliding arthroscopic knot was through a series of alternating post half-hitches applied after the sliding knot had been seated. The Duncan loop backed with alternating post half-hitches was shown to be the most secure arthroscopic knot of several tested in Loutzenheiser's paper and consequently has come to be one of the most commonly used arthroscopic knots. Several variations on the theme of placing locking knots behind a slip knot have since been described in search of a knot with the ideal qualities of ease of tying, tightness of tissue hold, and resistance to loosening.

Recently, attention has turned to 'locking' slip knots. 'Locking' slip knots are passed as slip knots, then the configuration of the knot is purposely changed once the knot is seated in order to convert the knot to a non-sliding configuration. This prevents the knot from loosening. Theoretically, this approach provides good tissue loop tension and knot security (resistance to loosening) with a small knot that can be rapidly tied. As discussed in greater detail below, locking slip knots do fulfill these objectives, but tying them can be difficult.

The development of arthroscopic implants has also influenced the evolution of arthroscopic knot tying. For example, as suture anchors have become more effective and easy to use, arthroscopists have been able to attempt more complicated procedures. With the advent of more complicated arthroscopic procedures, the need for and relevance on arthroscopic knot-tying skills has increased. Conversely, arthroscopic knot tying has also influenced the design of arthroscopic instrumentation. As manufac-turers have recognized that arthroscopic knot tying may not be a skill that all arthroscopists can master, devices have been devised to eliminate the need for knot tying. These devices have to date fallen into two categories: knot substitute devices such as the Y-Knot (Innovasive, Malborough, MA, USA) and knot elimination devices such as 'knotless suture anchors' (Mitek, Norwood, MA, USA; Arthrex, Naples, FL, USA and others). Knot substi-tute devices eliminate the need to tie knots when the surgeon places standard sutures, and knot elimination devices change the techniques of reconstruction such that no free suture ends need to be tied.[2]

Arthroscopic knot tying is indicated when there is a need to secure a suture repair intra-articularly and the arthroscopist has the technical expertise to tie a secure arthroscopic knot for fixation of that repair. Although knot-substitute devices or knotless suture anchors are available, it would be unwise to undertake a procedure known to require securing of suture intra-articularly if the surgeon does not have the technical expertise to tie knots arthro-scopically as a back-up. Knot-substitute devices or knotless anchors are useful adjuncts to arthroscopic knot tying, not substitutes for the ability to tie arthroscopic knots.[3]

Surgical principles

Arthroscopic knot tying is significantly more complex than open knot tying. Rather than simply memorizing knot configurations, a significant part of successfully tying knots arthroscopically is appropriate suture management.[4] It is critically important that the arthro-scopist understand the path of the sutures within the tissues being approximated, within the joint, and within the cannulas. This understanding is a prerequisite to tying and passing knots without tangling the sutures with each other, getting the sutures stuck in soft tissue, or breaking the sutures while tying. Paradoxically, most published information on arthroscopic knot tying focuses on the configuration of specific knots rather than the important issue of suture handling. Focusing on the fine points of arthroscopic knot configuration is analogous to debating the most efficient way to pack bundles of money into duffel bags and overlooking the issue of how you're going to get the bags into the bank vault. Certainly there is merit in finding the most effective arthroscopic knots, but the literature largely overlooks the issue that presents the greatest challenge to the vast majority of arthroscopists—avoiding problems that can preclude a knot of *any* configuration from being tied.

Surgical technique

In order to facilitate a more practical understanding of arthroscopic knot tying, we will consider the surgical technique as four distinct processes: preparation for arthroscopic knot tying; selection of the right arthroscopic knot; suture handling for arthroscopic knot tying; and configurations of specific arthroscopic knots.

Prior to developing the topic of arthroscopic knot tying, some knot terms should be clarified. The two free ends of any given suture are referred to as 'limbs'. A knot is made up of a series of loops passed around the 'post' limb. The limb that is not currently acting as the post is by default the 'non-post'. The post is not always the same limb and, in fact, it can be changed with every throw if desired—it is simply the limb the loops are being thrown around.

Preparation for knot tying

The basic foundation of learning to tie knots arthroscopically is practicing the techniques and knots involved. Materials for practice are inexpensive and readily available: a short segment of cord is really all that is needed to get started. When the surgeon is ready to progress on to tying with suture, the appropriate suture material, a knot pusher, and a cannula are needed. Either a commercially available or a makeshift knot-tying board is also required. The process of learning can be greatly accelerated by attending a teaching course that includes specific instruction in arthroscopic knot tying. Learning in a controlled environment with capable surgeons at hand to demonstrate the fine points is far more productive than on-the-job or at home trial and error learning. (Arthroscopic teaching courses are offered regularly in the United States by the Arthroscopy Association of North America (www.aana.org).)

Prior to tying knots arthroscopically in the operating room setting, it is critical to ensure that the necessary equipment and sutures are available. Being half way through an arthroscopic procedure and realizing that you don't have the piece of equipment you need to throw the knot is a very lonely feeling. Table 7.1 provides a general listing of the items needed.

What knot pusher is the best?

The answer is that it depends on what you're doing. In general, knot pushers are used for three purposes: (1) to check for suture twisting prior to knot tying; (2) to tie sliding knots; and (3) to tie non-sliding knots.

When checking for suture twisting prior to knot tying, a two-hole knot pusher is definitely the most reliable and easy to use.[5] There is no way for a suture twist to hide in the cannula when a two-hole knot pusher is used, whereas twists can occasionally remain undetected with a single-hole pusher. Any twisting detected can also be easily corrected with a two-hole pusher by simply rotating the pusher to untwist the suture under arthroscopic visualization. Once the suture has been untwisted, the two-hole pusher is withdrawn from the cannula without further rotation and the suture limbs are laid to the appropriate side of the cannula in their new, untwisted configuration. With regard to knot tying, two-hole pushers can be used to tie sliding knots but the increased bulk of the two-hole pusher is unnecessary and gives no advantage over the easier-to-use single-hole pusher. Using a two-hole knot pusher to tie non-sliding knots has been described, but there is no way to maintain tension on the tissue loop while subsequent throws are placed. This generally results in a loose and less effective knot. As a result, use of two-hole knot pushers to pass knots has now largely been abandoned.

For tying sliding knots, a single-hole knot pusher is the most commonly used and least complicated pusher. The single-hole design is relatively effective in checking for suture twists and allows easy passage of knots through cannulas and application of tension to seated knots. A modified one-hole knot pusher (Surgeon's 6th Finger, Arthrex) can also be used to check for suture twisting, pass knots through cannulas, and apply tension to seated knots. However, the modified one-hole pusher

Quantity	Description	Notes
	Table 7.1 Arthroscopic knot-tying equipment	
1 or more	Water-tight cannula(s)	Transparent cannulas are helpful[3,4] as are cannulas with differing inner diameters
1	Suture retriever	Suture graspers
		Crochet hook
1 or more	Knot pusher(s)	(see discussion in text)
N/A	Suture	27" for single or double-hole pusher
		36" for modified one-hole pusher

Table 7.2 A comparison of knot pusher types

Style	Ease of detecting twisting	Usefulness for sliding knots	Usefulness for non-sliding	Cost
One-hole	+/−	+	Don't use	One-time cost
Modified one-hole	+/−	+/−	+	Per-use charge
Two-hole	+	−	Don't use	One-time cost

is a bit bulkier than the standard one-hole pusher, requires use of a longer suture than the standard one-hole pusher, is associated with a per-use patient charge since it is disposable, and requires a certain technical expertise for proper use that can slow the inexperienced user. Proponents of the modified one-hole pusher cite greater 'loop security' than that obtained by a standard one-hole pusher by virtue of the pusher's ability to maintain tension in the initial knot loop while subsequent throws are placed.[6]

As discussed below, non-sliding arthroscopic knots are typically tied out of desperation rather than design. If one is forced to tie a non-sliding knot, the modified one-hole knot pusher is really the only good option since it is the only knot-tying device that can hold tension on the initial knot loop while subsequent throws are placed. Use of any other style of knot pusher relies on the friction of the suture against itself to hold the initial throw tight while another knot is thrown to secure the initial knot. This rarely results in a 'non-sliding' knot with satisfactory tissue loop tension.

To summarize, a one-hole knot pusher is the most commonly available and easiest pusher to use, a modified one-hole knot pusher should be available in case of the unexpected need to tie a non-sliding knot due to suture binding, and a two-hole knot pusher is the most effective when checking for suture twisting (Table 7.2).

Selecting the right arthroscopic knot

The basic objectives of tying an arthroscopic knot are to: (1) provide good tissue loop tension to approximate the desired tissues,[3,6] and (2) to maintain this tension as the tissues are loaded postoperatively.[3] The ideal knot is one that accomplishes these two objectives with the smallest bulk and greatest ease of tying.

Sliding versus non-sliding

Sliding knots inherently provide better tissue loop tension, but also inherently loosen more easily than non-

sliding knots. As arthroscopic knot tying has evolved, it has proven easier to devise techniques to keep a sliding knot from loosening than to get good tissue loop tension from a non-sliding knot. Consequently, sliding knots are preferred to non-sliding knots for all arthroscopic knot tying.

Non-locking versus locking

Two fundamentally different approaches to the prevention of loosening have been developed for sliding knots: throwing additional loops on top of the sliding knot after it is seated, and changing the sliding knot into a non-sliding knot after it is seated.

As demonstrated by Loutzenheiser et al,[1] the addition of just a few simple suture throws on top of a sliding knot can be very effective in preventing loosening. This approach is both easy to accomplish from a technical standpoint and very reproducible or predictable. Because of these benefits, the Duncan loop knot backed by alternating post half-hitches has become the workhorse of arthroscopic knots. Securing other types of sliding knots with additional suture throws has been described,[7] and has been shown to be effective as well.[3]

An alternative method of preventing sliding knots from slipping is the locking sliding knot. A locking sliding knot is one whose configuration can be selectively changed by applying tension to the suture limbs in the appropriate sequence. Theoretically, this is accomplished after the knot has been seated and good tissue loop tension has been achieved. The problem with this approach however, is that the knot can be inadvertently locked at any point in the tying process. Locking a knot in the cannula is one thing on a knot-tying board and quite another thing after working for 10 or 20 minutes in the operating room to get an anchor properly placed, pass the suture through the correct location in the correct tissue, and get the suture limbs back through the cannula without tangling. Locking knots are very attractive in theory but can be very unforgiving in practice.

For the average arthroscopist, the best knot to learn is probably the Duncan loop backed by alternating post half-hitches in light of the Duncan loop's proven effectiveness, relative ease of tying, and predictability.

Suture handling for arthroscopic knot tying

Tips and tricks: general

A good basic starting point when tying knots arthroscopically is to eliminate any distractions that may be present in the operating room.[4,8] Of course, a good view of the knot-tying field is also mandatory.[3,4,8,9] One should always check for twisting of the sutures prior to tying[4,10] (Figure 7.1) as a knot tied on twisted sutures will inevitably untwist after tying, thereby loosening the tissue loop.

It is a mistake to tie a sliding knot with a suture that does not slide freely.[4,10] At best, a knot with poor tissue loop tension results. At worst, the suture stops sliding altogether and the knot becomes firmly fixed about halfway down the cannula. If the knot does become stuck in the cannula you usually have to just cut the suture out and start over; such a knot can rarely be coaxed back up the cannula for untangling and retying. Which brings us to another important point—always have a back-up plan in case your arthroscopic knot tying is unsuccessful.[4,9,10]

Tips and tricks: the portals and cannulas

It is critical to ensure that both suture limbs being tied exit the joint through the same passage, with no soft-tissue bridge between the limbs. Clearly, it is not possible to seat a knot within the joint if a soft-tissue bridge blocks the knot's entry into the joint. Drawing the limbs to be tied through a cannula prior to tying ensures by default that there is no soft-tissue bridge.[4] Use of a cannula for tying also helps prevent interposition of stray soft tissue in the knot as it is seated. If the tip of the cannula is kept close to the area where the knot is to be seated the risk of soft tissue becoming entangled in the knot just prior to seating is minimized as well.[5] In effect, the less soft tissue the knot passes by the less likely the soft tissue is to become entangled in the knot.

Another approach that is very helpful is to use a third portal when tying knots arthroscopically.[4,9,10] Having a third portal allows the uninvolved sutures to be passed out of the joint clear of the tying process (Figure 7.2). This significantly reduces the likelihood of these other sutures becoming entangled within the knot. It is also generally easier to retrieve sutures from a third portal than from around the cannula in the tying portal, as is recommended by some authors (Figures 7.3 and 7.4).[11]

As discussed previously, an important part of successful arthroscopic knot tying is having an understanding of the suture's path within the tissues and cannulas. Having this understanding allows the surgeon to react appropriately and quickly when figuring out which limb to pull to tighten a knot, which limb to pull to draw the knot into the joint, and so on. One technique that is

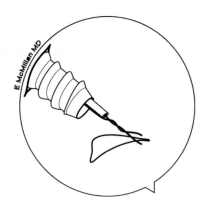

Figure 7.1
Knot pusher advanced to knot, revealing twisting.

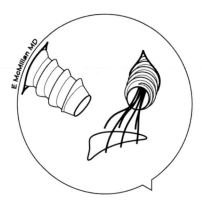

Figure 7.2
Uninvolved sutures passing out of accessory cannula, clear of the knot-tying process.

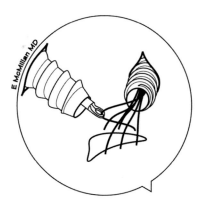

Figure 7.3
Suture being easily retrieved from accessory cannula.

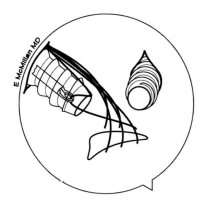

Figure 7.4

Suture binding at edge of cannula during retrieval when placed through tying portal adjacent to cannula.

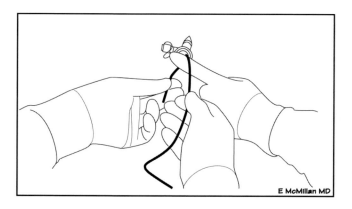

Figure 7.5

Assistant's finger placed between suture limb exiting cannula.

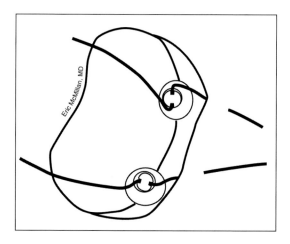

Figure 7.6

Top anchor has been placed such that suture must twist just to pass through desired tissue. Bottom anchor shows proper orientation to allow suture to slide freely.

very helpful in keeping the suture limb orientation straight is to classify the suture limbs in your own mind into two categories such as 'left' and 'right', 'anterior' and 'posterior', or similar. Once this informal classification has been assigned to the suture limbs, the limbs should be drawn out of the tying cannula without twisting and laid to the appropriate side of the cannula. In other words, the 'left' suture limb should be placed to the left side of the cannula, or the 'anterior' limb placed to the anterior side of the cannula and so on. Once the limbs have been separated in this fashion, the assistant or scrub nurse can place a finger between the limbs on top of the cannula (Figure 7.5).[4] This allows the surgeon to manipulate the suture limbs for knot tying while still maintaining the original orientation of the sutures within the cannula, thus preventing any suture twisting and maintaining a clear understanding as to which suture limb is the post. Knowing which suture limb is which and being able to access the desired suture limb without guessing will significantly speed and simplify your knot tying. Many surgeons also tag the post limb with a small hemostat in order to help themselves remember which limb is currently acting as the post.

Tips and tricks: the anchor

When using suture anchors, aligning the anchor such that the suture does not have to twist as it leaves the anchor will help ensure that the suture slides through the construct freely when it comes time to tie (Figure 7.6).[12] Also, be sure to avoid over-penetrating the anchor as sinking the anchor too far will introduce unwanted friction between the edge of the anchor hole and the suture. Above all, binding of the suture is to be avoided.

Tips and tricks: the suture—braided or monofilament?

Several factors deserve consideration when choosing a suture for arthroscopic knot tying—handling characteristics of the suture, initial strength of the suture, and changes in strength of the suture over time.

In terms of handling characteristics, monofilament sutures are generally easier to pass using currently available suturing instruments such as the Caspari Suture Punch (Linvatec, Largo, FL, USA) or the Spectrum Suturing System (Linvatec). Braided sutures tend to be easier to tie, and tend to loosen less than commonly used monofilament sutures.

If the surgeon prefers a non-absorbable suture but wants to use the Caspari suture punch or Spectrum Suturing System, two alternate methods are available: use of the Suture Shuttle Relay (Linvatec) or use of the Thal technique. The Suture Shuttle Relay is a twisted wire cable that is covered with plastic except at the center of its length where the wires can be separated. The Suture Shuttle is passed using the Caspari punch or Spectrum System, then once the Suture Shuttle has been removed

Table 7.3 Suture strength as a function of time[3]

Suture	Dissolve/non-dissolve	Mono/braided	Time (weeks)	Retained strength (%)
Monocryl	Dissolving	Monofilament	3	0
PDS II	Dissolving	Monofilament	3	80
			6	40
Maxon	Dissolving	Monofilament	3	67
			6	9
Vicryl	Dissolving	Braided	3	<10
Panacryl	Dissolving	Braided	3	95
			6	90
			12	80
Ethibond	Non-dissolving	Braided	3	100
			6	100

Monocryl, PDS II, Vicryl, Panacryl, and Ethibond are products of Ethicon, Inc (Somerville, NJ, USA). Maxon is a product of the United States Surgical Corporation (Atlanta, GA, USA).

from the suturing device a braided suture is placed between the wire strands in the center of the Shuttle Relay. The braided suture is drawn through the desired tissue by pulling the Shuttle Relay in the appropriate direction, thereby passing the braided suture retrograde through the tissues. A more gentle pull will limit the braided suture from stripping the plastic coating.

The other technique for passing braided suture using the Caspari punch or the Spectrum Suturing System is the Thal technique (R. Caspari, personal communication). A 2-0 or 3-0 monofilament suture is folded in half and the two free ends fed into the Caspari punch. The two free ends feed roughly the same as a single larger monofilament in most cases. Once the doubled monofilament suture has been placed through the desired tissues and retrieved from a cannula a braided suture is passed through the loop at the end of the doubled monofilament suture and drawn down into the joint and through the desired tissue by pulling on the free ends of the doubled monofilament suture. Alternatively, a suture punch specifically designed to accommodate braided suture (Arthrotek, Warsaw, IN, USA) can be used.

With regard to the strength of various sutures, non-dissolving braided sutures such as Ethibond (Ethicon, Mitek) tend to have higher failure strength than monofilament dissolving sutures such as PDS II (Ethicon).

As expected, dissolving and non-dissolving sutures vary significantly in their strength as time passes (Table 7.3).

Based on these data, it would seem prudent to use either Panacryl or Ethibond in an application where the suture was expected to be under greater tension (e.g. rotator cuff repair under tension) and in other circumstances the suture of the surgeon's choice.

With sliding knots, a significant disparity in the length of the limbs can result after the knot is seated if the limbs are not adjusted properly prior to tying. This length disparity can make it very difficult to continue the knot tying process and in extreme cases can even leave the surgeon with only one very long suture limb protruding from the cannula. Without access to both limbs, additional loops can not be thrown to back up a non-locking sliding knot and a locking sliding knot cannot be locked. For a sliding knot, leaving the non-post limb protruding about half the overall suture length farther than the post limb from the cannula provides limbs of roughly equal length once the initial sliding knot is seated (Figure 7.7).[4] For non-sliding knots, the post and non-post limbs should be about equal.

Tips and tricks: the knot pusher

With sliding knots, the knot pusher should be placed on the post limb only when seating the initial knot. This initial knot should be 'pushed' into place, keeping tension on the post in order to fully seat the knot and prevent its loosening once seated. Subsequently, the knot pusher is best placed on the non-post limb in order to 'pull' additional throws down onto the initial sliding knot. With non-sliding knots, the knot pusher should be placed onto the non-post limb for all throws.

When choosing the limb that will act as the post, choose the limb that passes through the tissue in the most out-of-the-way location.[11,12] For example, when securing a Bankart repair using a glenoid suture anchor, make the suture limb farthest away from the glenoid the post. This will tuck the knot out of the way and minimize the chance of knot interference with joint function after the repair is completed.

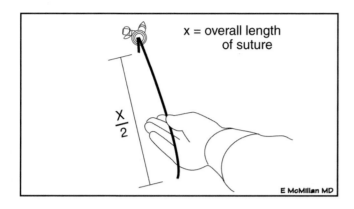

Figure 7.7

Non-post limb adjusted so it extends about half of overall suture length farther than post limb from cannula.

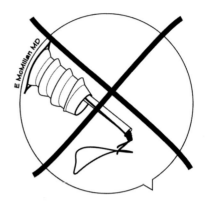

Figure 7.9

Knot pusher advanced obliquely, pulling suture.

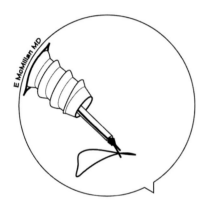

Figure 7.8

Knot pusher advanced directly toward knot.

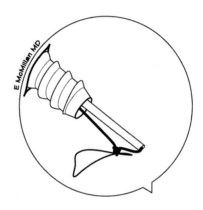

Figure 7.10

Past-pointing with the knot pusher to tighten the knot.

Even with the knot pusher correctly in place, it can be difficult to advance knots down the cannula and into the joint. The easiest way to facilitate advancement of knots is to gently alternate tension on the two limbs of suture in your hands.[4,5,10] Note that this technique should not be used on the throw immediately after the initial knot of a sliding knot because pulling on the non-post limb will usually loosen the initial suture loop. Advancing the pusher directly toward the knot (or the desired position of the knot if it is not already seated) relieves tension on the post limb and allows for easier passage of the knot (Figures 7.8 and 7.9).[4,5]

It is important to seat each knot fully under arthroscopic visualization prior to passing subsequent throws,[4,10,13] as the knot pusher can be inadvertently passed through the knot within the cannula. If the knot is left loose within the cannula and another knot is passed down, the two knots usually engage and lock. This can make for a long afternoon in the OR. Once a throw is seated, the knot pusher should be used to 'past-point' to gain additional tightness within the knot (Figure 7.10).[4,5,10,13] This is analogous to past-pointing commonly employed in open knot tying.

When holding the two suture limbs for knot tying, one easy technique to gain an 'extra' helping finger is to hold the two suture limbs slightly separated between the left thumb and middle finger. This leaves the left index finger free to help pass the non-post limb as it is thrown around the post to construct whatever knot is planned (Figure 7.11).

Arthroscopic knots

Sliding/non-locking

The Duncan loop (Figures 7.12–7.24) backed with alternating post half-hitches is a good basic sliding knot that is relatively easy to tie and provides good holding

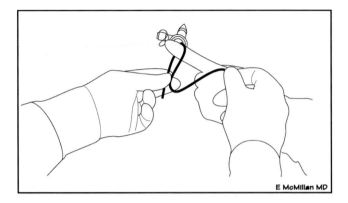

Figure 7.11

Suture being held between left thumb and middle finger, leaving the index finger free to help with knot tying.

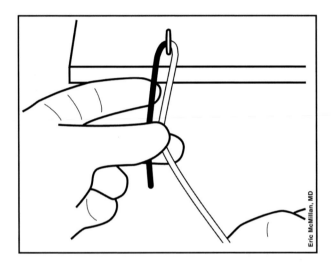

Figure 7.12

Adjust the suture limbs for a sliding knot and hold both limbs between the left thumb and middle finger.

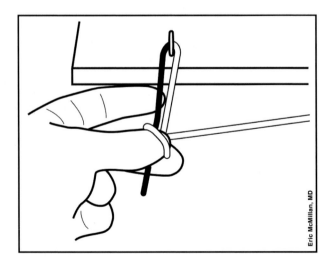

Figure 7.13

Throw an overhand loop over the tip of your thumb and subsequently over the post.

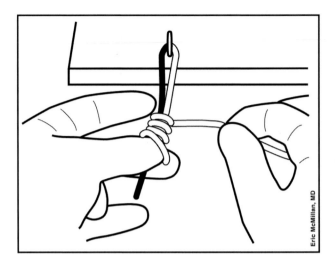

Figure 7.14

Throw three overhand loops on the post.

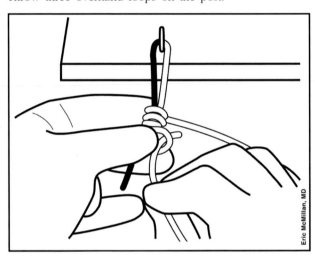

Figure 7.15

Move the loop that was over your thumb tip down and pass the end of the non-post limb through the loop in a downward direction.

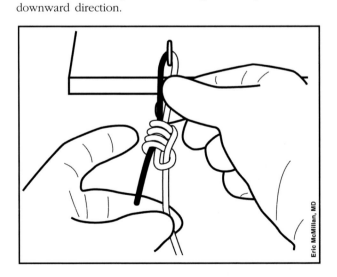

Figure 7.16

Apply tension to both ends of the non-post limb to snug the knot.

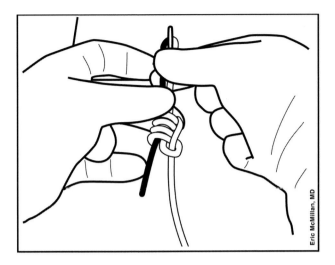

Figure 7.17

Hold both limbs with the right thumb and index finger, and apply a pull to the knot with the left thumb and middle finger to compact the knot. Use caution not to overtighten.

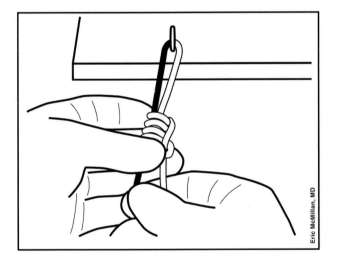

Figure 7.18

Apply a push to the knot to further compact it. Seat the knot by applying tension to the post and/or pushing the knot into the joint with a knot pusher on the post limb.

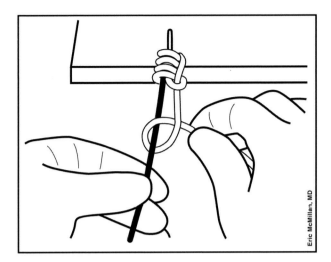

Figure 7.19

Throw an underhand loop on the post limb.

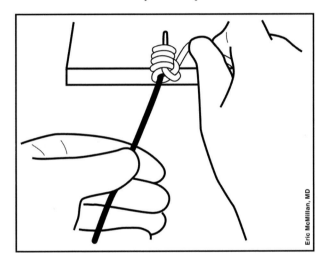

Figure 7.20

Pull the underhand loop down onto the knot and past-point to tighten. When using suture, the knot pusher should be on the non-post limb.

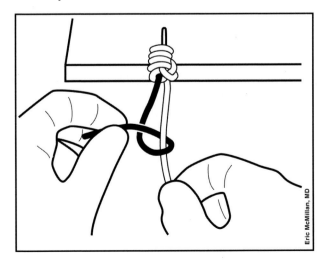

Figure 7.21

Switch posts and throw an overhand loop on the new post.

strength.[1] The only significant drawback to this knot is its relatively large size compared to other arthroscopic knots.

The Tennessee slider (Bunt-line hitch)[7] (Figures 7.25–7.29) is a knot that is easy to tie and has a comparatively low bulk. The Tennessee slider also has good holding strength.[3]

Sliding/locking

The tautline (or Midshipman's) hitch (Figures 7.30–7.37) is one of the more forgiving of the locking sliding knots.

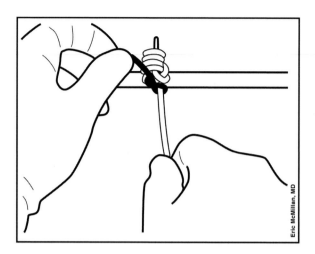

Figure 7.22

Pull the overhand loop down onto the knot and past-point to tighten.

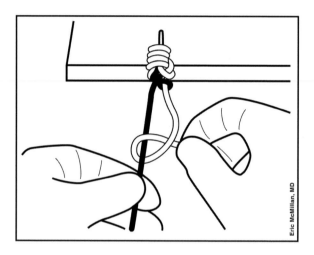

Figure 7.23

Switch posts again and throw an underhand loop on the new post.

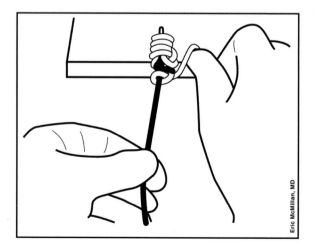

Figure 7.24

Pull the underhand loop down onto the knot and past-point to finish the knot.

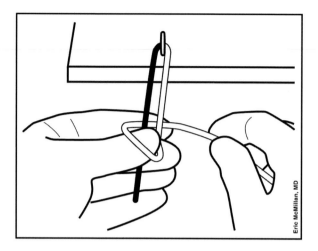

Figure 7.25

Adjust the suture limbs for a sliding knot and hold both limbs between the left thumb and middle finger. Throw an overhand loop over both limbs.

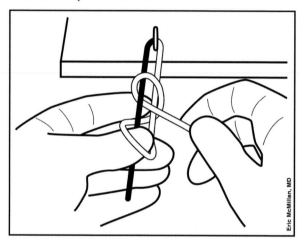

Figure 7.26

Throw an overhand loop on the post and pass the non-post suture back through the knot, as shown.

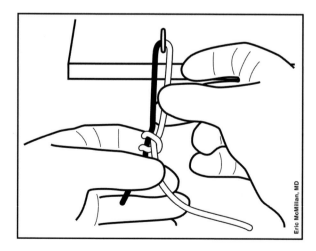

Figure 7.27

Apply tension to both ends of the non-post limb to snug the knot. Seat the knot by applying tension to the post and/or pushing the knot into the joint with a knot pusher on the post limb.

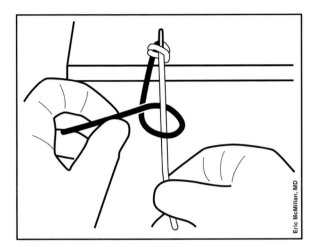

Figure 7.28

Switch posts and throw an overhand loop on the new post.
Pull the loop down and past-point to tighten.

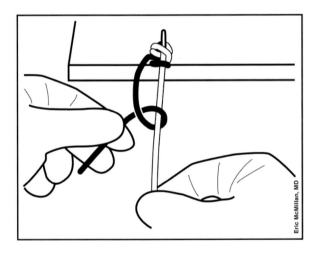

Figure 7.29

Switch posts and throw an underhand loop on the new
post. Pull the loop down and past-point to tighten.

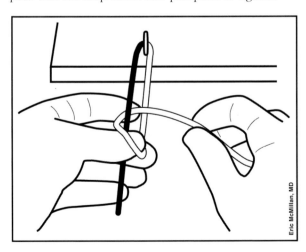

Figure 7.30

Adjust the suture limbs for a sliding knot and hold both
limbs between the left thumb and middle finger. Throw an
overhand loop on the post.

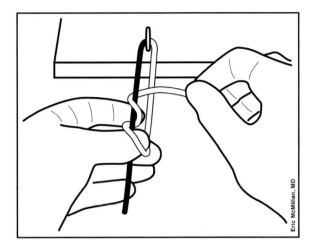

Figure 7.31

Throw another overhand loop on the post.

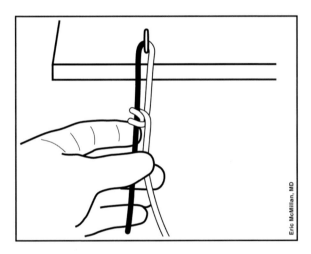

Figure 7.32

Slide your left thumb and middle finger down so that the
original loops are held under slight tension.

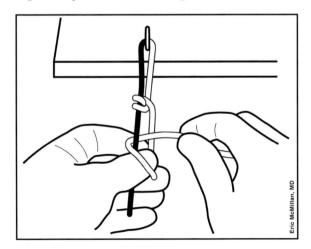

Figure 7.33

Throw an overhand loop on the post in this new position.

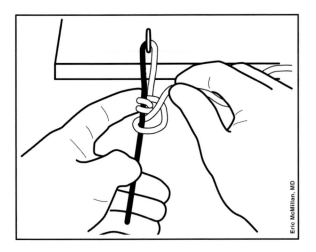

Figure 7.34

Pull the loop down to snug the knot.

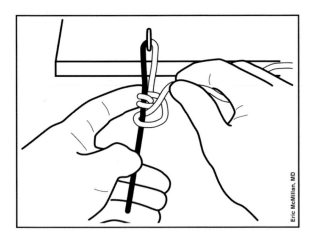

Figure 7.35

Seat the knot by applying tension to the post and/or pushing the knot into the joint with a knot pusher on the post limb.

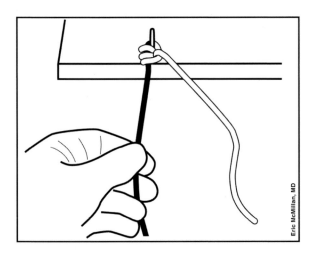

Figure 7.36

Release the post limb and grasp the non-post limb with your right thumb and index finger.

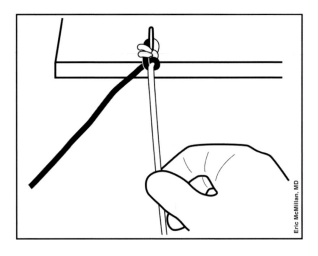

Figure 7.37

Change the knot to a non-sliding configuration by pulling on the non-post limb to finish the knot.

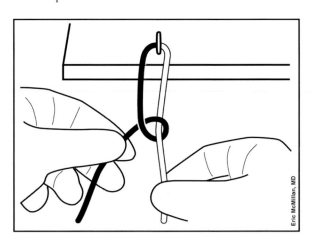

Figure 7.38

Adjust the limbs for a non-sliding knot and throw an underhand loop on the post. Pull the loop down to form the beginning of the knot and past-point to tighten.

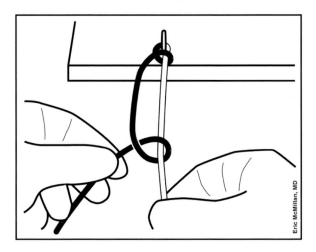

Figure 7.39

Throw another underhand loop on the post. Pull the loop down and past-point to tighten.

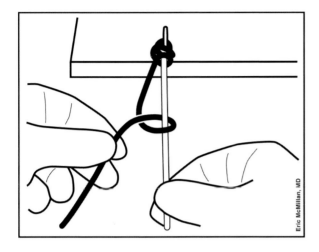

Figure 7.40

Throw an overhand loop on the post. Pull the loop down and past-point to tighten.

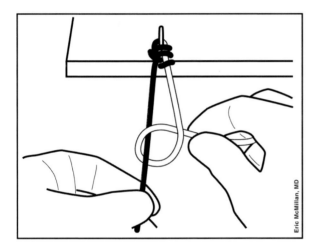

Figure 7.41

Switch posts and throw an underhand loop on the new post. Pull the loop down and past-point to tighten.

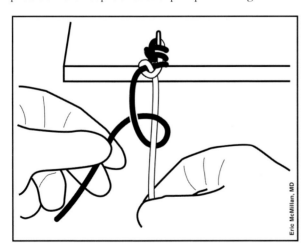

Figure 7.42

Switch posts again and throw an underhand loop on the new post. Pull the loop down and past-point to finish the knot.

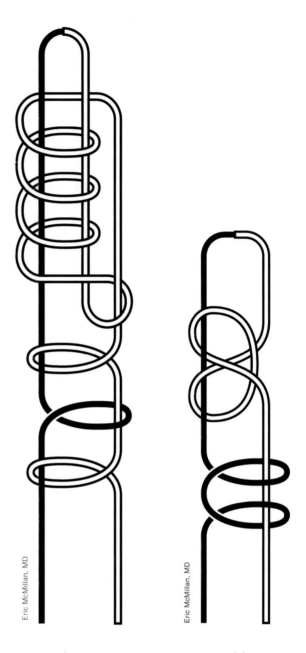

Figure 7.43

The Duncan loop knot backed with alternating post half-hitches—a non-locking sliding knot.

Figure 7.44

The Tennessee slider knot[7]—a non-locking sliding knot.

It has a small bulk and good holding strength empirically.

Non-sliding

The Revo knot (Figures 7.38–7.42) is a good choice when the need to tie a non-sliding knot arises. It is relatively easy to tie and has been shown to be very secure.[3]

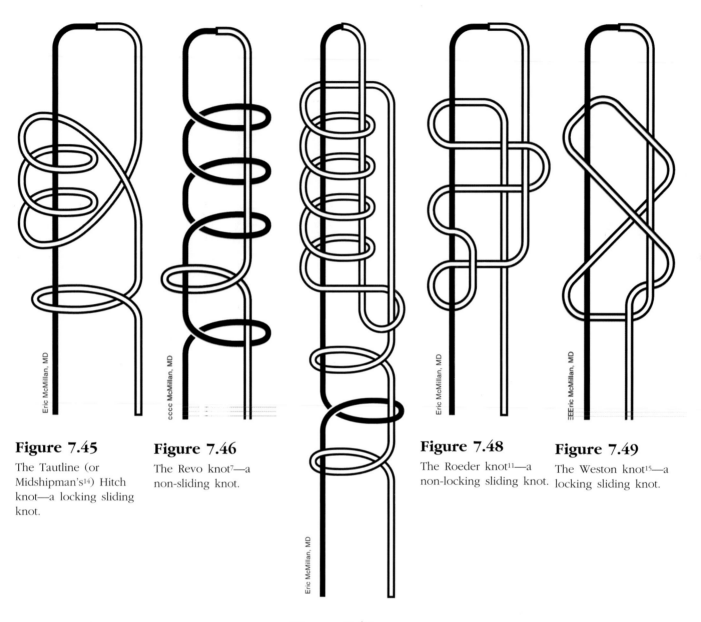

Figure 7.45

The Tautline (or Midshipman's[14]) Hitch knot—a locking sliding knot.

Figure 7.46

The Revo knot[7]—a non-sliding knot.

Figure 7.48

The Roeder knot[11]—a non-locking sliding knot.

Figure 7.49

The Weston knot[15]—a locking sliding knot.

Figure 7.47

The Hangman's loop knot backed with alternating post half-hitches—a non-locking sliding knot.

Knot diagrams (Figures 7.43–7.49)

Diagrammatic representations of all of the knots shown above as well as a few other common knots are included.

Conclusion

Arthroscopic knot tying is an exciting aspect of arthroscopy that significantly expands the arthroscopist's capabilities. Although technically demanding, observation of a few precautions and use of a few simple techniques can bring arthroscopic knot tying within the grasp of the interested arthroscopist.

References

1. Loutzenheiser TD, Harryman DT II, Yung SW et al. Optimizing arthroscopic knots. *Arthroscopy* 1995; **11**:199–206.
2. Thal R. A knotless suture anchor: technique for use in arthroscopic Bankart repair. Presented at the 18th Annual Meeting,

Arthroscopy Association of North America, Vancouver, BC, Canada, April, 1999.

3. Nottage WM. Suture, anchors, and knots. Presented at the 18th Annual Meeting, Fall Course, Arthroscopy Association of North America, Vancouver, BC, Canada, April, 1999.

4. McMillan ER. A simplified technique for suture handling during arthroscopic knot tying. *The 'Masters Experience' Knot Tying Manual.* Rosemont, IL: Arthroscopy Association of North America, 1999.

5. Nottage WM. Arthroscopic knot tying. Presented at the 15th Fall Course, Arthroscopy Association of North America, Palm Desert, California, 1996.

6. Burkhart SS, Wirth MA, Simonick M et al. Loop security as a determinant of tissue fixation security. *Arthroscopy* 1998; **14**:773–6.

7. Snyder SJ. Technique of arthroscopic rotator cuff repair using implantable 4mm Revo™ suture anchors, suture shuttle relays and #2 non-absorbable mattress sutures. Presented at the 18th Annual Meeting, Arthroscopy Association of North America, Vancouver, BC, Canada, April, 1999.

8. Abrams JS. Principles of arthroscopic stabilization. Presented at the 16th Fall Course, Arthroscopy Association of North America, Nashville, Tennessee, 1997.

9. Tauro JC. Arthroscopic rotator cuff repair: analysis of technique and results at 2- and 3-year follow-up. *Arthroscopy* 1998; **14**:45–51.

10. Fischer SP. Tying good knots arthroscopically. Presented at the Specialty Day Meeting, Arthroscopy Association of North America, San Francisco, California, 1997.

11. Nottage WM, Lieurance RK. Arthroscopic knot tying techniques. *Arthroscopy* 1999; **15**:515–21.

12. De Beer JF. Arthroscopic Bankart repair: some aspects of suture and knot management. *Arthroscopy* 1999; **15**:660–2.

13. Sweeney HJ. Knot tying. Presented at the 17th Fall Course, Arthroscopy Association of North America, Palm Desert, California, November, 1998.

14. Ashley CW. Hitches to spar and rail (right-angle pull). In: *The Ashley Book of Knots.* New York: Doubleday, 1944;296.

15. Chan KC. Classification of sliding knots for use in arthroscopic surgery. Presented at the 18th Annual Meeting, Arthroscopy Association of North America, Vancouver, BC, Canada, April, 1999.

Section III – Glenohumeral instability

8 Anterior shoulder instability: Transglenoidal technique

Franz Landsiedl

Introduction

Development of the procedure

Most arthroscopic transglenoidal shoulder stabilizing procedures are based on the Reider–Inglis[1] modification of the Bankart–Perthes procedure.[2,3] Reider used three mattress sutures to repair the capsule to the glenoid. These sutures are passed to the back of the shoulder using K-wires and are tied over buttons that are padded with felt. Early transglenoidal arthroscopic techniques were published by Caspari[4] who used one transglenoidal drill hole to deliver 6–8 simple sutures to the back, reattaching the labrum to the glenoid, whereas Morgan[5] fixed the labrum with a double mattress suture, which is passed through two transglenoidal drill holes. Similar techniques were developed by Benedetto and Glötzer[6] and Maki.[7] We started with our single-hole capsulorrhaphy technique in 1986 and have been using it since that time, with some modifications, in all patients with recurrent unidirectional dislocations of the shoulder.

In the last few years techniques using tissue anchors have become much more popular as they are technically easier and have no need for a transglenoidal passage with potential neurovascular complications. The drawback is that in the case of severely destroyed labrum–ligament complex (LLC) and capsule, fewer sutures to tighten the capsule can be applied.

Indications

The main indication for our capsulorrhaphy procedure is the posttraumatic anteroinferior instability of the shoulder with detachment of the LLC. Overstretched LLC or poor quality labrum are not contraindications as the labrum is only rarely addressed by the procedure and a capsulorrhaphy is part of the operation in every patient with recurrent dislocation. As a tight reattachment of the LLC can be achieved at the level of the glenoid, even a deep osteochondral Hill–Sachs lesion is no contraindication. Patients with bony Bankart fragments exceeding 10 × 4 mm are in our experience at much higher risk for redislocations than other patients.[8]

Patients suffering from unidirectional or multidirectional instability without detachment of the LLC should not be treated with this technique whereas patients with the anterior component of multidirectional instabilities with Bankart lesions have been successfully treated using this technique.

The procedure is technically very demanding and needs a skillful arthroscopist with a sound knowledge of the sometimes very difficult arthroscopic anatomy. The learning curve is very flat. My personal dislocation rate was 37% in the first 16 patients[9] and improved to 6% after more than 100 patients.[8]

Results

In our last follow-up evaluation of an unselected series of 48 traumatic and three non-traumatic recurrent undirectional anterior shoulder dislocations we found a redislocation rate of 6%.[8] Follow-up time was 36–61 months (average 43 months). Of 45 patients active in sports, 37 reached the preinjury level, nine were improved and three gave up sports. The average restriction of external rotation was 13° in 0° of abduction and 14° in 90° of abduction, respectively. Boszotta and Helperstorfer[10] reported a similar redislocation rate using the same technique in young first-time dislocators.

Surgical principles

In all transglenoidal repair techniques the detached capsulolabral structures are reattached by sutures that are brought out to the back via a transglenoidal passage. According to the extent of the capsular damage, three different transglenoidal techniques are used by us.

Detachment and widening of the anteroinferior LLC can be found in most recurrent dislocations. Therefore reduction of the patulous capsule and shortening of the overstretched inferior glenohumeral ligament (IGHL) is the main goal of the procedure in these cases, as in many multiple dislocators no reattachable labrum can be found (Figure 8.1). Therefore the stretched capsule[11] and not the labrum is the anatomical structure that should be addressed.

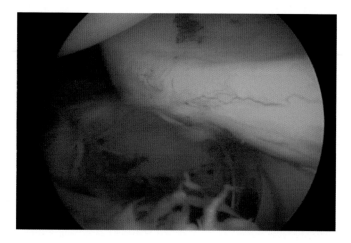

Figure 8.1

Right shoulder as seen from the anterior portal. Severely detached labrum–ligament complex. No reatttachable labrum.

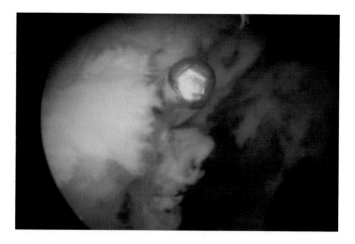

Figure 8.2

The abraded neck of the glenoid and the position of the transglenoidal K-wire are inspected from the anterior portal (left shoulder).

In order to re-establish a strong capsule, we try to achieve a capsular plication and reduction of the anteroinferior pouch by applying three to five sutures between the 3.30 and 6 o'clock position (referring to a right shoulder). These sutures are brought to the back through a transglenoidal drill hole. If these sutures are tightened, a significant reduction of the anteroinferior pouch with a superior shift of the inferior capsule and an impressive capsular plication can be observed.

The transglenoid drill hole to deliver the sutures posteriorly is positioned in the 4–4.30 o'clock position to achieve the maximum capsular reinforcement in the area of the anteroinferior glenoid, the hot spot where the dislocation takes place.[12]

If the capsular detachment extends cephalad beyond the 3 o'clock position in very unstable cases or if a SLAP (superior labrum, anteroposterior) lesion is present a second transglenoidal drill hole in the 2–3 o'clock position is created to perform one or two more superior sutures.

In first-time dislocations only the labrum is reattached using two, sometimes three, transglenoidal sutures and two transglenoidal passages.

Surgical technique

The patient is placed in the lateral decubitus position. The arm is suspended in a position of 35–45° of abduction and 10–20° of anteflexion, using 3 kg of traction. A rolled sheet with 20-cm diameter is placed in the axilla as a pulley. If the elbow is adducted, the humeral head is pulled off from the glenoid to improve the visualization of the joint.

The surgery is performed under general endotracheal anesthesia, using Ringer's solution with POR 8 (Sandoz, Novartis, Basel, Switzerland) (synthetic ornipressin) added to control bleeding (mixing ratio: 1 ampule of POR 8 to 1 liter Ringer's solution). If electrocautery is necessary in case of bleeding, the irrigation fluid is changed to Purisole SM (Sorbit 27.0 g and Mannit 5.4 g/liter) (Fresenius-Kabi, Graz, Austria).

Routine antibiotic prophylaxis with a single-shot dose of 4 g cefazolin is used nowadays. Prior to surgery, stability is tested. The arthroscope is inserted through a standard posterior portal. An anterior working portal is made just above the subscapularis tendon at the level of the glenoid, using an inside-out technique. Next, careful inspection and probing of the glenohumeral joint, especially of ligaments and the LLC, is always carried out from the anterior and posterior portals.

Repair begins with debridement of loose labral flaps only, avoiding damage to the capsule and bleeding. Next, the scapular neck is abraded in the area of the detached LLC down to bleeding bone using a motorized burr. This is a very important part of the technique and has to be checked by careful inspection from the anterior portal. A 2-mm K-wire is drilled at a distance of 4–5 mm off the anterior glenoid rim through the scapular neck from anterior to posterior, in the 4.30 o'clock position (referring to a right shoulder). The position of the K-wire should be checked from the anterior portal (Figure 8.2).

Angulation of the K-wire should be 30° inferior and 15–20° medial with respect to the glenoid articular surface. The K-wire will exit the skin posteriorly approximately 5–7 cm inferior to the posterior portal. At this location, a 2-cm skin incision is made, and the K-wire is overdrilled (after blunt preparation along the K-wire down to the bone) from posterior with a 5-mm cannulated drill, using a 7-mm sheath to protect the infraspinatus muscle. The edge of the drill hole should be very close to the anterior rim of the glenoid, so that after

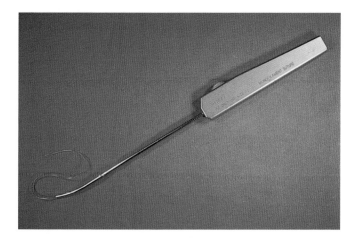

Figure 8.3

The Acufex shoulder stitcher.

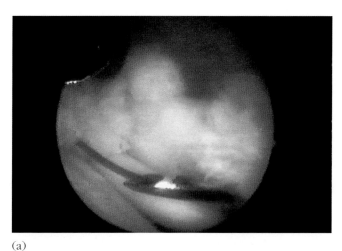

(a)

tightening of the sutures the reconstructed capsule will be in the same level as the surface of the glenoid cavity. A 5-mm working cannula with a 4-mm cannulated trocar is inserted from the posterior portal via the transglenoidal drill hole using the K-wire as guide until it can be seen in the joint. The trocar is removed. The working cannula facilitates the transglenoidal passage of the sutures. The IGHL is penetrated 15–20 mm away from the glenoid as inferiorly as possible, using the Acufex (Smith & Nephew, Andover, MA, USA) shoulder stitcher (Figure 8.3), which is inserted into the joint via the anterior portal. After a 10–20 mm passage through the LLC it is reinserted into the joint (Figure 8.4). Care should be taken to penetrate the whole thickness of the LLC and not superficial synovial tissue only. In the latter case the shoulder stitcher can be see under the thin synovial layer during the whole passage. A #1 Maxon thread is pushed into the joint through the shoulder stitcher and retrieved through the anterior cannula using a small grasper.

Both ends of the suture are delivered posteriorly through the transglenoidal working cannula using a K-wire with an eye. Both ends of the thread are secured with a clamp separately. The first suture is thus applied and a trial reduction of the joint and a superior shift of the IGHL can be observed by tensioning the suture (Figure 8.5). Depending on the area of damage, 4–7 divergent sutures are applied (Figure 8.6). In very patulous capsules, the desired maximum inferior position of the sutures is facilitated by tightening the applied sutures, thus shifting the capsule superior and enabling further inferior sutures down to the 6–6.30 o'clock position to achieve a maximum inferior to superior and lateral to medial shift of the capsule. In very unstable cases a final 'extra-articular' suture is applied. After having entered the joint through the anterior working cannula, the shoulder stitcher is passed outside the

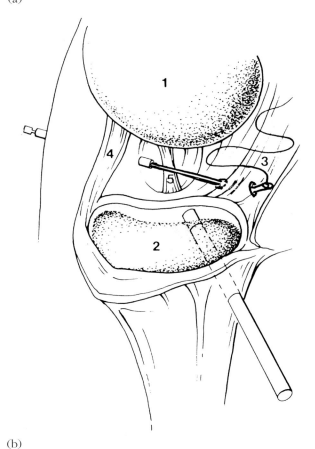

(b)

Figure 8.4

The shoulder stitcher re-enters the joint after a 15–20-mm passage through the LLC. (b) 1: Humeral head; 2: glenoid; 3: IGHL; 4: biceps tendon; 5: superior edge of the subscapularis tendon.

capsule from the superior margin of the subscapularis tendon to re-enter the joint in the 5.30 – 6 o'clock position after an extra-articular passage of 25–35 mm (Figure 8.6).

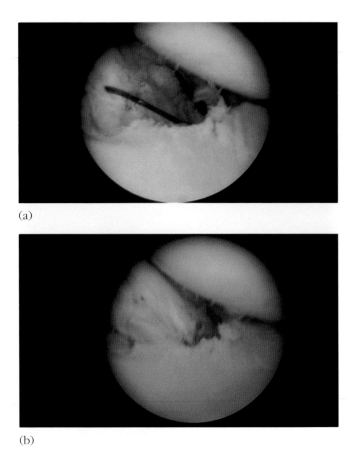

(a)

(b)

Figure 8.5

Right shoulder. (a) A suture through the anterior capsule before tightening. (b) Trial tightening of the suture results in superior and posterior translation of the humeral head and tight reattachment of the capsule to the glenoid.

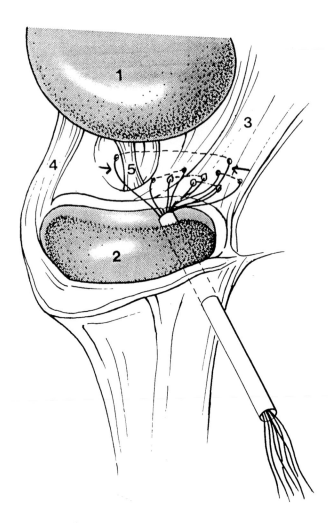

Figure 8.6

1: Humeral head; 2: glenoid; 3: IGHL; 4: biceps tendon; 5: superior edge of the subscapularis tendon. At the end of the procedure four to six sutures penetrate the IGHL. 'Extra-articular' suture is indicated by the arrow. Tightening of the sutures results in a superior and anterior to posterior shift of the LLC and capsulorrhaphy.

If this suture is applied great care must be taken to be in close contact with the capsule during the extra-articular passage to prevent damage to the axillary nerve. Tightening this suture results in an even better infero-superior and lateromedial capsulorrhaphy.

After all detached capsular structures have been grasped, the posterior working sheath is withdrawn. One bundle of the sutures is grasped with a clamp, the arm is lowered, and the strands of the other bundle are tightened. Individual suture tensioning is very important; because if the arm is adducted and brought in a neutral rotation for suture tightening, the distance at which the individual strands are in tension is much shorter for the sutures grasping the LLC close to the transglenoidal drill hole than for those grasping the IGHL or portions of the capsule more inferiorly (Figure 8.6). After tightening, all strands are tied in one knot on the fascia of the infraspinatus muscle on a 2-cm strip of woven 10-mm PDS band. The final result of the procedure is inspected from the posterior and anterior portals (Figures 8.7–8.10). No drain is inserted.

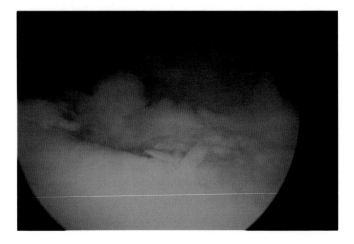

Figure 8.7

Destroyed LLC and patulous capsule as seen from posterior (left shoulder).

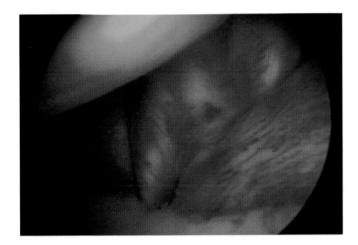

Figure 8.8

Result of the procedure as seen from the posterior portal (left shoulder).

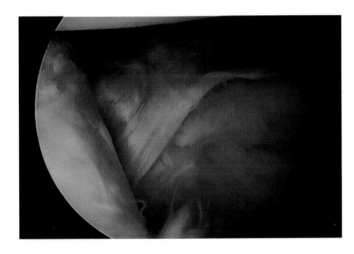

Figure 8.9

Detached LLC as seen from anterior (left shoulder).

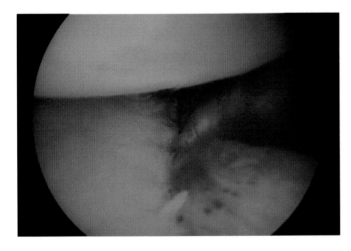

Figure 8.10

Result of the procedure as seen from the anterior portal (left shoulder).

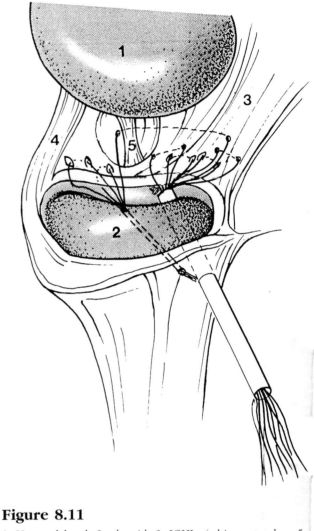

Figure 8.11

1: Humeral head; 2: glenoid; 3: IGHL; 4: biceps tendon; 5: superior edge of the subscapularis tendon. Double tunnel technique.

If the capsular detachment extends cephalad beyond the 3 o'clock position or if a SLAP lesion is encountered an additional 2.5-mm drill hole in the 2.30 o'clock position or higher can be used to apply one to three additional superior sutures. These sutures are delivered posteriorly through the same skin incision as the inferior sutures (Figures 8.11–8.13) using a K-wire with an eye or a shuttle thread. In this technique the superior sutures are tied with the inferior sutures over the posterior bone bridge between the two drill holes.

In most first-time dislocations a detachment of the labrum and only some elongation of the IGHL can be seen. If the anatomy of the anterior capsule is not destroyed in these cases the detached labrum is reinserted applying one suture in the 3 o'clock position and one suture in the 4.30 o'clock position. These sutures are brought out to the back using transglenoidal

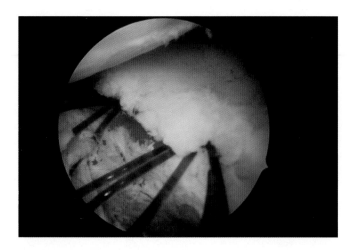

Figure 8.12

Double tunnel technique before tightening the sutures as seen from anterior (right shoulder).

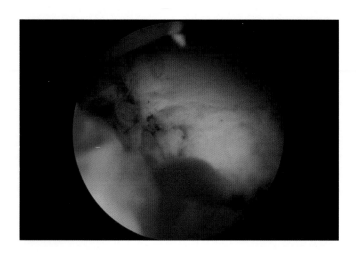

Figure 8.13

Double tunnel technique after tightening the sutures (right shoulder).

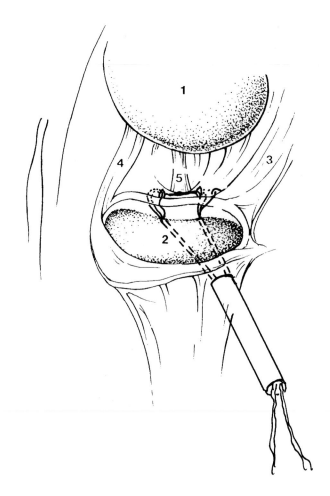

Figure 8.14

Transglenoidal reattachment of the labrum in first time dislocations with two simple sutures through the labrum and one mattress suture between the superior and inferior drill hole.

K-wires (Figure 8.14). Even better advancement of the labrum to the debrided neck of the scapula can be achieved by an additional mattress suture between the two K-wires as advocated by Morgan.[5] A #2 polyester suture is threaded through the eye of the superior and inferior pin and delivered together with the labrum sutures to the back (Figure 8.14).

This technique can also be used in some cases of recurrent dislocations if the anatomy of the anterior capsule is intact and the IGHL is not overstretched. In these cases two or three sutures should be applied in the IGHL region for a mild capsulorrhaphy and one or two sutures in the area of the superior drill hole.

Postoperative protocol

No drain is inserted. After application of skin sutures, the arm is placed in internal rotation in a flexible shoulder immobilizer for 4 weeks. The dressing may be removed to allow washing but patients are warned specifically against external rotation. Active physiotherapy is begun after 4 weeks with forward elevation and pendulum exercises. After 6 weeks abduction is encouraged. Internal and external rotation exercises are assisted by the physiotherapist after 8 weeks. Return to noncontact sports is allowed 3 months postoperatively. Vigorous activities such as high-speed (skiing, etc.), contact, shoulder, and overhead sports are not allowed for 6 months. Patients are examined 4 weeks after the operation, when the shoulder immobilizer is removed. Follow-up evaluations are made at 3, 6, and 12 months.

Pitfalls of the transglenoid technique

In the case of very hard bone it can be difficult to drill the transglenoid 2-mm K-wire as it can slip along the anterior neck of the glenoid and inner surface of the scapula. To avoid this inadvertant migration either a bony trough is made using a burr, or a short 4.5-mm Steinmann pin is tapped into the bone 2 or 3 mm, prior to drilling the K-wire. In some difficult shoulders a transsubscapularis approach is used to facilitate the inferior position of the transglenoid drill hole. After being inserted into the joint through the anterior working portal, a 5-mm sharp Steinmann pin is guided outside the subscapularis muscle downwards from the superior margin of the subscapularis muscle to re-enter the joint in the 5 o'clock position. A 6-mm working cannula is inserted into the joint via the Steinman pin. This anteroinferior portal makes precise transglenoidal drilling in the 4.30 or 5 o'clock positions much easier even in very tight shoulders. We have limited experience with drill guides such as the Concept drill guide (Figure 8.15) as advocated by Caspari[4] or other drill guides to facilitate the transglenoid drilling.

After the suprascapular nerve has passed the suprascapular notch, its main trunk runs in a lateroinferior direction directly to the base of the scapular spine. From the base of the scapular spine it curves medially and branches into the infraspinatus muscle within 1 cm. In this area it runs very close to the posterior exit of a medially directed transglenoidal drill hole. To avoid damage to the nerve the transglenoid K-wire should be drilled through the safe zone according to Bigliani et al (Figure 8.16), avoiding a too-medial angulation of the K-wire[13] as the distance of the nerve from the midline of the posterior glenoid rim averages only 18 mm (range 14–25 mm). Inferior angulation of the K-wire increases the distance of the posterior exit to the trunk of the suprascapular nerve, as it curves medially after having passed the base of the scapular spine.

By overdrilling the K-wire from posterior to anterior with a cannulated 5-mm drill bit the head of the humerus can be damaged if it is subluxated anteriorly. This can

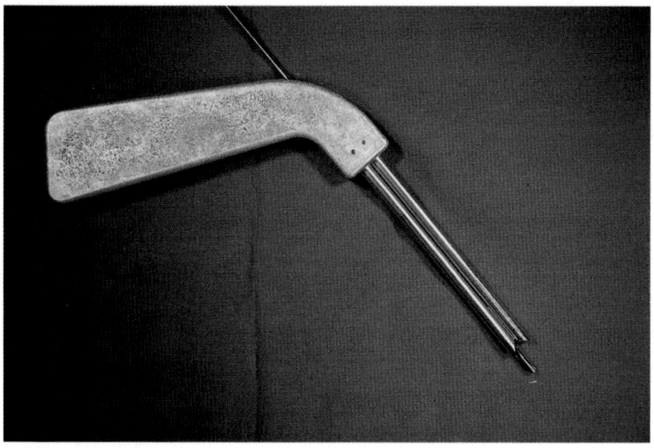

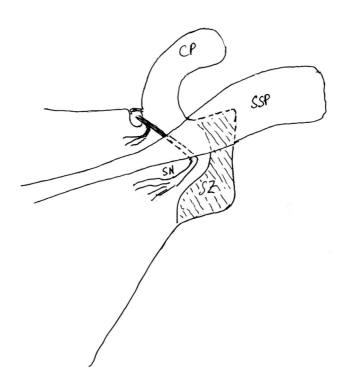

Figure 8.16

Safe zone of the posterior glenoid neck. SN: suprascapular nerve, CP: coracoid process, SSP: scapular spine, SZ safe zone.

Figure 8.15

The Concept drill guide facilitates positioning of the K-wire close to the edge of the glenoid.

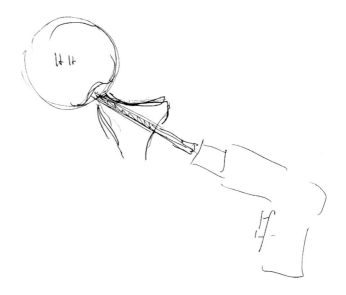

Figure 8.17

Humeral head is subluxated.

be prevented by reducing the humeral head posteriorly and pushing a 7-mm cannula from anterior over the 2-mm K-wire to protect the cartilage of the humeral head. In case of very inferior sutures in the 6 or 6.30 o'clock position the shoulder stitcher should be kept in close contact to the capsule during the extra-articular passage to avoid lesions of the axillary nerve.

Complications

In a retrospective analysis of 274 operations a complication rate of 5.1% (14 complications) was found. Six superficial wound healing problems in the area of the sometimes very large subcutaneous knot on the infraspinatus fascia healed uneventfully. In three patients a deep but extra-articular infection resulted in the formation of a sinus. All infections healed without revision or permanent impairment of the shoulder joint. As a consequence of this relatively high infection rate we have started routine antibiotic prophylaxis with 4 g cefazolin as a single-shot dose. No more infections have occurred since that time. Two cases of transient partial palsy of the radial nerve recovered fully as well as one case of complete palsy of the radial nerve. In the last case a traction injury was suspected, as at that time we used traction of 6 kg in this hypermobile and very unstable shoulder. It took 2 years to complete nerve recovery. Two cases of damage to the cartilage of the glenoid were sequelae of an inadvertent position of the drill hole. Both patients are stable and pain-free.

Other transglenoidal techniques

The most popular transglenoidal technique is the Caspari suture punch technique. The suture punch, a grasping instrument that allows passing sutures through soft tissue, is used to place from five to eight sutures into the detached labrum. The sutures are pulled out through a single transglenoidal 3.5–4-mm drill hole in the 2 o'clock position to shift the LLC cephalad. The sutures are tied on the fascia of the infraspinatus muscle. Failure rates (redislocation or subluxation) of 4–15% are reported.[4,14]

The modified (O'Neill) grasping stitcher mulberry knot technique (Maki) avoids tying a knot over the infraspinatus muscle.[7,15] The detached LLC is grasped by the grasping stitcher, a cannulated arthroscopic grasper, and shifted superiorly. Through the cannulated instrument, a 1.7-mm suture pin that penetrates the shifted LLC is

drilled from anterior to posterior. A #1 monofilament or braided suture is threaded through the eyelet of the pin. Pulling the pin out posteriorly, the suture is passed transglenoidally to the back to exit through a posterior 3–4 mm incision. The suture is cut and five knots are tied on each posterior suture end. The knots are advanced to the posterior cortex of the neck of the glenoid by retrograde pulling of the anterior end of the thread. A second thread is applied using the same technique. Both threads are tied anteriorly in the joint to create a mattress suture securing the LLC to the abraded neck of the glenoid. Two to three double sutures are applied (needing four or six transglenoidal passages). In a recent publication O'Neill[15] found a very low resubluxation rate of 5% using this technique, with no redislocations.

References

1. Reider B, Inglis AE. The Bankart procedure modified by the use of Prolene pull out sutures. *J Bone Joint Surg* 1982; **64A**:628–9.
2. Bankart ASB. Recurrent or habitual dislocation of the shoulder joint. *Br Med J* 1923; **2**:1132–3.
3. Perthes G. Über die Operation der habituellen Schulterluxation. *Dtsch Z Chir* 1906; **85**:191–227.
4. Caspari RB. Arthroscopic reconstruction for anterior shoulder instability. *Oper Tech Orthop* 1988; **3**:59–66.
5. Morgan CD. Arthroscopic transglenoid Bankart suture repair. *Arthroscopy* 1987; **3**:111–210.
6. Benedetto KP, Glötzer W. Die arthroskopische Bankart Operation mittels Nahttechnik – Indikation, Technik und Ergebnisse. *Arthroskopie* 1988; **1**:185–9.
7. Maki NJ. Arthroscopic stabilization: suture technique. *Oper Tech Orthop* 1991; **1**:180–3.
8. Landsiedl F. Arthroscopic therapy of recurrent anterior luxation by capsular repair. *Arthroscopy* 1992; **8**:296–304.
9. Landsiedl F, Meznik C. Operationstechnik und Frühergebnisse bei der arthroskopischen Behandlung der rezidivierenden vorderen Schulterluxation. *Arthroskopie* 1989; **2**:177–83.
10. Boszotta H, Helperstorfer W. Resultate der arthroskopischen ventralen Limbus Kapsel Refixierung nach primärer traumatischer Schulter Luxation. *Aktuelle Traumatol* 1993; **23**:239–43.
11. Speer KP, Xianghua D, Borrero S et al. Biomechanical evaluation of a simulated Bankart Lesion. *J Bone Joint Surg* 1994; **76A**:1819–26.
12. Turkel SJ, Panie MW, Marshall JL, Girgis RJ. Stabilizing mechanisms preventing anterior dislocation of the glenohumeral joint. *J Bone Joint Surg* 1981; **63**:1208–17.
13. Bigliani LU, Dalsey RM, McCann PD. An anatomical study of the suprascapular nerve. *Arthroscopy* 1990; **6**:301–5.
14. Torchia ME, Caspari RB. Arthroscopic transglenoid multiple suture repair: 2–8 year result in 150 shoulders. *Arthroscopy* 1997; **13**:609–19.
15. O'Neill DB. Arthroscopic Bankart repair of anterior detachments of the glenoid labrum. A prospective study. *J Bone Joint Surg* 1999; **81A**:1357–66.

9 Anterior shoulder instability: Extra-articular Bankart repair

Herbert Resch, Erwin Aschauer and Gernot Sperner

Introduction

The aim of the arthroscopic extra-articular Bankart operation is the step by step reproduction of the open Bankart procedure. The labrum–capsule complex, which has been detached from the edge of the glenoid, is reattached back onto the rim of the glenoid using an extracapsular technique.

Surgical principles

In carrying out this procedure special attention is given to the reattachment of the inferior glenohumeral ligament onto the lower third of the glenoid. Simultaneously this ligament is shifted in a mediocranial direction. The reattachment in the lower third of the glenoid is made possible by the so-called anteroinferior portal, which leads through the subscapularis onto the front lower third of the glenoid.

As anatomical studies[1,2] have shown, if the appropriate precautionary measures (see below) are taken, entry at this point is not dangerous to the bordering nerves and blood vessels. Depending on the expanse of the lesion, a variable number of implants are introduced with gaps of approximately 1 cm. The osseous edge of the glenoid is specially prepared by cutting shallow troughs in the edge of the glenoid into which the implants are placed. As a result of this preparation, despite the point fixation of the capsule, a watertight seal forms along the entire front area of the edge of the glenoid. This provides the prerequisite for the unhindered healing of the capsule along the complete edge of the glenoid. Indications for this technique are primary anterior shoulder dislocation and recurrent anterior shoulder dislocation and subluxation. Contraindications are atraumatic instability of the shoulder and a large chronic glenoid rim fragment.

Surgical technique

Typically the beach chair position is recommended. Furthermore, a special elbow holder (Lambert, Salzburg, Austria), capable of being sterilized, is placed over the drapes and holds the elbow in a 90° position, enabling shoulder rotation to be adjusted precisely during the operation. Approximately 2 kg of traction may be used over a pulley system to apply tension on the elbow holder. The pulley system is fastened to the table and holds the arm in a position abducted approximately 30°. The tension weight stabilizes the arm of the patient, which rests on the chest of the surgeon with 20–30° of external rotation so that both arms are free to carry out the operation. In the axilla of the shoulder to be operated on lies a roll of securely bound cloth approximately 10 cm thick, or a gas-sterilizable padded roll (Lambert, Salzburg, Austria) of synthetic material, which acts as a fulcrum. This permits distraction at the joint to be increased according to pressure exerted from the surgeon's hip to the cord of the weight (Figure 9.1). Two ventral portals are essential for the arthroscopic extra-articular reattachment technique.

The anterosuperior portal lies 1 cm above the coracoid process. It allows for the introduction of the probe as well as for the instruments for the preparation of the glenoid rim.

The anteroinferior portal (transmuscular entrance) lies 1.5 cm below the coracoid process on a line that begins at the palpable coracoid process and runs down parallel to the upper arm axis (Figure 9.2). Instruments used

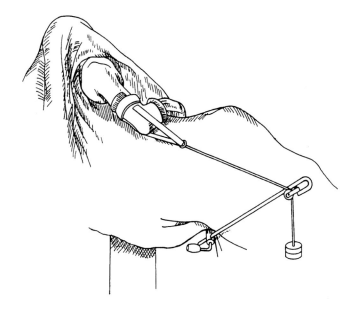

Figure 9.1

Beach-chair position for the patient: patient's arm is in a 90º elbow brace and a 2-kg traction weight is applied.

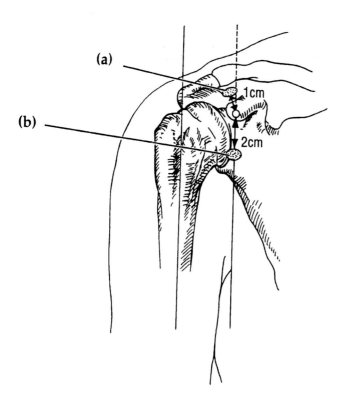

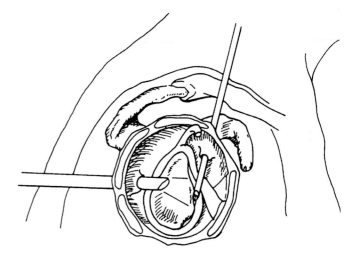

Figure 9.3

Preparation of the anterior glenoid rim: a 4.5-mm arthroplasty burr is used to cut two to three shallow notches in the glenoid rim in the 4, 3 and 1 o'clock positions so that the full width of the bony glenoid rim is visible as far as the cortex of the scapular neck.

Figure 9.2

Anterior portals: anterior portal (a) for arthroscopic instrumentation; anteroinferior portal (b) located on a line originating at the coracoid process and running parallel to the axis of the upper arm, 1.5-2 cm from the coracoid process.

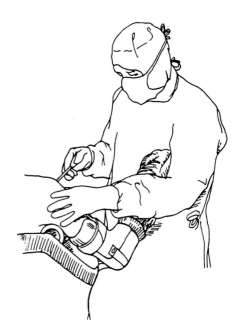

Figure 9.4

Positioning of the patient's arm for refixation in 30º of external rotation using a traction weight; the end of the weight passes round the surgeon's hip on the patient's side and ensures stable arm positioning leaving the surgeon with both hands free. A plastic roll of about 10 cm in diameter inplaces in the patient's axilla, which enlarges the joint space.

to prepare the edge of the glenoid are introduced through the anterosuperior portal through a cannula. The damaged labrum together with the capsule from the periosteal edge of the glenoid are detached using an elevator and moved deep into the neck of the scapula. The edge of the glenoid and the adjacent neck of the scapula are prepared using a 4.5-mm diameter burr. Finally, depending upon the extent of the lesion, two or three shallow troughs are cut into the edge of the glenoid, always beginning inferiorly in a position of about 5 o'clock (right shoulder). The trough is cut exactly to the point at which, with a 30° optic, the total width of the osseous edge of the glenoid, including the medial corticalis, is visible (Figure 9.3).

The surgeon is positioned in front of the patient. The patient's arm is placed close to the outer axilla of the surgeon. A roll is placed in the axilla of the patient. The cord for the weight is run around the inner hip of the surgeon (Figure 9.4).

The cannula with the blunt trocar (Smith & Nephew, Andover, MA, USA) is first introduced through the anteroinferior portal at about 45° in a dorsolateral direction, until it meets resistance (head of the humerus). The cannula is then swiveled into a dorsomedial direction and glides forward on the subscapularis tendon (slalom approach). The blunt end of the trocar is thereby contin-

ually pressed onto the head of the humerus below and moves automatically through the muscle tissue of the subscapularis until it bulges the capsule into the joint (Figure 9.5).

The cannula and trocar are moved through the muscle tissue of the subscapularis depressing the capsule into

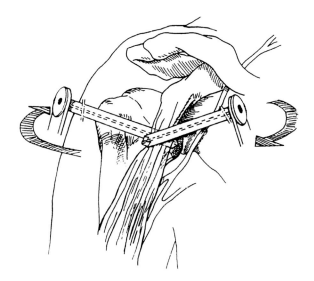

Figure 9.5

Slalom approach. The bracer is first advanced dorsolaterally (1) and then dorsomedially (2), sliding along the humeral head to the glenoid rim.

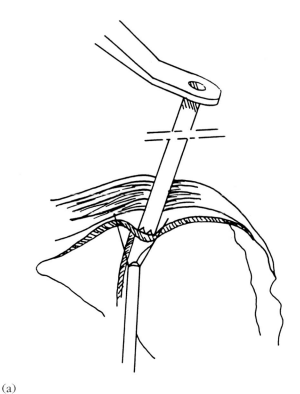

(a)

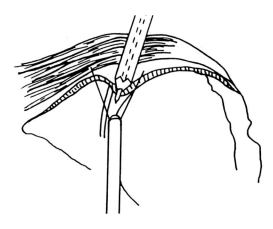

Figure 9.6

Depressing the capsule into the joint with the blunt end of the trocar; capsule perforated with the guidewire introduced.

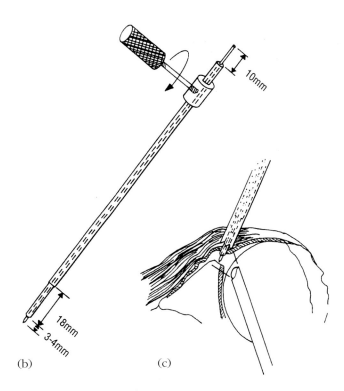

(b)   (c)

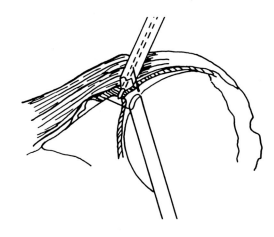

Figure 9.7

After tensioning the capsule medially and cranially, the tip is located in the inferiormost notch.

Figure 9.8

(a) After having located the ideal perforation point with the trocar, the sheath is advanced as far as possible and held in place. The blunt trocar with the guidewire is then removed. (b) Guidewire-drill combination. (c) The guidewire-drill combination is introduced and the capsule is perforated. The speared capsule is moved to the inferior notch and the tip of the wire is placed in the middle of the notch.

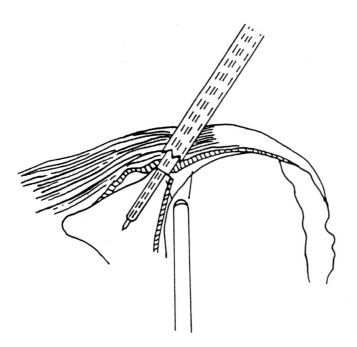

Figure 9.9

The guidewire-drill combination is drilled in up to the shoulder of the drill.

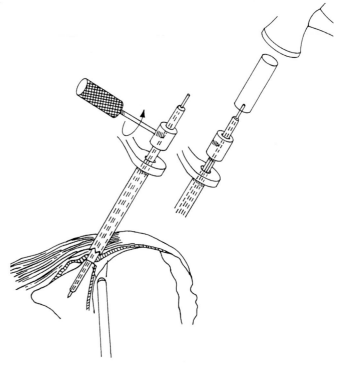

Figure 9.10

The guidewire is released and hammered home by the use of the wire handle.

the joint. The 1-mm guidewire is introduced through the cannula of the blunt trocar and the capsule is perforated at the desired spot (Figure 9.6).

The perforated capsule is led by the guidewire to the lowest prepared trough on the edge of the glenoid. The capsule should tighten in a superomedial direction. Should this not be the case, the process is repeated and the capsule is perforated in a more suitable (i.e. more lateral and distal) position (Figure 9.7). The cannula pushes the capsule forward as far as possible into the joint space and is held in position. This allows removal of the trocar together with the guidewire while the capsule remains in an unchanged position (Figure 9.8a).

The cannulated drill is introduced into the cannula together with the guidewire, which is locked in place with approximately 3 mm of the wire protruding from the point of the drill. The capsule is perforated by the wire and drill at the original site and the tip of the guidewire is placed at the center of the trough created in the bone (Figure 9.8b,c).

A power tool is used to advance the guidewire and drill into bone up to the shoulder of the drill. (The shoulder of the drill prevents overdrilling.) (Figure 9.9). After drilling, the power tool is removed from the drill and the guidewire locking mechanism is released. The wire handle is placed over the guidewire and is carefully tapped with a hammer to secure it firmly in bone (Figure 9.10). The drill handle is placed on the drill and locked in position. The drill is removed by hand leaving the guidewire in place. To prevent the guidewire from retracting (if not securely fixed in bone) when removing the drill, pressure should be applied to the wire (Figure 9.11).

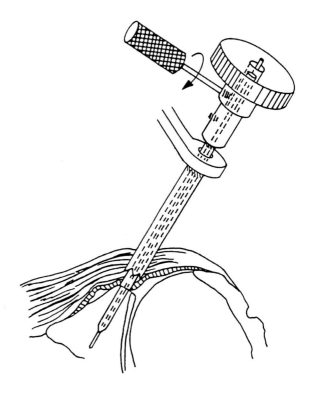

Figure 9.11

The drill is removed by the use of the drill handle, leaving the guidewire in place.

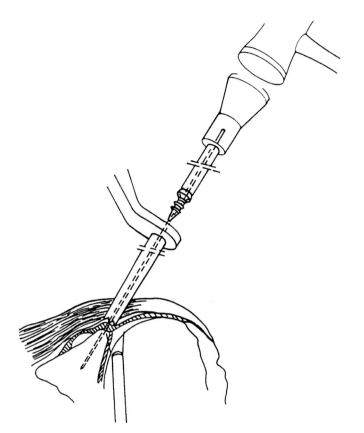

Figure 9.12

A Suretac II is introduced and hammered home till the capsule is pressed onto the edge of the glenoid.

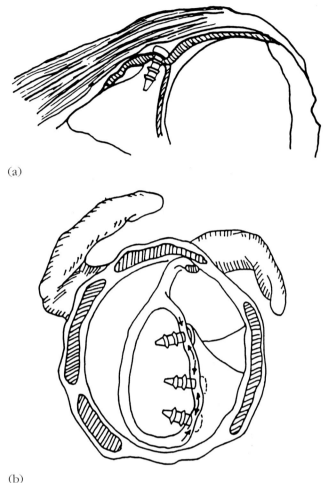

(a)

(b)

Figure 9.13

(a) The Suretac is placed in an extra-capsular (extra-articular) position. (b) Two to three Suretacs are introduced. Placing the implants in troughs also allows compression of the capsule between the implants.

A Suretac (Smith and Nephew) with a head of 8 mm diameter and spikes (Suretac II) on the undersurface of the head is introduced over the guidewire and hammered home by means of the Suretac driver (Figure 9.12).

The capsule is pressed onto the edge of the glenoid by the Suretac. If the capsule remains pressed against the glenoid when slightly withdrawing the driver and the cannula, then the Suretac has been inserted sufficiently. The guidewire is then removed using pliers to lever out the wire against the head of the cannulated blunt trocar, which is reinserted over the guidewire.

The head of the Suretac lies in an extra-articular (extra-capsular) position. Two or three implants are introduced, according to the extent of the lesion. The implant in the superior half of the glenoid is sometimes inserted intra-articularly, that is the cannula is introduced into the joint through the anterosuperior portal. Consequently, only the labrum is reattached. Placing the implants in troughs allows compression of the capsule between the implants, so that a watertight seal is formed against the edge of the glenoid (Figure 9.13).

Postoperative protocol

It is recommended that the arm be placed in a resting position on the body for 3 weeks. From the fourth to the sixth week the shoulder should be flexed no more than 90°. External rotation is allowed only up to the neutral position. After the sixth week the patient is requested to practice movements in all directions until a full range of motion is achieved. After 12 weeks sporting activities may be resumed, although sports involving throwing are not permitted until after the sixteenth week.

Results

An unbiased follow-up study was performed by two independent examiners from another country who had full access to all files and used their own inclusion and exclusion criteria. According to this study 72 out of 80 patients were followed-up (follow-up rate 90%) after an average follow-up time of 42.5 months (range 24–66). All patients were operated on according to the above described technique and all were suffering from recurrent anterior shoulder dislocation. Ninety-three per cent of the operated patients were sports enthusiasts (most of them snowboarders or skiers). The recurrency rate was 14% (seven redislocations, one subluxation and two positive apprehension tests). The average Rowe score was 97 points (range 51–100).[3] Eighty percent were excellent, 5% were good, 1% was fair and 14% were poor. The average loss of external rotation was 5°. Seventy-three percent (49/67) returned to former sports activities and reachieved the same level and 67% (28/42) returned to former overhead sports activities and also to the same level. The Constant score[4] was 94 points (range 56–100) compared with 97 points (range 80–100) on the uninjured side. There were no major intraoperative complications and there were no nerve or vessel injuries. Two patients (3%) have shown an increase in body temperature up to 38° for 3 days and an increased CRP value about 3 weeks after surgery. After 3 days all the symptoms were gone after non-steroidal treatment. This was seen as a foreign-body reaction to the Suretac material.[5] In 89% of patients at follow-up the drill holes were not or hardly visible. In the remaining 11% the visible drill hole was less than (one patient) or no more than (seven patients) 4 mm and in no case was it larger than 4 mm.

Dicussion

This technique is characterized by two criteria that differentiate it from all other arthroscopic stabilization techniques. One is the transmuscular approach through the subscapularis muscle that allows the insertion of the refixation device at the 7 o'clock position (left shoulder), which is directly in the center of the Bankart lesion. The second criterion is the extracapsular placement of the refixation device that allows an unlimited capsular shift. There were no patient selection criteria necessary for this technique except a large chronic Bankart fragment and a torn capsule.

When discussing the results of this technique it has to be taken into consideration that the follow-up study was performed by two independent examiners from another country with full access to all files of the patients. Also the inclusion and exclusion criteria were determined by these examiners. The follow-up time was a minimum of 2 years and the follow-up rate was 90%, which is very high and was very difficult to achieve.

Although the recurrence rate seems to be relatively high compared to open techniques, it has to be taken into consideration that a positive apprehension test was also seen as a failure. It should also be noted that 93% of the patients were athletes performing sports regularly at least once a week. Of these, 73% returned to their former sports activity level and 67% returned to their former overhead sports activity level. So far the study group has to be seen as a high-risk group for experiencing new dislocations.

A foreign-body reaction was seen in only 3% of the patients (two cases) with very moderate symptoms for about 3 days. No one needed surgical treatment such as arthroscopic irrigation.

In 89% of the patients the drill hole was not or hardly visible at follow-up which proves that osteolytic changes may not play a major role with the material used (polygluconate copolymer) as has been discussed in the past.[5] In no case was the visible tunnel larger than 4 mm.

We feel that for judging the quality of a stabilization technique, not only is the recurrence rate important but also the regained function. The difficulty is to find the right balance between these two contrary criteria. Taking both criteria into consideration we feel that the described technique is, while demanding, a safe and very successful procedure.

References

1. Resch H, Povacz P, Wambacher M et al. Arthroscopic extra-articular Bankart repair for the treatment of recurrent anterior shoulder dislocation. *Arthroscopy* 1997; **13**:188–200.
2. Resch H, Wykypiel HF, Maurer H, Wambacher M. The antero-inferior (transmuscular) approach for arthroscopic repair of the Bankart lesion: an anatomic and clinical study. *Arthroscopy* 1996; **12**:309–19.
3. Rowe CR, Patel D, Southmayd WW. The Bankart procedure: a long-term end-result study. *J Bone Joint Surg* 1978; **60A**:1–16.
4. Constant CR, Murley AH. A clinical method of functional assessment of the shoulder. *Clin Orthop* 1987; **214**:160–4.
5. Böstman OM. Osteolytic changes accompanying degradation of absorbable fracture fixation implants. *J Bone Joint Surg* 1991; **73B**:679–82.

10 Anterior–inferior labral tears: The new inferior portal (5.30 o'clock) and the FASTak/Bio-FASTak technique

Andreas Burkart and Andreas B Imhoff

Introduction

In the last few decades sports medicine and shoulder surgery have undergone a rapid technical evolution. With the advent of arthroscopic surgery, patient morbidity has significantly decreased. In the 1970s shoulder arthroscopy was used primarily as a diagnostic tool but by the 1980s it was utilized for therapeutic interventions.[1] With the development of special devices for arthroscopic surgery, attention was turned to the treatment of shoulder instability. The success of open surgical treatment for shoulder instability had been high, but the morbidity rate of such techniques combined with the loss of external rotation was a well-accepted consequence of open stabilization. Open surgical techniques permit repair of the medial capsulolabral complex through capsular tightening and appropriate tensioning of the capsular ligaments. A loss of external rotation may occur as a result of overtightening.[2] This has stimulated the interest in arthroscopic techniques.[2–4] Arthroscopic repair of the labrum could be anatomic and preserve external rotation. However a higher recurrence of instability was noted.[3,5]

Arthroscopic stabilization techniques are technically more demanding and have a higher learning curve than open techniques. On the other hand, the advantages of arthroscopic surgery include faster rehabilitation, decreased morbidity, improved cosmesis and diminished pain.[3,5,6] The arthroscopic techniques may be distinguished by the use of implantable fixation devices or the use of suture techniques. Arthroscopic staple capsulorrhaphy was originally introduced by L Johnson.[7] The goal was to arthroscopically reproduce the open technique of DuToit staple capsulorrhaphy. Although Johnson's arthroscopic technique had an overall failure rate of 10%, the occurrence of staple impingement on the humeral head with subsequent articular injury, staple loosening and migration, and staple breakage were associated problems with reported failure rates of around 30%.[8–12] However, the long-term results of the open DuToit technique are also disappointing, with a failure rate of up to 29%, removing the patients with a Putti–Platt procedure.[13]

Bioabsorbable devices like the Suretac (Smith & Nephew, Andover, MA, USA)[14] reduced the risks associated with metallic implants but the occurrence of postoperative synovitis and osteolysis have to be taken into account.[15] The Suretac is made of polyglycolic acid, which has a fast rate of reabsorption. In the late 1990s, several devices made of polylactid acid were developed, with promising short-term results. The advantage of using a bioabsorbable device is that it allows for an easier arthroscopic technique and placement of the device as close to the articular cartilage edge as possible.

Because of reported problems with implanted fixation devices such as the staple capsulorrhaphy, Caspari and Savoie,[16] Morgan,[17] and others[11,18,19] developed arthroscopic suture repair techniques. The sutures can be tied either externally or internally. The technique employed by Caspari, Savoie and Morgan is based on transosseous repair with placement of sutures through the inferior glenohumeral ligament complex (IGHLC) using a variety of suture-passing devices. A hole is drilled from the anterior scapular neck and out the infraspinata fossa, through which the sutures are gathered and then passed. The sutures are tied over the infraspinatus muscle. This technique requires an accessory posterior incision and there is a risk of injury to the suprascapular nerve by the transosseous pin placement.[20] Moreover, the suture should be taut over the infraspinatus muscle otherwise a gap may result at the repair site. Also the ideal orientation of the transosseous pin to create an anatomical capsulolabral repair is not easily achieved. In a rearthroscopy, Savoie found that by using the described point more than 5 mm medial to the articular surface, one creates an ALPSA (anterior labroligamentous periosteal sleeve avulsion) lesion.[21] As with the staple capsulorrhaphy, the results were variable, ranging from a success rate of 100%[22] to 53%.[23] The overall complication rate in shoulder arthroscopy (excluding recurrence) is very low. Small described the glenohumeral complication rate at 0.5%.[24]

Arthroscopic repair techniques with internal knots avoid the risks associated with transosseous passage of sutures. In 1991, Maki described a novel suture technique using internal knots.[25] He passed the sutures transosseously, but mulberry knots were tied in each suture so that the knot sat against the posterior scapula by pulling back. The remaining sutures were tied anteriorly also using an internal knot-tying technique. Other techniques, such as the FASTak™ (Arthrex, Naples, FL, USA), places the screw-in anchors along the glenoid rim. The sutures are tied down using different knot-tying techniques.[26] Suture anchors allow the capsule and ligaments to shift superiorly, bringing it close to the glenoid rim. In contrast to the Caspari technique, posterior drilling is avoided and soft-tissue fixation strength is improved. Specific pitfalls unique to this technique are that secure internal knot tying requires careful practice, and loosening of suture anchors or suture rupture during knot tying may occur. However, the reported success rate of using suture anchors with nonabsorbable sutures in 40 consecutive patients less than 20 years of age was 95%.[27] Kim et al also reported a high success rate with arthroscopic Bankart repair using a minimum of three suture anchors. He noted no differences in loss of external rotation and return to prior activity when comparing groups repaired arthroscopically and with open techniques.[28]

It is essential to determine whether the instability is purely traumatic or atraumatic, and whether it is anterior, posterior or multidirectional. The best candidate for an arthroscopic shoulder stabilization is an individual whose primary lesion appears to be capsulolabral separation of capsular and ligamentous tissue. This may have been due to a significant traumatic event with the arm in abduction, external rotation, or extension. Individuals with marked ligamentous laxity or injury may not be ideal candidates. Adolescents with a history of voluntary subluxations or dislocations of their shoulder and subsequent trauma which is now causing an involuntary shoulder dislocation, might be candidates for arthroscopic stabilization. The indication for the operation is always after the first dislocation since the recurrence rate of all unstable shoulders is high in the young patient.

Surgical technique

The anterior, inferior, and posterior labra are firmly attached to the glenoid, and separation of the labrum from the glenoid is pathologic. A Bankart lesion refers to an avulsion of the anteroinferior labroligamentous structures from the anterior rim of the glenoid. Although there is no single structure providing glenohumeral stability, the IGHLC is the structure of greatest interest.[29,30] The surgical techniques attempt to reestablish the continuity between the neck of the glenoid and the IGHLC. Reattachment of the wrongly-positioned healed ligament–labrum complex to the level of the articular surface is absolutely necessary for stability.

After the induction of general endotracheal anesthesia the patient is placed in a 'beach chair' position, which allows unrestricted access to the entire shoulder and permits free movement of the arm in all planes. A careful examination of the injured shoulder is performed under anesthesia for assessment of the degree and direction of instability. While the arm is held in various degrees of abduction and external rotation, a manual drawer test is performed in anterior, posterior and inferior directions. Laxity is graded as 0 if no translation of the humeral head in reference to the glenoid occurs, 1+ if translation occurs up to the glenoid rim, 2+ if the humeral head displaces over the glenoid rim with spontaneous reduction and 3+ if the humeral head dislocates and is locked over the glenoid rim.[31] The sulcus sign for inferior laxity is graded on the inferior displacement of the humeral head relative to the glenoid, measured in centimeters. The examination under anesthesia is compared with the unaffected contralateral extremity. The involved arm is placed in a mobile arm holder (McConnell Orthopedic Manufacturing Co., Greenville, TX, USA) in 45° of abduction and 45° of external rotation. After sterile prepping and draping of the shoulder the skin is marked to indicate the sites for the posterior portal, spine of the scapula, acromion, coracoid process and anterosuperior and anteroinferior portals (Figure 10.1). The arthroscopy is begun with a diagnostic look through the posterior portal (2 cm below and 2 cm medial to the posteroinferior edge of the acromion). If there are no contraindications, an irrigation solution with epinephrine (adrenaline) is used. With a spinal needle the anterosuperior portal is created in an outside-in technique. This portal should be located just anterior to the acromion and lateral to the acromioclavicular joint, so the needle enters just under the biceps tendon in a vertical orientation. An incision is made with a scalpel and the portal is created with a Wissinger rod. An 8-mm cannula (Arthrex) that 'screws in' permits repeated access for

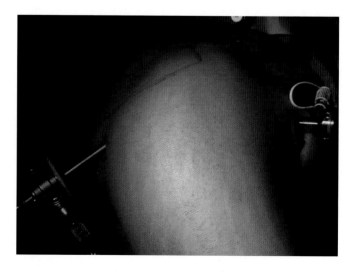

Figure 10.1

Patient in beach chair position with inserted cannulas.

passage of arthroscopic equipment and anchor devices. The superior portal is used for preparation and mobilization of the IGHLC. The use of clear cannulas is advantageous, because it allows direct visualization of the sutures and permits observation of the knot tied outside. Through this portal the capsulolabral complex is probed to judge the extent of its disruption. At this point the deep anteroinferior portal is created, also with an outside-in technique using a Wissinger Rod. We call it the 5.30 o'clock portal because this is the location in relation to the glenoid. This portal is located 8–10 cm distal to the coracoid process and lateral to the deltopectoral groove and in the axillary fold, going through the subscapularis muscle.[32] The cannula is oriented about 45°

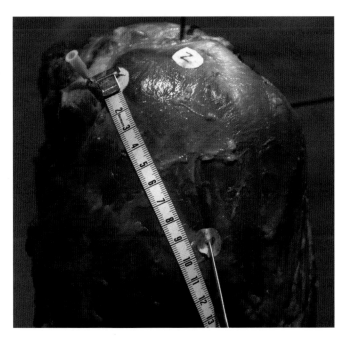

Figure 10.2

Left shoulder specimen locating the deep anteroinferior portal.

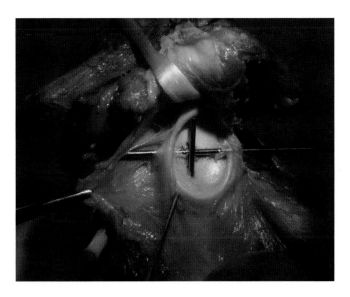

Figure 10.4

The anteroinferior portal direction at the glenoid is shown.

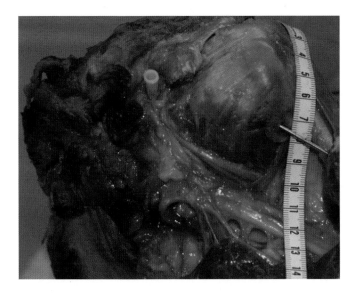

Figure 10.3

Axillary nerve showing distance to the anteroinferior portal.

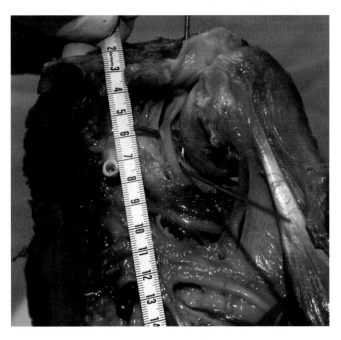

Figure 10.5

Distance between the axillary nerve and anteroinferior portal is shown, and direction and location of the anchor point at the glenoid rim.

in relation to the glenoid (Figure 10.1). This deep anteroinferior portal makes adequate placement of the suture anchor possible. Moreover, adequate shift of the IGHLC is achieved. According to our anatomic study the distance to the circumflex artery was on average 1.4 cm (range 0.5–2.5 cm), and to the axillary nerve on average 2.4 cm (range 1.5–5 cm) (Figures 10.2–10.5). It is crucial to place the superior and inferior portals as far apart from each other to prevent crowding of instruments.

Surgical principles

Poor patient positioning

Neurologic complication is the single most common complication reported in shoulder arthroscopy ranging from 0–30%. Brachial plexopathy is the most common complication, usually involving the musculocutaneous nerve, associated with improper arm position and traction use. One must pay close attention to positioning of the head, neck, trunk, and arm. It has also been reported that the beach chair position can produce a permanent quadriparesis when performed in conjunction with general anesthesia if care is not taken to position the patient properly. The critical issue is neck flexion in patients with variant spinal cord blood supply or canal stenosis producing cord ischemia.[33,34]

Poor portal placement

Anterosuperior portal

If the portal is too low, medial, or lateral, this results in problems with preparation of the glenoid. The motorized burr has to be used carefully in the region of the axillary pouch to prevent axillary nerve 'debridement'. Dissection of the glenoid too medially can damage the suprascapular nerve, and can also cause a direct injury from a superior portal that is too vertical.

Anteroinferior portal

If the portal is too high, lateral, or medial there may be difficulty placing the first anchor and achieving an inadequate capsular shift. A too inferior portal may cause damage to the musculocutaneous nerve and the circumflex vessels.

Posterior portal

The axillary nerve is at risk from a posterior portal placed too inferiorly or laterally. Also access to the joint with the arthroscope may be difficult.

Surgical technique

The Bankart lesion is prepared by initially mobilizing the labrum with a 'Bankart knife', rasp and motorized burr (Figure 10.6a–c). Usually, the IGHLC is displaced inferiorly and medially, possibly stretching to some degree. The capsulolabral separation and the IGHLC may scar in an inferior and medial position. It is important to mobilize this off the labrum of the glenoid to permit placement of the capsulolabral complex in the appropriate location and to reconstruct the IGHLC with the appropriate tension. The juxta-articular scapular neck must be debrided of soft tissue. When the labrum is elevated from the glenoid, a motorized burr is used to abrade the inferior and anterior glenoid at the 6 o'clock position. Decortication should be computed to approximately 1-cm medial to the cartilage edge. This preparation is very important because a vertical shift of the IGHLC can be achieved with good potential for healing. The rim of the glenoid is abraded adjacent to the articular cartilage until punctate bleeding bone is seen. Moreover it is important to enlarge the Bankart lesion and decorticate the glenoid rim down to the inferior glenoid. This preparation can be performed here through the anteroinferior portal. For any type of repair to be successful, the capsule must be completely released from the scapular neck, restoring the tension and advancing it laterally and superiorly. Additionally, about three or four 'target holes' are created for the FASTak at about 3.30 and 1.30 o'clock.

The 2.8 mm diameter FASTak anchor is armed with a No. 2 nonabsorbable braided suture. Through the anteroinferior portal, a 'spear' (Arthrex) loaded with the FASTak is inserted toward the 5 o'clock position. This anchor should be placed at the most inferior aspect of the glenoid, as close to the 6 o'clock position as possible. The 'spear' should be postioned immediately adjacent to the articular cartilage (Figure 10.7). This is crucial, because placing the anchor more than 1 mm medial to the glenoid rim is associated with a higher failure rate.[7] The back end of the cannulated power drill has two laser marks. The Jacob's chuck is positioned at the end of the second laser mark, so that the chuck has a mechanical stop on the guide sleeve during insertion. It is important not to stop during drilling, because the 2.4-mm FASTak anchor especially can break. The removal of the 'spear' should require one short pull.

After removal of the 'spear' the pull-out strength of the anchor should be assessed, otherwise the anchor may disengage from the bone during knot tying. Moreover the suture of the anchor should still slide. Next, the shuttle relay (Linvatec, Largo, FL, USA) is inserted with a right-angle needle at the tip of the shuttle relay. The elected area of the IGHLC has to be identified so that a medial and superior shift can be achieved. This step is the most critical step of the operation. The IGHLC should be pierced approximately 1-cm inferior and medial to the anchor placement. The tip of the shuttle relay with the

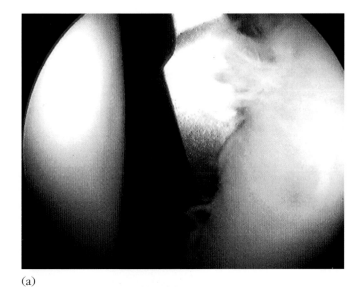

(a)

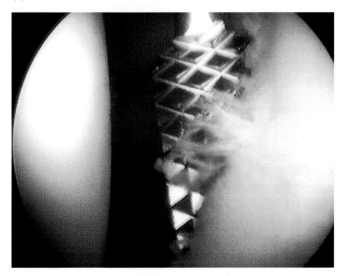

(b)

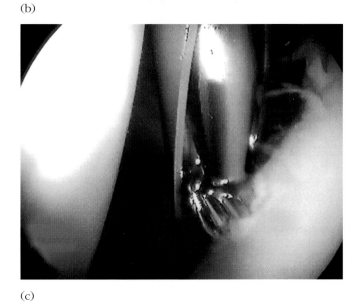

(c)

Figure 10.6

Preparation of the capsulolabral complex and the glenoid with (a) Bankart knife, (b) Bankart rasp and (c) motorized burr.

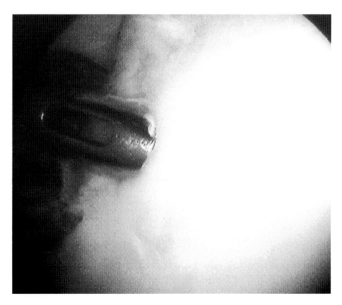

Figure 10.7

Cannulated guide at the articular margin.

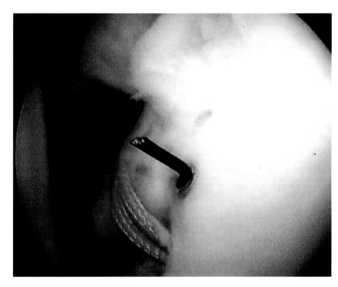

Figure 10.8

Inserted FASTak with braided, non-absorbable suture at the glenoid articular margin and inserted shuttle relay underneath the labrum.

pierced IGHLC comes under the labrum so that both together are rolled up, when the knot is tight (Figure 10.8). With that procedure the shift of the capsule can be achieved and a soft buttress along the glenoid rim can be created, thereby reconstructing the labrum. A suture retriever is brought into the anterosuperior portal and the shuttle relay is pulled back through the anterosuperior portal. In the same manner one limb of the anchor suture is pulled through the anterosuperior portal. The suture

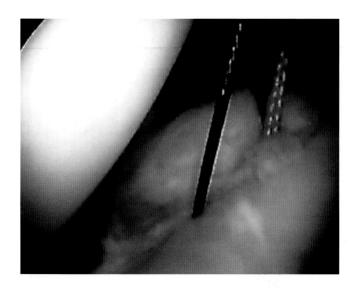

Figure 10.9

Shuttle relay system returning with the braided suture through the anteroinferior portal.

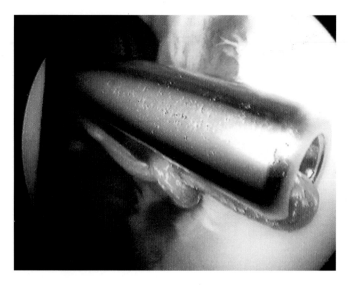

Figure 10.11

Knot tying with the sixth finger.

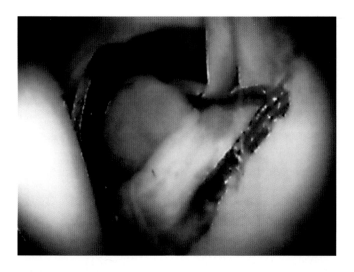

Figure 10.10

Suture is prepared for knot tying.

from the anchor is loaded onto the shuttle relay system and threaded through the capsulolabral complex, returning to the anteroinferior portal (Figures 10.9 and 10.10).

At this point arthroscopic knot tying follows with the use of the sixth finger knot pusher (Arthrex). The knot is advanced into the joint to the level of the Bankart lesion (Figure 10.11). Here one must ensure that no entanglements of the suture occur. Each suture should be clearly visualized. Two knots tied in the same direction should easily slide down and not slip. Otherwise, the repair of the IGHLC is not complete. When the second knot has been placed adjacent to the labrum, the suture may be

tightened and secured by 'past-pointing' the knot pusher into the joint. The third knot should be switched to create a knot that will not loosen. When the knot has been completed, the ends are cut with an arthroscopic suture scissors. When this most inferior anchor is in place, additional anchors are placed superior to it, for example at 3.30 and 1.30 o'clock in a right shoulder. At least three anchors should be placed. The technique for each additional anchor is the same. Placement of the first anchor is crucial to the success of the procedure, because this anchor is the first point of fixation which determines the tension in the IGHLC.

Common problems

Anchor-related problems include articular surface injury, loosening of the anchors and migrating of the anchors. These problems are minimized by adequate visualization at the time of passage of the anchors into bone and by directly viewing the anchor once seated well within the bone, and testing the anchor for pull-out before tying the suture.

Suture-related problems can include suture breakage, inadequately tied knots, and entanglements of the suture. Suture knot security is very important to maintain good apposition in the area of repair. Inadequately tied knots negatively impact the healing process and outcome. If suture breakage occurs, the FASTak anchor must be removed. This is possible by inserting the cannulated inserter without FASTak through the appropriate portal, placing it onto the inserted FASTak. In most cases it is possible to remove the 'empty' anchor

Problems with preparation are poor mobilization of IGHLC with inadequate superior shift, poor bony bed preparation with no healing of the capsulolabral complex to the bone, and medial placement of anchors with recurring instability.

Postoperative protocol

With the arthroscopic suture repair technique the initial strength of the repair does not allow early motion in all directions. The aim of the rehabilitation is to restore muscular strength, tone, endurance, and balance. After the operation the injured arm will be immobilized in a Gilchrist dressing (sling) for 24 hours. At the first postoperative day a rehabilitation program under the direction of a trained physical therapist is begun, focusing on rotator cuff strengthening and range of motion. A forceful stretching program is not allowed before 6 weeks. The rehabilitation program lasts for 3–6 months. Gentle pendulum exercises are started at the first postoperative day. Forty-five degrees of abduction is permitted immediately after the surgical procedure because experimental investigations have shown that there are no forces on the capsule and ligaments during abduction with the humerus in anatomic rotation and without external rotation.[35] External rotation is prohibited until the sixth postoperative week. After the sixth week, full external rotation is allowed. During the first 4 weeks the Gilchrist dressing is only important during the night. Patients are permitted to move their elbow and wrist without externally rotating the arm. In the first 4 weeks after surgery, we permit activities of daily living such as eating, writing, or working on a computer. Overhead activities, throwing and contact sports acitivities are not allowed for 6 months.

References

1. Stafford B, Del Pizzo W. A historical review of shoulder arthroscopy. *Orthop Clin North Am* 1993; **24**:1–4.
2. Rowe CR, Patel D, Southmayd WW. The Bankart procedure: a long-term end-result study. *J Bone Joint Surg* 1978; **60A**:1–16.
3. Cole B, Linsalata J, Warner JJ. Comparison of arthroscopic and open anterior shoulder stabilization. A two to six year follow-up study. *J Bone Joint Surg* 2000; **82A**:1108–14.
4. Jobe FW, Giangarra CE, Kvitne RS et al. Anterior capsulolabral reconstruction of the shoulder in athletes in overhand sports. *Am J Sports Med* 1991; **19**:428–34.
5. Abrams JS. Arthroscopic shoulder stabilization and repair. *Sports Med Arthroscopy Rev* 1999; **7**:104–16.
6. Green MR, Christensen KP. Arthroscopic versus open Bankart procedures: a comparison of early morbidity and complications. *Arthroscopy* 1993; **9**:371–4.
7. Johnson LL. *Diagnostic and Surgical Arthroscopy of the Shoulder.* St. Louis: CV Mosby, 1993, 304.
8. Zuckerman JD, Matsen FA. Complications about the glenohumeral joint related to the use of screws and staples. *J Bone Joint Surg* 1984; **66A**:175–80.
9. Matthews LS, Vetter WL, Oweida SJ et al. Arthroscopic staple capsulorrhaphy for recurrent anterior shoulder instability. *Arthroscopy* 1988; **4**:106–11.
10. Wiley AM. Arthroscopy for shoulder instability and a technique for arthroscopic repair. *Arthroscopy* 1988; **4**:25–30.
11. Gross RM. Arthroscopic shoulder capsulorrhaphy, does it work? *Am J Sports Med* 1989; **17**:495–500.
12. Detrisac D, Johnson LL. Arthroscopic shoulder capsulorrhaphy using metal staples. *Orthop Clin North Am* 1993; **24**:71–88.
13. O'Driscoll SW, Evans DC. Long-term results of staple capsulorrhaphy for anterior instability of the shoulder. *J Bone Joint Surg* 1993; **75A**:249–58.
14. Altchek JS. Arthroscopic shoulder stabilization using a bioabsorbable fixation device. *Instr Course Lect* 1996; **45**:91–6.
15. Burkart A, Imhoff AB, Roscher E. Foreign body reaction to bioabsorbable Suretac device. *Arthroscopy* 2000; **16**:91–6.
16. Caspari R, Savoie FH. Arthroscopic reconstruction of the shoulder: the Bankart repair. In: McGuinty J (ed.). *Operative Arthroscopy*, 1st ed. New York: Raven Press, 1991, 50.
17. Morgan CD. Arthroscopic transglenoid Bankart suture repair. *Op Techn Orthop* 1991; **1**:171.
18. Landsiedl F. Arthroscopic therapy of recurrent anterior luxation of the shoulder by capsular repair. *Arthroscopy* 1992; **8**:296–304.
19. Walch G, Boileau P, Levigne C et al. Arthroscopic stabilization for recurrent anterior shoulder dislocations: results of 59 cases. *Arthroscopy* 1995; **11**:173–9.
20. Shea KP, Lavallo JL. Scapulothoracic penetration of a beath pin: an unusual complication of arthroscopic Bankart suture repair. *Arthroscopy* 1991; **7**:115–17.
21. Savoie FH. Abstract: arthroscopic reconstruction of anterior shoulder instability. *AANA* 1993; **9**:358–9.
22. Morgan CD, Bodenstab AB. Arthroscopic Bankart suture repair: technique and early results. *Arthroscopy* 1987; **3**:111–22.
23. Mologne TS, Lapoint JM, Morin WD. Arthroscopic anterior labral reconstruction using a transglenoid suture technique. *Am J Sports Med* 1996; **3**:268–74.
24. Small NC. Complications in arthroscopic surgery performed by experienced arthroscopists. *Arthroscopy* 1988; **4**:215–21.
25. Maki NJ. Arthroscopic stabilization: suture technique. *Op Techn Orthop* 1991; **1**:180.
26. Wolf EM, Wilk RM, Richmond JL. Arthroscopic Bankart repair using suture anchors. *Op Techn Orthop* 1991; **1**:187.
27. Bacilla P, Savoie FH III, Field LD. *Arthroscopic Anterior Shoulder Reconstruction with Mitek Suture Anchor and Nonabsorbable Suture.* AANA, 4/1996, Washington.
28. Kim SH, Kwon-Ick HA, Sang-Hyun K. Suture anchor capsulorrhaphy in the traumatic anterior shoulder instability: open versus arthroscopic technique. AOSSM Specialty day, 2000, Orlando, FL, Abstract S. 70.
29. O'Brian SJ, Neves MC, Arnoczky SP et al. The anatomy and histology of the inferior glenohumeral ligament complex of the shoulder. *Am J Sports Med* 1990; **18**:449–56.
30. McMahon PJ, Dettling J, Sandusky MD et al. The anterior band of the inferior glenohumeral ligament. Assessment of its permanent deformation and the anatomy of its glenoid attachment. *J Bone Joint Surg* 1999;. **81B**:406–13.
31. Warner JJP, Janetta-Alpers C, Miller MD. Correlation of glenohumeral laxity with arthroscopic ligament anatomy. *J Should Elbow Surg* 1994; **3**(Suppl.): S32.
32. DeSimoni C, Burkart A, Imhoff AB. A new inferior portal for arthroscopic repair of the Bankart-lesion. *Arthroskopie* 2000; **13**:217–19.
33. Hitselberger WE, House WF. A warning regarding the sitting position for acoustic tumor surgery. *Arch Otolaryngol* 1980; **106**:69.
34. Wilder BL. Hypothesis: the etiology of midcervical quadriplegia after operation with the patient in the sitting position. *Neurosurgery* 1982; **11**: 530–1.
35. Debski RE, Wong EK, Woo SL et al. In situ force distribution in the glenohumeral joint capsule during anterior–posterior loading. *J Orthop Res* 1999; **17**:769–76.

11 Anterior shoulder stabilization with absorbable suture anchors

Frank Hoffmann

Introduction

The importance of the glenohumeral ligament labrum complex has been known since the first description by Broca and Hartmann in 1890.[1] In 1906 Perthes demonstrated that the detachment of the labrum is a reason for recurrent instability and emphasized refixation to regain stability.[2] This procedure was also described by Bankart in 1923 and became popular in the English-speaking world.[3]

Until the mid-1980s nearly all shoulder stabilizations were performed in an open manner. In 1986 Johnson[4] described his staple capsulorrhaphy and one year later Morgan and Bodenstab published an arthroscopic suture technique.[5] Since that time several other arthroscopic techniques have been described, including the use of screws, suture anchors, and tacks.[6–11]

We describe an arthroscopic shoulder stabilization technique using absorbable bone anchors (Panalok, Mitek-Ethicon, Norderstedt, Germany). Indication for this procedure is traumatic anterior or anteroinferior shoulder instability with a Perthes–Bankart lesion or an anterior labroligamentous periosteal sleeve avulsion (ALPSA) lesion with well-defined labrum or glenohumeral ligaments.[12] During the first anterior shoulder dislocation the glenohumeral ligaments are stretched before a Perthes–Bankart lesion occurs.[13] This elongation of the capsule and the ligaments increases with repetitive redislocation. Our experience shows that an arthroscopic stabilization with suture anchors is not successful after five dislocations. Other contraindications are multidirectional instabilities, loss of bone stock at the glenoid and the humeral avulsion of the glenohumeral ligaments (HAGL) lesion.[14]

Surgical principles

Similar to the open Bankart procedure, the torn labrum or the glenohumeral ligaments are fixed arthroscopically to the glenoid using an absorbable suture anchor molded from polylactic acid (PLA). PLA degrades through the process of simple hydrolysis which causes the polymer to breakdown to the soluble monomer L-lactide anion, which dissolves into the intercellular fluid. Total resorption time for PLA is typically between 2 and 4 years.

Besides normal arthroscopy equipment, instruments needed for this arthroscopic stabilization technique are a drill bit, a shaver system and the Mitek instruments for insertion of the anchor, perforation of the labrum and knot tying (Figures 11.1 and 11.2). The use of a fluid pump is helpful.

Special emphasis must be given in refixing the inferior glenohumeral ligament (IGHL) at the correct position of the glenoid. In comparison with transglenoid suture techniques there is no possibility of damaging the suprascapular nerve and because the implant is absorbable there is no need for anchor removal in a case of redislocation.

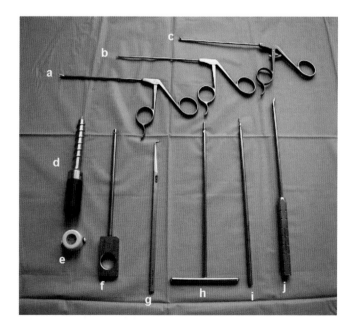

Figure 11.1

Instruments. (a) Suture retrieval forceps; (b) arthroscopic scissor; (c) grasper; (d) working cannula; (e) washer; (f) knot pusher; (g) suture hook; (h) reamer; (i) drill; (j) elevator.

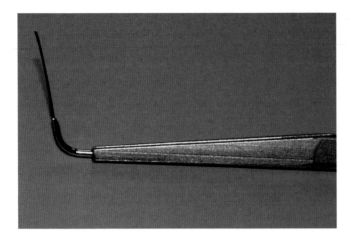

Figure 11.2

Suture hook (detail).

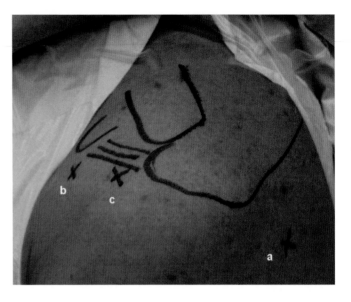

Figure 11.3

Landmarks and portals. (a) Posterior; (b) anteroinferior; (c) anterosuperior.

Surgical technique

The operation is performed under general anesthesia with the patient in the beach chair position. The forearm lies on a support in a neutral position. The operation is also possible with the patient in a lateral decubitus position and using a scalenus block. An examination under anesthesia is performed comparing the involved and uninvolved sides. After sterile draping and marking of the surface landmarks (scapular spine, acromion, acromioclavicular joint, coracoacromial ligament, and coracoid process) the arthroscope is introduced through the normal posterior portal (2-cm medial to the lateral edge of the scapular spine and 2-cm inferior; Figure 11.3). The fluid inflow runs through the trocar of the arthroscope. After routine arthroscopic inspection of the whole joint, the labrum and the glenohumeral ligaments are judged, followed by the assessment of the humeral translation in anterior, posterior, and inferior direction.

If a Perthes–Bankart lesion or a ALPSA lesion with medially displaced labroligamentous structures is found in combination with good quality of the IGHL, an anteroinferior working portal (AIP) is established. The skin incision for this portal is exactly lateral to the tip of the coracoid process and on the articular side above the superior border of the subscapularis tendon (Figure 11.4).[15] Prior to the incision the portal is located using a needle. An 8.5-mm reusable working cannula with a washer is inserted. For better visualization of the scapular neck, the arthroscope is changed to an anterosuperior portal, which is located lateral to the coracoacromial ligament in line with the base of the coracoid process. The entry point in the joint is the rotator cuff interval. Using a banana knife in the AIP, the ALPSA lesion is

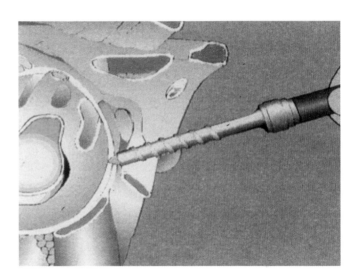

Figure 11.4

Placing of the anterior working cannula.

converted to a Perthes–Bankart lesion by dissection of the entire complex of fibrous tissue, labrum, glenohumeral ligaments and periosteum from the anterior scapula. Then a debridement and abrasion of the anterior rim of the glenoid cavity and scapula neck is accomplished with an aggressive meniscal cutter and a motorized burr. The drill guide and drill are inserted and drill holes (3.5-mm diameter, 18-mm depth) are created at the glenoid rim (Figure 11.5). To avoid any damage

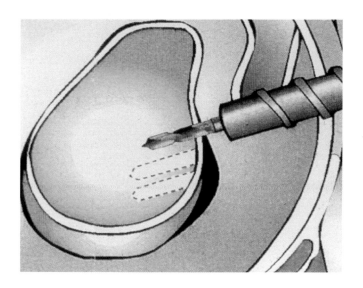

Figure 11.5

Creating drill holes.

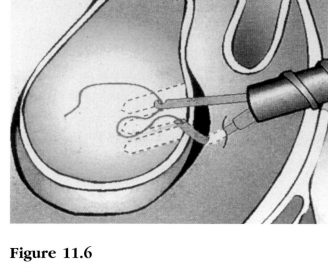

Figure 11.6

Perforation of the labrum using the suture hook.

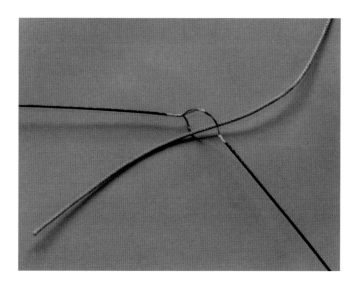

Figure 11.7

Shuttle relay suture passer.

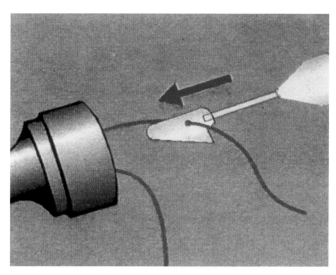

Figure 11.8

Insertion of the braided suture through the eyelet of the Panalok.

to the articular surface the drill must be angled 15–20° medially to the plane of the glenoid surface. The number of drill holes depends on the length of the labroligamentous detachment, usually two to four drill holes are sufficient. The distance between two drill holes should be at least 7 mm. The edges of the drill holes are chamferred with the T-handled reamer. For placing sutures in the detached labrum or IGHL we use a 90° suture hook (Mitek-Ethicon; Figure 11.6) and a shuttle relay suture passer (Linvatec, Largo, FL, USA; Figure 11.7). Because we prefer to use a slowly resorbable braided #2 suture (Panacryl, Mitek-Ethicon) for fixation

of the labrum, which cannot be pushed through the suture hook, we have to use the shuttle relay suture passer. Using a grasping forceps this device is drawn through the labrum; then the suture hook must be removed. The Panacryl suture is inserted in the eyelet of the shuttle and then pulled through the labrum. The first suture is inserted through the most inferior portion of the detached IGHL. The end of the suture which is nearer to the glenoid is armed with the Panalok anchor, which is fixed to the inserter (Figure 11.8). The anchor is passed down through the cannula and pushed into the first drill hole to full depth until the tapered portion

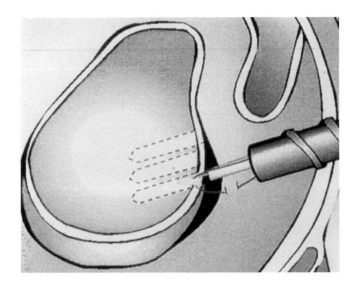

Figure 11.9

Insertion of the anchor.

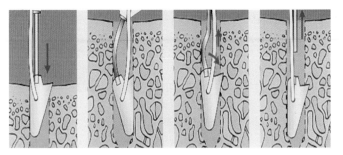

Figure 11.10

Locking mechanism of the Panalok in the bone.

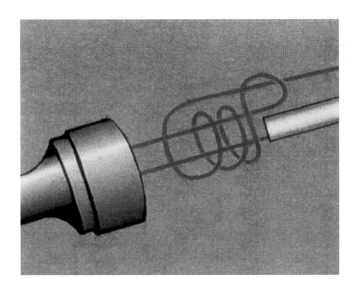

Figure 11.11

Fisherman's knot.

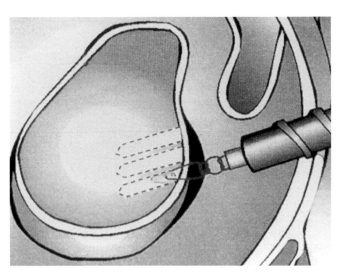

Figure 11.12

Knot tying.

of the inserter shaft bottoms against the bone or carti-lage surface (Figure 11.9). Because the anchor with its major diameter of 4.06 mm is larger than the drill hole with 3.5 mm the anchor inclines about 20° to fit the drill hole. When the anchor has been fully inserted the inserter handle must be removed by pulling in an axial direction. Afterwards both ends of the suture must be grasped and by applying tension on the length of the suture the anchor is fully engaged within the bone (Figure 11.10).

A common fishing knot is made and slid down the cannula with a knot pusher (Figures 11.11 and 11.12).

Two counterrunning knots complete the suture. The remaining threads are cut with the suture cutter. According to the length of the labral detachment this procedure must be repeated two or three times. For fixation of the proximal anchor it is sometimes helpful to switch the arthroscope to the posterior portal. The portals are closed by suture and an immobilizer and a Cryocuff (Aircast Europa, Stephanskirchen, Germany) is applied.

Another possibility that does not use a shuttle is to insert an anchor with the suture in the drill hole first and pull the threads through the labrum using a birdbeak, which is a specially designed suture grasper (Arthrex, Karlsfeld, Germany). Doing this twice, one creates a mattress suture on the outside of the labrum, which provides excellent stability of the knot without any impingement on the cartilage.

Postoperative protocol

The patients must wear the immobilizer for 4 weeks. The immobilizer may be removed for pendulum exercises and exercises to 70° flexion and 40° abduction, all in internal rotation. After 4 weeks the patient begins with flexion and abduction exercises without external rotation. After 6 weeks full range of motion exercises are allowed. Overhead sports are not allowed for 4 months and contact sports for 6–12 months after surgery.

References

1. Broca A, Hartmann H. Contribution à l'ètude des luxations de l'èpaule. *Bull Soc Anat Paris* 1890; **4**:312–36.
2. Perthes G. Über Operationen bei habitueller Schulterluxation. *Dtsch Z Chir* 1906; **85**:199–227.
3. Bankart ASB. Recurrent or habitual dislocation of the shoulder joint. *Br Med J* 1923; **2**:1123–33.
4. Johnson LL Shoulder arthroscopy. In: Johnson LL, (ed.) *Arthroscopic Surgery: Principles and Practice*. St Louis: CV Mosby, 1986.
5. Morgan CD, Bodenstab AB. Arthroscopic Bankart suture repair: technique and early results. *Arthroscopy* 1987; **3**:111–122.
6. Hoffmann F, Reif G. Arthroscopic shoulder stabilization using Mitek anchors. *Knee Surg Sports Traumatol Arthrosc* 1995; **3**:50–4.
7. Imhoff AB, Roscher E, König U. Arthroskopische Schulterstabilisierung. *Orthopäde* 1998; **27**:518–31.
8. Resch H, Wanitschek P, Sperner G. Die vordere Die Operation nach Bankart. *Hefte Unfallheilkd* 1988; **195**:205–10.
9. Resch H. Neuere Aspekte in der arthroskopischen Behandlung der Schulter-instabilität. *Orthopäde* 1991; **20**:273–81.
10. Wolf EM. Arthroscopic anterior shoulder capsulorrhaphy. *Tech Oper, Tech Orthop* 1988; **3**:67–73.
11. Wolf EM, Wilk RM, Richmond JC. Arthroscopic Bankart repair using suture anchors. *Oper Tech Orthop* 1991; **1**:184–91.
12. Neviaser TJ. The anterior labroligamentous periostal sleeve avulsion lesion: a cause of anterior instability of the shoulder. *Arthroscopy* 1993; **9**:17–19.
13. Bigliani LU, Pollock RG, Soslowsky LJ et al. Tensile properties of the inferior glenohumeral ligament. *J Orthop Res* 1992; **10**:187–97.
14. Wolf EM, Cheng JC, Dickson K. Humeral avulsion of glenohumeral ligaments as a cause of anterior shoulder instability. *Arthroscopy* 1995; **11**: 600–7.
15. Wolf EM. Anterior portals in shoulder arthroscopy. *Arthroscopy* 1989; **5**:201–8.

12 Anterior shoulder instability: FASTak/Bio-FASTak technique

Brian S Cohen and Anthony A Romeo

Introduction

Normal shoulder function represents a balanced relationship between mobility and glenohumeral stability. A large humeral head articulating with a small glenoid socket permits a wide range of motion at the glenohumeral articulation, but compromises the stability of the shoulder. Glenohumeral stability is imparted by both static (bony conformity, fibrous labrum, glenohumeral ligaments) and dynamic (muscles of rotator cuff and scapula stabilizers) structures.[1,2]

Anterior instability is the most common pattern of shoulder instability.[3] When the shoulder is in 90° of abduction and 90° of external rotation, anterior stability is derived mainly from the inferior glenohumeral ligament complex.[3] The middle glenohumeral ligament also contributes to anterior shoulder stability and is the primary ligamentous restraint when the arm is in 45° of abduction and external rotation. In the midranges of motion, when the ligaments are normally lax, the rotator cuff stabilizes the shoulder anteriorly by compressive forces across the glenohumeral joint. Recurrent anterior shoulder instability results in disability for the patient, both in terms of function and general health status. The risk of recurrence after a traumatic dislocation treated non-operatively is related to the age at which the initial injury occurred. Patients less than 20 years of age, treated 'conservatively,' have a higher risk of recurrent instability (greater than 90%) than patients over the age of 40 (less than 10%).[4,5] Therefore, a successful surgical reconstruction relies on identifying those patients who would best benefit from surgical treatment, having a complete understanding of the pathoanatomy that perpetuates anterior instability, and executing the steps necessary to restore the normal glenohumeral anatomy.

Surgical stabilization for patients with anterior instability has evolved over the past century as our understanding of the pathology has improved. Early procedures focused on approaches that are best described as non-anatomic solutions to the problem. Reconstructions such as the Putti–Platt, Magnuson–Stack, and Bristow procedure were successful in preventing recurrent instability but resulted in limited external rotation, compromising normal shoulder function.[6] Open anterior stabilization procedures that focus the reconstruction on the labrum and anterior ligaments have been more consistent in preventing recurrent instability while maintaining shoulder motion and function.[6]

Arthroscopic anterior stabilization procedures have evolved over the past 20 years. The advancements in the procedure have been driven by the improvements in the arthroscopic instrumentation, tissue fixation, and the surgeon's ability to interpret the arthroscopic findings. The primary goal has been obtaining an anatomic repair. Early results after arthroscopic stabilization procedures were less successful than those obtained with open procedures. Higher recurrence rates (15–40%) have been associated with failure to address the concomitant capsular injury, inability to anatomically repair the labrum, poor anterior tissue integrity, a lack of appreciation for the pathologic anatomy, and shorter periods of immobilization after surgery.[7,8] As a result of better understanding of the pathoanatomy, development of secure arthroscopic fixation devices, ability to address labral pathology and capsular laxity, and rehabilitation protocols that allow for appropriate tissue healing, more recent reports show results comparable to open stabilization procedures (recurrence less than 5–10%).[9,10] Arthroscopic stabilization has demonstrated 'significant improvements in operative time, perioperative morbidity, and complications when compared with the open technique for patients with anterior shoulder instability.'[11] The senior author (AAR) has performed the anterior arthroscopic stabilization procedure in more than 250 patients with traumatic, unidirectional anterior shoulder instability. The first 30 patients have been thoroughly analysed with a minimum follow-up of 2 years. There were no reports of recurrent dislocations, and 96% experienced good to excellent results.

Surgical principles

In general, the objective of an arthroscopic anterior stabilization procedure is to identify the pathoanatomy and perform an effective anatomic reconstruction. Information obtained prior to surgery is essential for understanding the etiology and pattern of instability. The patient's history, physical examination, diagnostic studies, and examination under anesthesia all contribute to the surgeon's ability to clearly define the pathoanatomy related to the unstable shoulder. The

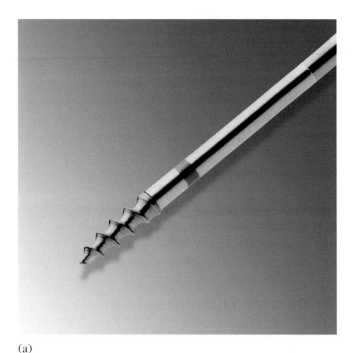

(a)

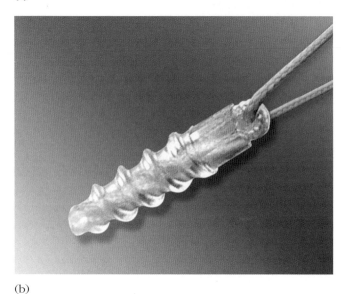

(b)

Figure 12.1

(a) FASTak suture anchor; (b) Bio-FASTak suture anchor (Arthrex, Naples, FL, USA).

arthroscopic technique attempts to restore the patient's normal anatomy by performing an anatomic reconstruction that mimics the procedure described by Thomas and Matsen[12] when there is a labral avulsion, or an anterior capsulolabral reconstruction or capsular plication as described by Jobe et al[13] when the labrum is intact. This is best accomplished by utilizing an 'anchor-first' suture anchor technique. The 'anchor-first' technique gives the surgeon the ability to first secure the anchor on the glenoid rim, and then perform the anatomic reconstruction. With other techniques available, the reconstruction

of the anterior structures may require the surgeon to simultaneously perform maneuvers related to the soft-tissue reconstruction as they are attempting to obtain secure anchor fixation.

While there are many effective anchors available, we prefer the 2.8-mm FASTak titanium suture anchor and the associated instrumentation for this anchor (Figure 12.1a). Attractive features include the 'self-drilling' suture anchor that can be placed by hand, an eyelet that allows the suture to slide for sliding knots, and a versatile instrumentation set. Furthermore, if the surgeon desires, an absorbable suture can replace the braided #2 non-absorbable suture. When an absorbable anchor is desired, the 3.0-mm Bio-FASTak is our anchor of choice (Figure 12.1b). The instrumentation for this anchor is surgeon-friendly and insertion of the anchor only requires hand-tapping of the glenoid with a specially designed 'ratcheting screwdriver handle'. The Bio-FASTak also has an eyelet that allows the suture to slide for sliding knots, and allows for the non-absorbable #2 braided stitch to be switched for an absorbable suture should the surgeon desire an absorbable suture.

Our primary goal during an arthroscopic anterior stabilization is to secure the labrum to the articular rim of the glenoid (Bankart repair) and locally plicate the capsule based on the concept and success of open anatomic repairs[12] (Figure 12.2a,b). We accept the concept that deformation of the capsule is a likely consequence of the initial dislocation, with further capsular laxity imparted after multiple, subsequent dislocations or instability events. Therefore, our second surgical goal is to shift the capsule and affected ligaments not just to the rim of the glenoid, but also in a distinctly cephalad (superior) direction. In general, these two critical goals are accomplished by placing the sutures through the tissue that is lateral and caudal (inferior) to the anchor ('anchor-first'). In order to accomplish these goals, it is important for surgeons to first understand the normal anatomy of the anterior glenohumeral ligaments. Secondly, they must have the skills to pass sutures arthroscopically and the ability to tie secure arthroscopic knots. Despite the variety of 'suture-less' fixation devices or tacks, the ability to pass sutures and tie them arthroscopically provides the most effective method to treat all aspects of shoulder instability. There are a variety of suture passing and knot-tying devices available and the surgeon needs to utilize those instruments, which allow performance of a successful, reproducible anatomic reconstruction.

The arthroscopic anterior stabilization procedure in general follows a stepwise approach to accomplishing its goal of an anatomic reconstruction. Therefore, the surgeon must pay close attention to detail and avoid excluding or performing the basic steps of the procedure out of order because this can lead to an inadequate reconstruction. The basic steps include: identifying the pathoanatomy (Bankart lesion; size and extent of Hill–Sachs lesion); proper portal placement including a

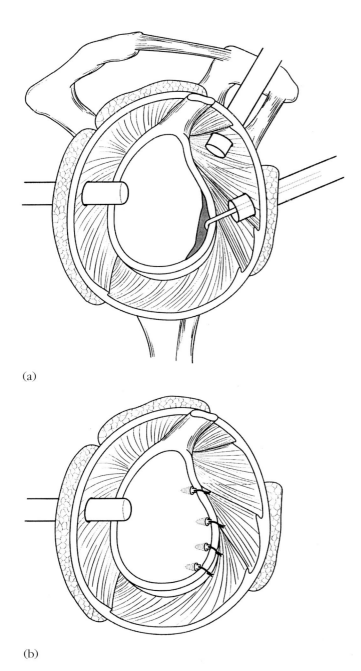

(a)

(b)

Figure 12.2

Schematic representation of (a) the Bankart lesion and (b) the Bankart repair.

standard posterior portal, a high anterosuperior portal and a low anteroinferior portal, which is essential for both tissue preparation and accomplishing an anatomic anterior reconstruction; mobilization of the anterior labrum without transecting the tissue; appropriate glenoid preparation to obtain an environment that will promote tissue healing; proper anchor placement on the glenoid rim, not on the anterior glenoid neck; pass sutures 'low and lateral' in order to obtain the proper tension within the anterior tissue structures to provide the appropriate capsular tension; and successful arthroscopic knot-tying

skills to appropriately secure the tissue, utilizing either a sliding or non-sliding knot, depending on the mobility of the suture.

Occasionally, the standard capsulolabral repair requires augmentation of the capsular plication. This can be accomplished by two additional techniques: plication of the posteroinferior capsule, and rotator interval plication. If the extent of the capsulolabral injury continues posterior to the 6 o'clock position, we establish a posteroinferior portal and perform a suture plication of the posteroinferior capsulolabral complex before proceeding with the anterior repair. Posteroinferior plication is very difficult, especially in the beach chair position, after the anterior capsulolabral repair.

Although the indications for rotator interval plication are still controversial, we use a rotator interval closure for the following indications: patients with a significant inferior component to their pathologic laxity, disruption of the rotator interval structures including the middle or superior glenohumeral ligaments, and revision stabilization procedures. Other relative indications include collision or high-contact athletes and the non-dominant shoulder of a patient with anterior instability and associated generalized ligamentous laxity.

The complications seen following open anterior stabilization procedures including neurovascular injuries (musculocutaneous and axillary nerve), 'over-tightening' of the shoulder, and subscapularis failure have been less common in patients who have been treated with an arthroscopic anterior stabilization. With proper placement of the anterior portals lateral to the coracoid process, injury to the musculocutaneous nerve is averted during arthroscopic stabilization procedures. The axillary nerve, however, can be at risk for injury when passing sutures through the inferior capsule (6 o'clock position), but this potential complication is rarely, if ever, seen with proper arthroscopic suture techniques. Although no prospective and truly randomized study has been performed comparing open versus arthroscopic anterior stabilization procedures, many surgeons believe that patients who are treated with an arthroscopic stabilization have less of a risk for 'over-tightening' of the shoulder than those patients treated with open techniques. Furthermore, since the subscapularis muscle is left intact during an arthroscopic approach, there is no risk of subscapularis failure.

One potential complication that is unrelated to the surgical approach is hardware failure. Anatomic reconstructions that utilize suture anchors or 'bio-tacks' run the risk of 'hardware failure.' Since utilizing the 2.8-mm FASTak and the 3.0-mm Bio-FASTak we have not experienced this problem. It is very likely that any metal anchor that is 'loose' on radiographs was probably never secure in the bone. Absorbable fixation devices may be associated with an inflammatory osteolysis and subsequent bone erosion or cyst, but we have not seen this complication using the Bio-FASTak. The most worrisome complication following a stabilization procedure is recurrent instability. Since more attention has been given to an appropriate anatomic reconstruction and a controlled rehabilitation program, the risk of recurrence following an arthroscopic stabilization has matched the results following open stabilization procedures.

Surgical technique

Obtaining the correct diagnosis is critical to the success of any type of stabilization procedure. The exam under anesthesia is crucial to a complete understanding of the direction of instability. All patients are examined after induction of general anesthesia. Both shoulders are evaluated beginning with the non-affected side. Humeral head translation is classified based on the following scale: 1+, the humeral head can be translated further in an anterior or posterior direction than the contralateral shoulder; 2+, the humeral head can be subluxated over the glenoid rim, but will spontaneously reduce when the applied force is removed; or 3+, the humeral head can be locked over the glenoid rim.[14] Examination for inferior instability is performed, and all findings are recorded and compared with the contralateral, normal shoulder.

When the surgeon is confident that the instability pattern is anterior, positioning for an arthroscopic anterior stabilization can begin. We have utilized the modified beach-chair position for this procedure (Figure 12.3). However, if there is a significant inferior component to the patient's pattern of instability, or a potential diagnosis of multidirectional instability with primarily anterior symptoms, our preference is to use the lateral position due to the improved access to the inferior and posterior capsuloligamentous structures. The patient is moved to the operative side of the table, exposing the posterior aspect of their symptomatic shoulder. All pressure points are padded appropriately, and the head is secured with three-inch cloth tape in the neutral position. We have not found the need to utilize any special equipment to position and secure the head, although their use has been advocated by many other surgeons. Before skin incisions, the shoulder and upper extremity are prepped and draped in the standard sterile surgical fashion. All bony landmarks are outlined around the shoulder utilizing a sterile marking pen, beginning with the notch formed by the scapular spine posteriorly and the clavicle anteriorly. The acromion, acromioclavicular joint and the coracoid process also are identified and marked for orientation throughout the procedure (Figure 12.4). Although skin markings seem to be a trivial point, the soft tissue distention of the shoulder during the surgical procedure can deceive the surgeon and lead to improper portal placement or inefficient use of instrumentation, which can be minimized with consistent orientation to the bony structures by means of the skin markings.

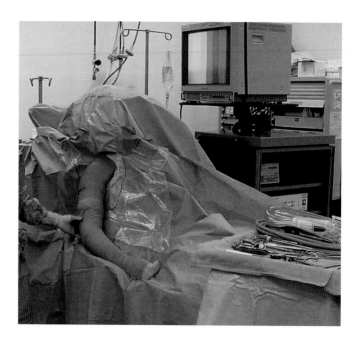

Figure 12.3
Modified beach-chair position.

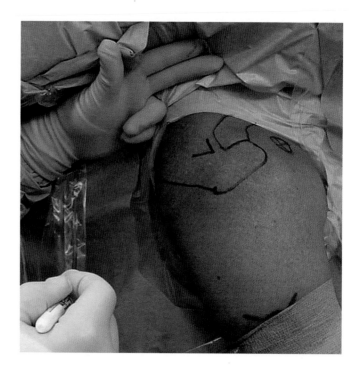

Figure 12.4
Anatomic landmarks.

A standard posterior portal is made after the subcutaneous tissue is infiltrated with 0.25% of a local anesthetic combined with epinephrine. This portal is positioned approximately 2 cm inferior and 1–2 cm medial to the posterolateral corner of the acromion in the 'soft-spot'. The arthroscope is introduced into the glenohumeral joint and a brief diagnostic evaluation is

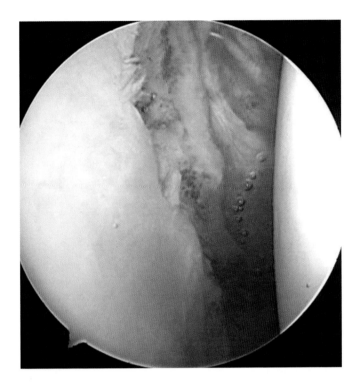

Figure 12.5
Bankart lesion.

Diagnostic arthroscopic evaluation of the shoulder

The diagnostic arthroscopy begins with a careful inspection of the biceps tendon and the biceps anchor. The posterior glenoid and posterior band of the inferior glenohumeral ligament are evaluated, followed by the posterior aspect of the humeral head. The bare area of the humeral head and the insertion site of the infraspinatus tendon are examined, as well as the posterolateral aspect of the humeral head to document the presence of the frequently seen Hill–Sachs lesion. The arthroscope is then brought over the top of the humeral head to evaluate the supraspinatus, the biceps tendon as it exits the shoulder and the superior portion of the subscapularis tendon. The arthroscope is then drawn back medially into the glenohumeral joint and the anterior structures are inspected.

The superior glenohumeral ligament is seen attaching on the glenoid anterior to the biceps anchor, then follows a course parallel to the biceps tendon leading over to its attachment anterior and inferior to the biceps as the bicep tendon exits the glenohumeral joint. The middle glenohumeral ligament can have a variable attachment and thickness, and occasionally be absent. When present, it traverses the upper border of the subscapularis tendon at a consistent 45° angle. The inferior glenohumeral ligament originates at or slightly above the glenoid equator marked by the subtle glenoid sulcus, which corresponds to the 3 o'clock position in a right shoulder (9 o'clock position, left shoulder). The inferior glenohumeral ligament complex is defined by the anterior band, a hammock-like axillary pouch inferiorly, and the posterior band.

A Bankart lesion is defined by a capsulolabral injury involving the anterior band of the inferior glenohumeral ligament complex with variable capsular deformity. The Bankart lesion can generally be assessed while viewing from the posterior portal, but substantial medial displacement of the capsulolabral complex requires a view from the anterosuperior portal for a complete evaluation. The diagnostic portion of the examination from the posterior portal is completed with an examination of the subscapularis tendon and its insertion on to the humerus, and an evaluation of the subscapularis recess looking for the presence of any osteochondral loose bodies.

Using a switching-stick technique, a smooth metal rod is placed under direct vision through the anterior cannula into the glenohumeral joint. The arthroscope is then removed from its sheath and a second metal rod is passed through the posterior cannula. Both cannulas are removed and placed into the shoulder over the opposite switching stick. The metal rods are removed, and the scope is introduced through the anterosuperior portal. The diagnostic portion of the procedure is completed with a re-evaluation of the Bankart lesion, the extent of the Hill–Sachs defect if present, and a

performed to confirm the presence of an anterior labral lesion (Bankart lesion) (Figure 12.5). Once the labral lesion is identified, attention is then directed towards creating an anterosuperior portal using an inside-out technique. This is executed by advancing the arthroscope superior to the biceps tendon and into the rotator interval. The arthroscope is then withdrawn from its sheath, and a Wissinger rod is advanced through the cannula. The rod is passed through the anterosuperior capsule of the rotator interval, below the coracoacromial ligament and into the subcutaneous tissue lateral to the coracoid process. The skin is infiltrated with the local anesthetic and epinephrine, and a skin incision is made over the Wissinger rod. An anterior cannula (5.7 mm; Arthrex) is then advanced over the rod and into the glenohumeral joint. The outflow tubing is switched to this anterosuperior cannula to establish directional flow of fluid. The Wissinger rod is removed, and the arthroscope is reintroduced into the shoulder through the posterior cannula. The anterior cannula is moved anterior then inferior to the biceps tendon. A complete diagnostic examination of the glenohumeral joint is performed. Patients with a history of a traumatic anterior shoulder dislocation can have additional intra-articular injuries other than a Bankart lesion, such as a large Hill–Sachs lesion, a superior labral tear (5–8% incidence with a Bankart lesion), a rotator cuff tear or an anterior glenoid rim fracture (bony Bankart).[15]

more thorough re-examination of the posterior structures including the posterior glenoid, posterior labrum and rotator cuff. The cannulas are then switched back to their original positions by using the switching-stick technique as described above.

After completion of the diagnostic examination of the shoulder, focus is shifted to the establishment of an anteroinferior portal. The approach to the anteroinferior aspect of the glenoid can be very challenging. The standard anteroinferior portal illustrated in most technique guides describes placement of this portal at the superior edge of the subscapularis tendon.[3] The angle of the portal above the subscapularis tendon makes placement of the arthroscopic fixation device at the anteroinferior corner of the glenoid very difficult, and possibly compromises the appropriate positioning of this crucial point of fixation. Furthermore, highly specialized instrumentation is required to pass suture through the tissue at the 6 o'clock position if the standard portal above the subscapularis is used. With the use of a trans-subscapularis portal, also known as the 5 o'clock portal, a direct approach to the antero-inferior corner of the glenoid can be achieved.[16] This portal is established using an 'outside-in' localization technique. We first localize the appropriate position of the portal with an 18-gauge spinal needle. The entry point into the glenohumeral joint should be 1–1.5 cm below the upper edge of the middle glenohumeral ligament. The skin is incised 3 cm below the standard anterior portal, and a small Wissinger rod is introduced into the glenohumeral joint at the previously documented position (Figure 12.6). The portal is established with increasing diameter cannulated dilation instruments (Arthrex) placed over the Wissinger rod until the appropriate soft-tissue dilation is obtained. A large screw-in disposable cannula is then advanced into the shoulder over the rod (8.25 mm; Arthrex). The cannula must be large enough to allow unimpeded positioning of the suture-passing instrument that the operating surgeon is most comfortable using. Establishing the 5 o'clock portal allows direct access to the Bankart lesion and anteroinferior quadrant of the glenohumeral joint.

Glenoid preparation

Glenoid preparation begins with mobilization of the capsulolabral avulsion. Adequate mobilization ensures that the avulsed labrum and capsule will be reparable back to their anatomic origin. An arthroscopic elevator is introduced into the shoulder through the antero-superior portal while viewing from the posterior portal (Figure 12.7). The elevator is positioned between the injured capsulolabral complex and the anterior glenoid. It is important to position the elevator parallel to the labrum to avoid transecting the labrum, which can dramatically complicate the surgical repair. The soft tissues are elevated beginning superiorly from the 3

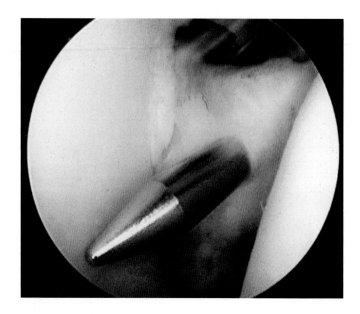

Figure 12.6
5 o'clock portal.

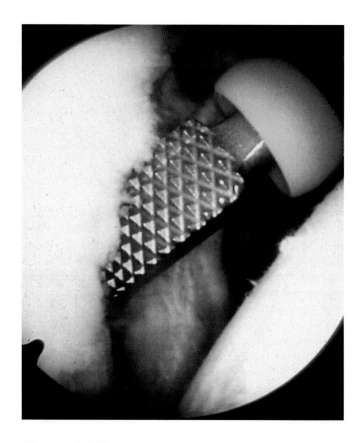

Figure 12.7
Mobilization of the anterior capsulolabral structures.

o'clock position in a right shoulder (9 o'clock position, left shoulder) and proceeding inferiorly to at least the 6 o'clock position. The dissection is continued medially along the anterior glenoid neck 1.5–2 cm until the muscular fibers of the subscapularis are visualized. To make certain the tissues are appropriately mobilized off the anteroinferior glenoid region to the 6 o'clock position, the elevator is instrumented through the anteroinferior portal to finalize the mobilization at the inferior aspect of the glenoid. If the capsulolabral injury continues past the 6 o'clock position, it may be necessary to establish an accessory posterolateral portal to access the posteroinferior quadrant of the glenohumeral joint.

A soft tissue grasper is introduced through the anterosuperior portal to assess the mobility of the capsulolabral complex and document that this structure can be repaired back to its anatomic position without excessive tension. A motorized shaver is used to remove soft tissue from the glenoid rim and neck, followed by a hooded arthroscopic burr to debride the anterior glenoid neck down to bleeding bone. Care should be taken to avoid damaging to the anterior capsulolabral structures. The area debrided should include the anterior glenoid neck from the articular cartilage to 1.5–2 cm medially, beginning at the 3 o'clock position and progressing to the 6 o'clock position in a right shoulder. Using the switching-stick technique as outlined above, the scope can be placed through the anterosuperior portal to assess the final glenoid preparation (Figure 12.8).

Suture anchor placement and Bankart repair

An anchor-first technique is used to repair the capsulolabral lesion. The advantage of this method is that it allows separation of anchor placement and tissue repair. Separating these two critical steps facilitates the goal of an anatomic repair of the labrum with a capsular shift in a superior and medial direction.

The first anchor is placed at the 5:30 o'clock position in a right shoulder (Figure 12.9). A targeting trochar within an anchor-specific cannula is placed through the

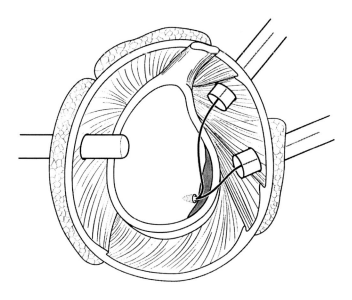

Figure 12.9

Schematic representation of first anchor placement, 5:30 o'clock or lower, in a right shoulder.

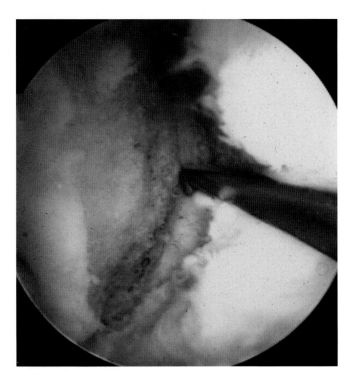

Figure 12.8

Completed glenoid preparation viewed from the anterosuperior portal.

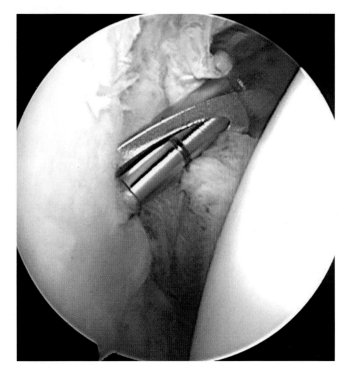

Figure 12.10

Proper anchor placement on the glenoid rim.

anteroinferior portal to ensure proper anchor placement. Correct positioning of the anchor on the glenoid articular edge is essential to the success of the procedure if a simple suture repair configuration is used. The anchor should enter the glenoid approximately 2 mm on the articular rim, with a medial inclination of 45° (Figure 12.10). Without traction on the arm, a gentle posterior force on the humerus using the targeting device allows for the optimal angle for anchor insertion. The anchor is manually screwed in until it is positioned well below the cortex of the glenoid bone, not just below the articular cartilage. For the 2.8-mm FASTak suture anchor, a laser mark on the insertion device assists in determining the correct depth of insertion. For the 3.0-mm Bio-FASTak suture anchor, the anchor is appropriately seated when the 'driver handle firmly contacts the insertion handle.' For both anchors, the inserter is disengaged from the anchor by pulling longitudinal traction on the handle. Close monitoring of the suture during this maneuver will avoid inadvertent unloading of the suture from the anchor. If the anchor needs to be withdrawn before it is properly seated, it should be unscrewed, rather than pulled out, to avoid inadvertently unloading the anchor from the insertion handle.

Once the anchor is implanted, the two suture limbs are separated. The inferior limb is retrieved through the anterosuperior portal (Figure 12.11a,b). This is accomplished by using a suture-retrieval device such as a crochet hook. It is important to pay close attention to suture management to avoid crossing or tangling of the sutures and to prevent unloading of the suture from the anchor. To appreciate the appropriate site to secure the capsulolabral tissue, a soft-tissue grasper is placed through the anterosuperior portal and the tissue is manually reduced to its anatomic position. A soft-tissue suture-retrieval device is then passed through the capsulolabral lesion at a position 5–10 mm inferior and 1.0–1.5 cm lateral to where the anchor is placed, depending on the amount of shift or capsulorrhaphy that is desired (Figure 12.12a,b). The suture from the anterosuperior portal is captured with the suture retrieval device, which is then pulled through the capsulolabral tissue. This limb of the suture will function as the post for the arthroscopic knot. Before tying the knot, a knot pusher is passed over one limb of the suture to ensure that the limbs are not tangled. The limb of the suture that will be the post is verified to maintain the knot on the non-articular side of the repair over soft tissue.

A sliding Duncan loop knot that is locked with switched-post, reversed direction half-hitches is our preferred technique (Figure 12.13). However, if the suture does not slide easily, a reversed direction,

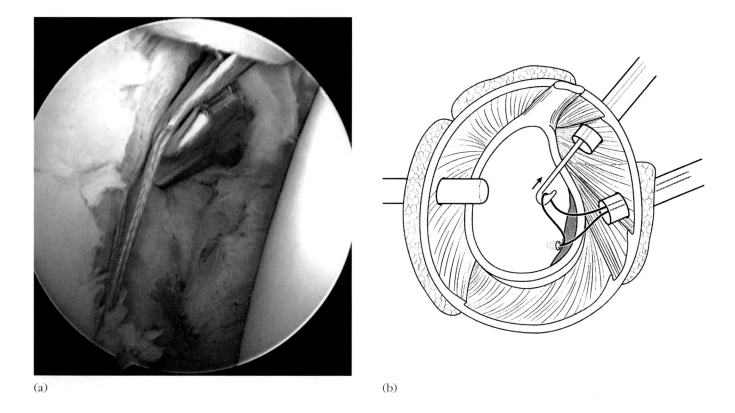

(a)

(b)

Figure 12.11

(a,b) Once the anchor is implanted, the two suture limbs are separated. The inferior limb is retrieved through the anterosuperior portal.

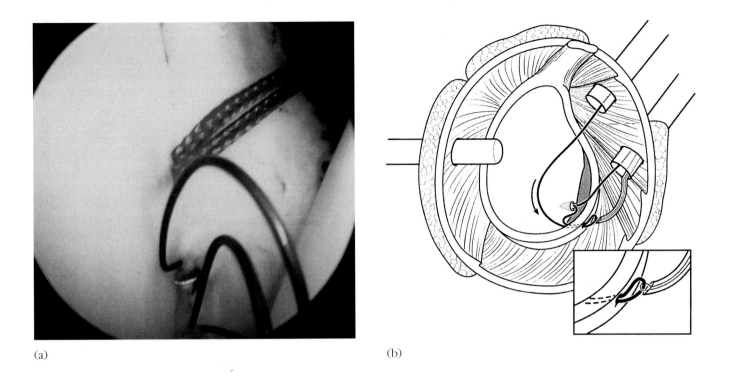

(a)   (b)

Figure 12.12

(a,b) Suture placement in capsulolabral tissue. A suture-retrieval device (or a suture-passing device) should be passed through the capsule and labrum inferior to the anchor and approximately 1–1.5 cm lateral to the medial edge.

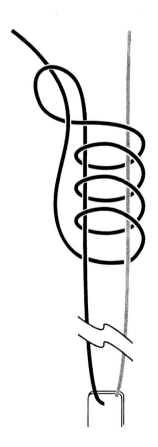

Figure 12.13

Schematic representation of the Duncan loop.

switched-post, multiple half-hitch knot (Revo knot) is also a very effective and secure method of tying the suture. Loutzenheiser et al[17] have shown that these two knots have the 'highest knot-holding capacity when compared with other knot configurations for braided suture.' They also showed 'no significant differences in the holding capacity between configurations tied by hand compared with those tied with a knot pusher.'

At least two more anchors are placed in a similar manner on the articular surface of the glenoid rim, using the same insertion techniques. The second anchor is placed at the 4 o'clock position and the third at the 2 o'clock position for a right shoulder. As each anchor is placed, the sutures are passed and the soft tissues tied down in their anatomic positions as described above. By securing the soft tissues to the anchor before seating an additional anchor, evaluation of the repair and appropriate adjustments are possible with subsequent anchors. Furthermore, suture management is easily accomplished. Once the repair is completed (Figure 12.14), the probe is introduced through the anterosuperior and antero-inferior portals to evaluate the quality of the repair. The repair is also evaluated with visualization from the anterosuperior portal.

The arthroscope and all cannulas are then removed and the shoulder is taken through a gentle range of motion. The post-stabilization change in external rotation, the resistance to anterior translation, and the ability of the humeral head to remain centered within

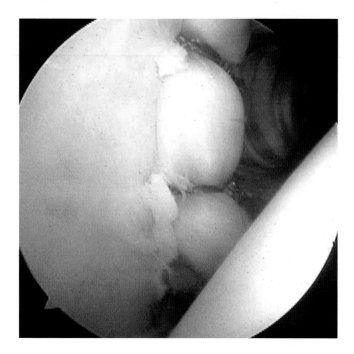

Figure 12.14

Arthroscopic view of the completed Bankart repair. Note the augmentation of the glenoid labrum producing a bumper effect.

the glenoid is evaluated and documented. The surgical incisions are closed with interrupted 3-0 monofilament suture. The glenohumeral joint is infiltrated with 20 cc of bupivacaine with epinephrine and the patient is placed in a sling or shoulder immobilizer.

Postoperative protocol

The patient is seen in the office 7–10 days after surgery for suture removal. During the first postoperative week, the patient may remove his or her sling for range of motion maneuvers of the elbow and wrist and grip strengthening. After 2–3 weeks of immobilization, the patient will begin a comprehensive rehabilitation program. Sling immobilization when not exercising continues for the first 4 weeks after surgery primarily for protection against an unexpected external rotation, especially at night. Shoulder motion movements are limited to active-assisted and active range-of-motion exercises for the first 8 weeks to avoid unnecessary and potentially harmful manipulation by anyone other than the patient. This guideline is adjusted depending on the experience of the therapist or athletic trainer and the ability of the patient to attain early range-of-motion goals. Range-of-motion goals by the end of 4 weeks are 140° of forward flexion, 45° of neutral abduction, and 45° of external rotation with the arm at the side. Internal

rotation can progress as tolerated. Shoulder strengthening is started at 2–4 weeks and is restricted to isometric exercises for the rotator cuff and deltoid with the patient's arm at their side. Scapula muscle strengthening such as shrugs, protraction and retraction can also begin. Fitness exercises are restricted to non-impact activities such as stair climbing or stationary bicycling.

After 4 weeks, the sling is discontinued. Goals for active shoulder motion by 8 weeks after surgery are increased to within 20° of the contralateral shoulder. Rotator cuff strengthening is advanced to isotonic strengthening with theraband tubing and light weights under strict control. These exercises are performed within the range-of-motion limitations. Strengthening exercises are expanded to include closed and eventually open chain exercises for the deltoid and scapular-stabilizing musculature. From weeks 8–12 after surgery, the motion goals for the shoulder are to regain greater than 90% of full motion comparable to the normal side. This is accomplished with both active and passive motion exercises. Manipulation to increase the combined motion of abduction and external rotation is avoided, unless an athlete requires this motion for his or her sports-related activity, or he or she lags substantially behind the range-of-motion goals. Strengthening of all muscles around the shoulder including the rotator cuff, deltoid, and scapula stabilizers are advanced as tolerated. To strengthen the muscles, we recommend 8–12 repetitions per exercise for three sets to the point of fatigue, but not complete loss of strength. Athletes should train with a well-intentioned partner or trainer. In general, strengthening exercises are performed three times per week, but can be reduced to two times per week if muscle recovery after the workout is delayed. We strongly discourage the popular practice in the USA of high repetition (greater than 30) strengthening exercises on a daily basis because this regimen does not allow the muscle to recover effectively between workouts. Fatigue gradually results in symptoms of tendonitis with activity and soreness at rest that slows the rehabilitation process down.

At 12 weeks after surgery, patients are allowed to return to pre-injury conditioning programs. Range-of-motion exercises are continued. Strengthening of the entire kinematic chain, including the lower extremities and torso musculature, is encouraged because this is essential for a successful recovery of sport-related abilities. Functional strengthening begins during this stage of rehabilitation and includes plyometric and proprioception training routines. A gradual resumption of sport-specific exercise, preferably under the tutelage of an experienced athletic or personal trainer, is recommended before a full return to sports is attempted. Return to non-contact sports and manual labor type vocations are possible for some at 3 months. Contact or collision sport participation is approved after 6 months if the athlete has been compliant with the rehabilitation program and has achieved adequate strength to safely participate in the sport. Most laborers and others with strenuous work responsibilities will be able to return to full duty without restrictions by 6 months after surgery. Maximum medical improvement is expected by 12 months after surgery.

References

1. Bowen MK, Warren RF. Ligamentous control of shoulder stability based on selective cutting and static translation experiments. *Clin Sports Med* 1991; **10**:757–82.

2. Howell SM, Galinat BJ. The glenoid–labral socket. A constrained articular surface. *Clin Orthop* 1989; **243**:122–5.

3. Warner JJP, Flatow EL. Anatomy and biomechanics. In: Bigliani LU, ed. *The Unstable Shoulder.* Rosemont, IL: American Academy of Orthopaedic Surgeons, 1996, 1–24.

4. McLaughlin HL, Cavallaro WU. Primary anterior dislocation of the shoulder. *Am J Surg* 1950; **80**:615–21.

5. Rowe CR. Acute and recurrent anterior dislocations of the shoulder. *Orthop Clin North Am* 1980; **11**:253–70.

6. Rokito AS, Namkoong S, Zuckerman JD, Gallagher MA. Open surgical treatment of anterior glenohumeral instability: an historical perspective and review of the literature. *Am J Orthop* 1998; **27**:723–5.

7. Grana WA, Buckley PD, Yates CK. Arthroscopic Bankart suture repair. *Am J Sports Med* 1993; **21**:348–53.

8. Green MR, Christensen KP. Arthroscopic Bankart procedure: two to five year follow-up with clinical correlation to severity of glenoid labral lesion. *Am J Sports Med* 1995; **24**:59–69.

9. Bacilla P, Field LD, Savoie FH III. Arthroscopic Bankart repair in a high demand patient population. *Arthroscopy* 1997; **13**:51–60.

10. Wolf EM, Wilk RM, Richmond JC. Arthroscopic Bankart repair using suture anchors. *Op Tech Orthop* 1991; **1**:184–91.

11. Green MR, Chistensen KP. Arthroscopic versus open Bankart procedures: a comparison of early morbidity and complications. *Arthroscopy* 1993; **9**:371–4.

12. Thomas SC, Matsen FA. An approach to the repair of avulsion of the glenohumeral ligaments in the management of traumatic anterior glenohumeral instability. *J Bone Joint Surg* 1989; **71A**:506–13.

13. Jobe FW, Giangarra CE, Kuitne RS. Anterior capsulolabral reconstruction of the shoulder in athletes in overhand sports. *Am J Sports Med* 1991; **19**:428–34.

14. Speer KP. Anatomy and pathomechanics of shoulder instability. *Clin Sports Med* 1995; **14**:751–60.

15. Lintner SA, Speer KP. Traumatic anterior glenohumeral instability: the role of arthroscopy. *J Am Acad Orthop Surg* 1997; **5**:233–9.

16. O'Brien SJ, Neves MC, Arnoczky SP et al. The anatomy and histology of the inferior glenohumeral ligament complex of the shoulder. *Am J Sports Med* 1990; **18**:449–56.

17. Loutzenheiser TD, Harryman DT III, Ziegler DW, Yung SW. Optimizing arthroscopic knots using braided or monofilament suture. *Arthroscopy* 1998; **14**:57–65.

13 Anterior shoulder instability: Laser-assisted capsular shrinkage (LACS)

Michael Kunz and Klaus Johann

Introduction

Laser arthroscopy operations on joints have become established since the end of the 1980s. The application of laser energy in the joint has shown that reasonable and good results in arthroscopy can be obtained with the holmium-YAG laser, which uses a wavelength of 2100 nm in the non-visible range. Owing to its very low depth of thermal penetration and the ability to control the energy, it proves to be clearly superior, for example to the neodymium-YAG laser when used in arthroscopy. Several studies have shown that with appropriate adjustment of the energy and exact targeting of the laser beam, there is no damage in the region of the joint.[1–3]

A special advantage of the holmium-YAG laser is the applicability of the energy by appropriate handpieces (infratomes), which can emit the laser beam in different directions. This enables even narrow areas of the joint to be easily reached, particularly since the laser probe has a diameter of approximately 1.5 mm. As a result, laser-assisted arthroscopy has been applied in many joints, so that laser-assisted operations can be performed today not only in all the large joints of the human body, but also in the smaller ones such as the wrist and the talocalcaneonavicular joint.

As there is less bleeding in laser application, postoperative rehabilitation can be much easier than after operations with mechanical instruments, especially in patients with shoulder conditions.[4] The intensity of pain after the operation is also very much less than in conventional arthroscopy.[3,5,6] Initially, laser technology was used only to ablate or to vaporize tissue, such as meniscus resections, synovectomies or cartilage–bone debridements. Since 1992, a further characteristic of laser energy has been utilized. It was shown by tissue investigations and animal experiments that the application of certain energies of the holmium-YAG laser leads to shrinkage of soft tissue. A study on the rabbit model showed that non-ablative laser application led to an energy-dependent contraction of the articular capsule tissue.[7,8] A change in the collagen fibril structure is responsible for this effect that is not due to the laser per se, but is based on the rise in temperature in the tissue. The shrinkage of the capsular tissue under the action of lasers cannot only be discerned under the microscope, but can also

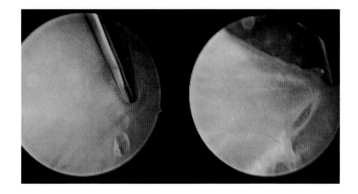

Figure 13.1

Laser capsular shrinkage.

be directly followed as an impressive effect in the clinical application to the joint capsule (Figure 13.1).

The ability of the holmium-YAG laser to shrink tissue was utilized clinically in an attempt to shorten the stretched capsular tissue in patients with recurrent shoulder luxations. The first multicenter study on laser-assisted capsular shift (LACS) was conducted in 1992 in the USA.[9] The encouraging results obtained at that time in treatment of recurrent shoulder luxations quickly led to widespread adoption of the method by laser users.[10]

This LACS method has been used in our hospital since 1994. Since our patients are mostly competitive athletes, the results of the operation were monitored with extreme care and caution. Initially, we also considered the danger of an excessive shrinkage of the capsule with subsequent restriction to movement of the shoulder. However, it has been shown in more than 150 operations performed on unstable shoulder joints that significant restrictions to movement of the operated shoulder are not likely when there is appropriate follow-up treatment. Studies published in the meantime by several other authors report similar results.[9,10]

Surgical principles

In principle, the arthroscope is introduced into the shoulder joint via the dorsal approach to detect all pathologic

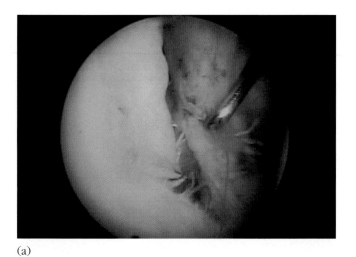

(a)

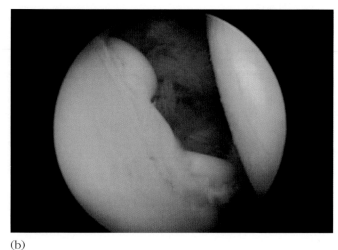

(b)

Figure 13.2

(a) and (b) Suretac fixation of the labrum.

processes within the joint and in the subacromial cavity. In particular, the objective is to diagnose additional lesions in the regions of the anterior labrum (Bankart lesion) or the various kinds of SLAP (superior labrum, anterior to posterior) lesions. These must be treated concomitantly in the arthroscopic operation. Depending on the nature of the lesion, refixations of the labrum are carried out with various fixation techniques. We prefer the Suretac (Smith & Nephew, Andover, MA, USA) fixation of the labrum or the biceps anchor (Figure 13.2). When there are degenerative changes in the labrum or lip ruptures that cannot be fixed, these can also be ablated or stabilized with the holmium-YAG laser (Figure 13.3). These additional operations in the region of the labrum will always be performed before the actual capsular shrinkage. Capsular shrinkage leads to an immediate

and noticeable constriction of the inner cavity of the shoulder and can make it much more difficult to apply anchor techniques to the labrum later. For this reason, the labrum operation is performed as the first stage.

In most cases, a laser handpiece is used for the capsular shrinkage itself. The laser handpiece emits the energy in a direction of 70° from the axis of the probe (Figure 13.4). This laser probe has the advantage that narrow locations in the joint can be readily reached and the danger of damaging the optical system of the arthroscope by direct action of the laser beam is avoided. In principle, the operation is carried out with an arthropump in order to keep the intra-articular pressure constant. Since the intra-articular pressure plays a considerable role in the observation of the capsular shrinkage process, a constant intra-articular pressure of approximately 50–70 mmHg is maintained.

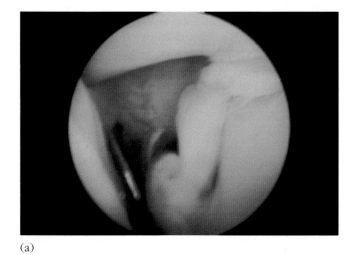

(a)

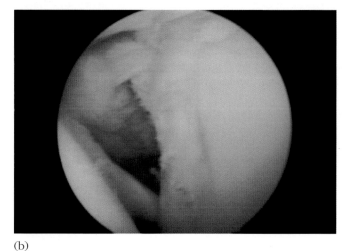

(b)

Figure 13.3

(a) and (b) Labrum stabilization with the holium-YAG laser.

Figure 13.4
70° Laser probe.

Surgical techniques

At our hospital, the operation is always performed in the beach-chair position under general anesthesia. It is also possible to operate on patients positioned on their side. However, since several access routes are frequently required from the front and from the back in multidirectional shoulder instabilities, we consider that the beach-chair position is the most favorable patient position for the surgical technique.

The process of shrinkage is initially started in the axillary recess with introduction of the 70° infratome. In most cases, this is where the most massive capsular slackening is found, so that shrinkage must be carried out very carefully in this region. Besides a ventral access with the infratome, the posterior parts of the axillary recess must sometimes be accessed dorsally. However, this can be achieved with no problems in view of the small diameter of the infratome. The process of shrinkage is continued from distal to proximal in the region of the ventral capsule and the intermediate glenohumeral ligament. Shrinkage is performed between the glenoid and the humerus insertion. In partial ruptures and slackening of the subscapular tendon, this is also included in the process of shrinkage. In cases with multidirectional instability or dorsal instability of the shoulder, an additional dorsal capsule shrinkage is effected by introducing the arthroscopic optical system from ventral. The capsule is shrunk with the 70° or 30° infratome handpiece, likewise beginning from distal to proximal. The shrinkage pattern has no effect on the result of the treatment and the contraction of the capsule. Both linear shrinkages and punctiform shrinkages can be performed (Figure 13.5). The energy setting of the laser generator that is applied is particularly important. Without exception, shrinkage is carried out with an output of 10 watts. Since the holmium-YAG laser is a pulsed laser, the pulse frequency is adjusted to 10 Hz and the energy to 1 joule per pulse. Higher energies lead to tissue ablation, lower energies are usually not sufficient to effect adequate capsule shrinkage (see accompanying video).

Postoperative protocol

Postoperatively, all patients receive an ultrasling bandage that holds the arm with the elbow bent in slight inward rotation position of the shoulder with abduction of about 20–30°. Additional abduction movements of 20–30° as

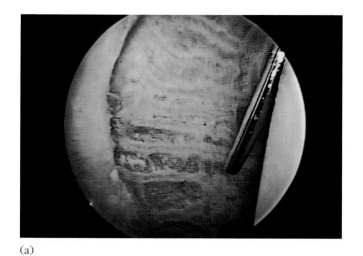

(a)

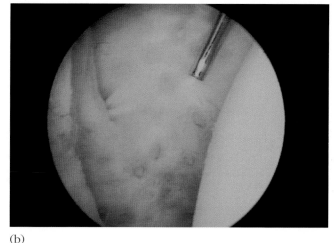

(b)

Figure 13.5
(a) and (b) Linear and punctiform shrinkage pattern.

well as anteversion and retroversion of the shoulder to the same extent are possible in the bandage, but it does not allow an outward rotation. The ultrasling bandage is worn for 2 weeks, and in cases with congenital multidirectional instability for 3 weeks. Afterwards, intensive physiotherapy starts with active and passive movement of the shoulder up to 90° abduction and elevation without practicing the rotation for a further 2–3 weeks. From the fifth to sixth week after the operation, there is mobility of the shoulder in all planes including rotation, and an intensive active and passive training. Sport is permitted 8–12 weeks after the operation.

Results

From 1994 to the beginning of 1999, 116 operations were performed. In the first year, only five patients were operated on. We monitored these cases for 6 months in order to be sure that no complications (especially restrictions of movement) occurred. Excellent results were observed in these five patients. The operation was then extended to all indications of shoulder instability. Besides traumatic recurrent luxations, patients with congenital multidirectional shoulder instability in which no operation had been possible with an adequate result were treated with this method of surgery. In the meantime, operations could be carried out successfully in five patients with instability in both shoulders. In addition, we have also included athletes with shoulder subluxations in surgical therapy using LACS. The athletic performance of these patients is substantially restricted by the pronounced instability in hand-over-head sport (handball, badminton, tennis).

Of these 116 cases, 107 could be followed-up several times after their operation. These patients comprised 31 women and 76 men. The right shoulder was involved in 73 cases, and the left shoulder in 34 cases. The average age of the patients was 26.9 years. The patients were investigated between 1 and 4 years after the operation. The average period of follow-up was 24.3 months. The patients were clinically evaluated using the score defined by Rowe and Zarins in 1982.[11]

There was a recurrent luxation including multidirectional instability in 68 cases. A fresh traumatic luxation was found to cause the instability in 21 cases and a recurrent subluxation was found in 18 patients (Figure 13.6).

The detection and treatment of concomitant injuries is particularly important. There was a Bankart lesion in 74 cases, a Hill–Sachs lesion in 67 cases, a degeneration of the labrum in 33 cases, and a different SLAP lesion in 24 cases (Figure 13.7). The labrum and Bankart lesions were treated with Suretac technique and laser stabilization.

Intraoperative or postoperative complications did not occur in any case. Above all, there were no nerve lesions or hemorrhages. The course of postoperative healing is

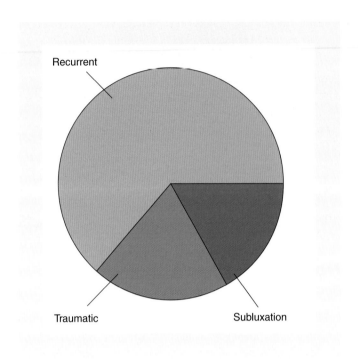

Figure 13.6

Type of instability.

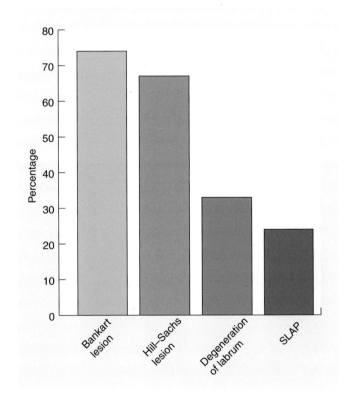

Figure 13.7

Concomitant injuries.

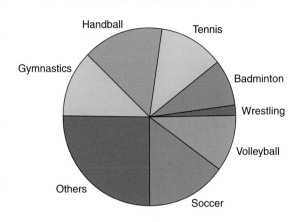

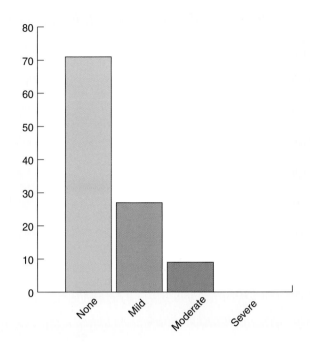

Figure 13.8

Types of sport.

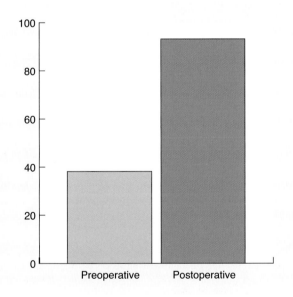

Figure 13.10

Score criterion: pain.

Figure 13.9

Rowe and Zarins score.

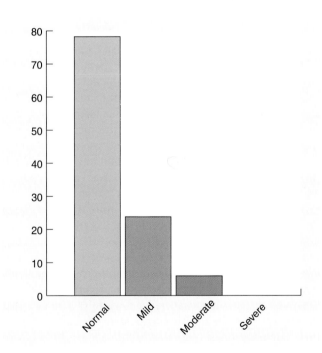

Figure 13.11

Score criterion: function.

characterized only by very slight pain and there is rapid restoration of the ability to engage in sport and to work. An average of 12 weeks after the operation, the competitive athletes were able to engage in their sport again at the level aspired to. Altogether, there were 80 competitive athletes from the highest German performance class. The most frequent kinds of sport were handball, football, tennis, and gymnastics (Figure 13.8).

In the period of observation, there were a total of six reluxations, corresponding to 5.6%. The Rowe score measured preoperatively improved postoperatively by an average of 38.2 points to 93.2 points (maximum number of points 100; Figure 13.9). The individual criteria of the score show in particular an appreciable improvement of the pain and function score (Figures 13.10 and 13.11).

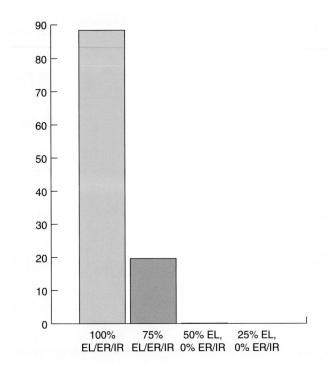

Figure 13.12

Score criterion: motion.

There was a slight restriction of external rotation compared to the contralateral side of not more than 20° in only 19 cases (Figure 13.12). This did not impede the athletes in practicing their sport in any instance. Considering the redislocations, it may be assumed that there was a true fresh traumatic luxation in one case, and there were errors in the surgical technique in two cases, as two multidirectional instabilities were treated only anteriorly. In a second operation, dorsal capsular shrinkage was carried out in addition, which led to stable shoulder joints.

Many open and arthroscopic techniques have been described for treatment of recurrent shoulder luxations and rates of reluxation of up to 49% have been published.[12,13] In view of these rates of reluxation, our rate of reluxation of 5.6% found in the group of patients treated with LACS can be regarded as a very good result. This was remarkable especially in view of the fact that these patients were mainly competitive athletes with very high demands on shoulder stability.

In addition, the possibility of a sufficient arthroscopic operation on a shoulder joint capsule that is too slack is available for the first time with the LACS technique. Until now, these patients were almost untreatable surgically because the results of the open and closed operations that were carried out were mostly poor. Use of the arthroscopic laser capsular shrinkage technique also shows very good results in these patients and can be recommended here. It is important that besides the mastery of the technique of shoulder arthroscopy the surgeon has a thorough training in the application of laser energy. This enables reliable avoidance of errors with a low-risk technique.

References

1. Brillhart A. *Arthroscopic Laser Surgery.* New York: Springer Verlag, 1994.
2. Siebert WE. Laseranwendung in der Arthroskopie. *Orthopäde* 1992; **21**:273–88.
3. Walker, Th. 2.1 nm Holmium:YAG arthroscopic laser surgery: prospective report of 100 cases. In: Brillhart A, ed. *Arthroscopic laser surgery.* New York: Springer, 1994; 269–73.
4. Imhoff A, Ledermann Th. Arthroscopic subacromial decompression with and without the Holmium:YAG laser: a prospective comparative study. *Arthroscopy* 1995; **11**:549–56.
5. Kunz M. Arthroscopical laser surgery in knee. A 2-year follow up presented at IMLAS International Congress, Lake Tahoe, 1995.
6. Lübers C, Siebert WE. Die arthroskopische Holmium-YAG-Laseranwendung im Vergleich zu konventionellen Verfahren am Kniegelenk. *Orthopäde* 1996; **25**:64–72.
7. Hayashi K, Markel MD, Thabit G et al. The effect of nonablative laser energy on joint capsular properties. *Am J Sports Med* 1995; **23**:432–87.
8. Hayashi K, Thabit G, Bogdanske JJ et al. The effect of nonablative laser energy of the ultrastructure on joint capsular collagen. *Arthroscopy* 1996; **12**:474–91.
9. Fanton GS. Schulterarthroskopie unter Verwendung des Holmium YAG Lasers. *Orthopäde* 1996; **25**:79–83.
10. Hardy P, Thabit G, Fanton GS et al. Arthroscopic treatment of recurrent anterior glenohumeral luxations by combining a labrum suture with holmium:YAG laser assisted capsular shrinkage. *Orthopäde* 1996; **25**:91–3.
11. Rowe CR, Zarins B. Chronic unreduced dislocation of the shoulder. *J Bone Joint Surg* 1982; **64A**:494–505.
12. Manta JP, Organ S, Nirschl RP, Pettrone FA. Arthroscopic transglenoid suture capsulolabral repair. *Am J Sports Med* 1997; **25**:614–18.
13. Walch G, Boileau P, Levigne C et al. Arthroscopic stabilization for recurrent anterior shoulder dislocation. *Arthrocopy* 1995, **11**:173–9.

14 Anterior shoulder instability: Electrothermally-assisted capsular shrinkage (ETACS)

Amir M Khan and Gary S Fanton

Introduction

Shoulder instability is one of the most common causes of functional limitation in recreational and competitive athletes. The essential lesion in nearly all cases of shoulder instability is attenuation of glenohumeral joint capsule, either as a result of high-energy failure (macrotrauma) or gradual tearing and stretching (repetitive microtrauma). In fact, it is now understood that capsule laxity from repetitive microtrauma is a common cause of shoulder pain in young overhead athletes, most notably throwers, swimmers, tennis players, and volleyball players.[1-3] The high tensile force generated in the glenohumeral ligaments, perhaps combined with weakness or fatigue of the rotator cuff, results in microscopic tearing of the capsule and gradual increase in humeral head translation. Tension failure of the undersurface of the rotator cuff and bicipital–labral complex tears (superior labrum anterior posterior (SLAP) lesions) often result.[4-6] Whether traumatic or atraumatic, aspects of pathology must be surgically addressed to assure a high success rate for return to sport.

Arthroscopic treatment of shoulder instability has evolved over the past 10 years. Initial attempts to address certain components of instability, such as reattachment of the capsule and labrum were achieved but recurrence rates were not comparable to open procedures.[7-9] Presumably, the stretched out capsule and ligamentous components were not successfully addressed with these arthroscopic procedures. Thermal capsulorraphy was introduced as a tool to arthroscopically address the capsuloligamentous component of shoulder instability. The concept of using heat to alter the structure of collagen and therefore effect changes in tissue structure has gained considerable interest in the past 15 years. In the early 1990s, the Holmium laser was found to be a useful tool for thermally contracting[10] the shoulder capsule and improving shoulder stability in the young active patient population.[11] Arthroscopic laser systems, however, have remained a small part of the surgeon's armamentarium because of lack of temperature control, the need for specialized training, and cost considerations. In the past few years, radiofrequency (RF) systems have been developed for arthroscopic use. There are two basic types of

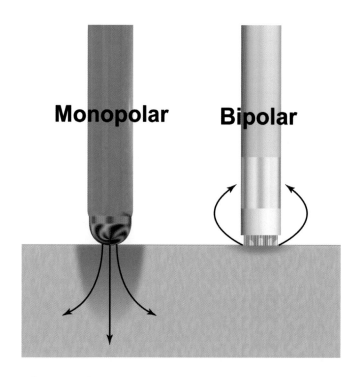

Figure 14.1
Monopolar versus bipolar tissue heating.

RF circuitry for use in orthopedic applications, monopolar and bipolar, and the tissue temperature profiles for these two different systems are vastly different (Figure 14.1). Monopolar RF systems utilize an alternating current between the treatment probe and the grounding plate. The high current density produces molecular friction, which heats the tissue to a desired temperature. Primary heating occurs in the upper layers of the tissue, which then heats the deeper layers of tissue.[12] The temperature is monitored 50 times per second, providing a constant feedback to the RF generator that automatically adjusts power output accordingly, much like the thermostat in a room. The gradient of thermal effect seen with monopolar RF arthroscopy is sufficient to achieve a full thickness capsule response if necessary.[13] In contrast, bipolar RF circuits create a current that follows a path of least resistance from the probe tip, through the

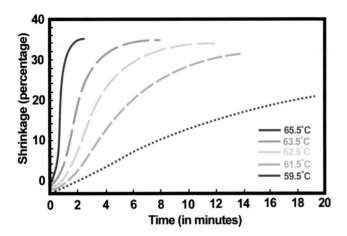

Figure 14.2

Shrinkage is a function of both time of exposure and applied temperature.

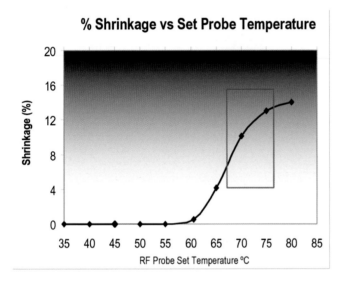

Figure 14.3

Ideal temperature for thermal shrinkage appears to be in the 65–75°C range.

conductive irrigating solution, and back to another conductive electrode a very short distance away. High temperatures between bipolar probe electrodes are reached as the current 'arcs' between them without producing molecular friction in the tissue. Therefore, bipolar RF circuits provide higher surface temperatures with lower tissue penetration that is less well suited for low-power temperature-controlled procedures. Thermal tissue penetration of only 1 mm or less is usually noted, which may only produce a synovial surface response.

Both in vitro and in vivo studies have demonstrated the ultrastructural and histologic changes that occur after treatment of capsular tissue.[13–19] Tibone et al[20] demon-

strated significant reduction in both anterior and posterior translation of the humeral head after thermal anterior capsuloplasty in cadavers. The percentage of tissue shrinkage is both time- and temperature-dependent (Figure 14.2).[21] Ideal temperature ranges for thermal shrinkage of mammalian collagen appears to be in the 65–75°C range in the tissue bath settings (Figure 14.3).[22] Initially, collagen contracts as the heat-sensitive bonds in the collagen molecule are broken and the molecule 'recoils' upon itself. As more and more intermolecular bonds are broken and as more molecules are treated the tissue begins to contract visibly. On this scaffold of shortened collagen molecules, new fibroblasts grow in and lay down new collagen to reconstitute the tissue. At higher energy applications, collagen molecules tend to hyalinize and lose their normal well-defined crossstriated appearance.

Early clinical results of RF energy in shoulder instability is promising, but careful patient selection and proper postoperative management are keys to a successful outcome. As more basic science data becomes available it will further our understanding of this technology and its uses in orthopedics.

Surgical principles

A careful history and physical examination is very important in evaluating patients for the possible need for surgical stabilization. A conservative program of rest, ice, anti-inflammatories, and rotator cuff and scapular strengthening and stabilization should be prescribed prior to considering surgical intervention. The entire dynamics of the scapulothoracic and glenohumeral mechanism should be evaluated and appropriately treated. Only when these conservative measures fail should arthroscopic surgical stabilization be considered. Preoperative studies including contrast magnetic resonance imaging and computed tomography arthrography may be helpful in elucidating the degree and direction of instability and determining whether any associated partial-thickness rotator tears or labral tears exist. The evaluation of shoulder pain in a young active athlete can be difficult and the physical findings are often subtle. It is important to determine preoperatively not only if instability exists, but also in which direction is the primary source of instability and whether it is unidirectional or multidirectional.

There are primarily two ways to use arthroscopic thermal stabilization techniques to enhance shoulder stability. The first is in patients with an attenuated but otherwise intact shoulder capsule. This type of patient usually develops symptomatic shoulder instability from repetitive microtrauma, such as in overhead throwing sports, racquet sports, and swimming. In some cases there is an underlying generalized ligamentous laxity that predisposes the patient to instability, which then becomes symptomatic during sports participation. As the glenohumeral ligament complex either acutely or gradually stretches out, more and more demand is placed on the rotator cuff and bicipital–labral complex to maintain a centralized humeral head. Aching, heaviness, or sharp pains associated with injury of the rotator cuff, biceps, or labrum are common presenting complaints. It is the underlying shoulder instability that is the primary pathology, and it must be addressed in the young overhead athlete to restore functional integrity of the joint.

The other main indication for thermal stabilization of the shoulder is as an adjunctive procedure to tighten a damaged shoulder capsule in association with arthroscopic capsulolabral repair. Capsule avulsion is usually the result of a high energy or traumatic event, and the patient can often identify the initial incident. It has been well recognized that secure repair of an avulsed glenohumeral capsule is necessary to achieve a stable shoulder, whether performed arthroscopically or through open techniques. However capsule detachment alone does not account for recurrent instability,[3] and anatomic reattachment of the capsule alone may not fully restore a secure and stable joint. In fact, the higher recurrence rates seen historically in arthroscopic repairs that only anchor or suture the capsule back to the glenoid margin may be explained by a failure to address the stretched out glenohumeral ligaments. Thermal capsulorrhaphy provides an excellent and technically easy approach to arthroscopically advancing the capsule in conjunction with arthroscopic reattachment procedures using anchors, sutures, or bioabsorbable tacks.

One non-laser system for tissue shrinkage in orthopedics incorporates an RF thermal feedback probe (Oratec Interventions, Inc., Menlo Park, CA, USA) and has been FDA-approved for the thermal treatment of soft tissues. The RF generator also has variable output that allows the surgeon to switch from temperature-controlled applications to high-power outputs that are necessary for tissue cutting, ablation, and vaporization (Figure 14.4). Finally, the capital outlay for RF equipment is substantially lower than for most arthroscopic laser systems and no special certification is required.

RF thermal stabilization is technically easy, but as in all surgical procedures attention to proper indications and avoidance of complications are priorities. Several cases of transient axillary neuropathy have been reported, including two sensory neuropathies in our patient population. The axillary nerve lies close to the inferior capsule at the 6 o'clock position. The surgeon must be careful if he or she elects to treat the axillary pouch, especially in multidirectional instability (MDI) patients with a thin capsule. We do not routinely treat the inferior capsule between the 5 o'clock and the 7 o'clock positions because the nerve is at risk in this area,[23] the inferior capsule has very little collagen, and adhesions of the axillary pouch can potentially cause a significant loss of motion. If this area is to be treated, access via an accessory posterior portal can be safely

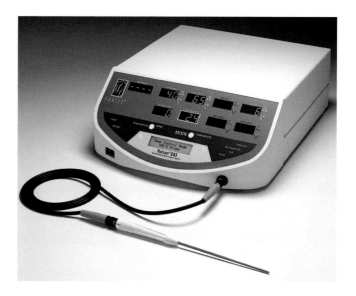

Figure 14.4

The Oratec Radiofrequency Generator and the attached TAC-S probe.

established[24] and it is recommended that the power settings be reduced to 30 watts and gradually increased to avoid excessive thermal penetration. Excessive abduction of the arm during this part of the procedure should be avoided because it places the axillary nerve at greater risk. Axillary neuritis is usually transient and recovers in 6–8 weeks, but recovery may take longer if there is associated motor weakness. We have not encountered any cases of axillary neuritis since we have utilized the 'grid' pattern of capsule treatment and employed the above precautions. Also, the new software algorithms for temperature control in the monopolar devices have improved significantly with much tighter temperature control and less risk of 'temperature overshoot' that might irritate the axillary nerve.

Most failures have probably been failures of judgement. It is appealing to think that all shoulder instabilities can be treated thermally, but such is not the case. We have seen higher failure rates in patients with large Hill–Sachs lesions, who lack bony congruity when the shoulder is fully externally rotated. Likewise, patients with a severally deficient capsule, a humeral-side avulsion of the capsule, or a bony avulsion of the capsule are probably best suited for open procedures. Although we have had some successes, patients who have previously undergone shoulder surgery are also poor candidates for thermal stabilization because of the lack of predictable thermal penetration into scar tissue and the non-linear alignment of the collagen bundles. Finally, in some patients with acute trauma to the joint or those who have a very thin capsule, there may not be very much response during thermal treatment. If raising the power and/or temperature settings on the RF

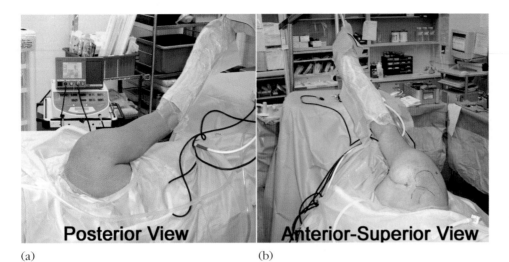

Figure 14.5

(a, b) Lateral decubitus position.

(a)   (b)

generator does not improve the capsule response, it may be better to consider other mechanical arthroscopic stabilization techniques or perhaps an open capsule shift procedure. It is not appropriate in these unresponsive capsules to continually paint the capsule over and over in hopes of achieving some response as this may do more than devascularize the capsule thereby making future surgery more difficult.

As with any shoulder operation, adhesive capsulitis will occasionally occur in patients with an inflammatory tendency. Close monitoring of the rehabilitation program and judicious use of anti-inflammatory medications will usually suffice to regain range of motion. The incidence of capsulitis in our patient population has been no greater than for other shoulder surgeries and to date only one patient has required postoperative manipulation.

Surgical technique

After induction of general anesthesia, the shoulder is examined for laxity. The degree and direction of translation of the humeral head relative to the glenoid socket is recorded with the scapula stabilized. The instability is recorded as mild (50% translation of the humeral head),

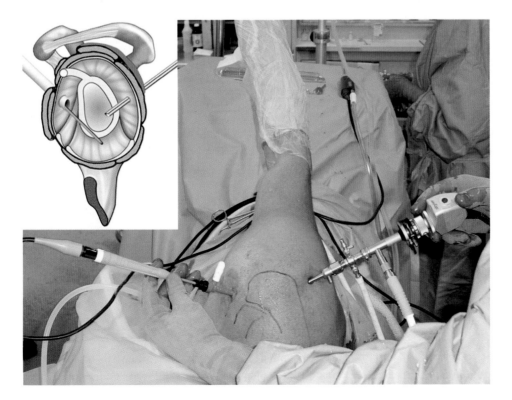

Figure 14.6

Standard anterior and posterior portals. Inset: for anterior capsular shrinkage the RF probe is placed anteriorly and the arthroscope is placed posteriorly.

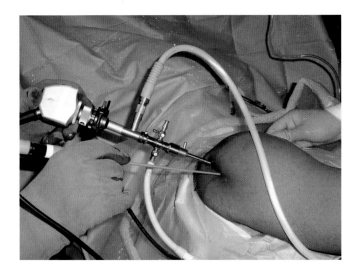

Figure 14.7

Accessory posterior portal. To reach the axillary recess the RF probe may be inserted through an accessory posterior portal as shown.

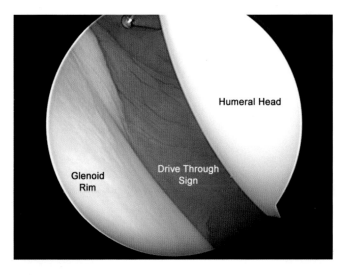

Figure 14.8

The drive-through sign implies anterior capsular laxity.

moderate (50–100% translation), or severe (subluxation beyond the glenoid rim). The primary direction of laxity and whether it is unidirectional or multidirectional is recorded. The opposite shoulder is examined for comparison. The patient is positioned in the lateral decubitus position (Figure 14.5) or the beach-chair position, based on the surgeon's preference. Rolling the patient's torso posteriorly 10–20° improves access to the anterior capsule.

A standard posterior arthroscopic portal is established at the posterior superior joint line near the lower border of the infraspinatus tendon. A second anterior portal is then established under direct visualization at the top of the subscapularis tendon (Figure 14.6). This portal is kept intentionally low to facilitate passage of the thermally assisted capsulorrhaphy (TAC) probe to the inferior portions of the capsule with less obstruction by the glenoid neck or humeral head. A spinal needle is helpful in localizing this portal. The portal is maintained with a disposable grommeted cannula through which standard instrumentation can be introduced. However, in some cases, an accessory posterior portal may be needed to reach the axillary recess between the area of 5 and 7 o'clock. The accessory portal is placed 1.5 cm below the standard posterior portal and introduced parallel to the arthroscope (Figure 14.7). Alternatively, the arthroscope can be placed in the anterior portal and the accessory portal can be placed under arthroscopic visualization with the help of a spinal needle.

Upon entering the shoulder joint, diagnostic arthroscopy is carried out with careful evaluation of the condition of the rotator cuff, articular surfaces, glenoid labrum, bicipital complex, ligaments and the capsule.

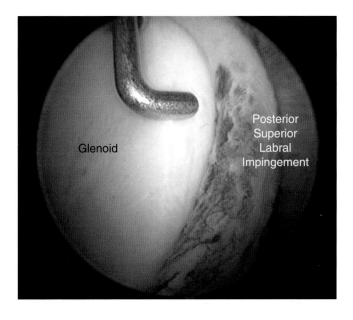

Figure 14.9

Internal impingement. The posterior superior labrum impingement as shown here often accompanies the posterior rotator cuff fraying seen in internal impingement.

Certain arthroscopic findings may support the diagnosis of recurrent instability. These patients often have softening of the articular cartilage of the anterior inferior portion of the glenoid socket. This area should be carefully probed and examined. Lateral displacement of

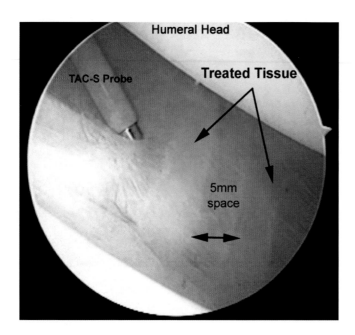

Figure 14.10

Grid technique. Application of RF energy can be done by utilizing a grid technique which leaves areas of untreated tissue between treated stripes.

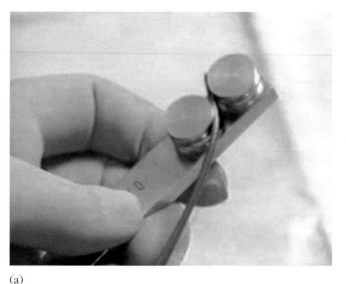

(a)

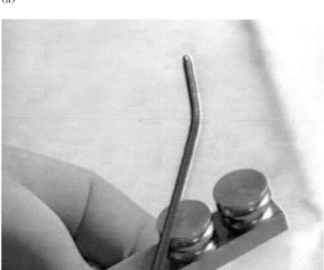

(b)

Figure 14.11

(a, b) Probe bender. Typically a 30° bend is placed at the tip of the probe.

the humeral head away from the glenoid socket with gentle traction, the so-called 'drive-through' sign, can usually be demonstrated in patients with anterior or multidirectional instability (Figure 14.8). Degenerative tears of the posterior superior glenoid labrum (Figure 14.9) or posterior rotator cuff are suggestive of internal impingement and can be seen in overhead throwing athletes with mild anterior instability. SLAP lesions are also suggestive of instability. Detachment of the capsulolabral complex from the glenoid margin below the equator of the glenoid is pathognomonic of instability. Upon completion of glenohumeral inspection and management of glenohumeral pathology, the subacromial space and the bursal surface of the cuff are inspected and addressed.

The technique varies depending upon the type of instability. For unidirectional anterior instabilility, the region from the middle glenohumeral ligament to the anterior inferior glenohumeral ligament is always addressed. However, in some cases additional shrinkage is needed and the axillary recess between the area of 5 and 7 o'clock is also treated including the posterior band of the inferior glenohumeral ligament complex. Since tissue tightening is both heat- and time-dependent, greater capsule contraction can also be achieved by leaving the probe stationary for 2–3 seconds until the desired amount of contraction is obtained. Likewise, an area that has been treated can be treated again if further tightening is desired. Surgical technique varies somewhat

between surgeons. However, in our practice we now exclusively employ a linear striking pattern to treat the various areas of the capsule. When the capsule is 'painted', much longer periods of immobilization are required. We feel there is a higher risk of thermal penetration and capsular devascularization. In addition, painting the capsule in some patients may result in a more intense inflammatory response. In all our patients, including overhead athletes, we now use a 'grid technique' (Figure 14.10). Thermally striping the capsule while leaving untreated areas in between treatment stripes creates nearly identical tissue contraction but a much faster healing response.[25]

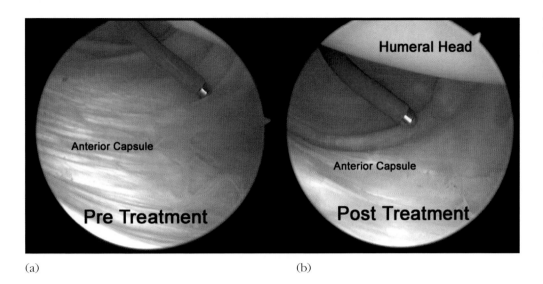

(a)   (b)

Figure 14.12

(a, b) Anterior capsule shrinkage during RF application.

For unidirectional *anterior instability*, the TAC probe is introduced through the anterior cannula and is directed toward the anterior capsule. Typically a 30° bend is placed about 1 inch from the tip using a probe bender (Figure 14.11). This allows the tip of the probe to reach around the curved surfaces of the humeral head and glenoid. The probe shaft can also be bent slightly if necessary. The capsule adjacent to the humeral head is treated first since this area is difficult to reach once capsule contraction has begun adjacent to the glenoid. An assistant who can rotate the arm as needed can also improve access to difficult areas of the capsule. The procedure is then continued towards the anterior inferior portions of the joint capsule including the inferior and middle glenohumeral ligaments. The surgeon sweeps the TAC probe in contact along the capsule in a back and forth motion while visualizing the capsule response. These areas of the capsule that have a higher collagen content will respond more dramatically. Typically, after a 1–2 second lag during which the treated tissue is heating up, the capsule dramatically shrinks and the anterior recess is drawn upward toward the joint, eliminating the capsular redundancy (Figure 14.12). Some areas of the axillary recess are fairly thin and will not respond as much. In addition, power settings should be reduced in these thin areas inferiorly to avoid irritation of the axillary nerve. In some cases, an accessory posterior portal may be used to reach the axillary recess between the area of 5 and 7 o'clock.

In patients with *posterior instability*, the entire posterior capsule is usually tightened. We like to shrink the region thermally including and above the posterior inferior glenohumeral ligament. This is usually performed by placing the arthroscope through the anterior portal and placing the TAC probe through the standard posterior portal (Figure 14.13). This provides good access to

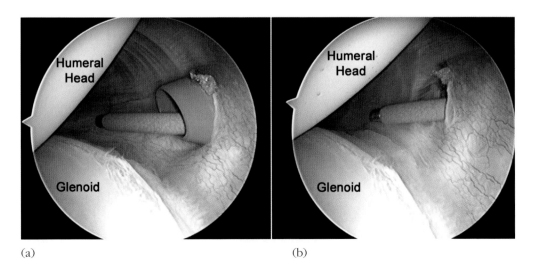

(a)   (b)

Figure 14.13

(a, b) Posterior capsule shrinkage. The RF probe is placed through the standard posterior portal and the arthroscope is placed through the standard anterior portal.

the middle and superior portions of the posterior capsule. An assistant who can internally or externally rotate the arm can also improve access to difficult areas of the capsule. Again, portions of the capsule may tighten variably depending on the collagen content. A grid or a paint technique can be used as needed. When the capsule has been tightened, the humeral head translation in internal and external rotation is rechecked and is compared to the preoperative condition.

For *multidirectional instability* (MDI), the TAC probe is introduced through the anterior cannula and is directed toward the anterior capsule. The region from the superior glenohumeral ligament to the anterior inferior glenohumeral ligament is always addressed. This includes shrinking the rotator interval. Additional shrinkage is often needed in the axillary recess between the areas of 5 and 7 o'clock. As mentioned earlier care is to be taken when shrinking in the axillary recess. If a component of posterior laxity is also present then the posterior capsule is also addressed. The techniques mentioned earlier are also employed here to address the degree of instability. The surgeon has to utilize his or her judgement to ensure that adequate capsular shrinkage is obtained by treating as much tissue as needed. Our patients with multidirectional instability, especially those with generalized ligamentous laxity, have presented a greater challenge. Rovner compared thermal and open capsule shift procedures in a cadaveric model.[26] His study showed that both procedures were successful in reducing capsule volume but that open capsule shift reduced volume by approximately 50% compared to 30% for the thermal capsulorrhaphy. Lyons et al[27] achieved excellent results with 96% success rate at 2-year follow-up performing laser-assisted thermal capsulorrhaphy of the shoulder with rotator interval closure for multidirectional instability. In these patients, especially those with severe laxity, thermal capsulorrhaphy alone may not provide enough capsule reduction to completely stabilize the joint and rotator interval closure may provide the additional stability required to achieve long-term success in this difficult patient population. We now consider adjunctive procedures, such as rotator interval closure or even open capsule shift, as necessary components to achieve the best results for patients with severe MDI.

Many patients with traumatic instability of the shoulder have a concomitant avulsion of the capsulolabral complex as well as attenuation of the glenohumeral ligaments. These patients are ideal candidates for arthroscopic fixation of the capsule to the glenoid and a thermally assisted shift. If the capsule separation from the glenoid rim is quite large, then arthroscopic repair of the capsule is performed first. This can be performed using any of the standard arthroscopic techniques such as suturing, anchoring, or bioabsorbable tack fixation. When anatomic restoration of the capsule to the glenoid rim is achieved, then electrothermal capsular shift procedure as described above is performed. If the capsule is

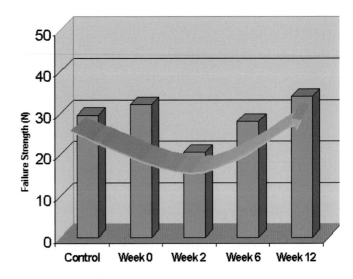

Figure 14.14
Recovery of tissue strength.

easily accessible and the area of avulsion is not widely displaced, then it is our preference to treat the attenuated capsule first and then address the capsule detachment. This is sometimes easier at the beginning of the procedure when there is less soft tissue swelling. Once the capsule shrinkage has been achieved, capsule fixation to the glenoid rim can be performed. Avoid heating the capsular tissue near the planned fixation to the glenoid in order to avoid weakening the capsulolabral repair.

Some patients with acute trauma to the joint and inflammation or patients who have had previous surgical procedures to the joint capsule may not have as much response during thermal treatment. If raising the power or temperature settings on the RF generator does not improve the capsule response, it may be better to consider other mechanical arthroscopic stabilization techniques or perhaps an open capsular shift procedure. As mentioned earlier, patients with severe instability and large rotator interval defects, a deficient capsule, a HAGL lesion, a large bony bankart, and engaging or large Hill–Sachs lesions, are probably best suited for open procedures.

Postoperative protocol

The postoperative program after a thermal stabilization of the shoulder is dependent on several factors including direction of instability, degree of preoperative laxity, tissue response, specific postoperative activity or sport, and whether supplemental fixation was used. The follow-

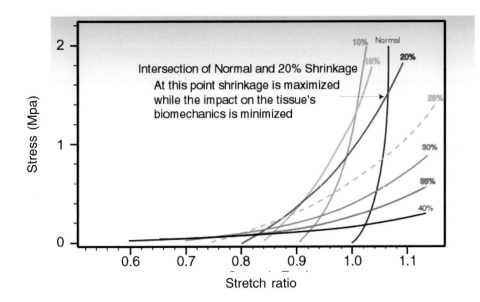

Figure 14.15

Percentage shrinkage versus biomechanics.

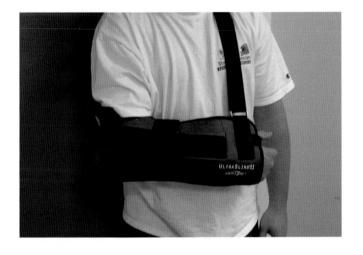

Figure 14.16

Immobilization of anterior thermal stabilization. The patient is primarily held in internal rotation for 2–4 weeks.

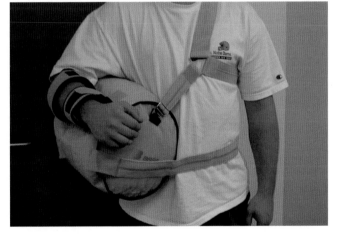

Figure 14.17

Immobilization of posterior thermal stabilization. The patient is primarily held in moderate abduction and neutral or slight external rotation for 4–6 weeks.

ing are guidelines that are useful in achieving postoperative goals with the least risk of recurrent instability or limitation of motion. Keep in mind that rehabilitation of any surgical procedure must take into account the patient's healing response, degree of postoperative inflammation, and strength of surgical repair. For thermal stabilization we know that the first 4–6 weeks after surgery are the most important to prevent restretching of the newly contracted capsule. During this time, vascular and cellular ingrowth occur, but it is not until new collagen deposition occurs that tensile strength begins to recover. Biomechanical studies (Figure 14.14)[19] have

shown that maximum capsule weakness is present during the first 2 weeks and may be reduced to 30% or less of normal. Recovery of mechanical strength is rapid and, by 6–8 weeks after surgery, 60% of the biomechanical properties are restored. By 12 weeks there is 80% restoration of biomechanical strength. Of course, the degree of tissue weakness and length of time to recover depend in large part on how much tissue is treated (Figure 14.15).[18] The recently described grid technique appears to create sufficient capsule contraction with an enhanced healing rate, perhaps because of the preservation of viable cells and vessels near the treated areas.

Phase 1 – Immobilization phase

For anterior instability, the patient is placed in a padded sling or shoulder immobilizer immediately after surgery. The patient returns for a recheck appointment, wound check, and dressing change during the first week. The shoulder immobilization is maintained for at least 14 days postoperatively. However, the determination of the actual length of postoperative immobilization is made at the time of surgery and is included as part of the postoperative instructions. This may depend on how loose the shoulder was before surgery and what other procedures were performed.

For an electrothermally assisted capsulorrhaphy (ETAC) procedure with supplemental capsule fixation (Suretac or capsule suturing) the immobilization phase will last for 2 weeks. Patients with unidirectional instability treated with ETAC procedure alone remain immobilized for 3 weeks (Figure 14.16). Patients with posterior instability are immobilized for 4 weeks in neutral to external rotation. This can include the use of a 'gunslinger' brace or an inflated pillow to maintain a humeral position in external rotation (Figure 14.17). This must be maintained for 4 weeks to allow the posterior capsule to heal in a more relaxed position. In patients with multidirectional instability treated with anterior and posterior capsule tightening, the immobilization is maintained for 4 weeks after surgery.

During this immobilization phase, all patients are allowed range of motion exercises of the wrist and elbow as well as gentle Codman exercises with the elbow supported. Shoulder abduction and flexion exercises are not allowed in any patient and external rotation past 0° is avoided in any patient treated for MDI or any type of anterior instability. In patients treated for posterior instability, no internal rotation is allowed during the immobilization period. After the period of immobilization, active abduction is allowed, as described below.

Phase 2 – Early range of motion

After the initial period of immobilization described above, limited range of motion is begun but the capsule is still protected for an additional few weeks. For anterior instability or MDI with a primary anterior component, external rotation is allowed to 45° with the elbow at the side and 45° with the arm abducted 90°. Forward flexion and abduction are limited to 90° each, and extension to 10° beyond the body plane. Within these range of motion restrictions, strengthening and progressive resistive exercises of the shoulder are encouraged but no passive stretches beyond these ranges are allowed. Shoulder shrugs and capsular retraction are encouraged to maintain the tone of the shoulder girdle. Progressive resistive elbow and wrist exercises are continued.

For posterior instability external rotation exercises are permitted but internal rotation is limited to avoid stretching the posterior capsule. These range of motion restrictions are maintained until 6–8 weeks after surgery.

Phase 3 – Intermediate rehabilitation

Depending on the amount of instability and the patient's postoperative goals, full rehabilitation of the shoulder is started between 6 and 8 weeks postoperatively. Patients who were treated for subluxation only or who plan to return to overhead throwing sports are started at 6 weeks. Patients with severe preoperative multidirectional instability or with posterior instability have their range of motion restrictions continued up to 8 weeks. Once full rehabilitation of the shoulder is begun, scapular patterns, internal and external rotation strengthening exercises, and deltoid strengthening are emphasized. Shoulder proprioceptive neuromuscular facilitation (PNF) patterns are continued. Resistive exercises can include manual resistance, elastic tubing, free weights, and shoulder strengthening equipment including wall pulleys. The only restriction to range of motion is that external rotation is limited to −15° compared with the opposite side for anterior instability and internal rotation is limited similarly for posterior instability. Although the patient may achieve rotation greater than this on his or her own, passive stretching should be stopped at 15° less than the opposite shoulder in forward flexion, abduction, and rotation. It is preferable to allow the patient to regain this last 15° on his or her own over time rather than push the capsule too early and risk stretching the repair. There should be a strong emphasis on continued scapular stabilization (protraction, retraction and elevation) as well as an extrinsic and intrinsic muscle endurance.

Phase 4 – Late rehabilitation

After 8 weeks, the patient proceeds with a self-directed gym program that emphasizes PNF shoulder patterns, chest presses, chest pulls, and a complete shoulder conditioning and endurance program. This may be monitored once a week by a physical therapist to make any necessary adjustments. The patient is not to return to strenuous overhead sports or work activities, including overhead flexion or throwing, until at least 16 weeks after surgery. At that time, the patient can continue to increase activities as tolerated with no limitations whatsoever.

Although the initial phase of rehabilitation for thermal stabilization procedures may be slower than with some open procedures, rehabilitation usually progresses quite rapidly and the patient often makes an excellent functional recovery far sooner than other surgical stabilization techniques. Although we do not know the ultimate tissue strength characteristics of any shoulder stabilization procedure, it is probably prudent to avoid any stress on the shoulder capsule in an overhead position until at least 16 weeks after surgery. Patients may feel more 'capable' of using the shoulder before that time, but precaution should be emphasized until we know more about the histologic and structural changes that occur after this type of shoulder surgery. As more information is gathered and our clinical experience grows, we may modify this program to encourage an even earlier return to work or sports.

Early clinical results

Our short to midterm (1–3 year) clinical results in over 120 patients treated have revealed an overall patient satisfaction rate of over 90%, but results do appear to correlate with type of preoperative instability.[28] The best results have been seen in those patients with mild to moderate unidirectional instability either alone or in combination with capsulolabral repair. In this group, the patient satisfaction rate and the ability to return to high level sports have been very high and less than 5% have required repeat surgery. Our patient population has included high demand collegiate and professional athletes involved in overhead sports such as water polo, volleyball, tennis and baseball. Patients with unidirectional posterior instability have also faired well, although at present we have only 12 patients with over 2 years of follow-up. Nevertheless, nine of these 12 patients have continued to participate in their activities at pre-injury level. Two patients have developed recurrent posterior instability but have not elected further surgery. Patients with a diagnosis of subluxation or dislocation did equally well provided that there was no large Hill–Sachs lesion (greater than 20% of the humeral head) or bony Bankart lesion. Anderson et al,[29] at the Hospital for Special Surgery, reported a failure rate of less than 10% in a preliminary follow-up of 80 patients, primarily throwers and overhead athletes. Levitz and Andrews[30] reported an 86% success rate in returning throwing athletes to very high levels of competition at 2 years' follow-up, a significant improvement in results when compared to a similar group of athletes without thermal capsulorraphy.

Our patients with multidirectional instability, especially those with generalized ligamentous laxity, have presented a greater challenge. Initial success rates at 1 year was nearly 90% but at 2 years declined to only 75%. These results have improved since the advocation of stricter postoperative immobilization for up to 4 weeks. Our more recent 2-year results for MDI patients now exceed 80%. Bradley[31] reported a 29% early failure rate in MIDI patients that likewise has since improved with longer periods of immobilization. Basamania[32] was able to achieve an 87% success rate in a review of 52 MDI patients treated with thermal capsulorraphy. He emphasized the need for complete treatment of the entire anterior and posterior capsule followed by strict immobilization for 4 weeks. While not as predictable as unidirectional instability, thermal capsulorraphy does appear to provide a treatment alternative for this very difficult patient population. Strengthening exercises to maintain 'dynamic' stability remain very important.

Summary

In summary, monopolar electrothermal stabilization of the shoulder shows considerable promise as a treatment alternative in athletes. Range of motion is preserved, recovery is faster than with open procedures, there is little disruption or alteration of inherent anatomy, and, most importantly, results at 2 years appear to equal or exceed other surgical procedures in this high-demand population. The procedure is technically easy to perform and the complication rate is low. Success, however, depends on proper patient selection, attention to the rehabilitation program, and patient compliance. Long-term follow-up will be necessary to determine if results for this procedure will deteriorate over time, especially in patients with MDI.

References

1. Bigliani LU, Pollock RG, Soslowsky LJ et al. Tensile properties of the inferior glenohumeral ligament. *J Orthop Res* 1992; **10**:187–97.
2. O'Brien SJ, Neves MC, Arnoczky SP et al. The anatomy and histology of the inferior glenohumeral ligament complex of the shoulder. *Am J Sports Med* 1990; **18**:449–56.
3. Speer KP, Deng X, Borrero S et al. Biomechanical evaluation of a simulated Bankart lesion. *J Bone Joint Surg Am* 1994; **76**:1819–26.
4. Wickiwicz TL. Glenohumeral kinematics in a muscle fatigue model: a radiographic study. *Orthop Trans* 1994; **18**:178–9.
5. Altchek DW. Shoulder instability in the throwing athlete. *Sports Med Arthrosc Rev* 1993; **1**:210–16.
6. Pollock RG, Bigliani LU. Glenohumeral instability: evaluation and treatment. *J Am Acad Orthop Surg* 1993; **1**:24–32.
7. Pagnani MJ, Warren RF, Altchek DW et al. Arthroscopic shoulder stabilization using transglenoid sutures. A minimum 4-year follow-up. *Am J Sports Med* 1965; **24**:459–67.
8. Lane JG, Sachs RA, Riehl B. Arthroscopic staple capsulorraphy: a long-term follow-up. *Arthroscopy* 1993; **9**:190–4.
9. Hawkins RB. Arthroscopic stapling repair for shoulder instability: a retrospective study of 50 cases. *Arthroscopy* 1989; **5**:122–8.
10. Hayashi K, Thabit G, Bogdanske JJ et al. The effect of nonablative laser energy on the ultrastructure of joint capsule collagen. *Arthroscopy* 1996; **12**:474–81.
11. Thabit G III. The arthroscopically assisted Holmium:YAG laser surgery in the shoulder. *Oper Tech Sports Med* 1998; **6**:131–8.
12. Hayashi K, Markel MD. Thermal modification of joint capsule and ligamentous tissues. *Oper Tech Sports Med* 1998; **6**:120–5.
13. Hect P, Hayashi K, Cooley AJ et al. The thermal effect of

monopolar radiofrequency energy on the properties of joint capsule. An in vivo histologic study using a sheep model. *Am J Sports Med* 1998; **26**:808–14.

14. Hayashi K, Thabit G, Massa KL et al. The effect of thermal heating on the length and histologic properties of the glenohumeral joint capsule. *Am J Sports Med* 1997; **25**:107–12.

15. Naseef GS, Foster TE, Trauner K et al. The thermal properties of bovine joint capsule. The basic science of laser and radiofrequency induced capsular shrinkage. *Am J Sports Med* 1997; **25**:670–4.

16. Vangsness CT, Mitchell W, Nimni M et al. Collagen shortening: an experimental approach with heat. *Clin Orthop* 1997; **337**:267–71.

17. Osmond C, Hecht P, Hayashi K et al. Comparative effects of laser and radiofrequency energy on joint capsule. *Clin Orthop* 2000; **375**:286–94.

18. Lopez MJ, Hayashi K, Fanton GS et al. The effect of radiofrequency on the ultrastructure of joint capsule collagen. *Arthroscopy* 1998; **14**:495–501.

19. Hecht P, Hayashi K, Lu Y et al. Monopolar radiofrequency energy effects on joint capsular tissue: potential treatment for joint stability. An in vivo mechanical, morphological, and biochemical study using an ovine model. *Am J Sports Med* 1999; **27**:761–71.

20. Tibone JE, McMahon PJ, Shrader TA et al. Glenohumeral joint translation after arthroscopic, nonablative, thermal capsuloplasty with a laser. *Am J Sports Med* 1998; **26**:495–8.

21. Wall MS, Deng XH, Torzilli PA et al. Thermal modification of collagen. *J Shoulder Elbow Surg* 1999; **8**:339–44.

22. Obrzut SL, Hecht P, Hayashi K et al. The effect of radiofrequency energy on the length and temperature properties of the glenohumeral joint capsule. *Arthroscopy* 1998; **14**:395–400.

23. Eakin CL, Dvirnak P, Miller CM, Hawkins RJ. The relationship of the axillary nerve to arthroscopically placed capsulolabral sutures. *Am J Sports Med* 1998; **26**:505–9.

24. DeFelice GS, William RJ, Warren RF, Cohen MS. The accessory posterior portal for shoulder arthroscopy: description of technique and cadaveric study. Arthroscopy Association of North America 18th Annual Meeting; April 18, 1999; Vancouver, BC, Canada.

25. Lu Y, Hayashi K, Edwards RB et al. The effect of monopolar radiofrequency treatment pattern on joint capsular healing: in vitro and in vivo studies using an ovine model. *Am J Sports Med* 2000; **28**:711–19.

26. Rovner AD. Volumetric change in the shoulder capsule after open inferior capsular shift versus arthroscopic thermal capsular shrinkage. Paper presented at ISAKOS Congress; May 14–18, 2001; Montreux, Switzerland.

27. Lyons TR, Griffith PL, Savoie FH III, Field LD. Laser-assisted capsulorraphy for multidirectional instability of the shoulder. *Arthroscopy* 2001; **17**:25–30.

28. Mishra DK, Fanton GS. Two year outcome of arthroscopic Bankart repair and electrothermal assisted capsulorraphy for recurrent traumatic anterior shoulder instability. Arthroscopy Association of North American 19th Annual Meeting; April 14, 2000; Miami, Florida.

29. Anderson K, McCarty EC, Warren RF. Thermal capsulorraphy. Where are we today? *Sports Med Arthrosc Rev* 1999; **7**:117–27.

30. Levitz CL, Andrews JR. The use of arthroscopic thermal shrinkage in the management of internal impingement. Arthroscopy Association of North America 18th Annual Meeting; April 18, 1999; Vancouver, BC, Canada.

31. Bradley JP. Thermal capsulorraphy for instability of the shoulders. Multidirectional (MDI) and posterior instabilities. AAOS 2000, Symposia: Thermal capsulorraphy for instability of the shoulder. March 19th, 2000, Orlando, Florida.

32. Basamania CJ. Surgical technique of RF thermally assisted shoulder stabilization. ISAKOS Congress. May 30, 1999; Washington, DC.

15 Arthroscopic suture capsulorrhaphy

Jeffrey S Abrams

Introduction

An unstable shoulder is a painful condition that produces dysfunction as a result of excessive glenohumeral translation. This may be due to trauma or overuse, or may be congenital: some individuals are predisposed to the problem because they are born with laxity. Surgical correction has emphasized reduction of glenohumeral joint volume by mobilizing and shortening the capsular ligaments. The robust inferior glenohumeral ligament has been transferred in a direction to reduce capsular redundancy and reinforce capsular-deficient areas depending on the direction of instability.[1] Excessive glenohumeral translation is corrected, and the humeral head can be centered on the glenoid. Labral detachment or a Bankart lesion is more commonly associated with a traumatic dislocation.[2] In order to prevent recurrence, the labrum is reattached to the glenoid and the capsule is retensioned to limit pathologic translation.[3] The arthroscope has become an effective instrument to plicate ligaments, advance and transfer the capsule, and close intervals or tears within ligaments. A balanced approach anteriorly, inferiorly, and posteriorly creates a stable concentric reduction.

Despite technical advances it is still difficult to estimate tissue redundancy and assess the amount of reduction needed to correct the problem.[4] The learning curve is steep, and a combination of techniques, restrictive rehabilitation, and muscular retraining creates the best opportunity for successful return to activities.

Arthroscopic stabilization techniques continue to evolve. Early on, Johnson used a staple placed into the glenoid neck for repair of the capsule labral avulsion. Subsequent concerns about exposed hardware led to the development of suture repairs. Multiple monofilament sutures were inserted through the labrum and capsule and passed transglenoid, shifting the structures up against an abraded glenoid rim.[5,6] The reattachment point approximated the articular surfaces and a capsule shift was achieved, but fixation was still felt to be vulnerable. Variations on this theme included the use of multiple drill holes and eventually articular knot tying was attempted.[7] Suture management and knot tying were challenging, and surgical thumb tacks of absorbable polymer were developed. Because of the size and shape of the implants, inferior quadrant positioning for fixation was not always possible.

Suture anchors and suture plication techniques have become the arthroscopic 'gold standard'.[8] Suture capsulorrhaphy can be accomplished using curved suture hooks (Linvatec, Largo, FL, USA). The angled hooks advance the capsule by creating a pleat (Figure 15.1). This transfer is oblique, and can shorten capsule ligaments side to side and advance the capsule 'south to

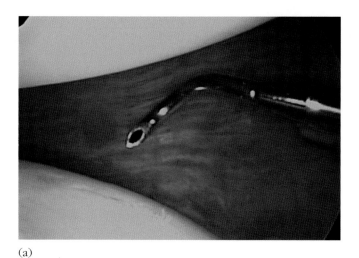
(a)

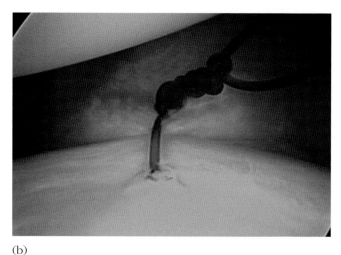
(b)

Figure 15.1

A curved suture hook can be introduced through a cannula, looking posteriorly and inferiorly, preparing for capsular advancement (a). A plication can be made by passing the hook through the capsule and then secondarily through the labrum. An absorbable monofilament suture can be retrieved and tied (b).

north'. Intervals or capsular defects can be closed, further reducing joint volume. Not only is the capsule adjacent to the direction of instability repaired, but in addition, the opposite capsular structures are sutured to maintain tension.[9] Both monofilament and braided sutures can be passed through the capsule and advanced to the labrum or to anchors with multiple points of fixation. Thermal capsular shrinkage may have a role in modifying the collagen, but so far has not replaced suture plication techniques. It is currently viewed as an augmentation technique that may further modify the capsule lateral to the plication. Capsular remodeling during the healing phase has led to concerns about the use of thermal shrinkage without sutures as an isolated treatment of instability.[10]

The indications for arthroscopic suture capsulorrhaphy include involuntary shoulder instability that has failed to respond to nonoperative treatment. A structured rehabilitation program including rotator cuff strengthening and scapular stabilization can be an effective way to manage instability in some cases. Capsular restraint is more important at the extremes of the range of rotation than in the middle range of movement. Dynamic factors have a greater role in stabilizing the glenohumeral joint, emphasizing the role of rehabilitation. Shoulder instability differs clinically from shoulder laxity, as patients are disabled and symptomatic from the excessive translation of the humeral head relative to the glenoid. Arthroscopic suture capsulorrhaphy is suitable for:

- primary capsule redundancy with symptomatic instability where there is an intact labrum;

- capsular redundancy associated with a Bankart lesion, when labral repair alone would be inadequate;
- revision surgery for failed stabilization due to capsular redundancy.

Although published reports of arthroscopic suture capsulorrhaphy are few, there have been several presentations regarding technique and personal results.[11–14] One of the difficult aspects of publication is classification of degree of instability. Patients present with pain and disability, but may have similar laxity in their asymptomatic shoulder. It is easier to define the pathologic condition when a locked dislocation is reduced and treated, or a Bankart lesion is present. Symptomatic microinstability or subluxations are more subtle and need individualized treatment. Experts have reported 79–89% successful treatment and return to activities. In a personal series, 34 of 38 patients (89%) were satisfied with pain levels after resumption of activities, but some of the younger patients had regained laxity without associated dysfunction on a 2-year follow-up examination.

Surgical principles

Symptomatic instability requires excessive translation that is both painful and disabling. It is important to assess glenohumeral translation and compare it with the asymptomatic shoulder. The examination under anesthesia consists of a 'load and shift' test and evaluation of a

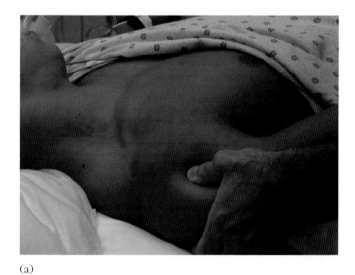

(a)

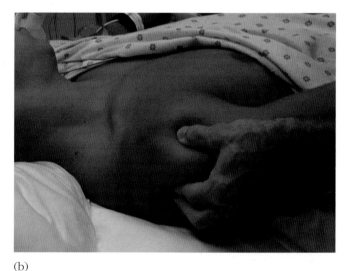

(b)

Figure 15.2

For the load and shift examination: (a) the examiner presses the humeral head into the glenoid and translates anteriorly and posteriorly to determine the amount of translation, palpable clicks, and possibly reproduction of symptoms; a sulcus sign (b) can be demonstrated by drawing the humerus inferiorly and palpating the humeral head as it translates beyond the inferior labrum.

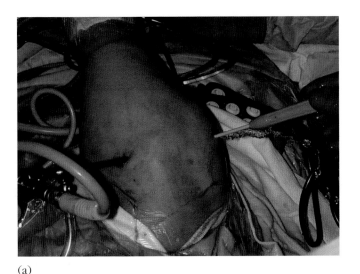

(a)

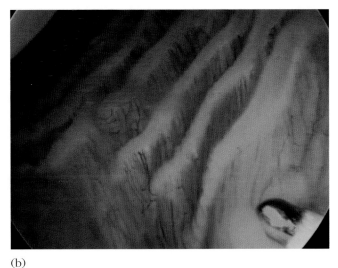

(b)

Figure 15.3

Anterior and posterior portals can be developed just lateral to the joint line (a), allowing for easy access to inferior, posterior, and anterior aspects of the shoulder. A thermal unit can be introduced through the posterior portal and the capsule is 'striped' from glenoid to humeral head (b) to stimulate the adjacent fibroblastic response.

sulcus sign (Figure 15.2).[15] By centering the humeral head into the glenoid and translating anteriorly, inferiorly, and posteriorly, glenohumeral translation and capsular laxity can be assessed. Further testing is performed by placing the arm in greater degrees of abduction and repeating the shift. This selectively tightens specific capsular structures to see if translation is reduced. Asymmetry in the two shoulders is significant, as well as continued luxation in spite of positioning the shoulder in a way that ordinarily tensions the capsular ligaments. In the awake patient, reproduction of symptoms can be a helpful diagnostic sign.

The surgical procedure can be performed with the patient in either the lateral decubitus or the beach-chair position. The lateral decubitus position allows greater access to the back of the glenohumeral joint. Arm abduction can be varied between 30° and 60° to improve visualization of the inferior capsular pouch. Although traction can be used for the diagnostic portion of the examination, it should be reduced to facilitate capsule mobilization. Reproducing the same scapular and humeral relationship is an important step in gaining experience in determining capsular length and volume.

A capsule plication is a technique to shorten the capsule and transfer it superiorly. Using curved suture hooks including left and right angles, a pass through the capsule followed by a second pass under and through the intact labrum can create a capsular pleat. The size of the capsule plication is dependent on the spacing of the two passes through the tissue. Multiple sutures are placed along the elongated ligaments. It is best to begin on the symptomatic side and work from inferior to superior. Overtensioning one side of a loose shoulder

without addressing the opposite side may create symptoms in the opposite direction. A balanced approach to shortening the capsule keeps the humeral head centered on the glenoid.

Capsular irritation should precede the plication. Shaving instruments, suction punches, and thermal devices can be used to alter the capsule and stimulate healing of the pleated capsule. The thermal probe should stripe the capsule rather than 'paint' an area, to avoid devitalizing large parts of the capsule. The stripes can extend laterally to the humeral head (Figure 15.3). This may be advantageous as the plication is medial, adjacent to the glenoid, and does not directly affect the lateral capsule.

The rotator capsular interval is the normal opening between the superior glenohumeral ligament and the middle glenohumeral ligament. This is deep to the interval between the subscapularis and the supraspinatus. The external aspect of this capsule includes portions of the coracohumeral ligament, which acts to limit inferior translation in the adducted shoulder.[16] Selective cutting and imbrication experiments have shown its importance in limiting posterior subluxation.[17] Closure or reduction of this interval may be important in cases of posterior and anterior subluxation, especially when there is a component of excessive inferior translation.

Surgical technique

The patient is transferred to the operating table and anesthesia is induced. The evaluation under anesthesia includes range of motion and load and shift examinations. The degree of translation and associated clicks or crepitus of the involved side are compared with those of the asymptomatic side. The shoulders are translated anteriorly, posteriorly, and inferiorly. The patient is then placed in the lateral decubitus position. A bean bag can be molded about the torso and chest wall. Allow the patient to roll back about 20° to position the glenoid parallel to the floor. Place the arm in 30–60° of abduction and apply a traction of 2.25–4.5 kg (5–10 lb). Secure the torso with tape and add a warming blanket to the patient's covers.

The posterior portal is positioned first. Palpate the spine of the scapula, the acromion, the acromioclavicular joint, and the coracoid process. Place a spinal needle 2 cm inferior to the junction of the lateral margin of the acromion with the spine of the scapula, and enter the joint space with gentle distraction of the humerus. Inflate the joint with 30 ml of saline and observe the angle of the needle prior to creating the portal. If this is favorable, create a puncture with a #11 blade. The blunt trocar and cannula can be introduced by a twisting motion. The anterior portal is created halfway between the acromion and coracoid by placing a spinal needle and entering the joint above the subscapularis and below the biceps. A cannula should be placed in the anterior quadrant, removing air bubbles, debris, and blood.

The diagnostic examination is sequentially performed. Begin by identifying the biceps and look medially to its insertion on the superior labrum. Visualize and probe the entire circumference of the labral attachment to the glenoid. Look for glenoid articular changes at the margin of the labral attachments, as well as pathologic changes in the substance of the labrum. Examine the capsule including the anterior capsular ligaments, inferior pouch, and posterior capsule. Global laxity is often coexistent with a capacious capsule and a large view of the entire glenohumeral joint. Visualize the rotator cuff beginning with the superior border of the subscapularis. Rotating the arthroscope, examine the insertion of the supraspinatus, infraspinatus and teres minor. The shoulder can be released from traction to help identify coexistent internal impingement.

Remove the arthroscope and place it in the anterior portal. Visualize the position of the humeral head relative to the glenoid with minimal traction. Slight anteroinferior luxation is not uncommon. Inspect the anterior capsule labral attachment medially and visualize laterally to the humeral head attachment. Further reduction of traction combined with internal rotation will improve visualization, and can be accomplished manually or by using a second traction sling. The posterior and posteroinferior labrum and capsule are examined and palpated. Maintain access to the front and back of the shoulder to allow for further evaluation intraoperatively.

The capsulorrhaphy is started on the primary direction of symptomatic instability. In cases of posterior subluxation, the arthroscope is left in the anterior portal and the posteroinferior pouch is approached. In cases of anterior subluxation, the posterior viewing portal is used and hooks can be introduced into the anteroinferior pouch. In cases of multidirectional instability, the posterior viewing portal is used and the inferior pouch is visualized. Irritation of the capsule can be accomplished using a shaver blade, a punch, or a thermal probe. If

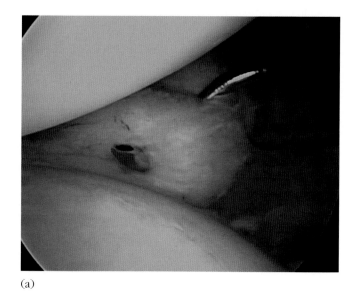

(a)

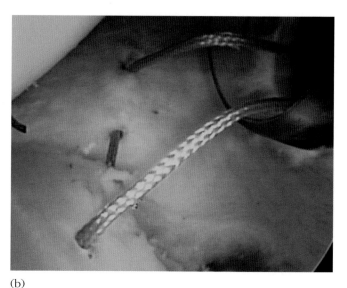

(b)

Figure 15.4

A suture hook (a) can be passed through the capsule and secondarily through the intact labrum. Suture anchors can be used when labral detachment or deficiency is present. (b) The capsule can be plicated against the edge of the glenoid, shortened, and superiorly transferred.

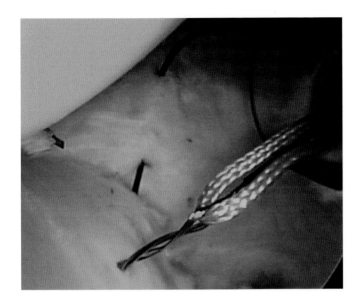

Figure 15.5

A suture shuttle can be used to assist the transfer of a braided suture from the edge of the glenoid through the capsule.

thermal shrinkage is selected, stripe the capsule from the glenoid to the humeral head. Viable islands of capsule are an important aspect of capsular regeneration and can possibly shorten the remodeling phase.[18]

A variety of curved suture hooks can be helpful in creating the plication. Beginning inferiorly, take a full-thickness pass with the appropriate hook, draw the tissues superiorly, and pass the hook under and through the intact labrum (Figure 15.4). If a labral detachment has occurred, a series of suture anchors can be used to repair the detached labrum and secure the advanced capsule. Absorbable monofilament or braided sutures can be used. Each has its advantages and the choice depends on the surgeon's preference. If a braided suture is chosen, an additional step is required to draw the suture through the capsule labral tissues. Using a suture hook, create a pleat and introduce a suture shuttle (Linvatec) or pass a monofilament suture. Retrieve the free end out of the cannula and make sure the suture or shuttle can slide back and forth. Introduce a #2 braided suture and use the shuttle to draw it through the capsule and under the labrum (Figure 15.5).

Sliding knots can simplify the intra-articular fixation. Suture management eliminates tangles, twists, and soft tissue interposition. Using a simple slider knot is a consistent way of placing a knot that is secure (Figure 15.6). The knot-tying instrument is placed on the 'post' limb of the suture (the limb around which the knot will be tied). This is the suture arm that exits through the capsule away from the glenoid. Shorten the post limb and use the nonpost limb of the suture to create an underhanded hitch followed by an overhanded hitch. Dress the knot by removing unnecessary slack and let the nonpost limb of the suture go to avoid premature locking. Pull on the post and use the knot pusher to direct the knot to its destination. To lock the knot, grasp the other suture limb with your free hand and apply equal traction on both limbs. 'Past-point' with the knot pusher to evert the second throw. To do this, loosen

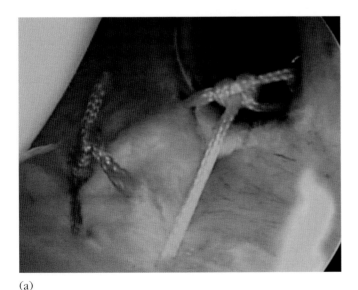
(a)

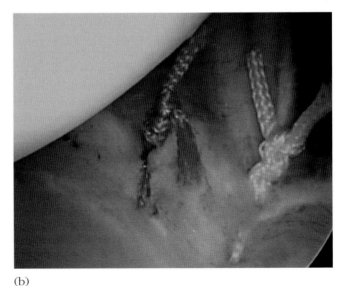
(b)

Figure 15.6

To tie a simple slider knot, (a) the underhanded pass followed by an overhanded pass can be advanced down the post, transferring the soft tissue to the labrum; 'past-pointing' with a knot tyer can bend the post and secure the knot. Multiple half-hitches (b) can follow the sliding knot to prevent any potential loosening, creating a secure knot.

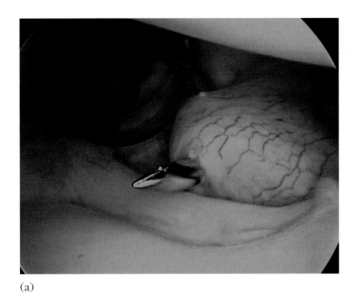

(a)

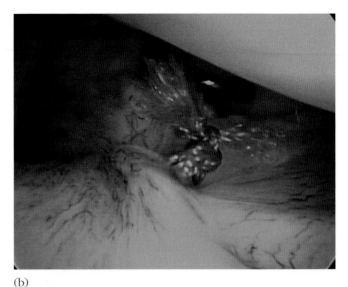

(b)

Figure 15.7

For rotator interval capsular closure. (a) Using a suture hook introduced through the anterior portal, the middle glenohumeral ligament can be advanced to the superior glenohumeral ligament or superior labrum. (b) Beginning medially and working laterally, close the capsular interval to provide additional stabilization.

hand tension and back the knot-tying instrument up about 5 cm. Then push the knot tyer past the knot – pulling the second hitch, causing it to flip and kink the post. This will prevent the knot from backing up. Follow this with a series of half-hitches. Switching the knot tyer to the other suture limb may apply additional friction, reducing the possibility of the knot loosening.

Sutures are placed 5–10 mm apart, fixing the capsule in an oblique direction to the glenoid, beginning inferiorly and working superiorly. Labral detachments that are not felt to be congenital can be repaired as well.

Remove the arthroscope and replace it in the opposite portal. Plication along the opposite capsule is used to create symmetrical shortening of the ligaments. Thermal shrinkage is not often needed to supplement the asymptomatic direction. Begin inferiorly and proceed up the opposite side. Minimal plication is needed if the condition is asymptomatic, and larger pleats are created if multidirectional laxity is present.

With the arthroscope in the posterior viewing portal, the rotator capsule interval can be closed. Use a suture hook that can advance the middle glenohumeral ligament superiorly (Figure 15.7). For the right shoulder use a right hook, and for the left shoulder use a left hook. Grasp the middle glenohumeral ligament at the superior border just lateral to the labrum. Draw this superiorly and advance the hook to pass into the superior labrum, or superior glenohumeral ligament. Tie a sliding knot and repeat these steps, working in a medial to lateral direction, until the cannula obstructs the passage of the last knot. Knot tying can be completed while visualizing from the bursae, and the suture is cut.

Revision surgery can be done arthroscopically in many cases. It is essential to evaluate the reasons for failure preoperatively. Unidirectional corrective operations often fail to address and correct the excessive translation symmetrically. Pouch obliteration and interval closure are important steps that are often overlooked. Rather than performing an arthrotomy, one can consider arthroscopic evaluation and correction with an inside-out approach. If one direction has been overtensioned, consider dividing the capsule and creating equal tension anteriorly and posteriorly. One of the major advantages of an arthroscopic approach is the global correction that can be achieved. Ligament shortening, rather than transfer, can be achieved without rotator cuff division.

Use both portals to evaluate the repair. The traction can be removed and the arm rotated while visualizing ligament tensioning. Viewed from the anterior portal, the anterior capsular ligaments should demonstrate tension at 30° of external rotation, and the posterior capsular ligaments should demonstrate absence of a pouch. Additional plication sutures can be added to tension the capsule further if need be. After the arthroscope is removed, confirm reduction of the sulcus sign. The portals are closed with simple sutures, and dry dressings are applied followed by immobilization.

Postoperative protocol

The patient's arm is placed in a sling (Ultrasling, DJ Ortho, Carlsbad, CA, USA) for 4–6 weeks. The sling places the glenohumeral joint in a more neutral orientation and provides superior support to avoid inferior capsular strain. It can be removed for bathing, dressing, and gentle exercises.

The initial exercises emphasize scapular stabilization. Shoulder shrugs and scapular retraction should be done twice daily. Elbow motion with biceps and triceps exercises can be started. Stretching is limited with a restrictive range of motion. Generally, more than 20° of external rotation and internal rotation behind the back should be avoided. Forward elevation to the face will allow many daily functions to be achieved without jeopardizing the repair.

At week 4, tightness is reassessed. Patients whose shoulder cannot easily achieve these movements are instructed in new flexibility exercises with the assistance of physical therapy. Limits of 30° external rotation and forward elevation below 120° are enforced. Shoulders that have attained these movements should be left in the sling for another 2 weeks.

At 6–8 weeks more emphasis is placed on protective stretching, rotator cuff strengthening, and continued scapular stabilizing exercises. Seated rows, wall push-ups in a neutral grip, and light resistive exercises can be started. Latissimus dorsi, rhomboid, pectoralis, trapezius, and serratus anterior muscle strengthening and endurance exercises can be performed with a daily schedule. Low-resistance and high-repetition activities are started, with special advice to the patient on avoiding inferior traction.

At 12 weeks, near-normal motion allows greater emphasis on strength. Sport-specific exercises and training can be started when motion is complete and strength testing suggests that functional activities can be started. Critical evaluation of biomechanics as well as addressing other potential liabilities is important. Poor mechanics due to hamstring tightness, low back and torso weakness continues to place the shoulder at increased risk. Many noncontact athletic activities can be resumed at 4–6 months and contact sports at 6–8 months. The return to sport needs to be individualized, depending on the patient's preoperative morbidity and the nature of the activity that is expected postoperatively. Patient selection, a balanced and symmetric surgical approach, and a protective return to activities ensure the greatest chance of success. Many patients, including athletes and those receiving worker's compensation, have been able to return to their desired activities.

References

1. Neer CS, Foster CR. Inferior capsular shift for involuntary inferior and multidirectional instability of the shoulder. *J Bone Joint Surg* 1980; **62A**:897–908.
2. Rowe CR, Patel D, Southmayd WW. The Bankart procedure: a long-term end result study. *J Bone Joint Surg* 1978; **60A**:1–16.
3. Thomas SC, Matsen FA. An approach to the repair of avulsion of the glenohumeral ligaments in the management of traumatic anterior glenohumeral instability. *J Bone Joint Surg* 1989; **71A**:506–13.
4. Abrams JS. Arthroscopic shoulder stabilization for recurrent subluxation and dislocation. *J Shoulder Elbow Surg* 1993; **2**:25.
5. Caspari RB. Arthroscopic reconstruction for shoulder instability. *Tech Orthop* 1988; **3**:59–66.
6. Morgan CD, Bodenstab AB. Arthroscopic Bankart suture repair: technique and early results. *Arthroscopy* 1987; **3**:111–22.
7. Maki NJ. Arthroscopic stabilization suture technique. *Oper Tech Orthop* 1991; **1**:180–3.
8. Abrams JS. Shoulder stabilization and evolving trends in arthroscopic repair. *Sports Med Arthrose Rev* 1999; **7**:104–16.
9. Wolf EM. Capsular plication techniques for anterior, posterior or multidirectional instability. AANA Specialty Day, 1996, Atlanta, Georgia, 21–25.
10. Abrams JS. Thermal capsulorrhaphy for instability of the shoulder: concerns and applications of the heat probe. *Instr Course Lect* 2001; **50**:29–36.
11. Treacy SH, Savoie FH, Field LD. Arthroscopic treatment of multidirectional instability. *J Shoulder Elbow Surg* 1999; **8**:345–50.
12. Wichman MT, Snyder SJ, Karzer RP et al. Arthroscopic capsular plication for involuntary shoulder instability without a Bankart lesion. *Arthroscopy* 1997; **13**:377.
13. Tauro JC. Arthroscopic inferior capsular split and advancement for anterior and inferior shoulder instability: technique and results at 2 to 5 year follow-up. *Arthroscopy* 2000; **16**:451–56.
14. Weber SC. Arthroscopic suture capsulorrhaphy in the management of type 2 and type 3 impingement. *Arthroscopy* 2000; **16**:430–1.
15. Hawkins RJ, Abrams JS, Schutte JP. Multidirectional instability of the shoulder: an approach to diagnosis. *Orthop Trans* 1987; **11**:246.
16. Warner JS, Deng XH, Warren RF et al. Static capsuloligamentous restraints to superior–inferior translation of the glenohumeral joint. *Am J Sports Med* 1992; **20**:675–85.
17. Harryman DT, Sidles JA, Harris SL et al. The role of the rotator interval capsule in passive motion and stability of the shoulder. *J Bone Joint Surg* 1992; **74A**:53–66.
18. Lu Y, Hayaski K, Edwards RB et al. The effect of monopolar radiofrequency treatment pattern on joint capsular healing. *Am J Sports Med* 2000; **28**:711–19.

16 Multidirectional shoulder instability

Uwe König, Jens D Agneskirchner and Andreas B Imhoff

Introduction

Strategies in operative and non-operative treatment of shoulder instability have changed enormously in recent years. In addition to the aims of restoring stability and minimizing the rate of redislocation, treatment methods increasingly focus on restoring range of motion and strength, especially in young and active patients. It has been recognized that this can be accomplished by an exact reconstruction of capsulolabral anatomy in open procedures such as Neer's capsular shift and Bankart repairs, or by the newer arthroscopic procedures.[1]

A more complex problem with respect to diagnosis and therapy, however, is that of non-unidirectional or multidirectional instability (MDI). As these conditions are relatively rare (2% of all forms of instability), mainly conservative management rather than operation has been advocated as their appropriate treatment. With the increasing identification of transitional forms between unidirectional and multidirectional instability, operative treatment has come more and more to the fore.[2–12] Differentiation between 'laxity' and 'instability', and identification and classification of the different degrees of instability, are mandatory in order to determine the appropriate treatment.

Laxity and instability

Laxity is the degree of humeral head translation in the glenoid fossa without rotation, and can be assessed using the clinical 'shift and load' test. A certain amount of laxity is required for every shoulder to function in its large range of motion. By definition, instability means the lack of ability to retain the humeral head within the glenoid during normal and active shoulder function.[6] Hawkins and colleagues described four degrees of laxity:[13,14]

0   no translation at all;
1   the humeral head rides on the glenoid rim (translation of up to 1 cm);
2   subluxation with spontaneous reduction (translation of up to 2 cm);
3   complete dislocation (translation of more than 2 cm).

Pathological findings (instability) are mostly to be found among grades 2 and 3.

Thus, differentiating between laxity and instability means that the diagnosis of instability can only be made clinically, not by test manoeuvres under anaesthesia.[15,16] In particular, young and active athletes frequently have lax (subluxating, Hawkins 2) shoulder joints that are not necessarily unstable.

Classification of shoulder instability

In classifying shoulder instability four different criteria need to be focused on: *aetiology, degree, frequency* and *direction*. This classification also covers the complex types of instability including MDI. Moreover, it facilitates individual management for every patient.[13,17]

Aetiology

Five different aetiologies of shoulder instability can be distinguished: traumatic, atraumatic, repetitive microtrauma (overuse), congenital and neuromuscular. Thomas and Matsen used the terms 'TUBS' and 'AMBRI' to describe the two outermost points of the whole spectrum of instability.[11] The term 'TUBS' describes the traumatic, unidirectional type of instability, often comprising a classic Bankart defect which is open to surgical management. The other extreme – AMBRI – is an atraumatic, mostly multidirectional (often bilateral) form of instability that should initially be treated with rehabilitation, with surgical therapy (inferior capsular shift) only indicated if this treatment fails.[8,9,18] However, these types only exemplify two clearly distinguishable types of instability and oversimplify the variety of all the other forms. Moreover, they do not take into account transitional forms with a hyperlaxity component. For example, the degree of capsuloligamentous hyperlaxity that is necessary for 'overhead' sports such as throwing, swimming and climbing, can – through repetitive microtrauma – lead to symptomatic instability.[15,19–22] Congenital instability such as increased anteversion or retroversion of the glenoid, dysplasia or neurologic disease (e.g. Erb's palsy) is relatively rare.[23]

Differentiation between voluntary and non-voluntary dislocation (or subluxation) is another important point. *Voluntary* dislocation means that the patient, using only the muscles of the shoulder girdle, is capable of dislocating the head of the humerus anteriorly, inferiorly or posteriorly. This is often associated with psychiatric disease and should not be treated surgically. Non-voluntary dislocations always occur when the arm is held in a certain position, which the patient tries to avoid; these cases are usually accessible to operation.

Degree of instability

The degree of instability can be divided into subluxation (spontaneous reduction of the humeral head back into the glenoid) and complete dislocation.

Frequency

The frequency of instability can be acute, chronic or recurrent. Acute instability occurs within 24 hours of the first dislocation; it is chronic if the time to humeral head dislocation is longer than that. Recurrent instability is the appropriate term if there is more than one occurrence of subluxation or dislocation. A special case is the form of dislocation in which closed reduction is impossible; these are called 'locked' dislocations and often coincide with a large impression fracture of the humeral head (Hill–Sachs or reversed Hill–Sachs lesion).

Direction

Directions of instability can be anterior, inferior, posterior or superior, combinations of these, or multidirectional. Anterior instability is the most common form (95%). Superior instability has only recently been identified, and is mostly found in young patients complaining about impingement pain. This kind of impingement is called secondary impingement and is predominantly produced by superior labral or biceps pathology such as superior labrum anterior to posterior (SLAP) lesions, or hyperlaxity.[24–28] While SLAP lesions can be caused by macrotrauma, more often they result from repetitive microtrauma causing degeneration at the origin of the long head of the biceps tendon. Proper treatment for this kind of impingement is elimination of the instability originating from the unstable biceps insertion (arthroscopic refixation of SLAP), not a subacromial decompression.[1,29,30]

Multidirectional instability

MDI is defined as a symptomatic form of glenohumeral instability occurring in more than one direction: anteriorly, inferiorly and posteriorly.[2,9,31–35] This kind of instability is frequently bilateral and can be found in young

patients who often have psychiatric difficulties. This is why a voluntary component always has to be looked for in these patients.[36,37] There is still debate as to whether there is a clear definition of MDI at all.

Like Bigliani et al[38] and Walch et al,[16] we believe that MDI is only one extreme appearance of general hyperlaxity of different degrees. We prefer to speak of *multidirectional hyperlaxity* showing additional anterior, inferior or posterior instability, rather than multidirectional instability. Besides multidirectionally unstable shoulders in children, symptomatic instabilities can often be found in athletes participating in overhead sports and usually result from a combination of recurrent microtrauma and hyperlaxity.[16]

Both types can be the source of a secondary impingement syndrome. Furthermore, patients with hyperlaxity can naturally experience anterior dislocations resulting from macrotrauma which generate a miscellaneous type of instability with both traumatic and atraumatic components.[15,20–22,39]

Pathomorphology

Anatomically, the decisive structural abnormalities causing instability are to be found at the capsulolabral ligamentous complex. Posttraumatic instabilities result from the typical Bankart lesion representing a detachment of the labrum and anterior capsule from the glenoid rim with or without a chondral or osseous avulsion of the glenoid.[1,40–47] Recurrent dislocations more often produce Perthes lesions (subperiosteal anterior capsulolabral disruptions reaching onto the scapular neck), anterior labrum periosteal sleeve avulsion (ALPSA) lesions[1,29,30] or capsuloligamentous distensions into the direction of dislocation.

Rather than by capsuloligamentous disruptions or avulsions, multidirectional instabilities are characterized by the abnormal quality of the capsular tissue. General capsular redundancy anteriorly, inferiorly and posteriorly, as well as weak, poorly developed glenohumeral ligaments together with an enlarged rotator interval, cause increased humeral translation in all directions with the arm abducted and adducted.[17] The situation of an enlarged capsule together with a hypoplastic labrum is a non-Bankart lesion.[1,48,49]

Clinical appearance

Clinically, patients with MDI complain about recurrent subluxations and subjective instability rather than real dislocations.[17] In cases of actual dislocation, more often minor traumatic events rather than adequate macrotrauma are the reason for injury. Reduction mostly occurs

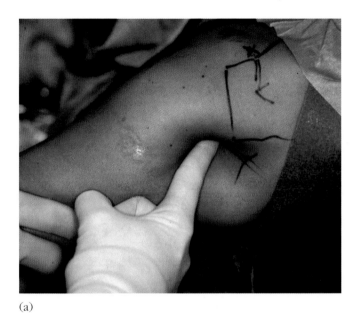

(a)

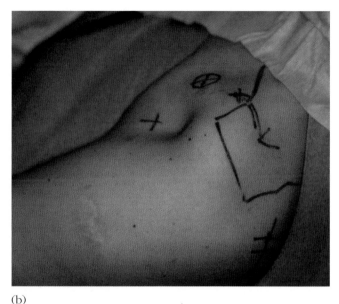

(b)

Figure 16.1

Examination under anaesthesia in multidirectional instability: (a) anterior dislocation of the humeral head; (b) posterior dislocation of the humeral head.

spontaneously. A voluntary component must always be considered.[36]

Mostly there is one dominant direction of instability. This is why in cases of anterior instability the patients feel pain or discomfort with the internally and externally rotated and abducted position, whereas in cases of posterior instability pain is felt in the flexed and internally rotated position. Problems (pain or discomfort) caused by inferior instability can be seen during the carrying of heavy weights; superior instability causes a secondary impingement (see above). Some patients experience instability while sleeping.[6] It is important always to examine the patients for general joint laxity and systemic disease such as Ehlers–Danlos syndrome, as well as obtaining a family history.[23,50–52]

Diagnosis

A careful and thorough examination of the shoulder includes the exact recording of the range of motion and muscular strength. Instability must be assessed separately using special stability tests.[1,39] Anterior and posterior humeral head translation is examined using the drawer test with the arm adducted and 90° abducted and the scapula in a fixed position. For description, the Hawkins classification should be used (see above). Inferior translation can be assessed using the *sulcus sign*: grade 1 is a distance of up to 1 cm between the undersurface of

the acromion and humeral head, grade 2 is a distance of up to 2 cm, and grade 3 is a distance of more than 2 cm. An important test is the anterior and posterior *apprehension test* which – performed in three specific arm positions (60°, 90°, 120° abduction and external rotation) – can be used for testing of the individual anterior glenohumeral ligaments as well as for assessment of subjective patient instability (apprehension). In addition, the shift and load test and the relocation test can be performed, the latter being important in the diagnosis of posterosuperior glenoid labral lesions.[1]

Additionally, SLAP lesions can be found.[27] Tests for clinical diagnosis are the Crank test (palpable clicking in passive rotation of abducted arm), the O'Brien test and the 'Slapprehension' test (pain felt in flexion and internal rotation).[26,53] Preoperatively translation in any direction should be tested under anaesthesia (Figure 16.1).[13,14]

Radiographic examination

Three standard radiographs (true anteroposterior, axial, Y-view or supraspinatus outlet view) should always be taken in order to exclude bony Bankart lesions or large Hill–Sachs defects, but often are normal in MDI.

The 'gold standard' investigation is magnetic resonance arthrography (arthro-MRI). Not only the capsulolabral structures but also the glenohumeral ligaments and the volume of the joint capsule (typically widened in MDI)

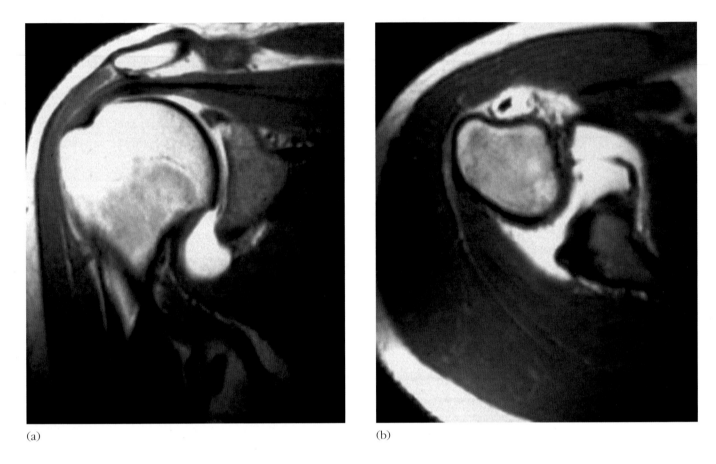

(a)   (b)

Figure 16.2

Arthro-MRI with intra-articular gadolinium: (a) frontal plane, showing a wide axillary recess in a patient with multidirectional instability; (b) horizontal plane (same patient), showing a wide anterior and posterior capsule; anteriorly the capsuloligamentous tissue is detached.

can be assessed (Figure 16.2). Arthro-MRI is of special importance in diagnosing instability since it has better sensitivity than conventional magnetic resonance imaging[54,55] or computed tomographic arthrography. The latter imaging technique is indicated in situations of osseous injury or abnormalities, such as large Hill–Sachs or Bankart defects, or pathologically increased glenoid anteversion or retroversion, if operative correction is planned.

Conservative treatment

Multidirectional shoulder instability should primarily be treated conservatively. A physiotherapeutic rehabilitation programme should be initiated to strengthen the rotator cuff and improve coordinative abilities. Patients with instability *and* hyperlaxity have been shown to have a significant deficit of coordinative and proprioceptive capacities in the muscles of the shoulder girdle, giving this therapeutic regimen its scientific rationale.[56–60]

Furthermore, activities in which dislocations or pain might happen should be avoided. In all MDI patients operative management should not be considered before 6 months of thorough physiotherapy. Patients younger than 16 years should not be operated on at all since juvenile hyperlaxity sometimes improves spontaneously within years.[61] Surgical treatment is contraindicated also in MDI patients who through voluntarily dislocating their shoulders have a secondary psychological benefit from their disease. In this case redislocation within 1 year of operation is very likely.[25,37,39]

Operative treatment

The indications for surgical management of MDI have gradually been extended as new and better operative techniques in shoulder surgery – in particular arthroscopy – have been developed. Candidates for operation are patients in whom a specific arm position almost always leads to a dislocation. This type of patient tries to avoid the specific trigger situation. Their form of instability is by definition non-voluntary and is almost always of traumatic origin.

Patients with a unidirectional instability but multidirectional hyperlaxity are also suitable for surgery. These patients characteristically cannot voluntarily dislocate their shoulders. The direction of instability often is anterior, and sometimes on arthroscopy a SLAP lesion can be found in addition to hyperlaxity.[1]

Open surgical approach

Neer's inferior capsular shift is the classic surgical treatment for multidirectional instability;[8] it comprises a three-dimensional reduction of capsular volume (anterior, inferior, posterior).

Like anterior capsulorraphy, this technique requires an anterior approach to the shoulder joint. Incision of the capsule is performed along the anatomic neck from anterior to posterior up to the 3 o'clock position (in a right shoulder). After mobilization of the anterior and inferior capsule, the anterior capsule is duplicated, resulting in an anterior shift of the axillary pouch that leads to increased tension of the posterior capsule. Neer called this technique 'inferior capsular shift' since by approaching from only one (anterior) side and by shifting the inferior part of the capsule, both the anterior as well as the posterior capsular tissue can be reduced. This is why the technique can be performed equally well from the posterior approach.[2,39,62–68] It is up to the surgeon to choose the appropriate technique in each individual case. Cooper and Brems recommend working on the side where clinically the major direction of instability is found, on the grounds that scarring in the duplicated tissue increases stability.[4] Occasionally the decision can only be made by clinical examination under anaesthesia. The operation is difficult, not least because manipulation at the inferior recess takes place in direct proximity to the axillary nerve.

The outcome after inferior capsular shift is promising. In a series of 43 patients Cooper and Brems reported that 91% had a satisfactory result without redislocation after 2 years.[4] In a study by Bigliani et al, 52 patients were followed up at an average of 5 (range 2–11) years after operation, 94% of whom were satisfied with the outcome.[2,38]

Typically the inferior capsular shift procedure should be performed if capsular redundancy is the main pathological problem. If – and this is most likely to be the case – additional lesions are present, alternative techniques have to be applied. In case of a Bankart lesion, Altchek et al recommend the classic Bankart procedure in combination with a modified inferior capsular shift procedure.[19] Altchek et al reported encouraging results, but Hawkins et al's series of 31 patients had a more discouraging outcome: 39% of his patients were not satisfied and had redislocations after a follow-up period of 2–5 years.[62]

Arthroscopic technique

Arthroscopic shoulder stabilization has become a reliable treatment method in the management of unidirectional, posttraumatic instability and in the treatment of superior glenoid labral disorders.[1] The development of fixation systems (suture anchors) and capsular shrinking techniques (electrothermal or laser-assisted) are enlarging the spectrum of indications.

Following failed conservative treatment of multidirectional instability, arthroscopic management largely depends on the capsulolabral anatomy. Osseous abnormalities such as increased glenoid anteversions or retroversions or large Bankart lesions have to be excluded.

A typical Bankart lesion in combination with an increased capsular volume can be treated by arthroscopic capsular shrinkage of the posterior and inferior capsule, while anteriorly the capsulolabral ligamentous complex is reattached to the glenoid by means of suture anchors. Anteriorly, before suture anchor fixation, thorough debridement of the glenoid and subperiosteal mobilization of the capsulolabral tissue and ligaments are mandatory. By performing a shift of the tissue from inferior to superior, 'new' tissue for formation of the anteroinferior labrum is obtained, and additionally the inferior capsule is stretched. Ideally the most superior suture anchor is placed in the 1 o'clock position. It is important to give the anterior band of the inferior glenohumeral ligament enough strength and stability since it is one of the major stabilizing factors.[1,21] In case of an additional SLAP lesion we recommend its refixation.[26,29,30]

Several techniques of arthroscopic capsulolabral reconstruction have been advocated. Staples and transglenoid sutures should be avoided because of their high complication rate.[69] Refixation of the labrum and capsule can be performed using bioabsorbable tacks (Suretac; Smith & Nephew, Andover, MA, USA)[46,70] or suture anchors; absorbable (Bio-FASTak, Arthrex, Naples, FL, USA; Panalok, Mitek, Westwood, MA, USA) or nonabsorbable (FASTak, Arthrex) suture anchors are available (Figure 16.3a). For laser-assisted capsular shrinkage the holmium-YAG laser is used;[42,71–73] systems for electrothermally assisted capsular shrinkage (Figure 16.3b) are available from Arthrocare (Sunnyvale, CA, USA), Oratec (Menlo Park, CA, USA) and Mitek (VAPR).[1,39,68,74–79]

First results from arthroscopic operations of MDI using the techniques described above were published by McIntyre et al.[72] In 19 patients only one recurrent subluxation was noted after an average follow-up of 34 months. All the other patients were content with the result and most of them even returned to a high level of sporting activity. The outcomes of our patients treated arthroscopically for MDI confirm these positive results. However, the decisive prerequisite is the correct patient selection and indication.[1,39]

An alternative to the suture anchor technique in combination with capsular shrinking is the suture punch

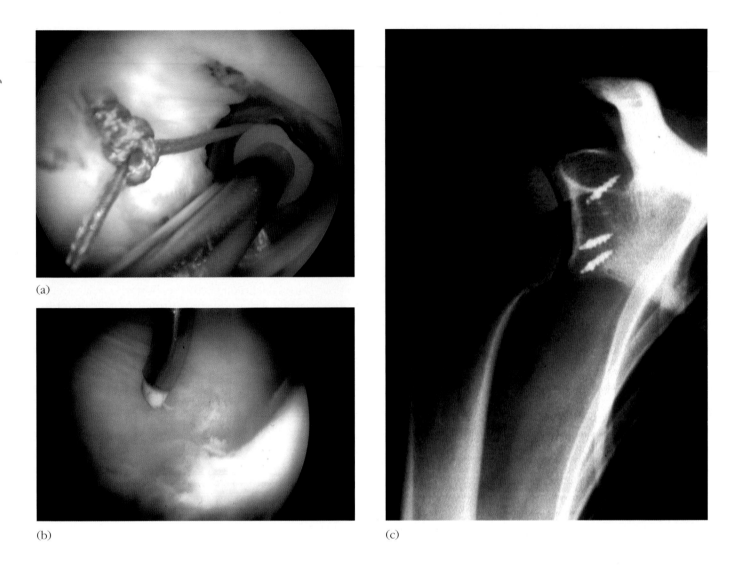

(a)

(b)

(c)

Figure 16.3

Capsulolabral reconstruction. (a) A suture anchor equipped with a polyester suture is used for anterosuperior refixation of the middle glenohumeral ligament. The suture is tied with the 'sixth finger' knot pusher (Arthrex, Munich, Germany). (b) Electrothermally assisted capsular shrinkage of the anterior band of the inferior glenohumeral ligament (ArthroCare®). (c) Postoperative radiograph showing three suture anchors FASTak (Arthrex, Naples, FL, USA) in correct position.

technique. These patients are managed by an arthroscopically-assisted inferior capsular shift. Duncan and Savoie presented a report of this arthroscopic method.[5] This technique involves extending the dissection and capsular freeing for the Bankart reconstruction inferiorly and posteriorly past the 6 o'clock position to approximately the 8 o'clock position. In patients with no detachment, an arthroscopic knife or end-cutting shaver is used to create a capsular detachment from the glenoid. The capsule is incised along a line projected from the rim of the glenoid. Sutures are then placed into the posterior middle and anterior point of the inferior glenohumeral ligament, and anterior middle and anterosuperior glenohumeral ligaments. This requires approximately 10–12 sutures (20–24 strands). These sutures are then pulled through one or two drill holes through the glenoid neck, eliminating the redundancy of the posterior capsule, inferior pouch, and reconstructing the ligamentous tissues.

Caspari's group has reported on a combined arthroscopic anterior and posterior capsular reconstruction for multidirectional instability.[72] In this procedure, a 5-mm portion of the inferior glenohumeral ligament is left attached at approximately the 6 o'clock position. The anterior aspect of the shoulder is reconstructed as with a normal Bankart reconstruction in Caspari's method except

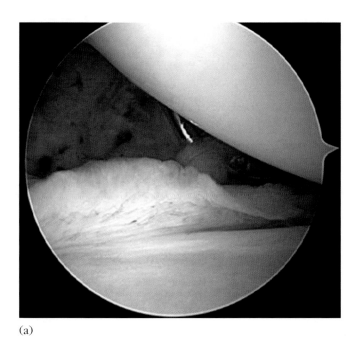

(a)

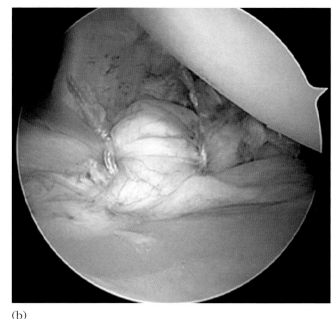

(b)

Figure 16.4

Arthroscopic capsular plication (suture plication) without suture anchors. (a) Panacryl sutures are pulled through the capsular tissue by means of a curved suture hook. (b) The completed procedure for the reduction of capsular volume with sutures are in place (Courtesy of Dr Craig Buttoni, Tripley Army Medical Center, Honolulu, HI, USA).

that the 6 o'clock attachment of the capsule is maintained. The Caspari sutures are placed and then pulled out of the posterior aspect of the shoulder. The arthroscope is then placed anteriorly, and a posterior reconstruction as described by Duncan and Savoie is accomplished. The arm is placed in a position of neutral rotation and adduction and the anterior and posterior sutures are tightened until central stability of the humeral head on the glenoid is achieved and the sutures are tied in this position.

Duncan and Savoie[5] have reported 91% satisfactory results for the arthroscopic inferior capsular shift procedure. In their patient population no complications were noted. Caspari's group has reported on the anterior and posterior capsular shift for multidirectional instability. In a series of 40 patients followed up after 2–5 years, 36 (90%) satisfactory results were noted.[72]

Another technique for the reduction of capsular volume is arthroscopic capsular plication without the usage of suture anchors (suture plication; Figure 16.4). The technique can be applied anteriorly and posteriorly and can also be used for augmentation of a suture anchor reconstruction. The capsule is tightened with sutures that are pulled through the tissue 'inside in' by means of a curved suture hook. Either polydioxanone sutures (PDS; Ethicon, Rutherford, NJ, USA) or braided synthetic absorbable sutures (Panacryl, Ethicon) can be used. The sutures are placed vertically or horizontally through the

capsular tissue and tied inside the joint (Figure 16.4). Ideally, before tying, all sutures should have been inserted; if not, handling of the suture hook may become difficult because of the narrowed joint space. Moreover, a 'spider's web' of sutures inside the joint may confuse the surgeon. To avoid this, Snyder recommends the use of 'suture savers' (angiocatheters without hubs) for identification and separation of the different suture strands.

Postoperative protocol

In both open and arthroscopic shoulder stabilization procedures we recommend 24 hours of immobilization (Gilchrist sling), followed immediately by initiation of passive physiotherapy with the sling worn only while sleeping for 3 weeks. During this period we advise against exercise involving more than –45° of external rotation and 45° of flexion and abduction. After 3 weeks the amount of external rotation can be extended to 0°, and from the sixth week the full range of external rotation is permitted but with only 90° of abduction and flexion. It is important to remember that after operative treatment of MDI a comprehensive physiotherapeutic programme of at least 3 months' duration is required for an optimal outcome.

References

1. Imhoff AB, Roscher E, König U. Arthroskopische Schulterstabilisierung: differenzierte Behandlungsstrategie mit Suretac, Fastak, Holmium:YAG-Laser und Elektrochirurgie. *Orthopäde* 1998; **27**:518–31.

2. Bigliani LU. Anterior and posterior capsular shift for multidirectional instability of the shoulder. *Orthop Trans* 1989; **13**:680–1.

3. Bigliani LU, Pollock, RG, Owens JM et al. The inferior capsular shift procedure for multidirectional instability of the shoulder. *Orthop Trans* 1993–1994; **17**:576.

4. Cooper RA, Brems JJ. The inferior capsular-shift procedure for multidirectional instability of the shoulder. *J Bone Joint Surg* 1992; **74A**:1516–21.

5. Duncan R, Savoie FH. Arthroscopic inferior capsular shift for multidirectional instability of the shoulder: a preliminary report. *Arthroscopy* 1993; **9**:24–7.

6. Flatow EL, Warner JP. Instability of the shoulder: complex problems and failed repairs. *J Bone Joint Surg* 1998; **80A**:122–40.

7. Jobe FW, Giangarra CE, Kvitne RS, Glousman RE. Anterior capsulolabral reconstruction of the shoulder in athletes in overhand sports. *Am J Sports Med* 1991; **19**:428–34.

8. Neer CS, Foster CR. Inferior capsular shift for involuntary inferior and multidirectional instability of the shoulder. A preliminary report. *J Bone Joint Surg* 1980; **62A**:897–908.

9. Neer CS. Involuntary inferior and multidirectional instability of the shoulder: etiology, recognition, and treatment. *AAOS Instr Course Lect* 1985; **34**:232–8.

10. Rowe CR, Patel D, Southmayd WW. The Bankart procedure. A long-term end-result study. *J Bone Joint Surg* 1978; **60A**:1–16.

11. Thomas SC, Matsen FA. An approach to the repair of avulsion of the glenohumeral ligaments in the management of traumatic anterior glenohumeral instability. *J Bone Joint Surg* 1989; **71A**:506–13.

12. Warner JJ, Kann S, Marks P. Arthroscopic repair of combined Bankart and superior labral detachment anterior and posterior lesions: technique and preliminary results. *Arthroscopy* 1994; **10**:383–91.

13. Silliman JF, Hawkins RJ. Classification and physical diagnosis of instability of the shoulder. *Clin Orthop* 1993; **291**:7–19.

14. Hawkins RJ, Bokor DJ. Clinical evaluation of shoulder problems. In: Rockwood CA, Matsen FA, eds. *The Shoulder*, vol. 1. Philadelphia: WB Saunders, 1990; 149–77.

15. Emery RJH, Mulli AB. Glenohumeral joint instability in normal adolescents. Incidence and significance. *J Bone Joint Surg* 1991; **73B**:406–8.

16. Walch G, Agostini JY, Levigne C, Nové-Josserand L. Recurrent anterior and multidirectional instability of the shoulder. *Rev Chir Orthop Repar Appar Mot* 1995; **81**:682–90.

17. Warner JJP, Schulte K, Imhoff AB. Current concepts in shoulder instability. *Adv Oper Orthop* 1995; **3**:217–48.

18. Lusardi DA, Wirth MA, Wurtz D et al. Loss of external rotation following anterior capsulorrhaphy of the shoulder. *J Bone Joint Surg. Am* 1993; **75A**:1185–92.

19. Altchek DW, Warren RF, Skyhar MJ et al. T-plasty modification of the Bankart procedure for multidirectional instability of the anterior and inferior types. *J Bone Joint Surg* 1991; **73A**:105–12.

20. Dowdy PA, O'Driscoll SW. Shoulder instability. An analysis of family history. *J Bone Joint Surg* 1993; **75A**:782–4.

21. Speer KP, Deng X, Borrero S et al. Biomechanical evaluation of a simulated Bankart lesion. *J Bone Joint Surg* 1994; **76A**:1819–26.

22. Warner JJ, Miller MD, Marks P, Fu FH. Arthroscopic Bankart repair with Suretac device. Part I: clinical observations. *Arthroscopy* 1995; **11**:2–13.

23. Jerosch J, Castro WH. Shoulder instability in Ehlers–Danlos syndrome. An indication for surgical treatment? *Acta Orthop Belg* 1990; **56**:451–3.

24. Jobe FW, Kvitne RS, Giangarra, CE. Shoulder pain in the overhand or throwing athlete: the relationship of anterior insta-

bility and rotator cuff impingement. *Orthop Rev* 1989; **18**:963–75.

25. König U, Barthel T, Imhoff AB. Anatomie und Histologie des Labrum-Kapsel-Komplexes. In: Imhoff AB, König U, eds. *Schulterinstabilität, Rotatorenmanschette*. Darmstadt: Steinkopff, 1999; 30–40.

26. Oettl G, Imhoff AB, Merl T, Keydel M. Physical examination. MRI, MRA and arthroscopy of SLAP-lesions – a prospective comparison. Eighth Congress of the European Society of Sports Traumatology, Knee Surgery and Arthroscopy (ESSKA), Nice, France. 29 April–2 May, 1998; 422.

27. Snyder SJ, Karzel RP, Del Pizzo W et al. SLAP lesions of the shoulder. *Arthroscopy* 1990; **6**:274–9.

28. Walch G, Liotard JP, Boileau P, Noel E. Postero–superior glenoid impingement. Another impingement of the shoulder. *J Radiol* 1993; **74**:47–50.

29. Imhoff AB, Agneskirchner JD, König U et al. Superior labrum pathology in the athlete. *Orthopäde* 2000; **29**: 917–27.

30. Barthel T, König U, Gohlke F, Löhr J. Anatomie und Histologie des Labrum glenoidale unter besonderer Berücksichtigung des sublabralen Foramen und der SLAP-Läsionen. *Orthopäde* 1999.

31. Cordasco FA, Pollock RG, Flatow EL, Bigliani LU. Management of multidirectional instability. *Oper Tech Sports Med* 1993; **1**: 293–300.

32. Flatow EL. Multidirectional instability. In: Kohn D, Wirth CJ, eds. *Die Schulter: Aktuelle operative Therapie*. Stuttgart: Thieme, 1992; 180–7.

33. Foster CR. Multidirectional instability of the shoulder in the athlete. *Clin Sports Med* 1983; **2**:355–68.

34. Mallon WJ, Speer KP. Multidirectional instability: current concepts. *J Shoulder Elbow Surg* 1995; **4**:54–64.

35. Neer CS. *Shoulder Reconstruction*. Philadelphia: WB Saunders, 1990; 273–341.

36. Huber H, Gerber C. Voluntary subluxation of the shoulder in children. A long-term follow-up study of 36 shoulders. *J Bone Joint Surg* 1994; **76B**:118–22.

37. Rowe CR, Pierce DS, Clark JG. Voluntary dislocation of the shoulder. A preliminary report on a clinical, electromyographic, and psychiatric study of twenty-six patients. *J Bone Joint Surg* 1973; **55A**:445–60.

38. Bigliani LU, Kurzweil PR, Schwartzbach CC et al. The inferior capsular shift procedure for anterior–inferior shoulder instability in athletes. *Am J Sports Med* 1994; **22**: 578–84.

39. König U, Imhoff AB. Die multidirektionale Schulterinstabilität. In: Meyer P, Gächter FA, eds. *Schulterchirurgie in der Praxis*. Heidelberg: Springer, 1999; 87–110.

40. Bateman JE. *The Shoulder and Neck*, 2nd edn. Philadelphia: WB Saunders, 1978; 515.

41. De Palma AF. *Surgery of the Shoulder*, 2nd edn. Philadelphia: JB Lippincott, 1973; 425.

42. Imhoff AB, Debski RE, Warner JJP et al. Biomechanical function of the glenohumeral ligaments – a quantitative assessment. AOSSM, 16–19 July 1995, Toronto, Canada.

43. Hardy P, Thabit G, Fanton GS et al. Arthroscopic management of recurrent anterior shoulder dislocation by combining a labrum suture with an antero–inferior holmium:YAG laser capsular shrinkage. *Orthopäde* 1996; **25**:91–3.

44. Fu F, Ticker JB, Imhoff AB. *An Atlas of Shoulder Surgery*. London: Martin Dunitz, 1997. 1–140.

45. Imhoff A, De Simoni C. Die arthroskopische Schulterstabilisierung mit Suretacs – eine Komplikationsanalyse. 2. Zentraleuropäischer Unfallkongress 29.5.–1.6.1996, Davos. *Swiss Surg* 1996; **2**:30.

46. Imhoff A, Perrenoud A, Neidl K. MRI bei Schulterinstabilität – Korrelation zum Arthro-CT und zur Arthroskopie der Schulter. *Arthroskopie* 1992; **5**:122–9.

47. Resch H, Povacz P, Wambacher M et al. Arthroscopic extra-articular Bankart repair for the treatment of recurrent anterior shoulder dislocation. *Arthroscopy* 1997; **13**:188–200.

48. Rowe CR, Zarins B. Recurrent transient subluxation of the shoulder. *J Bone Joint Surg* 1981; **63**:863–72.

49. Warner JJ, Deng XH, Warren RF, Torzilli, PA. Static capsuloligamentous restraints to superior–inferior translation of the glenohumeral joint. *Am J Sports.Med* 1992; **20**:675–85.

50. Belle RM. Collagen typing in multidirectional instability of the shoulder. *Orthop Trans* 1989; **13**:680–1.

51. Carter C, Sweetnam R. Recurrent dislocation of the patella and of the shoulder. Their association with familial joint laxity. *J Bone Joint Surg* 1960; **42B**:721–7.

52. Finnsterbush A, Pogrund H. The hypermobility syndrome. Musculoskeletal complaints in 100 consecutive cases of generalized joint hypermobility. *Clin Orthop* 1982; **168**:124–7.

53. Berg EE, Ciullo JV. A clinical test for superior glenoid labral or SLAP-lesions. *Clin J Sports Med* 1998; **8**:121–3.

54. Friedman RJ, Bonutti PM, Genez B, Norfray JF. Cine magnetic resonance imaging of the glenohumeral joint. *Orthop Trans* 1993–1994; **17**:1018–19.

55. Jalovaara P, Myllylä V, Päivänsalo M. Autotraction stress roentgenography for demonstration anterior and inferior instability of the shoulder joint. *Clin Orthop* 1992; **284**:136–43.

56. Burkhead WZ, Rockwood CA. Treatment of instability of the shoulder with an exercise program. *J Bone Joint Surg* 1992; **74A**:890–6.

57. Kronberg M, Broström LA, Nemeth G. Differences in shoulder muscle activity between patients with generalized joint laxity and normal controls. *Clin Orthop* 1991; **269**:181–92.

58. Lebar RD, Alexander AH. Multidirectional shoulder instability. Clinical results of inferior capsular shift in an active-duty population. *Am J Sports Med* 1992; **20**:193–8.

59. Lephart SM, Warner JJP, Borsa PA, Fu FH. Proprioception of the shoulder joint in healthy, unstable, and surgically repaired shoulders. *J Shoulder Elbow Surg* 1994; **3**:371–80.

60. Rockwood CA. Management of patients with multi-directional instability of the shoulder. *Orthop Trans* 1994; **18**:328.

61. Flatow EL. Multidirectional instability. In: Bigliani LU, ed. *The Unstable Shoulder*. Rosemont: The American Academy of Orthopaedic Surgeons, 1996; 79–90.

62. Hawkins RJ, Kunkel SS, Nayak NK. Inferior capsular shift for multidirectional instability of the shoulder: 2–5 year follow-up. *Orthop Trans* 1991; **15**:765.

63. Jobe C. Symposium on anterior instability. Fourth Congress of the European Society for Surgery of the Shoulder and the Elbow, 4 October 1990, Milan, Italy.

64. Jobe CM. Anatomy and surgical approaches. In: Jobe FW, ed. *Operative Techniques in Upper Extremity Sports Injuries*. St Louis: CV Mosby, 1996; 124–53.

65. Mizuno K, Itakura Y, Muratsu H. Inferior capsular shift for inferior and multidirectional instability of the shoulder in young children: report of two cases. *J Shoulder Elbow Surg* 1992; **1**:200–6.

66. Warner JJP, Johnson DL, Miller MD, Caborn DNM. The concept of a 'selective capsular shift' for anterior–inferior instability of the shoulder. *Orthop Trans* 1994–1995; **18**:1183.

67. Welsh RP, Trimmings N. Multidirectional instability of the shoulder. *Orthop Trans* 1987; **11**:231.

68. Fanton GS, Wall MS, Markel MD. *Electrothermally assisted capsule shift (ETACS) procedure for shoulder instability.* Menlo Park: Oratec, 2001.

69. Zuckerman JD, Matsen FA. Complications about the glenohumeral joint related to the use of screws and staples. *J Bone Joint Surg* 1984; **66**:175–80.

70. Burkart A, Imhoff AB, Roscher E. Foreign-body reaction to the bioabsorbable suretac device. *Arthroscopy* 2000; **16**:91–5.

71. Fredrich H, Imhoff AB, Höfler H. Biomechanische und histomorphologische Untersuchungen zur Laserwirkung an der Schultergelenkskapsel. *Z Orthop* 1998; **136**:A119–20.

72. McIntyre LF, Caspari RB, Savoie FH. The arthroscopic treatment of multidirectional shoulder instability: two-year results of a multiple suture technique. *Arthroscopy* 1997; **13**:418–25.

73. Thabit G. Laser-assisted capsular shift for treatment of glenohumeral instability. *Orthop Spec Ed* 1994; **3**:10–12.

74. Field LD, Warren RF, O'Brien SJ et al. Isolated closure of rotator interval defects for shoulder instability. *Am J Sports Med* 1995; **23**:557–63.

75. Imhoff A. The use of lasers in orthopaedic surgery. Controversial topics in sports medicine. *Oper Tech Orthop* 1995; **5**:192–203.

76. Imhoff A, Ledermann T. Arthroscopic subacromial decompression with and without Holmium:YAG-Laser – a prospective comparative study. *Arthroscopy* 1995; **11**:549–56.

77. Imhoff AB. Arthroscopic shoulder stabilisation and capsular shift with Fastak and laser assisted capsular shift procedure (LACS). Fifth Symposium of the Korean Arthroscopy Association, 20 June 1997, Seoul, Korea.

78. Imhoff AB. The role of capsuloligamentous structure in the unstable shoulder – a biomechanical and arthroscopical approach. 24th Annual Meeting of the Japan Shoulder Society, 31 October–1 November, 1997, Kyoto, Japan.

79. Imhoff AB, Burkart A, Roscher E. Adverse reactions to bioabsorbable suretac device in arthroscopic shoulder stabilisation and SLAP-refixation. Eighth Congress of the European Society of Sports Traumatology, Knee Surgery and Arthroscopy (ESSKA) 29 April–2 May 1998, Nizza, France.

17 Posterior shoulder instability: Arthroscopic management

Eugene M Wolf and William T Pennington

Introduction

Many authors have commented on the difficulty in treating the patient with recurrent posterior shoulder instability.[1-6] In contrast to anterior instability, the surgical results have been less consistent, with higher failure rates and various complications reported. The historical lack of differentiation between dislocations and subluxations, voluntary versus involuntary instability, traumatic versus atraumatic causes, and unidirectional versus multidirectional conditions has added to the confusion in trying to define and treat this relatively uncommon and ill-defined entity. Our increasing knowledge of the stabilizing anatomic structures and mechanisms of the shoulder, as well as an improving ability with diagnostic arthroscopic examination, has led to a better understanding of the pathology of posterior shoulder instability.

The applications of arthroscopy in the diagnosis and treatment of shoulder pathology are rapidly expanding. There are several advantages of an arthroscopic approach in the treatment of shoulder pathology. Arthroscopic surgery produces less morbidity with minimal violation of skin, fascia, capsular ligaments and musculotendinous units, and usually results in an easier recovery. Arthroscopy allows the intra-articular pathology to be more clearly viewed and more precisely defined with minimal morbidity. Finally, arthroscopy is the gold standard in the diagnosis of intra-articular lesions. It allows complete visualization of the entire glenohumeral joint as well as the subacromial bursal space. This thorough evaluation permits identification of any associated pathology that can be remedied at the same time. The surgical decision and approach can be modified based on the intra-articular pathology. We have previously reported our results of arthroscopic capsular plication for posterior shoulder instability.[7] In our patient group after a minimum of 2-years' follow-up all patients were satisfied with their results. One patient had a recurrence that responded to a second arthroscopic posterior capsular reconstruction. McIntyre et al recently reported results of their technique of arthroscopic treatment of posterior instability with a 25% recurrence rate in their patient population.[8]

Subsequent to our initial report on the treatment of patients of the arthroscopic treatment of posterior shoulder instability, we have modified the technique to better address new concepts of global capsular attenuation that is felt to be present in these patients. The 'circle concept'

of shoulder stability proposed by Pagnani and Warren[9] theorizes that shoulder instability requires capsular deformation on both sides of the joint. Strain gauge analysis by Blaiser et al[10] and Terry et al[11] confirmed strain in both the anterior and posterior shoulder capsule with translation of the humeral head upon the glenoid. In addition, Harryman et al[12] described the role of the rotator interval capsule in shoulder stability. In this anatomic study the rotator interval capsule was sectioned and posteroinferior instability was noted. Field et al[13] reported isolated rotator interval closure in 15 patients with isolated inferior instability and rotator interval defects. All 15 of these patients had good to excellent results at an average 3.3 year follow-up. These authors stressed the importance of recognizing this entity in stabilization procedures and repairing these lesions when present.[13] Speer et al,[14] in a cadaveric study, created simulated Bankart lesions and noted only very small increases in anterior translation with the creation of a simulated Bankart lesion alone. It was their hypothesis that the injury to the anterior part of the inferior ligament at the level of the glenoid is not soley responsible for the glenohumeral translation necessary to produce an anterior dislocation of the shoulder.[14] In an extensive review of stabilizers of the glenohumeral joint, Pagnani and Warren[9] confirmed the contribution of all the aforementioned theories and recommended that operative treatment of shoulder instability should be directed at the restoration of the capsulolabral disruption or the reduction of abnormal capsular laxity. Since 1995 we have addressed all patients with glenohumeral instability, including posterior instability, with the 'Triad technique' of stabilization. This technique not only addresses the primary direction of instability, but also addresses any more diffuse capsular deficiency that is present in many patients in the spectrum of pathology called shoulder instability. This arthroscopic technique places the surgical emphasis in area of the primary direction of instability, but also addresses any redundancy in the axillary pouch and closes the superior capsular ligaments (superior and middle glenohumeral ligaments) in the rotator interval.

This chapter describes this author's Triad technique to treat posterior shoulder instability arthroscopically. This approach has been developed to address glenohumeral instability of all directions. The previous cited references establish a complex interaction of various regions of the shoulder capsule on both sides of the joint and in the rotator interval that when intact, provide stability to the glenohumeral joint. The Triad approach to the patient with shoulder instability is designed to address any capsular attenuation that is present outside of the primary area and direction of instability, as well as to repair those lesions of the primary direction.

Surgical principles

No single lesion has been demonstrated to be responsible for the development of posterior shoulder instability.[6] Many reports contend that the primary anatomic feature in posterior shoulder instability consists of a patuluous or redundant posterior capsule.[1,3,5,6,13–16] Several studies have also pointed to the importance of the inferior glenohumeral ligament as a primary stabilizing force against posterior subluxation and dislocation.[4,17,18] There are several reports on the importance of maintaining capsular integrity for stabilization of humeral head on the glenoid.[3,19] In addition, Warren et al[20] have suggested that the anterosuperior glenohumeral ligament, arising from the anterosuperior neck of the glenoid, may function to prevent posterior instability.

The role of the posterior labrum in posterior instability is less well defined. It has been thought that posterior labral avulsions from the glenoid, the so-called 'reverse Bankart lesion', are rather uncommon in posterior shoulder instability except in cases involving a significant isolated traumatic episode.[3,5,6,21] Several recent studies suggest that the posterior labrum may provide a significant degree of stability against posterior migration of the humeral head.[22–24] A study by Cordasco et al[22] noted 100% of patients with isolated posterior or inferior labral tears and no clinical symptoms of instability nevertheless had instability on examination under anesthesia.[22] These authors did not report on the capsular findings at arthroscopy. Lippitt et al[24] found that the labrum contributes approximately 20% to the concavity–compression stabilization of the glenohumeral joint, with a greater contribution of the labrum to inferior and posterior inferior stability.[24] Rowe and Yee[25] noted posteroinferior labral detachment in two shoulders with posterior instability, and stability and full function in both cases was restored with reattachment of the posterior capsule to the glenoid rim.

The surgical principle in the arthroscopic treatment of posterior shoulder instability involves first confirming the existence of this entity with a thorough examination under anesthesia. When the examination confirms primarily a posterior component of shoulder instability, surgical treatment emphasizes arthroscopic evaluation of the joint followed by addressing posterior capsular laxity with capsulorrhaphy and reconstruction of any posterior labral lesion that exists. We treat our patients with posterior instability similarly to patients with anterior instabil-

ity; that is, although the primary direction of instability is posterior, there is often a component of anterior and inferior capsular laxity that may be addressed with capsular plication. Rotator interval capsular closure performed by suturing the inferior border of the superior glenohumeral ligament to the superior border of the middle glenohumeral ligament is performed to provide additional capsular volume depletion. Addressing the entire capsular ring in this manner has been a successful technique in restoring stability to patients with complaints of and examination findings consistent with posterior glenohumeral instabilty.

Portal placement during the procedure is of essential importance. The posterior portal placement is more lateral and distal than the standard posterior portal thus facilitating access to the posterior glenoid and axillary pouch. If this portal is not created in this manner, access to these regions will be difficult for the surgeon prohibiting the procedure from proceeding in a fluid manner. Another potential pitfall faced by the surgeon is overtightening of the shoulder capsule resulting in a stiff shoulder postoperatively. This potentially can occur during capsular plication. After the initial capsular plication suture is placed at a distance of 1 cm from the glenoid rim, a fold of plicated capsule is created as it is advanced to the labrum. It is important that the subsequent sutures follow the same fold and not take in additional capsule length with each advancing stitch.

Surgical technique

The surgeon should enter the operating theater with the diagnosis of posterior shoulder instability already made through a good history and clinical examination. Most patients with posterior shoulder instability will tell you that 'it's going out the back'. On clinical examination, the standard posterior drawer sign is helpful, but not reliable. For those patients who cannot precisely define their posterior instability, the posterior relocation test is most diagnostic. It is performed with the patient standing, the affected arm internally rotated and adducted so that the back of the forearm rests on the patient's brow. The examiner stabilizes the scapula with one hand and applies a posteroinferior translation force on the flexed elbow (Figure 17.1). This should subluxate the humeral head posteriorly and inferiorly. It will reduce with a clunk as the arm is brought into external rotation and abduction. Unfortunately a significant proportion of patients can voluntarily produce the posterior subluxation. It is amongst this group that we must decipher which of them really want to permanently change this pathologic picture and which of them actually thrive on its existence. Look for some tell-tale sign of trouble: the subtle smile during the maneuver and the obsessed parent or loved one who is taking in every bit of it. The one minute psychiatric/orthopedic assessment is usually

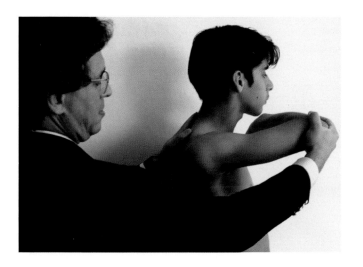

Figure 17.1

The jerk test for posterior instability is performed with the arm in forward flexion, adduction, and internal rotation. The examiner's left hand stabilizes the scapula, while the right hand applies a posterior force that subluxes the humeral head over the posterior labrum.

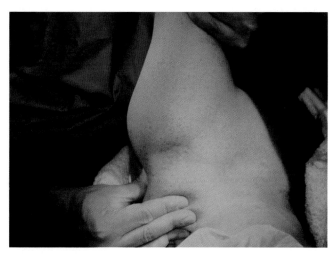

Figure 17.2

The maneuver performed in the operating room during the examination under anesthesia. Note the posterior subluxation of the humeral head over the examiner's thumb which is stabilizing the scapula during the maneuver.

enough to weed out these potential problem patients, but no psychiatric evaluation is perfect.

Once the diagnosis of posterior instability is made, the next step is to determine the presence, degree or absence additional directions of instability. A clinical examination of the opposite side will usually produce the same type of instability although it is usually and suprisingly asymptomatic.

The examination under anesthesia is performed to confirm the diagnosis of posterior shoulder instability and the degree of any anterior and inferior instability. (This examination is performed with the patient in the lateral decubitus position.) An accurate determination of posterior humeral translation necessitates that the glenoid be stabilized while the humeral head is forced posteriorly. This is accomplished by stabilizing the scapula (i.e. the glenoid) with one hand while the other applies a posterior translational stress to the humerus (Figure 17.2). In the patient with posterior instability the convexity of the humeral head can be felt to slide over and beyond the posterior rim of the glenoid. More importantly, the head will then reduce with a significant clunk with external rotation and abduction. (The examination is always performed on the contralateral shoulder and the results compared.) Anterior and inferior translation is also assessed and compared to posterior translation.

We generally utilize three portals in all instability cases (Figure 17.3). The working portals include a posteroinferior portal (PIP) and an anteroinferior portal (AIP), while an anterior superior portal (ASP) accommodates the arthroscope. The posterior inferior portal is placed more lateral and distal to the standard posterior portal in shoul-

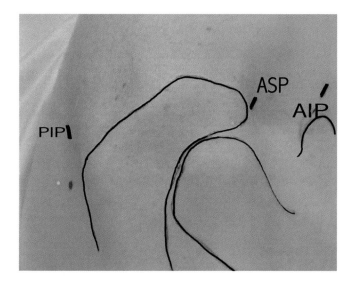

Figure 17.3

Three portals are generally utilized for our arthroscopic stabilization procedures.

der arthroscopy. The procedure begins by making the PIP 3 cm directly distal to the posterolateral corner of the acromion. It is this portal that allows appropriate angular access to the posterior glenoid rim, axillary pouch, and posterior capsule. The AIP is placed with an outside-in approach by first marking it with a spinal needle. Care should be taken by the surgeon to ensure an appropri-

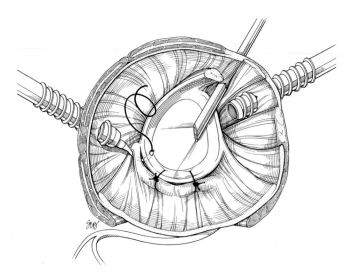

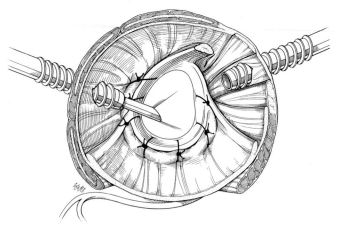

Figure 17.4

The inferior and posterior capsule is addressed initially. While viewing from the ASP the capsule is plicated starting from the 6 o'clock position and progressing posteriorly.

Figure 17.5

Sutures are placed in the anterior capsule to provide an additional decrease in capsular volume after plication. The arthroscope is placed through the PIP and the AIP is utilized as the working portal to plicate the anterior band of the inferior glenohumeral ligament.

ate distance between the ASP and AIP to allow enough room to utilize the AIP as a working portal.

A large (8.4 mm) threaded cannula is placed in the AIP. The ASP is created immediately adjacent to the anterior margin of the acromion and enters the joint at the level of the biceps tendon. This portal is most optimally created with the aid of an 18-gauge spinal needle. Switching sticks are used to take the scope from the PIP and move it to the ASP. An 8.4-mm cannula is then placed over a switching stick into the PIP.

The procedure always begins with the use of a slotted whisker blade to gently abrade the synovial surface of the entire capsule. A more aggressive shaver blade will quickly ablate the normally thin posterior capsule and leave nothing to work with. The capsular abrasion is necessary to stimulate a fibroblastic response in the capsule to be plicated so that it will heal to itself once it is folded onto itself.

The plication begins with the most inferior stitch at the 6 o'clock position (Figure 17.4). With the large threaded cannula in the posterior portal, a #1 PDS (Ethicon, Rutherford, NJ, USA) suture is placed through the lax capsule with the use of an 'angled' suture hook (Linvatec Corp., Largo, FL, USA). A 25% capsulorrhaphy is obtained by passing through the capsule a selected distance (approximately 1 cm) from the labrum. An anatomic study by Eakin et al[26] demonstrated that arthroscopic capsular sutures placed 1 cm from the glenoid rim are safe with regard to the axillary nerve. The hook is first

pointed down and pushed through the capsule. There is a perceptible 'pop' as it goes through the capsule. Once through the capsule the crescent hook is turned and lifted up, and pushed through the capsule so the tip re-enters the joint. The tip of the hook and the capsule are then brought up to the 6 o'clock position on the glenoid labrum. The tip of the hook is then passed through the labrum. As much of the suture as possible is fed into the joint and the suture hook is withdrawn from the labrum and capsule, and pulled from the cannula. The suture is then retrieved with a suture grasper (Linvatec Corp.). A slip knot (Duncan loop) is created outside the cannula and slid down into the joint with a knot pusher. As the knot is closed the capsule is thus folded on itself to the posterior labrum. Two square knots are used to ensure that the knot does not slip back. As many as eight sutures may be used to achieve the posterior capsulorrhaphy and adequate reduction of general capsular volume. The suturing always begins in the axillary pouch and continues up the posterior band and posterior capsule. Each stitch shifts the capsule proximally on the posterior glenoid labrum (Figure 17.4).

Most cases of shoulder instability do not have true posterior Bankart lesions. They often have a split and frayed labrum in the posteroinferior quadrant, but these are secondary lesions that do not require reattachment to the glenoid. In those cases where there is significant labral detachment, suture anchors may be used to fasten the capsulolabral complex directly to the posterior bony

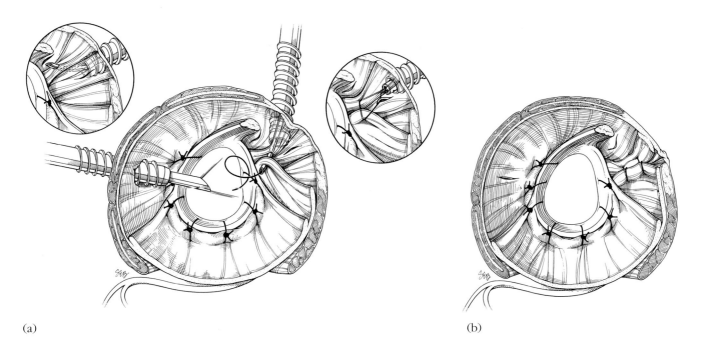

(a) (b)

Figure 17.6

The anterior threaded cannula is withdrawn to a position that is just extracapsular. A crescent hook is then passed through the inferior edge of the superior glenohumeral ligament and the superior edge of the middle glenohumeral ligament (a). The suture is retrieved and tied blindly, extracapsullarly. An additional suture is placed through the rotator interval capsule providing complete closure of the rotator interval capsule (b).

rim of the glenoid. A burr is used to freshen the glenoid rim and drill holes are made on the edge of the rim to accommodate the anchors. The sutures and anchors are placed and tied one at a time. In this case the suture hook is passed through the capsule, then through the detached labrum. The anchor is then threaded onto the retrieved suture limb, slid down the cannula, and inserted into a drill hole in the edge of the glenoid. The slip knot is then made in the usual fashion. Any additional posterior labral irregularities are debrided.

Upon completion of the posteroinferior repair, attention is then directed towards the anterior shoulder capsule and labrum. An element of ligamentous attenuation in the anterior half of the inferior glenohumeral ligament is addressed by the same suture capsulorrhaphy in the anterior half of the inferior glenohumeral ligament (Figure 17.5). This capsule is then brought proximally to a point on the anterior labrum where the hook is passed through and the suture is passed. Knot tying is performed in a similar manner.

The final component of the procedure involves closure of the rotator interval capsule. The anterior threaded large cannula is withdrawn to a point just outside the shoulder capsule. The crescent hook is then utilized to suture the inferior margin of the superior glenohumeral ligament to the superior margin of the middle glenohumeral ligament. This may be repeated placing two sutures in this manner. These sutures are tied extra-articularly with the knot remaining extracapsular (Figure 17.6).

Postoperative protocol

The patient is placed in a standard shoulder immobilizer and is discharged to home the day of the procedure with instructions to remain immobilized until seen in the office 5–7 days postoperatively. When the patient is seen in the office, the sutures are removed and depending on the degree of pathology, the security of the repair and the confidence in the patient, education on the limitation to function in the 'nose to toes' triangle is explained. They are allowed out of the immobilizer to eat and shower, with the remainder of the time being spent in the shoulder immobilizer. At 6 weeks postoperatively the patient is allowed to begin a shoulder exercise program with active and passive motion exercises as well as a strengthening program. Return to activities is activity dependent, but ranges from 4 to 6 months.

References

1. Fronek J, Warren RF, Bowen M. Posterior subluxation of the glenohumeral joint. *J Bone Joint Surg* 1989; **71A**:205–16.
2. Hawkins RJ, Kippert G, Johnston G. Recurrent posterior instability (subluxation) of the shoulder. *J Bone Joint Surg* 1984; **66A**:169–74.
3. Pollock RG, Bigliani LU. Recurrent posterior shoulder instability. Diagnosis and treatment. *Clin Orthop* 1993; **291**:85–96.

4. Schwartz E, Warren RF, O'Brien SJ, Fronek J. Posterior shoulder instability. *Orthop Clin North Am* 1987; **18**:409–19.

5. Tibone JE, Bradley JP. The treatment of posterior subluxation in athletes. *Clin Orthop* 1993; **291**:124–37.

6. Tibone JE, Ting A. Capsulorrhaphy with a staple for recurrent posterior subluxation of the shoulder. *J Bone Joint Surg* 1990; **72A**:999–1002.

7. Wolf EM, Eakin CL. Arthroscopic capsular plication for posterior shoulder instability. *Arthroscopy* 1998; **14**:153–63.

8. McIntyre LF, Caspari RB, Savoie III FH. The arthroscopic treatment of posterior shoulder instability: 2-year results of a multiple suture technique. *Arthroscopy* 1997; **13**:426–32.

9. Pagnani MJ, Warren RF. Stabilizers of the glenohumeral joint. *J Shoulder Elbow Surg* 1994; **3**:173–90.

10. Blasier RB, Guldberg RE, Rothman ED. Anterior shoulder stability: contributions of rotator cuff forces and the capsular ligaments in a cadaver model. *J Shoulder Elbow Surg* 1992; **1**:140–50.

11. Terry GC, Hammon D, France P, Norwood LA. The stabilizing function of passive shoulder restraints. *Am J Sports Med* 1991; **19**:26–34.

12. Harryman DT 2nd, Sidles JA, Harris SL, Matsen FA 3rd. The role of the rotator interval capsule in passive motion and stability of the shoulder. *J Bone Joint Surg* 1992; **74A**:53–66.

13. Field LD, Warren RF, O'Brien SJ et al. Isolated closure of rotator interval defects for shoulder instability. *Am J Sports Med* 1995; **23**:557–63.

14. Speer KP, Deng X, Borrero S et al. Biomechanical evaluation of a simulated Bankart lesion. *J Bone Joint Surg* 1994; **76A**:1819–26.

15. Bigliani LU, Pollock RG, McIlveen SJ et al. Shift of the posteroinferior aspect of the capsule for recurrent posterior glenohumeral instability. *J Bone Joint Surg* 1995; **77A**:1011–20.

16. Boyd HB, Sisk TD. Recurrent posterior dislocation of the shoulder. *J Bone Joint Surg* 1972; **54A**:779–86.

17. Bowen MK, Warren RF. Ligamentous control of shoulder stability based on selective cutting and static translation experiments. *Clin Sports Med* 1991; **10**:757–82.

18. O'Brien SJ, Neves MC, Arnocaky SP et al. The anatomy and histology of the inferior glenohumeral ligament complex of the shoulder. *Am J Sports Med* 1990; **18**:449–56.

19. Gibb TD, Sidles JA, Harryman DT 2nd et al. The effect of capsular venting on glenohumeral laxity. *Clin Orthop* 1991; **268**:120–7.

20. Warren RF, Kornblatt IB, Marchand R. Static factors affecting posterior shoulder instability. *Orthop Trans* 1989; **8**:1.

21. Caspari RB, Geissler WB. Arthroscopic manifestations of shoulder subluxation and dislocation. *Clin Orthop* 1993; **291**:54–66.

22. Cordasco FA, Steinman S, Flatow FL, Bigliani LU. Arthroscopic treatment of glenoid labral tears. *Am J Sports Med* 1993; **21**:425–30.

23. Habermeyer P, Schuller V, Wiedemann E. The intra-articular pressure of the shoulder: an experimental study of the role of the glenoid labrum in stabilizing the joint. *Arthroscopy* 1992; **8**:166–72.

24. Lippitt SB, Vanderhooft JE, Harris SL et al. Glenohumeral stability from concavity-compression: a quantitative analysis. *J Shoulder Elbow Surg* 1993; **2**:27–35.

25. Rowe CR, Yee LBK. A posterior approach to the shoulder joint. *J Bone Joint Surg* 1944; **26**:580.

26. Eakin CL, Dvirnak P, Miller CM, Hawkins RJ. The relationship of the axillary nerve to arthroscopically placed capsulolabral sutures. An anatomic study. *Am J Sports Med* 1998; **26**:505–9.

18 Superior instability: SLAP lesions

Ralph Wischatta, Franz Kralinger and Karl Golser

Introduction

Pathology of the superior labrum of the glenoid was first described by Snyder et al in 1990.[1] He classified it as a SLAP lesion (superior labrum anterior to posterior), which describes a detachment of the labrum from the superior neck of the glenoid. The long head of the biceps originates from the superior pole of the glenoid at the supraglenoid tubercle (Figure 18.1). It is an important stabilizer in the shoulder joint and it also plays a role as a depressor of the humeral head. A detachment of the long head of the biceps from the superior pole of the glenoid thus causes superior instability of the humeral head. Andrews et al[2] described a 'popping' phenomenon caused by incarcerations of the detached labral–biceps–tendon complex in the glenohumeral joint. Patients report pain on activity, especially with flexion and elevation and external rotation motion. The apprehension test at and above 90° mostly causes discomfort or pain. Also, in a high percentage of patients, both the palm-up and the O'Brien test are positive due to the tension on the tendon on long head of the biceps. Physiotherapy usually does not have any effect on the symptoms of this pathological entity. The majority of SLAP lesions occur in young, active patients, who primarily engage in overhead activities. For this reason an unstable SLAP lesion calls for surgical refixation.

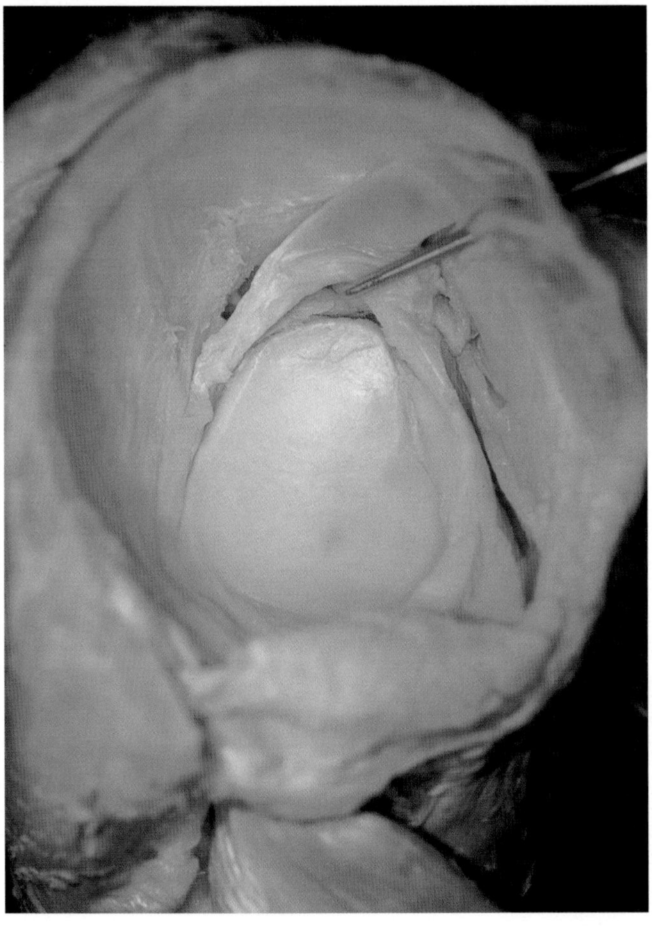

Surgical principles

Arthroscopic refixation of a SLAP lesion is a demanding surgical procedure. Generally two experienced arthroscopists are needed to complete the procedure, because many steps require simultaneous working. Numerous techniques for SLAP refixation have been published (suture anchor techniques, transglenoid sutures, staples).[3–8] Labrum refixation with the Suretac device (Suretac, Smith & Nephew Endoscopy, Inc., Andover, MA, USA) is a well-established technique and can be performed fairly easily through standard arthroscopic portals. However, the technique contains some crucial steps and thus some potential complications, such as breakage of the device, if not tapped in correctly (Figure 18.2) or lesion of the articular cartilage due to drilling in the wrong direction.

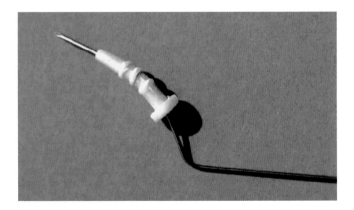

Figure 18.1

Cadaveric specimen showing the glenoid with detachment of the superior portion of the labrum anterior and posterior of the biceps anchor (type II SLAP).

Figure 18.2

Broken Suretac due to misalignment of the punch used for Suretac fixation.

Surgical technique

The set-up for this procedure is an arthroscopic standard. The patient is positioned in a beach-chair position.[9] The arm of the injured side is put in a special elbow holder (Atlantech Medical Devices Ltd, N Yorkshire, UK; Figure 18.3), which ensures both free movement of the arm and secure positioning in every desired arm position. The patient's head is placed in a special head support, which is height adjustable.

After sterile washing and draping, it is advisable to mark out the landmarks for the arthroscopy: the acromion, the acromioclavicular joint and the coracoid process (Figure 18.4). For the first part of the procedure we use two standard portals. The posterior portal for the arthroscope is approximately 1–1.5 cm inferior and medial of the angulus acromialis. The anterior portal for the instruments is created by introducing a rod into the

joint at the superior edge of the subscapularis tendon under arthroscopic control. It is advisable to use a canula for the instrument portal in order to maintain constant intra-articular pressure.

Anesthesia is usually induced endotracheally. This permits controlled intraoperative blood pressure reduction. Systemic blood pressure should not exceed 110 mmHg because otherwise visibility could be impaired by bleeding from the surrounding tissue. A pressure pump is advisable and can compensate for fluctuations in blood pressure for short periods by increase of the inflow pressure.

Diagnostic arthroscopy is performed first. With the help of a hook probe the entire labrum is palpated, so that partial or complete disruptions can be easily visualized. According to Snyder et al,[1,6] type II and type IV SLAP lesions have to be reattached to the glenoid rim (Figure 18.5). The first step of the arthroscopic SLAP refixation is

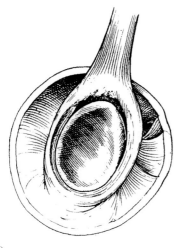

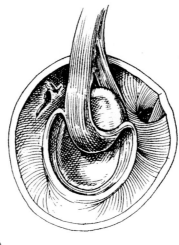

Figure 18.3

Set-up for shoulder arthroscopy with the patient in the beach-chair position and the arm fixed in the adjustable elbow holder.

Figure 18.4

Landmarks for shoulder arthroscopy with incisions for the arthroscope (posterior), the lateral standard incision, and the transacromial incision, along with various anterior portals.

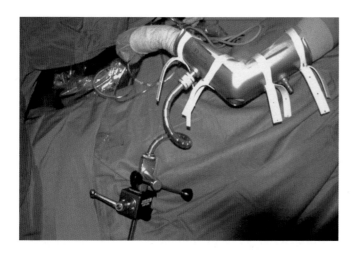

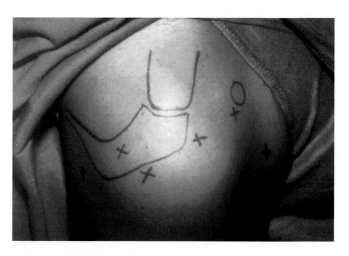

Figure 18.5

(a, b) Type II and type IV SLAP lesions.

(a)   (b)

the preparation of the glenoid rim. The superior glenoid neck is debrided of soft tissue. Abrasion of the glenoid neck is performed with an arthroscopic shaver-abrader to create a bleeding bony surface (Figure 18.6).

In order to place the Suretac anchors, an additional portal is created close to the lateral tip of the acromion.

Care must be taken throughout the entire process of drilling. In some patients the acromion extends too far laterally and causes a too small angle of the drill when positioned at the superior neck of the glenoid. In these cases a transacromial portal has to be created (Figure 18.7).

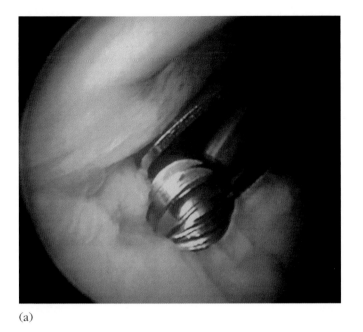

(a)

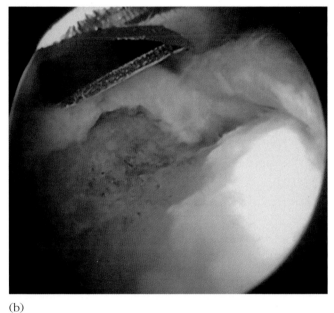

(b)

Figure 18.6

(a, b) Arthroscopic picture of the superior neck of the glenoid. Soft tissue and subcortical bone abrasion is needed for labrum reattachment.

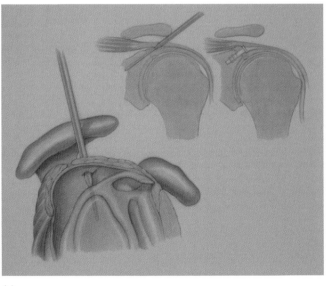

(a)

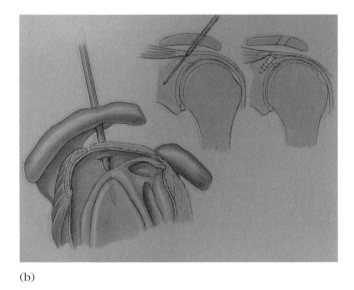

(b)

Figure 18.7

Schematic representation of (a) the normal approach for SLAP refixation and (b) the transacromial approach if the patient has a wider acromion that extends more laterally.

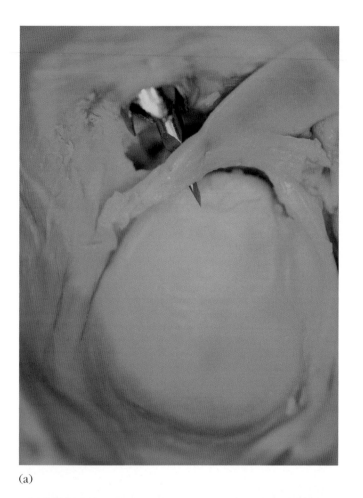

(a)

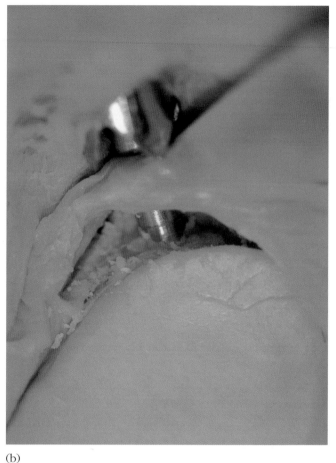

(b)

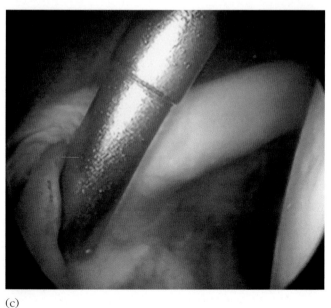

(c)

Figure 18.8

(a) Cadaveric specimen showing the drill with the central pin that is used to load the labrum and to reattach it to the glenoid neck. (b) Same cadaveric specimen with the drill advanced into the glenoid neck. Note the step in the drill indicating the stop. (c) Same situation as in (b). The step in the drill indicates the necessary depth.

The transacromial approach was first described by Resch et al in 1993.[7] After palpating the borders of the acromion, a skin incision is made in the center of the acromion. A 7-mm diameter drill bit is used to create this portal. After a longitudinal split of the supraspinatus tendon, ideal access to the superior labrum is possible. Fracture of the acromion as a possible complication has been reported. To avoid this complication the hole has to be drilled in the center of the acromion. The special drill for the Suretac is brought in through the appropriate portal. These drills are cannulated and a highly flexible 1-mm diameter pin is engaged centrally and protrudes from the drill by 2–3 mm. With this pin the labrum is then loaded and brought to the correct position, to which it should be reattached (Figure 18.8).

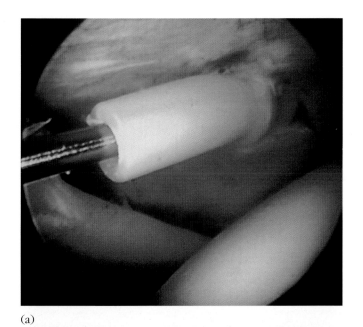

(a)

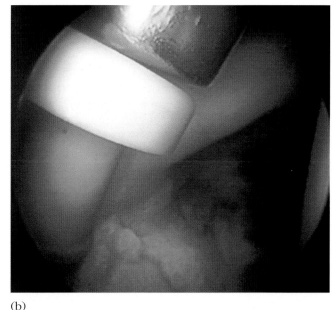

(b)

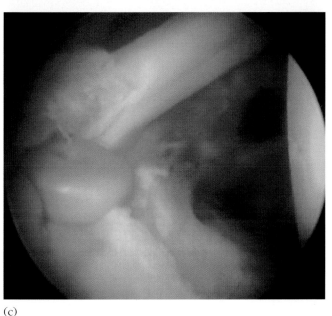

(c)

Figure 18.9

(a) Arthroscopic image showing a Suretac that is brought in through the lateral standard approach after longitudinal split of the supraspinatus tendon. (b) Arthroscopic image of the Suretac and the punch. Care must be taken that the central pin, the Suretac and the punch are aligned correctly to prevent damage of the Suretac. (c) Arthroscopic image with the Suretac in position at the posterior aspect of the biceps anchor showing a sufficient refixation of a type II SLAP lesion.

The direction of the drill should be double-checked (it should run in a lateromedial oblique direction of approximately 30–40°) The drill is advanced into the superior glenoid neck to a depth of 1.8 cm indicated by a step in the drill. The central pin is then disengaged and tapped in gently to provide a secure fit, before the drill is pulled back. Care must be taken not to pull out the central pin during this maneuver. A second pin can be pushed in through the central hole of the drill to keep the first pin in position, while the drill is pulled back. After removal of the drill the Suretac device is then advanced along the guiding pin to the labrum. The Suretac is tapped in with the help of a cannulated punch and a mallet. With the last few taps the broad head of the Suretac presses the labrum onto the glenoid neck (Figure 18.9).

A hook probe is used to check the secure fit of the reattached labrum. Finally the guiding pin is removed from the joint. A diagnostic look and a wash-out of the arthroscopic fluid finishes the procedure. The arthroscope is removed. A suction drain is inserted into the joint. Single sutures are used to close the incisions, which are covered with sterile adhesive wound dressings. Postoperatively the operated arm is put in a special shoulder sling in neutral position (Figure 18.10).

Postoperative protocol

The drainage tube is removed from the joint on the second day postoperatively. Regular changes of dressings

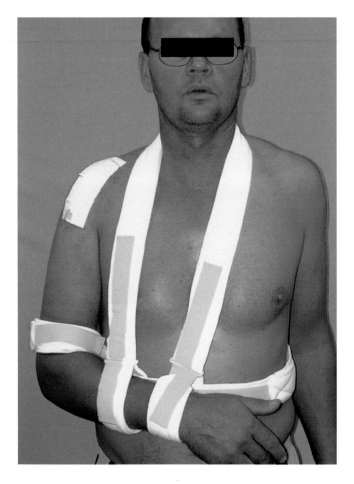

Figure 18.10

Postoperative immobilization in a shoulder sling in neutral position (after 3 weeks).

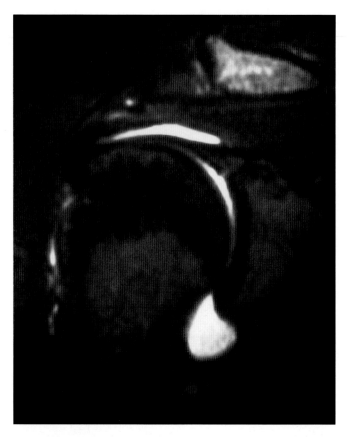

Figure 18.11

Magnetic resonance imaging of a right shoulder with intra-articular application of gadolinium showing a refixed type IV SLAP lesion 6 months postoperatively.

should monitor the uneventful wound healing. The sutures are usually removed between the eighth and tenth day postoperatively. To provide secure healing of the superior labral complex with the glenoid rim, immobilization of the operated shoulder for 3 weeks in a shoulder sling is necessary. Physiotherapy usually starts in week 4 with gentle passive and active motion exercises restricted to 90° of flexion, 70° of adduction and 0° of external rotation. From week 7 postoperatively, mobilization exercises without restriction are allowed. We advise our patients not to return to demanding sports such as tennis, volleyball or snowboarding for at least 4 months after the surgery (Figure 18.11).

References

1. Snyder SJ, Karzel RP, Del Pizzo W et al. SLAP lesions of the shoulder. *Arthroscopy* 1990; **6**:274–9.

2. Andrews JR, Carson WG, McLeod WD. Glenoid labrum tears related to the long head of the biceps. *Am J Sports Med* 1985; **13**:337–41.

3. Habermeyer P, Wiedemann E. Arthroscopic suture repair for SLAP-lesions of the shoulder. Paper presented at the 5th Congress of the European Society for Surgery of the Shoulder and the Elbow, Würzburg, Germany, June 6–8, 1991.

4. Yoneda M, Hirooka A, Saito S et al. Arthroscopic stapling for detached superior glenoid labrum. *J Bone Joint Surg* 1991; **73B**:746–50.

5. Field LD, Savoie FN III. Arthroscopic suture repair of superior labral detachment lesions of the shoulder. Presented at the AAOS Specialty day, 59th Annual Meeting, American Academy of Orthopedic Surgeons, Washington DC. 1992.

6. Snyder SJ. Labral lesions and SLAP lesions. In: Snyder SJ, ed. *Shoulder Arthroscopy.* New York: McGraw-Hill. 1993; 115–31.

7. Resch H, Golser K, Thöni H, Sperner G. Arthroscopic repair of superior glenoid labral detachment. *J Shoulder Elbow Surg* 1993; **3**:1147–55.

8. Golser K, Wambacher M, Resch H. Arthroscopic treatment of SLAP lesions: transacromial aproach. In Fu FH, Ticker JB, Imhoff AB, eds. *An Atlas of Shoulder Surgery.* London: Martin Dunitz, 1998; 105–11.

9. Skyhar MJ, Aldchek DW, Warren RF et al. Shoulder arthroscopy with the patient in the beach chair position. *Arthroscopy* 1988; **4**:256–9.

19 SLAP lesions: Suture fixation

Julious P Smith III, Felix H Savoie III and Larry D Field

Introduction

The variability of the anatomy of the superior aspect of the glenohumeral joint can make assessment of injuries in this region quite difficult. Many of the anatomic variations that occur in the superior labrum and the capsular ligaments can be easily confused with pathologic lesions of these structures. The development of arthroscopy has allowed better evaluation of this anatomy and provided a method of carefully defining the different types of pathology. Snyder et al[1] used this technology in 1990 to describe lesions involving the superior labrum in conjunction with the biceps tendon anchor. He termed these injuries SLAP lesions (superior labrum anterior and posterior), and he described four types based on the characteristics of the lesion (Figure 19.1).

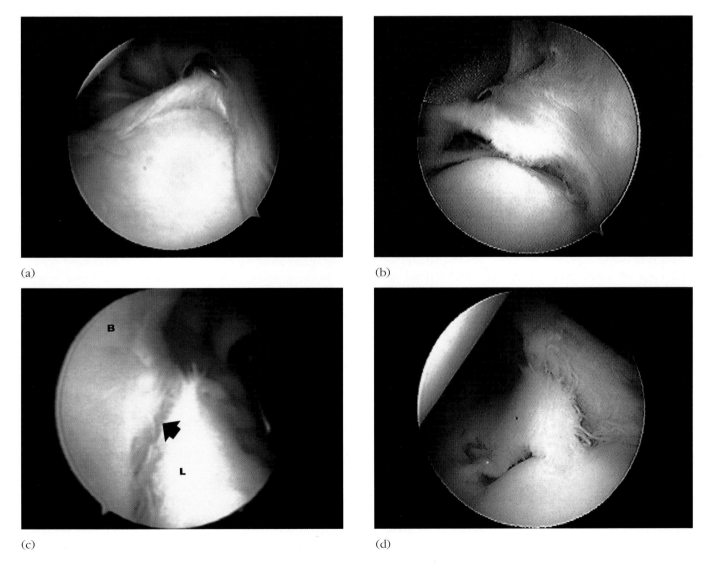

(a)

(b)

(c)

(d)

Figure 19.1

The four types of SLAP lesions as described by Snyder. (a) Type I: degenerative fraying of the superior labrum. (b) Type II: avulsion of the superior labrum and biceps tendon from the superior glenoid. (c) Type III: bucket handle tear (arrow) of the superior labrum without involvement of the connection of the labrum to the glenoid. B = biceps tendon; L = labrum. (d) Type IV: a type II or III lesion with extension into the biceps tendon.

As surgeons have gained more experience with SLAP lesions, the treatment of these injuries has evolved. Treatment of stable type I and III lesions still consists of simply debriding the frayed or torn labral tissue. Treatment of the unstable type II and IV lesions has changed with improving arthroscopic technology. The original treatment of these injuries involved debridement of the damaged labrum with abrasion of the underlying glenoid to encourage the lesion to heal back to bone. When unsatisfactory results were obtained using this technique, direct fixation of the labrum to the glenoid became the treatment of choice.[2,3] Procedures involving transglenoid drilling, absorbable tacks, and suture anchors have since been described. This chapter will focus on the various suture repair techniques.

Indications for SLAP repair are dependent upon the correct diagnosis of the lesion. In 1992, Cooper et al[4] showed this area of the labrum to be very loosely and peripherally attached to the glenoid. They also demonstrated that there is often a small recess beneath the biceps and superior labrum due to the proximal insertion of the complex. Occasionally there is even a communication beneath the labrum between the superior recess and the rotator interval. Each of these variants can easily be confused for a type II SLAP or other anterosuperior labral lesion.

Because of the difficulty encountered in diagnosing SLAP lesions, it is important to obtain a good preoperative history and physical exam. Patients with SLAP tears will usually present with shoulder pain and catching. Most will also have a history of a throwing injury, traction injury, or a fall involving the affected extremity.[5,6] Physical examination techniques that are helpful in identifying SLAP lesions include the SLAP test as described by Field and Savoie[7] and the O'Brien test. Superior labral lesions that are found unexpectedly on arthroscopic examination should be examined carefully to ensure that they are pathologic. Some arthroscopic findings that are suggestive of pathology are the following: sublabral hemorrhage; chondromalacia of superior glenoid; bucket handle labral tear; gap between edge of articular cartilage and superior labral/biceps tendon insertion; more than 3–4-mm gap between labrum and glenoid when biceps is under tension. These findings will be further discussed in the technique section below.

Surgical principles

Suture fixation of SLAP lesions was originally described using transglenoid fixation, but this procedure has been greatly simplified by the evolution of the suture anchor. Both surgical techniques will be described in this chapter. The arthroscope is placed in the posterior portal to begin both types of suture reconstruction. A spinal needle is then used to localize and establish the anterior portal. The lesion is identified and debrided to further

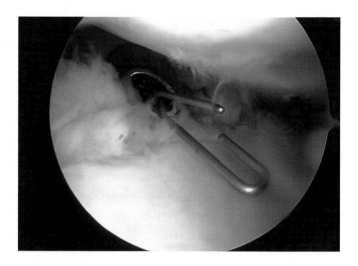

Figure 19.2

The suture retriever used for arthroscopic SLAP repair.

delineate the pathology. Decisions about reconstruction are then made. If an anchor is to be used, the anchor is placed on the anterior glenoid in a high superior position. The limbs of the suture are then retrieved through the superior labrum, using either a suture retriever (we use the Suture Grasper, Mitek, Norwood, MA, USA; Figure 19.2) or a Caspari suture punch. A mattress suture is used to properly buttress the labrum and to avoid putting knots on the articular surface. If the lesion extends posteriorly, a second anchor can be placed through a posterosuperior portal and a similar technique used to repair the posterior labrum.

If the Caspari technique is used, sutures are placed into the superior labrum using a suture punch. Suture placement is begun at the posterior extent of the lesion and then continued more anteriorly. One suture is placed into the biceps tendon itself to take tension off the repair. Additional sutures are placed in the superior glenohumeral ligament and the superior labrum as needed. A Beath pin is then passed across the glenoid as described in the Caspari reconstruction for anterior instability,[8] and the sutures are passed through the glenoid and tied over the fascia of the medial scapula.

Both techniques are complicated and contain many potential pitfalls. Placement of the anterior portal is essential to both procedures. Improper portal placement can greatly restrict access to the superior shoulder and make reconstruction much more difficult. By using a spinal needle to localize the portal, access to the various regions of the shoulder can be assessed before the portal is created. Suture placement is difficult with both the Suture Grasper device and the suture punch. Care must be taken when using both so as not to damage the articular surface or cut or score the suture. The surgeon should have extensive laboratory experience with both devices before they are tried in vivo. Placement of the

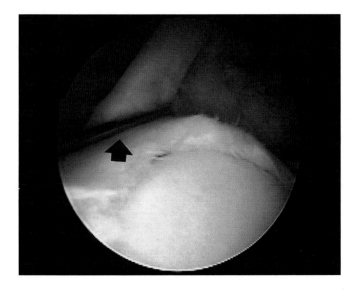

Figure 19.3

A spinal needle (arrow) placed through the rotator interval for localization of the anterior portal. The needle can be manipulated to ensure access to the superior labrum.

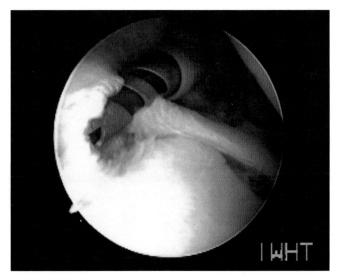

Figure 19.4

Debridement of the labrum using an arthroscopic shaver. Thorough debridement is necessary to define the lesion and to remove all degenerative tissue.

Beath pin is also difficult. Care must be taken during insertion to prevent the pin from sliding over the superior aspect of the glenoid neck and damaging the suprascapular nerve. Once the starting point of the pin has been established, orientation is very important. It should be directed inferomedially to exit in the infraspinatus fossa of the medial scapula. Aiming the pin too laterally can cause articular or neurovascular injury. Aiming too medially can cause thoracic injury.[9]

The most common complication from these procedures is residual shoulder instability. This can result from mistakenly diagnosing a normal anatomic variant as a SLAP lesion or from failure to identify additional instability in the shoulder.[10] The results of the preoperative examination should be used in conjunction with the arthroscopic findings to ensure that all instability is corrected. If proper indications are used, results of arthroscopic techniques have approached a 90% success rate.[7]

Surgical technique

The patient is placed in the lateral position and rolled posteriorly 30°. Five to 10 pounds of traction is applied to the arm and draping is completed to allow access to the entire shoulder. When using transglenoid fixation, it is important to include the entire scapula in the surgical field so that the exit point of the Beath pin is exposed. A posterior portal is then established and the joint is distended. Gravity flow of lactated Ringer's with epinephrine is used for fluid inflow. Use of a pump is avoided to prevent the shoulder from swelling too quickly.

Diagnostic arthroscopy is performed initially. As mentioned previously, it is important to perform a good preoperative examination and have an expected diagnosis at the time of arthroscopy. The entire shoulder should then be thoroughly inspected arthroscopically in a systematic fashion. If a SLAP lesion is found, it is still important to evaluate the remainder of the labrum and capsular ligaments for other instability patterns. It is especially important to examine the anterior labrum and middle glenohumeral ligaments, as injury to these structures has been seen to occur in up to 75% of SLAP lesions. The rotator cuff should also be carefully examined, as partial or full thickness tears have been described with up to 50% of SLAP lesions.[11] Injuries to the rotator interval are also common. If a superior labral lesion is discovered unexpectedly, it is even more essential to inspect the shoulder for further pathology, because the 'SLAP' may not be the cause of the patient's symptoms.

An anterior portal is placed upon the discovery of a superior labral lesion. This second portal allows examination and debridement of the labrum to better define any pathology. When creating the anterior portal, as mentioned previously, it is important to be sure that it is located in a position that allows access to the superior shoulder. This access will be essential if reconstruction is necessary. It is best to place this portal by using a spinal needle to localize its position. The needle should be placed into the shoulder through the rotator interval and manipulated to be sure that all areas can be reached (Figure 19.3). When a suitable location is established, the portal is created from outside in.

Frayed labral tissue should be removed with the shaver to further expose the underlying attachment (Figure 19.4). Minimal suction should be used during this

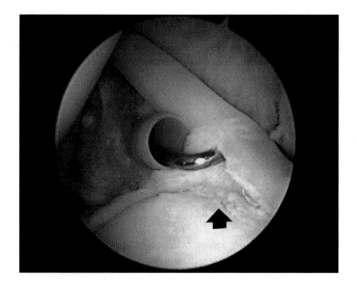

Figure 19.5

Superior glenoid chondromalacia (arrow) seen with a type II SLAP lesion.

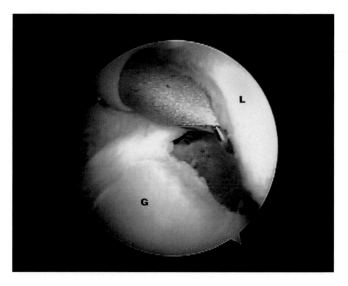

Figure 19.6

Abrasion of the superior glenoid using an arthroscopic burr. Abrasion should begin along the articular surface and continue medially down the glenoid neck. G = glenoid; L = superior labrum.

part of the procedure, and debridement should be done with the shaver blade facing away from the articular surface. This will prevent damage to the articular cartilage and the surrounding normal labrum. Suspected unstable type II and IV lesions must be examined carefully due to the variable anatomy. Certain normal variants that have a large superior recess can be difficult to differentiate from SLAP lesions.

Despite the anatomic variation that is seen in the shoulder, there are certain specific findings that suggest a pathologic separation of the superior labrum. Although a superior pouch may exist, articular cartilage normally extends over the top of the glenoid to the insertion of the labrum and biceps. In contrast, SLAP lesions will usually have an area of exposed bone beneath them that is not covered by articular cartilage. This area is also often hemorrhagic in response to the injury that has occurred, especially in the acute setting.[12,13] The superior instability that occurs with a SLAP lesion[14] will also cause wear of the superior glenoid articular cartilage and result in chondromalacia of this area (Figure 19.5).

Once it has been established that a lesion is an unstable SLAP tear, reconstruction is undertaken. The first steps in this process are debridement of the lesion and abrasion of the underlying glenoid rim. The suction and debris from the abrasion can make visualization difficult, and it is sometimes necessary at this point to insert a larger inflow cannula through the posterior portal. If all frayed or degenerative tissue was not debrided from the labrum during the initial inspection of the lesion, it should be done at this time.

Abrasion of the glenoid should be carried out along the full extent of the tear and must be performed

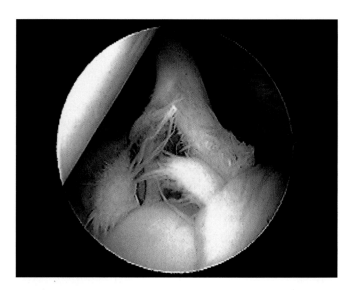

Figure 19.7

Assessing a type IV SLAP lesion using a spinal needle. The amount of tendon and labral involvement should be assessed before debridement of the lesion to help determine how the lesion will be treated.

medially along the glenoid neck as well as along the edge of the articular surface (Figure 19.6). A burr, full radius resector, or other aggressive shaver blade can be used for this portion of the procedure. Care should be taken not to damage the articular surface along the superior margin of the glenoid during the abrasion

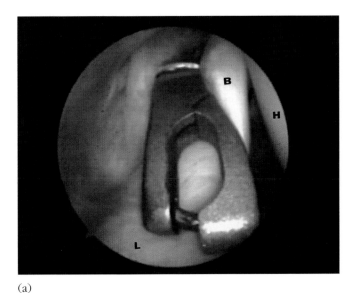

(a)

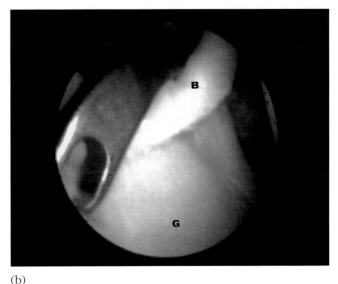

(b)

Figure 19.8

(a) The suture punch positioned above the biceps tendon for suture repair. B = biceps; L = labrum; H = humeral head. (b) Placement of the initial suture in the most posterior portion of the tear. G = glenoid.

process. If anterior reconstruction is to be done then the anterior glenoid should also be prepared at this time. When thorough debridement and abrasion is completed, the reconstruction is carried out.

If a type IV lesion is found, the amount of biceps tendon involvement should be assessed before the flap is debrided (Figure 19.7). Degenerative tears of less than 30% of the tendon should simply be removed. For lesions involving 30–50% of the tendon, especially in younger patients, the complex can be repaired or included in the reconstruction. Tears involving more than 50% of the biceps may be treated with repair, release, or biceps tenodesis. Unstable labral lesions will need reconstruction regardless of how the biceps lesion is treated.

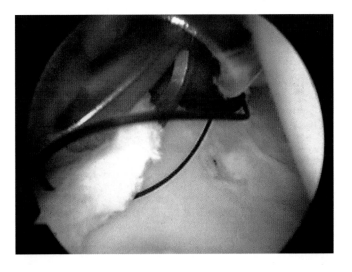

Figure 19.9

Placement of a suture at the base of the biceps tendon insertion.

The Caspari transglenoid technique

The transglenoid technique was the first to be described for arthroscopic repair of SLAP lesions. To begin this reconstruction, the anterior cannula should be exchanged for a suture punch cannula. The curved suture punch is inserted first, and it should be single-loaded with an absorbable #2 suture (i.e. #2-0 PDS, Ethicon, Somerville, NJ, USA). The suture punch is passed over the biceps tendon superiorly and positioned at the posterior aspect of the lesion (Figure 19.8a). The first stitch is placed into the posterior corner of the tear (Figure 19.8b). Both limbs of the suture are then brought with the suture punch over

the biceps and out of the anterior cannula. When removing the suture punch, it is essential to keep the jaws separated so as not to cut the suture. Both ends of the suture are then brought together and clamped using a hemostat or mosquito clamp. If there is significant posterior extension of the tear, a second stitch can then be placed in similar fashion with the suture punch positioned over the biceps tendon. This second suture is placed slightly anterior to the first one, but still posterior to the insertion of the biceps. The stitch is again brought out of the anterior cannula and clamped.

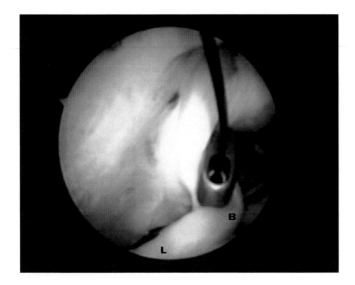

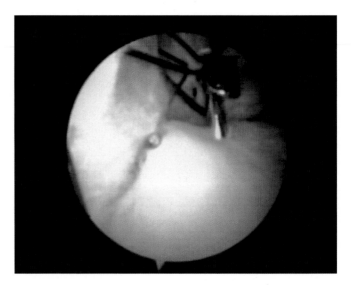

Figure 19.10

Placement of a suture into the biceps tendon in a right shoulder. The biceps suture should be placed 5–7 mm distally along the tendon. B = biceps; L = labrum.

Figure 19.11

Placement of the transglenoid Beath pin in a right shoulder. The starting point should be at the 1 o'clock position, just off the articular surface.

The next suture is placed in the labrum directly inferior to the biceps tendon at approximately the 12 o'clock position on the glenoid (Figure 19.9). A suture is then placed into the biceps tendon itself to protect the repair during healing. This tendon stitch is placed approximately 5–7 mm more distally along the tendon than the labral sutures are (Figure 19.10). A larger suture is used for the tendon stitch to give further support to

the repair (we use #0 PDS). Suture placement is then continued anteriorly along the labrum in sequential fashion until the entire defect has been spanned. Four to seven sutures are usually required, and the superior glenohumeral ligament is included in the repair. A second biceps tendon anchor stitch can also be placed if it is necessary. All sutures are brought out of the anterior cannula.

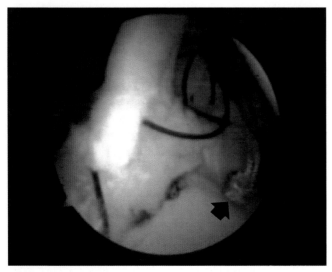

(a)

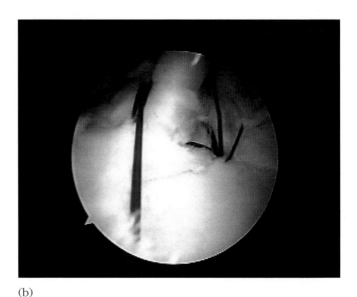

(b)

Figure 19.12

(a) The loop of the Ticron suture can be seen (arrow) after the Beath pin has been pulled through the glenoid. This Ticron is used as a shuttle to pull the sutures of the repair through the tunnel from the Beath pin across the glenoid. (b) View of the repair after the sutures have been pulled through.

Once all of the sutures have been placed, the transglenoid Beath pin is drilled. The pin is placed through the anterior portal and the tip is positioned at the 1 o'clock position (for a right shoulder) on the neck of the glenoid, approximately 3–5 mm medial to the articular surface (Figure 19.11). It is important to ensure that the starting point is correctly placed, visualizing the tip of the pin on glenoid bone if possible. The pin is directed medially and inferiorly and oriented so as to exit in the infraspinatus fossa on the scapula. Misdirection of the pin in the superior, medial, or lateral direction can lead to neurovascular damage, so it is essential to correctly orient this pin.

A small incision is made at the exit site of the Beath pin and dissection is done to expose the tip of the pin as it penetrates through fascia of the medial scapula. Both ends of a #2 Ticron (Davis and Geck, St Louis, MO, USA) suture are then passed through the eyelet of the Beath pin and pulled through the transglenoid tunnel, leaving a loop of suture out of the anterior portal (Figure 19.12a). The ends of all of the labral sutures are placed through the loop in this Ticron, and the Ticron is then used as a shuttle to pass the sutures through the glenoid neck and out of the posterior aspect of the shoulder (Figure 19.12b).

After they are brought through the fascia the individual sutures are again identified and both ends are marked. The sutures are then appropriately tensioned, and the repair is evaluated with the arthroscope. If it is adequate, the sutures are divided into two equal bundles posteriorly, and each bundle is passed through the thick fascia independently. After again properly tensioning the sutures, traction is removed from the arm and the two bundles are tied over the fascia (Figure 19.13).

As the sutures are tensioned, the initial sutures placed in the posterior labrum will wrap around the biceps and cross the labrum to enter the transglenoid tunnel (Figure 19.12b). The biceps anchor sutures will do the same. Do not be concerned by this. These sutures are absorbable and act to temporarily augment the superior/biceps anchor portion of the repair.

Suture anchor technique

The development of suture anchors has simplified the technique for suture repair of SLAP lesions, allowing the surgeon to attach the labrum back to bone without many of the difficulties that were previously faced. In most circumstances a suture punch is not necessary, and the dangers of transglenoid drilling are avoided. With new absorbable anchors, permanent implants are no longer required either. The technique is still technically difficult, however, and requires previous experience with the anchors as well as a suture retriever or suture punch. The surgeon must also have experience with arthroscopic knot tying in order to ensure a tight repair.

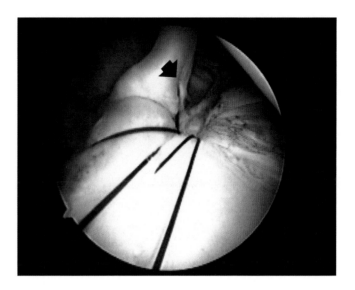

Figure 19.13
A view of a SLAP repair after the sutures have been tied. An older technique is depicted in which the posterior sutures crossed the articular surface. Note the tension on the biceps tendon suture (arrow) to take stress off of the repair.

As with transglenoid fixation, the procedure begins with debridement of the lesion and glenoid abrasion. When this is completed, a 7-mm plastic cannula is placed in the anterior portal and preparation for anchor placement is made. We use the absorbable Panalok anchor (Mitek). The guide is placed at the 12.30–1 o'clock position (for a right shoulder) on the glenoid. The drill is started slightly up on the face of the glenoid to position the completed repair onto the abraded surface on the glenoid rim (Figure 19.14a). The anchor is drilled and placed (Figure 19.14b). All needles should be removed from the anchor sutures. A hemostat or mosquito clamp should then be placed at the tip of each end of the suture to prevent the suture from being pulled out of the anchor.

A 30° Suture Grasper retriever is then placed through the anterior portal. The retriever is guided superiorly above the biceps tendon (Figure 19.15a) as was done with the suture punch in the early portions of the Caspari technique, and the tip of the retriever is brought down through the biceps anchor and superior labrum. The superior/posterior-most limb of the suture anchor is retrieved through this portion of the labrum (Figure 19.15b). Retrieval of this suture can be difficult. It is sometimes easier if the suture limb is pushed into the posterosuperior portion of the joint with a knot pusher or arthroscopic grabber before the retriever is inserted. It is important to identify and unclamp the limb of the suture that has been grasped before the retriever is withdrawn. If the limb is not identified then the suture can be inadvertently pulled out of the anchor while being retrieved. After the correct limb of the suture is

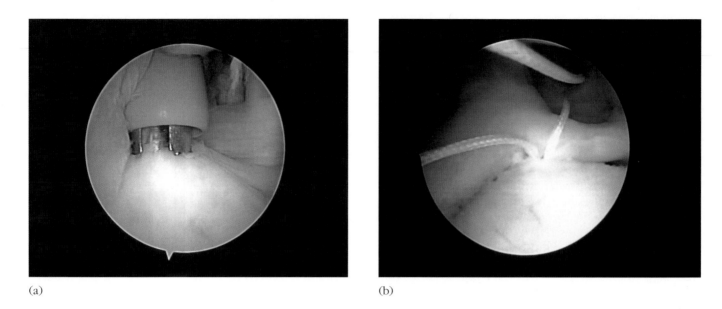

(a)   (b)

Figure 19.14

Placement of a suture anchor. (a) Drilling the pilot hole for the anchor. The guide is placed at the 12.30–1 o'clock position on the glenoid, just slightly up onto the articular surface. (b) The anchor in place.

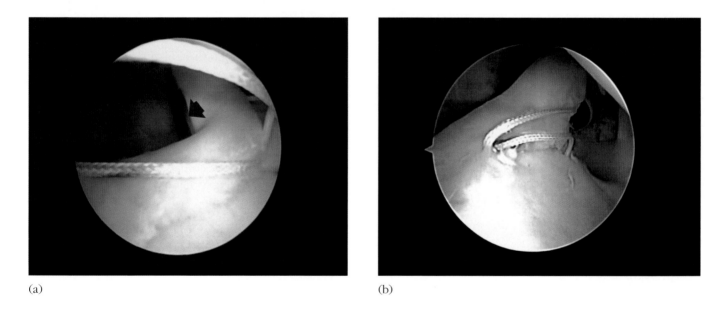

(a)   (b)

Figure 19.15

(a) The retriever (arrow) is positioned superior to the biceps tendon for retrieval of the first limb of the suture. (b) The suture being retrieved through the superior labrum.

identified, it is brought out of the anterior portal with the retriever and clamped again.

The retriever is then placed back through the anterior portal and passed through the superior labrum near the anterior extent of the tear. The superior glenohumeral ligament should be included in this stitch. The inferior/anterior-most limb of the suture anchor is then retrieved and brought out of the anterior portal (Figure

19.16). Care should be taken to avoid twisting or crossing the two limbs of the suture during retrieval, as this will complicate knot tying and compromise the repair.

If the surgeon does not have access to a suture retriever or is not experienced with its use, then the suture punch can also be used to place the sutures for this technique. The suture punch should be loaded with either a shuttle device or a double-loaded #2-0 PDS that can be used to

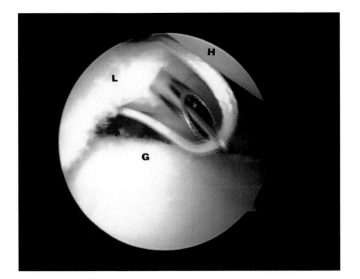

Figure 19.16

Retrieval of the second limb of the suture through the anterior labrum. G = glenoid; L = labrum; H = humeral head.

guide the limb of suture from the anchor through the labrum. The remainder of the technique is the same.

After both limbs of the suture have been brought out, the two limbs are tied using arthroscopic knot-tying techniques. We use a mattress suture because it pulls the labrum down to bone over a broader area than a simple suture and it buttresses the labrum up onto the edge of the glenoid. It also keeps the knots off the articular surface. We have found the modified Roeder knot to be the most effective for tightly securing the torn labral tissue back to bone (Figure 19.17). The knot position can be difficult to visualize, but it is important to ensure that a secure knot is tied so that the repair does not loosen. We use the Roeder knot because it will slide to tighten and can be locked when it is in the correct position. Other slip knots and half hitches can be used if the surgeon feels more comfortable tying them. Any other knot that is used should tightly approximate the labral tissue to the glenoid. If the Roeder knot is used, a second half-hitch should be used to back the stitch up.

We have found that most unstable SLAP lesions require only one anchor to create a stable repair. If there is significant anterior or posterior extension, a second anchor can be placed to further secure the labrum. Additional anterior and inferior anchors can be placed through the anterior portal. If a posterior anchor is required, it can be placed through a posterosuperior portal made through the interval between the supraspinatus and infraspinatus tendons. This portal should also be created with the use of a spinal needle for localization. The skin position is usually just posterior and medial to the posterolateral corner of the acromion. Once the portal is established, the technique used is the

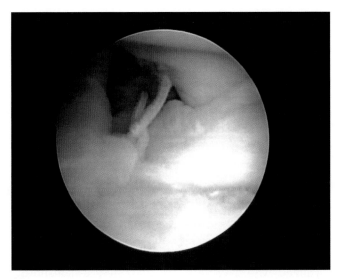

(a)

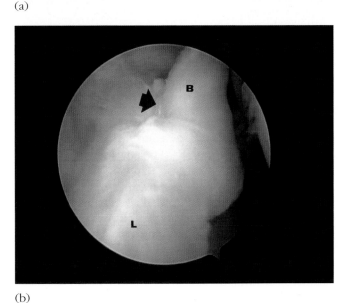

(b)

Figure 19.17

(a) A Roeder knot securing the SLAP repair to the glenoid.
(b) A superior view of the Roeder knot (arrow). B = biceps; L = labrum.

same as for the anterior anchor except that the camera is placed through the anterior portal and the anchor and retriever are placed through the posterior portals. After the SLAP repair is done, then additional work on the rotator cuff, rotator interval, and subacromial space can be performed.

Postoperative protocol

The postoperative protocol for both types of arthroscopic suture repair is basically the same. The shoulder is placed into a shoulder abduction sling before the patient awakens from anesthesia, and most patients are discharged home on the day of surgery. Patients are told to wear this immobilizer at all times except while showering, which is allowed beginning postoperative day 2. Patients are kept in an immobilizer for a week and then placed in a sling for an additional 3 weeks. During the period in which they are in the sling, patients are encouraged to do shoulder shrugs and to start passive forward flexion and external rotation. They are told to sleep in their immobilizer for this period. At 4 weeks postoperatively the sling and immobilizer are removed and waist level active exercises are begun. At 6 weeks pain-free active therapy is begun and at 8 weeks full therapy is started. At 12 weeks patients begin plyometrics.

Patients who have jobs with low physical demand on the involved upper extremity are allowed to return to work as tolerated. Athletes involved in contact sports and those individuals who have jobs involving heavy lifting are held out for at least 3 months. They are then allowed to return to their activity when the operated arm has full range of movement and 90% of the strength of the opposite arm.

Throwing athletes are begun on a strict return to throw program at 3 months postoperatively. This protocol is based upon the program of Dr James Andrew et al,[15] which gradually progresses the throwing distance as the shoulder allows. Warm-up jogging and stretching should always be done before throwing is begun. Using the Crow-hop method the athlete should then begin warm-up throws at a comfortable distance and progress to the distance indicated for their phase of the program. Patients start out throwing at 45 feet and progress to 60, 90, 120, 150 and then 180 feet as they can tolerate. Progression from level to level is based on the ability to make 75 throws at a distance without pain. Symptoms in the shoulder indicate that the progression is too rapid. All throwing should be done under the supervision of a pitching coach and/or therapist and strict adherence to the mechanics of throwing should be followed.

After the athlete can throw 50 times at 180 feet without pain, then he or she is ready to return to their position or begin throwing off the mound. From here progression to unrestricted throwing should still be slow and as tolerated by the patient. Pitchers should begin with only fastballs at 50% and progress to fastballs at 75% and

100% before throwing the more stressful breaking pitches. Position players should do simulated game situations and also progress from 50% to 100%. Any time that the athlete develops pain or swelling then the program should be backed-off and then advanced again as tolerated.

References

1. Snyder SJ, Karzel RP, Del Pizzo W et al. SLAP lesions of the shoulder. *Arthroscopy* 1990; **6**:274–9.
2. Snyder SJ, Banas MP, Karzel RP. An analysis of 140 injuries to the superior glenoid labrum. *J Shoulder Elbow Surg* 1995; **4**:243–8.
3. Altcheck DW, Warren RF, Wickiewicz TL et al. Arthroscopic labral debridement: a three year follow-up study. *Am J Sports Med* 1992; **20**:702–6.
4. Cooper DE, Arnoczky SP, O'Brien SJ et al. Anatomy, histology, and vascularity of the glenoid labrum: an anatomical study. *J Bone Joint Surg* 1992; **74A**:46–52.
5. Snyder SJ, Banas MP, Belzer JP. Arthroscopic evaluation and treatment of injuries to the superior glenoid labrum. *Instr Course Lect* 1996; **45**:65–70.
6. Savoie FH, Field LD. Lesions of the superior aspect of the shoulder. In: Norris TR, ed. *Shoulder and Elbow Orthopaedic Knowledge Update*. Rosemont, IL: AAOS, 1997;269–76.
7. Field LD, Savoie FH. Arthroscopic suture repair of superior labral detachment lesions of the shoulder. *Am J Sports Med* 1993; **21**:783–90.
8. Caspari RB, Savoie FH. Arthroscopic reconstruction of the shoulder: the Bankart repair (suture technique). In McGinty JB, ed. *Operative Arthroscopy*. Philadelphia: Lippincott-Raven, 1996;695–707.
9. Savoie FH, Caspari RB. Instability of the shoulder: superior, posterior, and multidirectional. In McGinty JB, ed. *Operative Arthroscopy*. Philadelphia: Lippincott-Raven, 1996;709–23.
10. Warner JJP, Kann S, Marks P. Arthroscopic repair of combined Bankart and superior labral detachment anterior and posterior lesions: technique and preliminary results. *Arthroscopy* **10**:383–91.
11. Maffett MW, Gartsman GM, Moseley B. Superior labrum–biceps tendon complex lesions of the shoulder. *Am J Sports Med* 1995; **23**:93–8.
12. Snyder SJ. *Shoulder Arthroscopy*. New York: McGraw-Hill, 1993.
13. Karzel RP, Snyder SJ. Labral lesions. In McGinty JB, ed. *Operative Arthroscopy*. Philadelphia: Lippincott-Raven, 1996;663–75.
14. Pagnani MJ, Deng X-H, Warren RF et al. Effect of lesions of the superior portion of the glenoid labrum on glenohumeral translation. *J Bone Joint Surg* 1995; **77A**:1003–10.
15. Andrews JR, Carson WG Jr, McLeod WD. Glenoid labrum tears related to the long head of the biceps. *Am J Sports Med* 1985; **13**:337–41.

20 Arthroscopic treatment of SLAP lesions: Types III, IV and V

Vladimir Martinek and Andreas B Imhoff

Introduction

The diagnosis of superior labrum anterior posterior (SLAP) lesions was first made possible with the advent of shoulder arthroscopy. Snyder et al classified the partial or complete detachment of the superior glenoid labrum at the area of the long biceps tendon insertion into four distinct types (Figure 20.1a).[1] This classification was later extended by Maffet et al, who added three further types of labral defects (Figure 20.1b): type V lesions consist of a classical anterior Bankart lesion that extends superiorly to include the separation of the biceps anchor from the superior glenoid; type VI lesions consist of an unstable flap tear of the labrum in addition to the biceps anchor separation; and type VII lesions are SLAP tears that extend anteriorly and laterally beneath the middle glenohumeral ligament.[2] In this chapter, treatment of type V lesions is addressed.

The SLAP lesion is frequently a source of significant pain and disability, especially in active participants in 'overhead' sports.[3] As the long head of the biceps and the superior labrum function as a static stabilizer of the

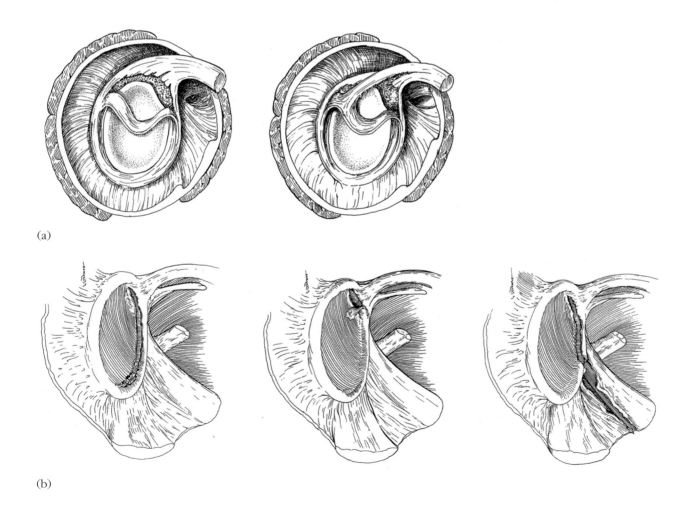

(a)

(b)

Figure 20.1

(a) Types III and IV SLAP lesions according to Snyder et al; and (b) types V, VI and VII by Maffet et al.

glenohumeral joint,[4,5] unstable SLAP lesions are an indication for surgical refixation whenever it is technically possible. Particular attention should also be given to extended lesions with involvement of the superior, anterior and inferior labrum (SLAP V).[6]

Surgical principles

The operative management of SLAP lesions, which is exclusively performed as an arthroscopic technique, has been described by several experienced authors.[6–9] As the simple debridement of a SLAP lesion showed deteriorating long-term results,[10] this procedure today can be recommended only for type I lesions. The role of the glenoid labrum in the shoulder can be thought of as comparable to that of the meniscus in the knee joint. For this reason, labral tears in lesions of types II to VII, where the biceps anchor is unstable and separated from the glenoid rim, are best treated by arthroscopic refixation.[6,11,12] However, the treatment of types III and IV lesions depends on the extent of labral tissue disruption and involves either debridement or suture repair.[8] An exception can be made in older patients with degenerative changes of the biceps tendon, in whom a primary biceps tenodesis with debridement of the torn labral cartilage is performed.

The refixation of the superior labrum can be a difficult operative procedure, requiring considerable arthroscopic experience. A large variety of metal and bioabsorbable suture anchors or tacks are available for the SLAP repair. We prefer the FASTak anchor (Arthrex, Naples, FL, USA), a threaded suture anchor that is screwed into the glenoid rim, offering the benefit of being retrievable for cases of suture failure or intraoperative false positioning of the anchor. A newly introduced poly-L-lactic acid suture anchor (Bio-FASTak, Arthrex), offers the advantage that no intra-articular hardware remains after the material has been absorbed.

The key point of the procedure is the placement of the working portals. The portals normally used for shoulder arthroscopy do not permit the necessary perpendicular access to the superior glenoid rim. Therefore, we use an accessory portal just lateral to the middle of the acromion to reach the superior rim of the glenoid (Figure 20.2). Inserting the instruments directly without using a cannula through this trans-rotator cuff portal limits the harm to the supraspinatus tendon. For the refixation of the anteroinferior labrum in type V SLAP lesions, we have introduced an inferior portal midway between the 5 and 6 o'clock positions, allowing perpendicular access to the anterior–inferior parts of the glenoid rim for the Bankart repair (Figure 20.3).[13]

In cases where the Bankart lesion is combined with a SLAP tear (type V), the repair starts with the posterosuperior labrum, continues with the anteroinferior labrum and ends with the anterosuperior labrum. In this sequence, the technically most challenging steps of the stabilization are performed before swelling of the shoulder makes the repair difficult.

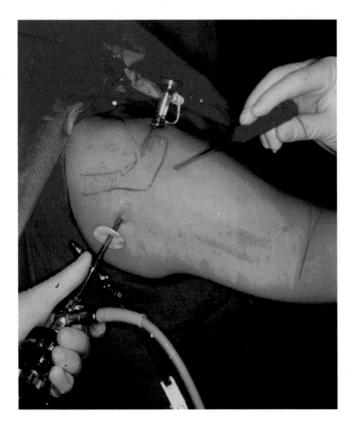

Figure 20.2

Arthroscopic portals for the SLAP repair procedure

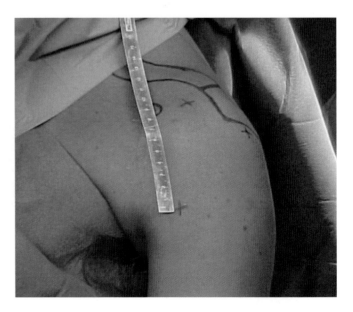

Figure 20.3

Inferior portal midway between the 5 and 6 o'clock positions for refixation of the anteroinferior labrum.

Surgical technique

Following induction of general anaesthesia or regional anaesthesia with an interscalene block, both shoulders are examined under relaxed conditions for increased glenohumeral translation. The arthroscopic procedure is performed in the beach-chair position with the table at 70°, and with the arm wrapped and attached to a sterile, articulated arm-holder (McConnell Orthopedic Manufacturing Co., Greenville, TX, USA). This positioning allows free movements in all planes, as well as traction of the shoulder, while avoiding possible neuropraxia of the brachial plexus associated with traction of the arm in the lateral decubitus position.

Prior to the incisions, all arthroscopic portals are infiltrated with diluted epinephrine (adrenaline) solution to improve haemostasis and visualization. Using the standard posterior portal at a position 2–3 cm inferior and 1–2 cm medial to the posterolateral corner of the acromion, an arthroscopic examination of the glenohumeral joint is performed. The entire labrum and the long biceps tendon are carefully examined to judge the true extent of the labral detachment and of the involvement of the long biceps tendon. The second anterior portal is placed just in front of the acromioclavicular joint, introducing the cannula anterior to the biceps tendon. This access allows for the preparation of the superior glenoid rim, and of the anteroinferior glenoid rim in cases of type V lesions. We use a sharp Bankart rasp and then a motorized round burr (3.5 mm) to remove remaining tissue from the anterior scapular neck and to prepare a bleeding bony surface at the superior and anterior glenoid rim for the repair. To improve visualization and to keep the torn and displaced superior labrum away from the working instruments, a holding suture is passed around the superior labrum using a needle, which is introduced from the supraspinous fossa (Figure 20.4).[14] During the decortication procedure of the glenoid rim, care must be taken to avoid damage to the articular cartilage. Torn labral and biceps tendon tissue is also carefully debrided with a shaver without capturing the remaining labrum.

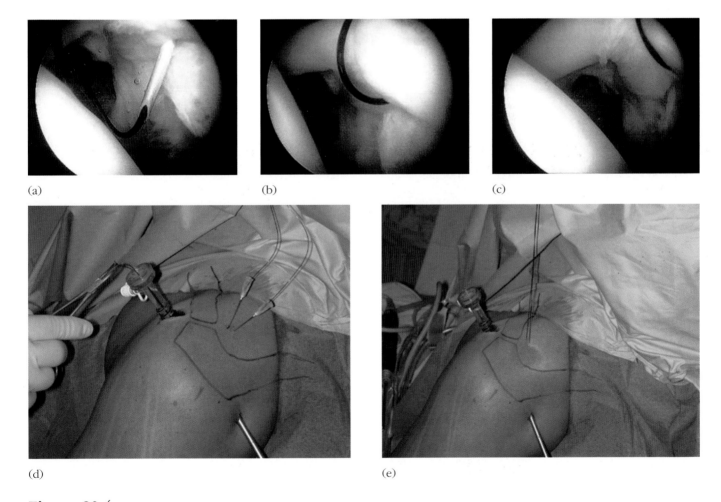

(a)   (b)   (c)

(d)   (e)

Figure 20.4

Suture passed through the supraspinous fossa holding the torn and displaced superior labrum medially and superiorly, improving a better visualization of the superior glenoid rim.

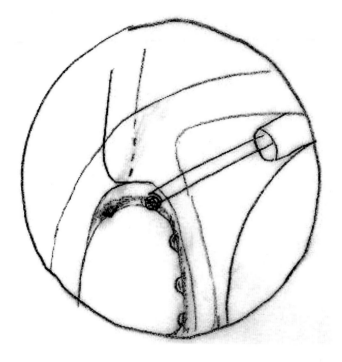

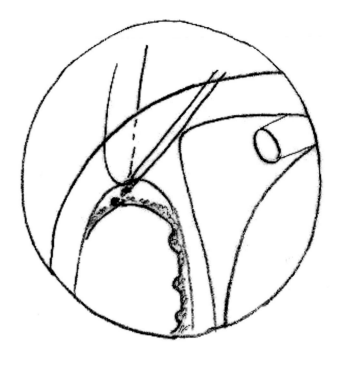

Figure 20.5

The soft tissue along the superior and anterior labrum is removed and the bone along the glenoid rim is lightly decorticated to a bleeding surface. Pilot holes are created with a burr along the glenoid rim at the locations where the suture anchors will be implanted.

Figure 20.6

A suture anchor loaded with #2 non-absorbable braided polyester suture is drilled into the glenoid rim using a cannulated speer guide.

After preparation of the glenoid is complete, pilot holes are created with a burr along the glenoid rim at the locations where the suture anchors will be implanted (Figure 20.5). For reparable type III and type IV lesions, one pilot hole is located just anterior and another posterior to the biceps tendon insertion. For type V lesions, an additional three pilot holes are created at the 5.30, 4, and 2.30 o'clock positions (for a right shoulder). In cases of a Bankart lesion in combination with a SLAP type V lesion, the posterosuperior labrum is always repaired first. For the placement of the anchors at the superior glenoid rim, an additional portal just laterally to the middle portion of the acromion is created in order to reach the upper glenoid rim at an angle of 135° (see Figure 20.2). The anteroinferior portal, 8–10 cm distal to the coracoid process and lateral to the deltopectoral sulcus (see Figure 20.3) is used for the placement of three suture anchors at the anterior glenoid rim.

A cannulated speer guide (Figure 20.6) is placed in the pilot hole at the planned position on the glenoid rim in 135° angulation to the plane of the glenoid and then used for the drilling of the suture anchor. The FASTak suture anchor is loaded with #2 non-absorbable braided polyester suture (Ethibond, Ethicon, Sommerville, NJ, USA) and inserted exactly to the level of the stop mark (Figure 20.6). Avoid shallow placement of the anchor,

which can cause chondral damage to the humeral head, as well as deep placement, which can result in suture failure. Once the anchor is seated, and its stability tested by pulling on the sutures, the labrum is caught by a suture hook (Arthrex) or suture passer (Linvatec, Largo, FL, USA; Figure 20.7a) or cuff stitch angulated 30–45° (Smith & Nephew, Andover, MA, USA) and the suture is passed with a shuttle relay (Linvatec) medially (Figure 20.7b). Alternatively, a penetrator (Arthrex) or an epidural needle placed through the anterosuperior portal can be used for passing the suture through the labrum. One limb of the suture is passed and a simple knot is created using an arthroscopic knot pusher or 'sixth finger' (Arthrex) (Figure 20.8). The placement of the suture anchors and the refixation of the labrum should be started posteriorly for type III and IV lesions and be continued inferiorly in cases of type V lesions (Figure 20.9). Type III lesions are repaired only in cases of a strong bucket-handle tear of the labrum. In some cases, especially in older patients with degenerative changes of the labrum, a simple resection and debridement of the loose labral fragment may be sufficient. In cases of type IV lesions, the torn biceps tendon has to be sutured additionally to the labral refixation to the glenoid. The suture of the biceps tendon can be performed percutaneously using a 17-gauge epidural needle placed through the split portion of the tendon and

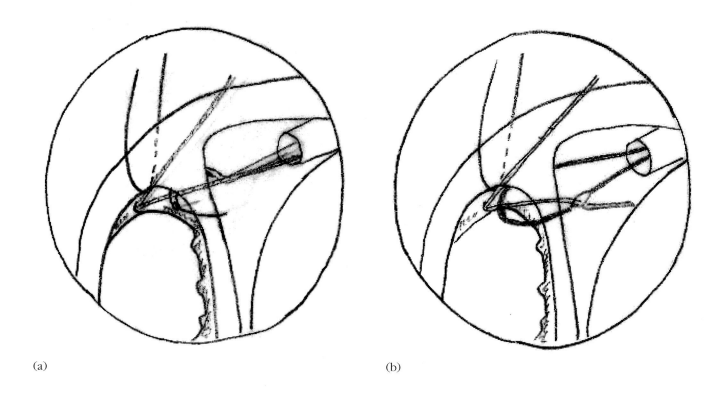

(a)   (b)

Figure 20.7

(a) The detached labrum is caught by a hooked needle and (b) one limb of the suture is passed with a shuttle relay medially.

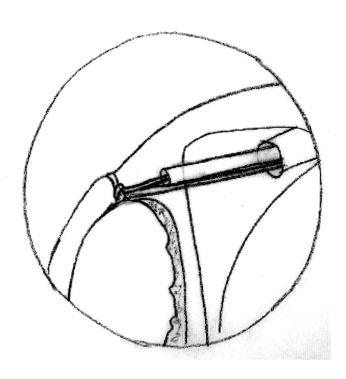

Figure 20.8

Sutures are tied with an arthroscopic 'sixth finger' knot pusher.

then the arthroscopic knot pusher for the tying of the #2 Ethibond sutures. However, in cases of a fragmented and degenerative biceps tendon, a debridement of the labrum and a biceps tenodesis or a biceps tenotomy in elderly patients should be considered.

Postoperative protocol

The majority of the patients with an arthroscopic SLAP lesion repair are admitted for approximately a week to enable us to control the postoperative rehabilitation. The shoulder is immobilized with a Ultrasling (Donjoy, Irving, TX, USA) or Shoulder Sling II (Medi, Bayrenth, Germany) for the first 24 hours postoperatively. After that, the patient is allowed to remove the sling during the daytime and to swing the arm gently in a hanging position. Passive and active exercises are performed at the range of motion 45° flexion, 45° abduction and 45° internal rotation, except for active elbow flexion and supination, which should be avoided for 6 weeks to protect the healing biceps insertion from strong traction. The external rotation can be extended to 0° between weeks 4 and 6 and then allowed beyond 0° between weeks 7 and 12. Non-contact overhead activities are possible after 3 months, and contact sports are permitted after 6 months.

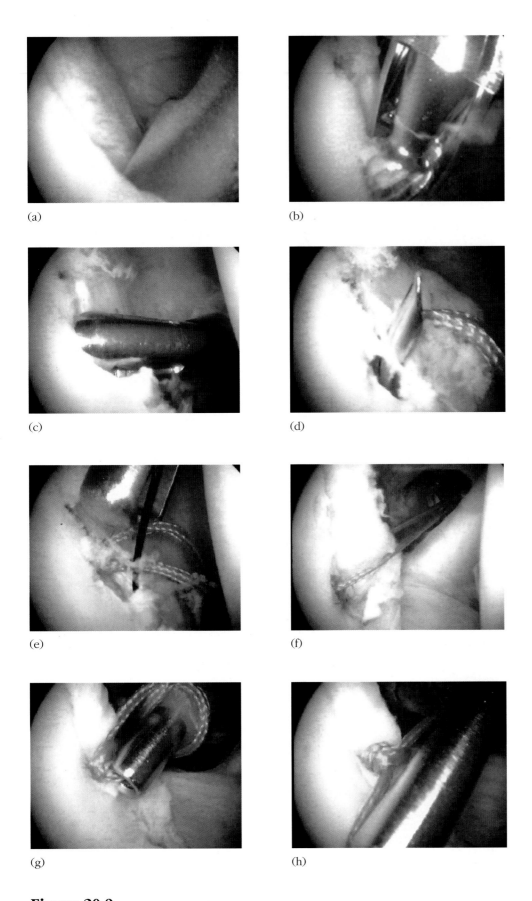

Figure 20.9

Arthroscopic reattachment of the anteroinferior labrum with a suture anchor. (a) Rim preparation with a sharp rasp. (b) Pilot holes placed. (c) Angle and position of anchor placement using the inferior portal. (d–f) Suture limb passage using a shuttle relay for a simple knot configuration. (g) Knot tying with the sixth finger knot pusher. (h) Past-pointing to ensure knot strength.

References

1. Snyder SJ, Karzel RP, Del Pizzo W et al. SLAP lesions of the shoulder. *Arthroscopy* 1990; **6**:274–9.

2. Maffet MW, Gartsman GM, Moseley B. Superior labrum–biceps tendon complex lesions of the shoulder. *Am J Sports Med* 1995; **23**:93–8.

3. Andrews JR, Carson WG, McLeod WD. Glenoid labrum tears related to the long head of the biceps. *Am J Sports Med* 1985; **13**:337–41.

4. Itoi E, Kuechle DK, Newman SR et al. Stabilising function of the biceps in stable and unstable shoulders. *J Bone Joint Surg* 1993; **75B**:546–50.

5. Rodosky MW, Harner CD, Fu FH. The role of the long head of the biceps muscle and superior glenoid labrum in anterior stability of the shoulder. *Am J Sports Med* 1994; **22**:121–30.

6. Warner JJ, Kann S, Marks P. Arthroscopic repair of combined Bankart and superior labral detachment anterior and posterior lesions: technique and preliminary results. *Arthroscopy* 1994; **10**:383–91.

7. Burkhart SS, Fox DL. SLAP lesions in association with complete tears of the long head of the biceps tendon: a report of two cases. *Arthroscopy* 1992; **8**:31–5.

8. Snyder SJ, Banas MP, Karzel RP. An analysis of 140 injuries to the superior glenoid labrum. *J Shoulder Elbow Surg* 1995; **4**:243–8.

9. Imhoff AB, Agneskirchner JD, König U et al. Superior labral pathology in sports. *Orthopäde* 2000; **29**:917–27.

10. Cordasco FA, Steinmann S, Flatow EL, Bigliani LU. Arthroscopic treatment of glenoid labral tears. *Am J Sports Med* 1993; **21**:425–30.

11. Field LD, Savoie FH. Arthroscopic suture repair of superior labral detachment lesions of the shoulder. *Am J Sports Med* 1993; **21**:783–90.

12. Resch H, Golser K, Thoeni H. Arthroscopic repair of superior glenoid labral detachment. *J Shoulder Elbow Surg* 1993; **2**:147–55.

13. De Simoni C, Burkart A, Imhoff AB. A new inferior (5.30 o'clock) portal for arthroscopic repair of Bankart lesions. *Arthroskopie* 2000; **13**:217–19.

14. Burkart A, Imhoff AB. Arthroscopic fixation technique of SLAP II lesions. *Arthroskopie* 2000; **13**:226–8.

21 Rotator interval: Closure with sutures

Dann C Byck, Larry D Field and Felix H Savoie III

Introduction

In this chapter we discuss the importance of the rotator interval to glenohumeral stability and how closure of the interval may be performed arthroscopically. Rotator interval closure may be used to augment other instability procedures or simply to tighten the anterior ligaments when a 'lesion' is not present. It has been shown both experimentally and clinically that an incompetent rotator interval can lead to posteroinferior, as well as superior, instability.[1] Upon first glance, this may seem contradictory. However, the clinical circumstance dictates the direction of patholaxity an individual might develop. Patients with an isolated rotator interval tear may develop posteroinferior instability due to the inability of that portion of the rotator cuff to compensate. Conversely, patients with very large interval tears, particularly those with concomitant rotator cuff tears, may experience abnormal superior humeral head translation. As with a large rotator cuff tear, the humeral depressing forces of the supraspinatus tendon are diminished and the patholaxity results in superior humeral head migration.[2]

Understanding glenohumeral instability mandates a thorough knowledge of both the static and dynamic restraints to glenohumeral motion. Prosection, clinical and intraoperative observations have proved invaluable in defining glenohumeral pathology. Prior to the advent of arthroscopy, the interval capsular tissue joining the superior border of the subscapularis muscle with the anterior border of the supraspinatus muscle was noted in the literature. Neer and Foster[3] and Rowe and Zarins[4] described interval closure with regard to their open inferior capsular shift for glenohumeral instability, but the functional importance of the rotator interval was not defined until later. Recent anatomic studies have defined the role of the rotator interval in resistance to humeral head translation. Harryman et al demonstrated that sectioning the rotator interval capsule, as well as the superior glenohumeral ligament and the coracohumeral ligament, permitted a 50% increase in posterior translation of the humeral head and a 100% translation inferiorly.[1] This study also showed that imbricating the rotator interval produced shoulders with significantly less posterior and inferior translation. Schwartz et al demonstrated that for posterior dislocation to occur in the flexed, abducted and internally rotated position, the anterosuperior capsule, as well as the posterior capsule,

had to be incised.[5] Ovesen and Nielsen were the first to report that the rotator interval contributed significantly to the prevention of inferior humeral head subluxation in the abducted shoulder.[6]

Additional reports of rotator interval capsule closure or imbrication performed to supplement other stabilization procedures or as isolated procedures have been published. Rowe and Zarins identified full-thickness defects in 20 of 37 patients operated on for recurrent subluxation of the shoulder.[4] Nobuhara and Ikeda identified 84 shoulders that had an extensive inflammation of the rotator interval associated with their instability.[7] In each study both groups of patients underwent closure of this interval as part of their reconstruction, with excellent overall results reported. More recently, Field et al reported on 15 patients with recurrent instability of the shoulder, where the only pathologic condition noted at surgery was an isolated defect in the rotator interval.[8] Closure of this interval provided adequate intraoperative stability, and no other stabilization procedure was performed. All of these patients had good or excellent results after an average 3.3 years of follow-up. Itoi et al looked at the role of the capsular interval with respect to superior and inferior glenohumeral translation in cadavers. They found that by sectioning the interval, the humeral head developed both superior and inferior instability. This was particularly evident when the arm was in neutral or internal rotation.[2] Dumontier et al have suggested that some rotator interval lesions may be a result of coracoid impingement syndrome. After interval closure the authors state that all shoulders improved, but more than half of the patients at a follow-up of 4 years still lacked strength and internal rotation.[9]

Both cadaveric sectioning data and clinical follow-up support rotator interval capsule imbrication as an effective and important intervention in selected glenohumeral instability cases. If inferior or posteroinferior translation is present, the surgeon should consider such rotator interval tightening. We also suggest that in every case of symptomatic instability of the shoulder, capsular repair or imbrication should be considered either as a supplement to more standard stabilization procedures or as an isolated procedure in the appropriate individuals.

To date, most reported techniques for closing the rotator interval capsule have been performed through open approaches.[3-8] These approaches include the deltopectoral, modified deltopectoral, the Neer approach and mini-open approaches to the rotator cuff (both in line with Langer's lines as well as transverse to Langer's lines). Arthroscopic methods have been described for capsular shift procedures and Bankart reconstructions in the shoulder.[10,11] Treacy et al, however, described the first arthroscopic rotator interval capsule closure.[12] In that paper the principles of arthroscopic surgery were applied to the patholaxity and they reported a technically easy yet very effective method of imbricating the rotator interval. Further study will be required to produce long-term results of this procedure. Gartsman et al followed with a description of an arthroscopic interval closure technique that is performed entirely within the glenohumeral joint.[13] In this chapter we describe two methods for the arthroscopic closure of the rotator interval capsule.

Surgical principles

Imbrication of the rotator interval capsule is performed using one to three sutures. The sutures are placed in the lateral to medial direction. The decision to use absorbable or non-absorbable sutures is determined by the clinical indications of the procedure. If closing the rotator interval is performed to augment another instability procedure then absorbable sutures may be used. We prefer Panacryl (Mitek, Norwood, MA, USA) sutures due to increased time interval to failure as Panacryl sutures retain 80% of their strength for at least 3 months. Otherwise, we prefer non-absorbable braided sutures for isolated closure of the rotator interval.

Our arthroscopic techniques demonstrate how sutures placed through standard portals can encompass the rotator interval defect and repair it with the use of simple suture imbrication and knot tying. Nonetheless, care must be taken with regard to the placement of the sutures. Incorporating the capsule at the superior surface of the subscapularis and the anterior border of the supraspinatus tendon is critical. Also, avoidance of the biceps tendon by proper placement of the intra-articular sutures must be adhered to. The type of knot the surgeon employs is not as important. What is important is the ability to secure the repair with a knot that does not loosen. We use and recommend the Roeder knot for its ease of tying and holding power.

Surgical technique

Prior to indicating a patient for surgery, a thorough history and physical examination must be performed. A detailed understanding of the etiology of the instability as well as provocative maneuvers, position of the shoulder and neurologic symptoms is crucial to a proper diagnosis.

Operative arthroscopy is performed in either the lateral decubitus position with the arm in 10–15 pounds of traction or in the beach chair position. A standard operating table is used and if the beach chair position is selected then one of several positioners can be employed. Once the patient is anesthetized, a careful re-examination is performed on both shoulders. Without the disadvantage of patient guarding, a more precise examination may be possible. A posterior portal is established in the interval between the glenoid and the humeral head at the equator of the humeral head. The glenohumeral joint is then insufflated with normal saline using gravity flow and under direct visualization a diagnostic arthroscopy is performed. The entire joint is evaluated paying careful attention to the labrum, capsule, insertion of the supraspinatus tendon, biceps anchor, articular surface and, of course, the anterosuperior quadrant within which the rotator interval capsule is found.

The rotator interval is carefully assessed for laxity either in the interval itself or in the superior glenohumeral ligament. One might see a discrete tear of the capsule within the interval or more commonly, an outpouching of the interval is visualized. If associated with bicep tendon pathology, the interval may be obscured by a subluxed biceps tendon. Chondromalacia of the superior glenoid similarly is evaluated as evidence of anterosuperior instability. Inferior laxity in the capsule or a subluxation of the humeral head inferiorly is also an indication of rotator interval pathology. The diagnostic arthroscopy is also used to carefully evaluate the attachments of the middle glenohumeral ligament and inferior glenohumeral ligament, including its anterior and posterior bands.

Once the patholaxity is confirmed, an anterior instrument portal is established in the rotator interval just superior to the subscapularis tendon, avoiding damage to either the superior or middle glenohumeral ligaments. A 6-mm cannula with a dam is placed through the anterior portal. A pathologic condition within the glenohumeral joint is addressed systematically from the inferior to superior repairing or reconstructing any anterior or posterior Bankart lesions or any inferior capsular laxity first.

We sometimes utilize radiofrequency capsular shrinkage techniques at this point. For a redundant anterior capsule, the shrinkage probe is placed through the anterior portal and beginning as inferior and posterior as possible, the shrinkage is performed in a linear fashion from posterior to anterior. When there is posterior laxity the arthroscope is placed in the anterior portal and the shrinkage probe is placed in the posterior portal. Similarly, the shrinkage proceeds from anterior to posterior in linear fashion. Shrinkage superior to the posterior portal is considered unnecessary. Once the entire arthroscopic reconstruction is completed, attention is then turned to the rotator interval (Figure 21.1).

Rotator interval laxity may be reconstructed by one of two methods. Prior to either technique, the tissue is

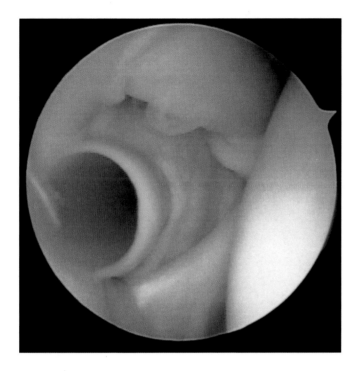

Figure 21.1

The rotator interval defect is visualized within the glenohumeral joint of the right shoulder between the supraspinatus and subscapularis tendons.

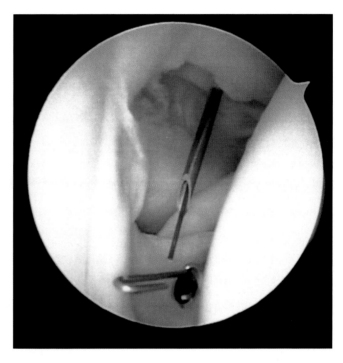

Figure 21.2

Initiation of intra-articular rotator interval repair. Note the suture retriever device pierces the subscapularis tendon and middle glenohumeral ligament; then it is advanced anterior to the biceps tendon. The spinal needle passes through the anterior margin of the supraspinatus tendon and adjacent capsule. A Prolene suture is being advanced through the spinal needle.

lightly rasped or abraded with a motorized shaver to promote bleeding. We feel this step induces more rapid healing. In the first technique, the arthroscope is maintained in the posterior portal, a Suture Grasper (Mitek) is inserted through the anterior portal. The anterior cannula is pulled back just through the capsule so that the Suture Grasper will pierce the capsule anterior to the subscapularis muscle. The capsule adjacent to the subscapularis tendon, the middle gleno-humeral ligament as well as a small portion of the subscapularis tendon, are included in this repair. The Suture Grasper is then manipulated superiorly and carefully passed anterior to the biceps tendon. This is very important in order to avoid capturing the biceps tendon as the suture is tightened.

A spinal needle is then placed through the antero-superior shoulder adjacent to the inferolateral corner of the acromion and through the capsule including the anterior margin of the supraspinatus tendon. A #1 absorbable (Panacryl) or #1 Prolene (Mitek) suture is then passed through the spinal needle and retrieved out of the anterior portal using the Suture Grasper device (Figure 21.2). In cases where the rotator interval imbri-cation is utilized to augment an instability procedure, we use the Panacryl suture. This type of suture was selected because of its extended dissolution time, and its coating

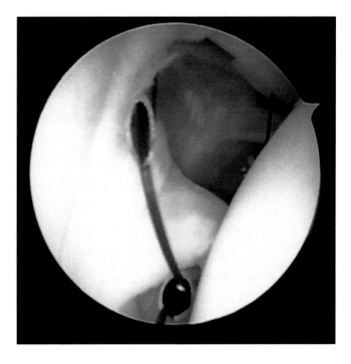

Figure 21.3

A lateral plication suture is seen in place. A second, more medial suture is being completed as the suture retriever device retrieves the suture out of the anterior portal.

that facilitates knot tying. Gentle traction on this suture will close or plicate the more lateral portion of the rotator interval and this will be visualized through the arthroscope. The suture retriever is then placed back into the anterior cannula and through the capsule medial and superior to the previous suture. By design, the Suture Grasper should penetrate the superior glenohumeral ligament anterior to the glenohumeral joint. The spinal needle is again placed in similar fashion through the anterior margin of the supraspinatus, but more medially than the initial suture. The suture is then placed through the spinal needle and retrieved out the anterior cannula, using the Suture Grasper (Figure 21.3). A third suture may be placed more medially if necessary. Utilizing this technique, two to three sutures may be placed from lateral to medial across the rotator interval. Once the sutures have been properly positioned, they can be tensioned to obtain adequate closure of the rotator interval and thus reduce the intra-articular instability.

The arthroscope is then removed from the posterior portal and reinserted into the subacromial bursa. Repositioning of the anterior cannula into the bursa following the line of sutures facilitates identification of the anterior sutures. The superior sutures should be readily visualized in the anterior margin of the supraspinatus tendon. Often an arthroscopic bursectomy is necessary to obtain adequate visualization. A crochet hook is then used to retrieve the more lateral of the sutures out through the anterior cannula, and an arthroscopic knot is tied tightening the more lateral aspect of the rotator interval. Arthroscopic scissors are then employed to cut the sutures leaving a 3–4-mm tail.

In similar fashion, the second and third sutures are retrieved and tightened arthroscopically. The adequacy of each knot can be assessed arthroscopically in the bursa. Replacement of the scope into the posterior glenohumeral portal confirms adequate plication and capsular tensioning.

Alternatively, once comfortable with this technique, the sutures may be tied blindly through the anterior portal while leaving the arthroscope in the glenohumeral joint to visualize the repair. Manipulation of the cannula to the area of the superior suture will facilitate the crochet hook technique of bringing the superior suture through the anterior portal. Once both limbs of the suture are brought through the cannula in the anterior portal, an arthroscopic knot is secured and the repair is completed. This technique obviates the need for an additional bursectomy.

A second method of closing the rotator interval can be performed exclusively on the bursal side of the rotator cuff and capsule. After an adequate assessment of the rotator interval from within the glenohumeral joint has been performed, the arthroscope is placed into the subacromial bursa. The bursa is then resected using a motorized shaver device, allowing adequate visualization of the rotator interval. A standard curved Caspari suture punch is threaded with the #0 Prolene suture and intro-

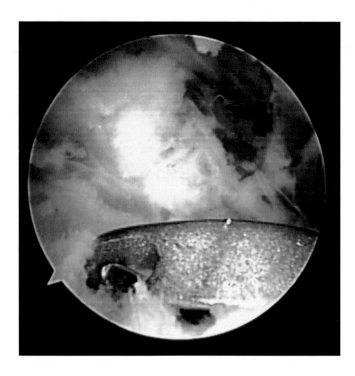

Figure 21.4

The suture punch technique involves dual biting with the suture punch to plicate the rotator interval. Here, the initial bite through the subscapularis tendon is made with the curved suture punch.

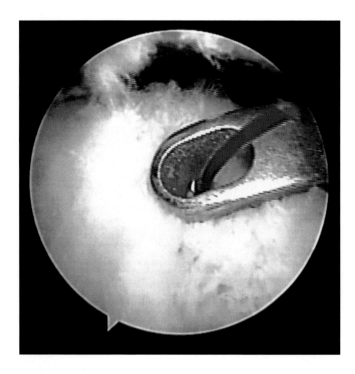

Figure 21.5

The second bite with the suture punch is made through the supraspinatus tendon, facilitating closure of the rotator interval. Here, the second bite has been completed, and a #0 Prolene suture is being passed through the suture punch, and will be retrieved out the lateral portal.

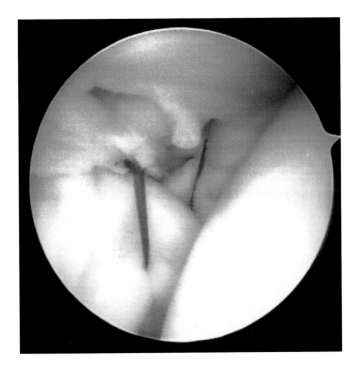

Figure 21.6

Intra-articular visualization of the rotator cuff interval assures adequate interval closure has been achieved.

duced into the bursa through the lateral portal. The arm is slightly externally rotated and a small portion of the most superior aspect of the subscapularis tendon and/or capsule adjacent to the tendon is taken. The suture punch is then opened but the needle is contained through this anterior capsule and in the tendinous structure (Figure 21.4). The arm is internally rotated bringing the anterior margin of the supraspinatus into the open drawer of the suture punch. Closure of the suture punch at this point creates a second bite through the most inferior aspect of the supraspinatus tendon. The suture is then threaded through the bursa and drawn through the lateral portal by an arthroscopic grasper (Figure 21.5). The efficacy of the suture in plicating the rotator interval can be assessed under direct visualization. If the plication is thought to be adequate, an arthroscopic knot is then tied, tightening the more lateral aspect of the rotator interval. In this case, the steps are repeated, placing two to three sutures across the rotator interval from lateral to medial. The initial suture tightens the rotator interval facilitating placement of the next suture in a more medial position. Plication of the rotator interval can be checked from both the intra-articular and bursal sides to insure adequate stability. Direct visualization of the rotator interval plication ensures that an adequate stabilization procedure has been performed (Figure 21.6).

References

1. Harryman DT, Sidles JA, Harris LS, Matsen FA. The role of the rotator interval capsule and passive motion and stability of the shoulder. *J Bone Joint Surg* 1992; **74A**:54–66.
2. Itoi E, Berglund LJ, Grabowski JJ et al. Superior–inferior stability of the shoulder: role of the coracohumeral ligament and the rotator interval capsule. *Mayo Clin Proc* 1998; **73**:508–15.
3. Neer CS, Foster CR. Inferior capsular shift for involuntary inferior and multidirectional instability of the shoulder. *J Bone Joint Surg* 1980; **62A**:897–908.
4. Rowe CR, Zarins B. Recurrent transient subluxation of the shoulder. *J Bone Joint Surg* 1981; **63A**:863–71.
5. Schwartz E, Ward RF, O'Brien SJ. Posterior shoulder instability. *Orthop Clin Med Am* 1987; **18**:409–19.
6. Ovesen J, Nielsen S. Experimental distal subluxation in the glenohumeral joint. *Arch Orthop Trauma Surg* 1985; **104**:78–81.
7. Nobuhara K, Ikeda H. Rotator interval lesion. *Clin Orthop* 1987; **223**:44–50.
8. Field LD, Warren RF, O'Brien SJ et al. Isolated closure of rotator interval defects and shoulder instability. *Am J Sports Med* 1995; **23**:556–63.
9. Dumontier C, Sautet A, Gagey O, Apoil A. Rotator interval lesions and their relationship to coracoid impingement syndrome. *J Shoulder Elbow Surg* 1999; **8**:130–5.
10. Duncan R, Savoie FH. Arthroscopic inferior capsular shift for multidirectional instability of the shoulder: a preliminary report. *Arthroscopy* 1993; **9**:24–7.
11. Caspari RB, Savoie FH. Arthroscopic reconstruction of the shoulder: Bankart repair. In: McGinty JB, ed. *Operative Arthroscopy* New York: Raven Press, 1991;507–15.
12. Treacy SH, Field LD, Savoie FH. Rotator interval capsule closure: an arthroscopic technique. *Arthroscopy* 1997; **13**:103–6.
13. Gartsman GM, Taverna E, Hammerman SM. Arthroscopic rotator interval repair in glenohumeral instability: description of an operative technique. *Arthroscopy* 1999; **15**:330–2.

Section IV – Impingement pathology and acromioclavicular joint

22 Subacromial impingement

Guido Engel and Andreas B Imhoff

Introduction

In many publications the pathomechanism of impingement is still closely linked to Charles S Neer and his first report in 1972. His general explanation that impingement of the supraspinatus tendon occurs in the narrow space under the coracoacromial arch is still valid. His proposed treatment of impingement – a subacromial decompression – is nowadays only one therapeutic option. In the last 30 years the 'Neer Impingement' has evolved into just one differential diagnosis of several completely independent etiologies of subacromial impingement. The ongoing discussion of acromion morphology as a primary cause of impingement (extrinsic) or a secondary sign of primary rotator cuff insufficiencies (intrinsic) is not decided.[1-3]

Budhoff et al see the primary source of impingement pain in a loss of humeral head centralization due to an eccentric tendon overload. This leads to intratendinous degeneration or tendinosis and a secondary spur formation (traction spur) in the coracoacromial ligament.[1] A confirming observation is the statistical evaluation of the location of partial rotator cuff lesions. According to the primary impingement hypothesis, most partial ruptures should be at the bursal aspect of the cuff, but clinical documentation and cadaver studies have revealed a higher prevalence of partial articular side defects.[4,5]

Our classification of subacromial impingement (Table 22.1) includes primary (extrinsic and intrinsic) and secondary factors. Primary are all forms of osseous subacromial stenoses (extrinsic) and relative entrapment by chronic changes of the rotator cuff and the bursa (intrinsic). As described above, the extrinsic forms of a primary impingement are only present in a small number of patients, most forms are based on the intrinsic tendon failure. Our main interest is to differentiate these primary forms from the heterogenic group of secondary forms, which mimic a subacromial impingement. One cannot stress enough the necessity of a thorough clinical work up. Subtle instabilities and the dorsal capsular contracture are the most difficult to diagnose.

In 1983 Ellman established the arthroscopic version of Neer's open anterior acromioplasty as an alternative method and reported first results in 1987.[6] The advantages of performing the subacromial decompression arthroscopically include avoiding the detachment of the deltoid muscle from the acromion and avoiding a muscle dehiscence, major cuts of the skin or denervation postoperatively. Generally, the arthroscopic exploration of the glenohumeral joint as well as of the subacromial space preceding the operative treatment has to be regarded as an advantage in contrast to the open method.

Surgical principles

Indications and contraindications

Indications for the arthroscopic subacromial decompression (ASD) are the mechanical outlet-impingement (stage II and III described by Neer), as well as a less than 3 mm malunited greater tuberosity. Acromioclavicular (AC) joint pathologies, i.e. AC joint arthritis and osteolysis or stenotic AC joint osteophytes, can be

Table 22.1 Impingement etiologies

Primary		Secondary
Extrinsic	*Intrinsic*	
Acromion morphology	Hypertrophic bursitis	Instability
Os acromiale	Rotator cuff tendinitis	Frozen shoulder
Dislocated greater tuberosity	Partial rotator cuff lesions	Posterior capsular restraints
AC joint arthritis	Calcifying tendinitis	Neurologic disorders

addressed by this technique in either partial (co-planing) or complete resection of the AC joint. We treat rotator cuff tears up to a size of 3 cm (Bateman II) in mini-open technique, which includes an ASD and a deltoid splitting open rotator cuff repair that preserves the deltoid insertion.

Contraindications are basically all forms of secondary impingement with the exception of the above mentioned malunited greater tuberosity fracture less than 3 mm. The most frequent contraindication is the so-called instability-impingement, which occurs in young athletes who participate in overhead sports. Their loss of humeral head centralization can be due to hyperlaxity, a superior labrum anterior to posterior (SLAP) lesion or injuries of the labrum-ligament complex. After a conservative rehabilitation, the treatment of choice is an operative stabilization of the glenohumeral joint. Rotator cuff lesions larger than 3 cm (> Bateman II) are treated by open acromioplasty with the reinsertion of the detached deltoid and coracoacromial ligament after reconstruction of the rotator cuff.

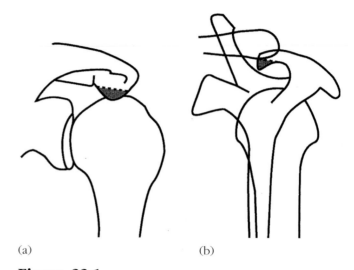

(a)   (b)

Figure 22.1

(a) Rockwood anteroposterior view with 30° tilt and (b) lateral outlet view.

Clinical examination

After taking a thorough history, a number of tests should be performed to detect the cause of impingement and to differentiate it from concomitant pathologies, i.e. radicular origin. Both the impingement test by Hawkins–Kennedy (internally rotated with the elbow flexed) and by Neer (examiner brings the arm passively in full flexion) lead to an entrapment of the supraspinatus tendon (major tubercle and lateral acromion) with characteristic pain. These two tests have the highest sensitivity.[7,8] After ruling out any underlying rotator cuff lesion, i.e. ultrasound, it is very useful to perform a subacromial injection test with 10 ml of 1% lidocaine. The prior positive impingement signs should now become negative. Significant relief of pain under provocation provides further confirmation of the presence of impingement. Persisting painful movement localized in the AC joint, accompanied by a positive horizontal adduction test, requires an infiltration of the AC joint to differentiate the source of the pain.

In younger patients the instability tests are most valuable as part of secondary impingement lesions, i.e. anterosuperior Bankart lesion, SLAP lesion, or/and hyperlaxity. Using these examination and injection tests routinely will lead to a fairly exact diagnosis of localization and cause.

Radiographic evaluation

We start with a standard set of routine radiographs in three planes: true anteroposterior view, supraspinatus

outlet view, and axillary view. These may reveal a loss of centralization of the humeral head, mostly superior migration, and/or sclerosis with spur formation on the antero-lateral edge of the acromion (Figure 22.1). In addition, corresponding subchondral cysts or sclerosis of the greater tuberosity can be seen and interpreted as an indirect sign of a rotator cuff lesion.[6] The standard X-ray examination helps to identify other impingement-causing pathologies, i.e. calcium deposits or an os acromiale. The supraspinatus outlet view shows us the inferior prominence of the anterolateral acromion. Care has to be taken not to over interpret these radiographs, because minor changes in the technique can change the appearance of the acromion spur drastically. In our hands these three radiographs are a minimum for diagnostic work-up and provide information about the degree of acromial resection. Accompanying or isolated AC joint symptoms need special X-ray projections.

For the evaluation of the acromion's prominence which projects anteriorly to the clavicle border, we recommend the anteroposterior view with a 30° caudal tilt as described by Rockwood (Figure 22.1).[9] Another very helpful plane offers the AC joint view for evaluation of the joint space, spur formation, and cysts.

For verifying a rotator cuff lesion magnetic resonance imaging (MRI) has gained increasing popularity. With MRI, we prefer the application of an intra-articular contrast medium (gadolinium) to detect higher graded partial lesions of the rotator cuff, which are difficult to demonstrate by ultrasound. Also, lesions of the biceps pulley and origin can be better visualized.[10]

Technical variations

Some operative publications focus only on one resection plane of the acromion. Mostly by using the anterolateral portal for instrumentation, they do not switch with the arthroscope from posterior to anterior in order to check the resection plane. We believe that the two-plane resection from antero-lateral and from posterior, as described below, ensures a much safer way of subacromial decompression.

For partial resection of the bursa and debridement of the undersurface of the acromion the new radio-frequency devices are most helpful (VAPR II, Ethicon, Mitek). Without causing bleeding the bursa can be resected in a much faster way and in one step without the fear of bleeding at the deltoid insertion or at the fat pad below the AC joint.

Complications

Generally we find a low rate of complications associated with ASD. A compromised view caused by either wrong penetration of the subacromial bursa or by bleeding is the most common complication. Another point is the insufficient debridement of the undersurface of the acromion prior to resection. Fractures due to excessive resection as well as infections or nerve damage are very rare. Nerve damage is generally not caused by wrong portal placement, but by wrong positioning of the patient. Unphysiologic flexion of the spine (cervalgia), traction force at the arm holder (brachialgia), or compression of the superficial branch of the radial nerve at the styloid process can be the reasons. The soft tissue edema, which sometimes causes the shoulder to look monstrous, vanishes usually within 24 hours and does not result in a compartment syndrome.

Surgical technique

Instruments

The arthroscopic standard equipment consists of an optic system, which includes a 3 CCD-chip camera (width 4 mm) with 30° wide angle optic and a 5.5 mm arthroscopy shaft that is wired to a cold light source via a light conductor. The image is transmitted to a monitor. For documentation a picture print-out or video system is mandatory. The integrated pump system runs with Ringer solution, which allows for one less regulation step. For bursectomy and acromioplasty we use a standard shaver system with either an incisor blade or burr ('acromionizer'). Another option for

debridement and especially hemostasis is an electrothermal system. We favor the bipolar systems with minimal heat penetration (Conlation™, ArthroCare™, Sunnyvale, CA, USA; VAPR™, Ethicon, Mitek, Norwood, MA, USA).

Patient positioning

Today the standard positioning for subacromial decompression is the beach-chair placement. The lateral decubitus once the preferred positioning in our hands, has been largely abandoned due to the faster set-up of the beach-chair and the easy access to the shoulder joint with a freely moveable arm. In addition the possible switch to an open surgery can be done at any time without replacement of the patient. Generally the upper body should be tilted 60–70° relative to the horizontal plane. The elimination of the shoulder restraint also lowers the risk of complications such as neuropraxia of the brachial plexus or damage of the ulnary nerve.[11] Besides the possibility of a freely movable arm held by an assistant, we place the arm in a McConnell positioner (McConnell Orthopedics, Greenville, TX, USA) which is fixed to a special armholder. The armholder can be adapted in all three planes. Furthermore, to perform an intraoperative impingement test, the system ensures easy disconnection and reconnection from the armholder.

Examination under anesthesia

Preceding any operative intervention on the shoulder, physical examination of the shoulder in the relaxed and 'pain free' state should be performed. Thereby an important evaluation of the passive range of motion and the degree of instability can be carried out and documented.

Landmarks and portal placement

After careful disinfection and coverage of the operative field we outline the bony landmarks for orientation (clavicle, spina scapulae, acromion, coracoid). Marking the bony landmark on the shoulder is very helpful in order not to lose the orientation for portal placement once the arthroscopy has begun and the water slowly distends the tissues. Three portals can be recommended for subacromial arthroscopy: Posterior, anterolateral and anterosuperior in case an AC joint resection is necessary (Figure 22.2). Prior to portal placement we infiltrate the shoulder with 0.5 ml epinephrine in 20 ml physiologic saline using a spinal needle.

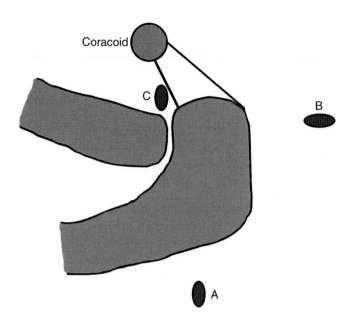

Figure 22.2

Arthroscipic portal placement: (A) posterior portal; (B) anterolateral portal; (C) anterosuperior portal.

Posterior portal

Any arthroscopic procedure is started with the 'diagnostic' portal in the so-called soft spot through the infraspinatus muscle. This soft spot is located approximately 2 cm medial and 2 cm inferior to the posterolateral corner of the acromion. As described above, we use a spinal needle to fill the glenohumeral joint and check the orthograde position regarding the joint space. This prevents us from placing the posterior portal to lateral, in which case the humeral head could block our anteroinferior view.

Anatomical structures at risk are the suprascapular artery and nerve when the portal is placed too high (incisura scapulae, spinogleniodal notch) and the axillary nerve when the portal is placed too low.[12]

Lateral portal

This portal is located in the anterior third of the acromion and approximately 4 cm lateral to the acromion border. It provides ideal access to the subacromial space. Different placement techniques exist concerning the exact anterior and posterior orientation of the portal in the anterior third. The preferred option is to make the incision in line with the anterior edge. In our hands this anterior placement offers a direct approach to the anterolateral corner of the acromion, which is one of the essential structures to address by the acromioplasty. Another advantage is that the incision for the mini-open approach runs through this portal and only one scar will result.

The nerve structure prone to damage is the axillary nerve about 5 cm lateral to the acromion border. In general the axillary nerve is not in danger during portal placement. More importantly, the mini-open and classic open incisions should not exceed the 4 cm distance from the acromion without special operative preparation.

Anterosuperior portal

In cases with symptomatic AC joint arthritis we perform as a last step the AC joint resection (see the later section entitled 'Bony resection of AC joint osteotypes (co-planing) and AC joint resection'). For adequate access an anterosuperior portal is necessary and located directly anterior to the AC joint and above the coracoid. By marking the tip of the coracoid, one cannot place the portal too low and therefore any nerve damage is prevented.

Diagnostic glenohumeral arthroscopy

We recommend a standardized systematic diagnostic examination. A systematic step-by-step procedure ensures the complete visualization of all parts of the joint. The surgeon is obligated to document his diagnostic evaluation with special regard to the following structures: biceps tendon, labrum, glenohumeral ligaments, rotator cuff, cartilage structures, and synovia.

We start with the puncture of the glenohumeral joint via the posterior approach with a spinal needle directed toward the coracoid process. After injecting 20 ml of physiologic saline + 0.5 ml epinephrine a free backflow confirms the intra-articular placement. A small stab incision is made at the injection point and the arthroscopic cannula with the blunt trocar is used to enter the glenohumeral joint while distending the joint by slightly pulling the humeral head laterally. Especially in dislocated shoulders with a Hill–Sachs lesion one has less trouble finding the penetration point when the arm is in internal rotation and the humeral head defect is rotated out of the way. The loss of resistance after penetrating the capsule between the humeral head and the glenoid, and the backflow of the injected solution after withdrawal of the blunt trocar confirm the correct intra-articular placement.

The so-called 'starting position' of the diagnostic examination is the insertion of the long head of the biceps (LHB) at the supraglenoidal tubercle with the glenoid rim in vertical position and the humeral head next to it. Due to the penetration force the camera usually has to be pulled back to find this landmark.

This view allows evaluation of the LHB origin and the superior labrum to rule out any pathologic detachments, i.e. SLAP lesions, as an important differential diagnosis of mechanical impingement in younger patients. A biceps tendinitis or synovitis is caused by a primary pathology, for example rotator cuff lesions and most forms of instability. By turning the optical lens almost

180° looking downward, the cartilage of the glenoid and the humeral head can be inspected. To evaluate the labrum and the glenohumeral ligaments we push the arthroscope slightly forward and then downward between the glenoid rim and the humeral head. If the scope can slide down the joint space all the way, the joint capsule is lax (positive drive-through sign). Inferiorly the anterior band of the inferior glenohumeral ligament (IGHL) attaches at the glenoid rim. The IGHL forms the axillary recesses and completes its hammock structure with the posterior band and contributes decisively to the stabilization of the humeral head. In case of a questionable detachment of the labrum it might be necessary to introduce a probe through an antero-superior portal in order to check the structure by manipulation.

The most prominent anterior landmark is the horizontal extension of the superior border of the subscapularis tendon. Between the medial and middle third of the subscapularis tendon runs the medial glenohumeral ligament at an angle of 60° up to its varying insertion at the anterior edge of the glenoid. The triangular-shaped space bounded by the subscapularis tendon and the superior glenohumeral ligament (SGHL), which runs from the supraglenoidal tubercle to join the subscapularis insertion at the lesser tuberosity, is called rotator interval or Foramen of Weitbrecht. Following the subscapularis to its insertion, the pulley system of the LHB is visualized. This sling consists of the superior subscapularis tendon, the SGHL, the coracohumeral ligament, and the supraspinatus tendon.

The rotator cuff needs a thorough inspection, starting with the subscapularis insertion up to the supraspinatus at the greater tuberosity, following the greater tuberosity to the infraspinatus insertion downward. If an articular side tear of the rotator cuff is present, fibers will hang down and can be easily identified using a probe. To measure the depth of an articular tear one difference between the insertion of the supraspinatus and the infraspinatus has to be taken into account. The supraspinatus tendon inserts directly at the cartilage joint surface whereas the infraspinatus tendon inserts behind the bare area approximately 6–8 mm behind the cartilage surface. Complete ruptures of the rotator cuff are easily identified. The arthroscopic examination is especially helpful in detecting ongoing horizontal tears at the edges, which in some cases are complete splits of the upper and lower layer. These defects are difficult to detect by open techniques.

Arthroscopic decompression

The diagnostic examination is as demanding an operation as the subacromial decompression and we prefer to perform it under total anesthesia. Experience and secure handling of the instruments are essential in order to stay within the time limits; otherwise swelling of the soft tissues due to fluid uptake can compromise further surgical steps, especially in case of a mini-open rotator cuff repair. Other technical difficulties arise through the varying amount of bursal adhesions and possible repeated bleeding. The following important principles have to be taken into account.

To avoid bleeding during the procedure the mean systolic pressure should be lowered to approximately 90 mmHg perioperatively, the inflow pressure is set at about 50 mmHg with maximum flow. Unless medically contraindicated epinephrine is added to the arthroscopic fluid (3 ml epinephrine to a 3-l bag of saline). The aim is to keep the pressure in the subacromial space constant to avoid further bleeding by sudden loss of pressure. Persistent bleeding should not be stopped by increasing the inflow pressure. Early application of a radiofrequency device (RF-wand, electrothermal wand) or electrocautery are more helpful. The resection of bursal tissue medial of the AC joint as well as the superomedial part of the coracoacromial ligament should be avoided as strong bleeding from the branches of the thoracoacromial vessels is to be expected. It is our aim to differentiate the following structures: acromion with anterolateral and anterior borders; coracoacromial ligament; AC joint; rotator cuff with impingement region.

Using the posterior portal again, the blunt trocar and cannula are directed to the posterior acromion ridge. By sliding down the ridge, the tip of the blunt trocar follows the bony undersurface of the acromion and is pushed through the bursal layer. The free hand is placed at the anterior acromion to prevent a too forceful protrusion with the danger of perforating the deltoid fascia inside. With a side-to-side movement of the trocar small adhesions are detached and visibility is facilitated. If there is no luminous effect of the light source at the anterior border of the acromion the cannula is probably still too posterior and the view is blurred by the bursa. After correct placement of the cannula the subacromial space can be inspected without prior debridement. For better orientation the anterolateral acromion border as well as the AC joint can be marked by a needle (Figure 22.3). In this way we define reproducible orientation points comparable to the systematic procedure in arthroscopy of the glenohumeral joint. To start debridement the position of the anterolateral instrumentation portal should be checked by a needle, which imitates the shaver system coming from the lateral direction. With the shaver or RF-system the debridement starts from the anterolateral corner in a medial direction. For orientation it is strongly recommended that contact is kept with the acromion so as not to risk any injury to the deltoid or supraspinatus muscle. After partial bursectomy the entire anterior third of the undersurface of the acromion including the medial position of the AC joint should be visible. Starting at the anterolateral corner we use a high-speed shaver system or a special round burr called acromion-

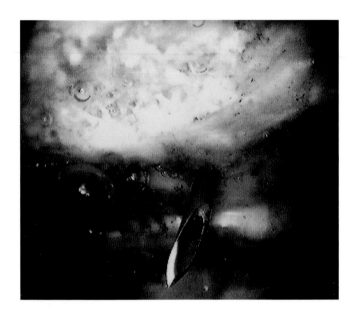

Figure 22.3

The anterolateral corner of the acromion is marked by a needle.

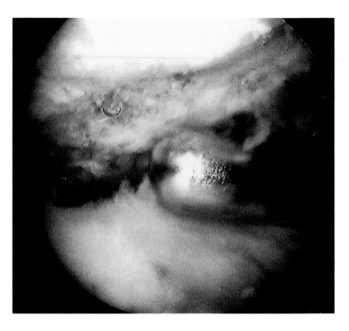

Figure 22.4

Anterolateral starting point of the resection plane.

izer for resection (Figure 22.4). Depending on the acromion morphology about 4–6 mm are resected. The width of the shaver system is 6 mm and this is a very useful given depth measure. Another option is the use of a laser system which achieves, with higher energy settings, a bony resection with ablation.[13] The enormous investment costs of the laser are a definite disadvantage.

Going from the anterior ridge posteriorly we create a plane by gradually decreasing the resection depth. The complete rectangular area (approximately 20 × 15 mm) of the undersurface of the acromion is treated (Figures 22.5 and 22.6). To finish the resection we flatten the anterior acromion by switching working portals. Coming from a posterior direction, the shaver can level the sometimes irregular step off along the acromion which can result by only a one-plane decompression from lateral (Figure 22.7). The other advantage is the second angle for evaluating the resection plane. By taking 4–6 mm off the bony anterior ridge the insertion of the coracoacromial ligament is only partially detached and the main superficial layers are preserved.

To achieve an exact resection two main areas have to be addressed – the anterolateral corner and the medial portion as part of the AC joint. The medial portion can be especially problematic, because it is not always possible to spare the inferior AC joint capsule even though the patient has no AC joint symptoms. In these inevitable cases we follow two basic rules. If the opening is like a puncture (minimal point-like opening) the AC joint is not touched. In case of a longitudinal opening we perform a co-planing of the distal clavicle (see next section).

Bony resection of AC joint osteophytes (co-planing) and AC joint resection

A thorough clinical examination determines if pathology of the AC joint is present and which of the two treatment options for the AC joint is necessary. The surgical resection of the inferior osteophytes of the distal clavicle is called co-planing, because the resection plane of the medial acromion is carried further medially. This procedure is not a treatment option if the examiner can elicit definite AC joint symptoms. Indications are the necessary sacrifice of the joint capsule by acromial debridement and radiologic osteophytes as part of a mechanical outlet-impingement.

The AC joint is opened inferiorly by the lateral approach and the complete inferior dimension of the distal clavicle should be visible. Using the acromial resection plane as orientation, the inferior osteophytes are taken away and the intra-articular disc is debrided. Several studies have demonstrated that the outcome shows no statistical differences although violation of the AC joint capsule and partial distal clavicle resection may increase the motion of the remaining AC joint.[14,15]

If significant AC arthritis with its typically clinical symptoms is present, we perform a complete distal claviculectomy. The first two steps as described above (acromioplasty, removal of inferior capsule) are completed with a third step – the actual resection of the distal clavicle. Using the acromionizer as depth measure

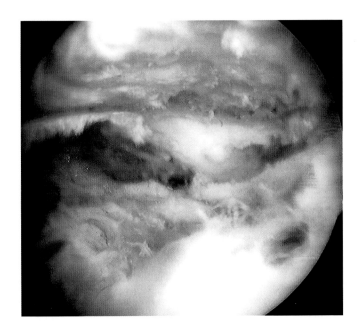

Figure 22.5

Posterior view after anterolateral resection.

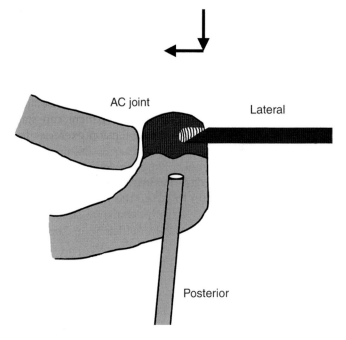

Figure 22.6

Starting at the anterolateral corner the acromion is resected in lateral to medial and anterior to posterior directions.

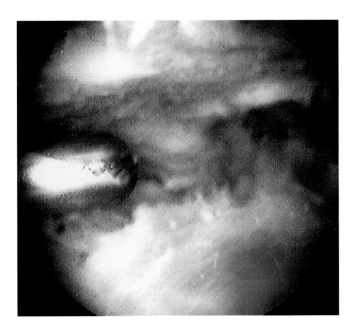

Figure 22.7

Anterolateral view with shaver system through the posterior portal, which offers the second resection plane.

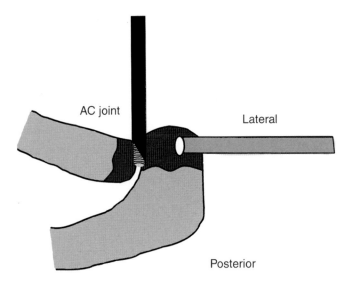

Figure 22.8

After standard arthroscopic acromioplasty the anterosuperior working portal is used for AC joint resection.

we resect about 6 mm of the clavicle without violating the posterosuperior capsule, which is the strongest capsular restraint. In our opinion the ideal working portal is the anterosuperior portal offering a direct approach in line with the joint space (Figure 22.8). Starting from inferior to superior, the bone is taken off layer by layer until completion. Finally by switching the arthroscope to the anterosuperior portal the amount of resection can be evaluated.

At the end the joint must be thoroughly irrigated to eliminate all debris and, after wound closure, a sterile bandage is applied.

Postoperative protocol

As well as in conservative treatment, postoperatively, centralization of the humeral head is the foremost aim in physiotherapeutic treatment. An intact rotator cuff allows the patient to discontinue using the Gilchrist sling on the first postoperative day and the patient can start with pendulum exercises. Isometric tension exercises for the rotator cuff muscles, as well as for the deltoid muscle within the pain-free range of motion, may start on the second postoperative day. Passive mobilization should be exerted in a range up to 90° in the first 2 weeks and then gradually increased actively. Oral non-steroid anti-inflammatory drugs are usually sufficient in the early postoperative phase.

It is mandatory to use the arm for all activities in every day life to regain satisfying function and range of movement within 3–6 weeks.

References

1. Budhoff JE, Nirschl RP, Guidi EJ. Debridement of partial-thickness tears of the rotator cuff without acromioplasty. *J Bone Joint Surg* 1998; **80**:733–748.
2. Bigliani LU, Morrison DS, April EW. The morphology of the acromion and its relationship to rotator cuff tears. *Orthop Trans* 1986; **10**:216.
3. Neer CS. Anterior acromioplasty for the chronic impingement syndrome in the shoulder. A preliminary report. *J Bone Joint Surg* 1972; **54**:41–50.
4. Uhthoff HK, Hammond DJ, Sarkar K et al. The role of the coracoacromial ligament in the impingement syndrome. A clinical, radiological and histological study. *Int Orthop* 1988; **12**:97–104.
5. Payne LZ, Altchek DW, Craig EV et al. Arthroscopic treatment of partial rotator cuff tears in young athletes. A preliminary report. *Am J Sports Med* 1997; **25**:299–305.
6. Ellman H. Arthroscopic subacromial decompression: analysis of one- to three-year results. *Arthroscopy* 1987; **3**:173–81.
7. Calis M, Akgun K, Birtane M et al. Diagnostic values of clinical diagnostic tests in subacromial impingement syndrome. *Ann Rheum Dis* 2000; **59**:44–7.
8. MacDonald PB, Clark P, Sutherland K. An analysis of the diagnostic accuracy of the Hawkins and Neer subacromial impingement signs. *J Shoulder Elbow Surg* 2000; **9**:299–301.
9. Rockwood CA, Matsen FA (eds.) *The Shoulder*. WB Saunders 1990. 178.
10. Imhoff AB. In: TD Bunker, A Wallache, eds. *MRT-Diagnostik an der Schulter*, in *Schulterarthroskopie*. Stuttgart: Thieme Verlag. 1992, 167–72.
11. Imhoff AB. N. axillaris-Schädigung bei Schulterarthroskopie und Mobilisation. In: H Contzen, ed. *Komplikationen bei der Arthroskopie. Fortschritte in der Arthroskopie*. Stuttgart: Enke Verlag, 1989.
12. Bigliani LU, Dalsey RM, McCann PD et al. An anatomical study of the suprascapular nerve. *Arthroscopy* 1990; **6**:301–5.
13. De Simoni C, Ledermann T, Imhoff AB. Holmium:YAG-Laser beim Outlet-Impingement der Schulter. *Orthopaede* 1996; **25**:84–90.
14. Barber FA. Coplaning of the acromioclavicular joint. *Arthroscopy* 2001; **17**:913–17.
15. Weber SC. Coplaning the acromioclavicular joint at the time of acromioplasty: A long-term study. *Arthroscopy* 1999; **15**:555 (abstr).

23 Posterosuperior impingement

Gilles Walch and Laurent Nové-Josserand

Introduction

In 1991 Walch and colleagues[1-3] and Jobe and colleagues[4-7] simultaneously developed the concept of posterosuperior impingement. This internal impingement is produced between the articular surface of the supraspinatus and the glenoid when the arm is abducted and externally rotated in the late cocking phase (Figure 23.1). Furthermore Jobe et al[8] recognized this internal impingement as being a cause of pain in throwing athletes, rather than external impingement and they also reported that this was always related to subtle anterior instability. The problem is now to find out whether pain in throwing athletes is related to mechanical intra-articular impingement, or to anterior instability. Since internal contact is observed in each individual during abduction– external rotation, and since the internal impingement was described initially by Jobe et al in cadaver specimens with no instability, we think that pain in the throwing athlete is related to lesions (deep part of the cuff, posterosuperior labrum and glenoid rim) secondary to repetitive hard throwing even with no anterior instability.

Lesions from posterosuperior impingement are very frequent in throwing athletes, and can be tolerated by subjects in so far as they manage to adjust their activity level and modify the cocking motion. In case adaptation fails, conservative treatment is proposed consisting of rest, non-steroid anti-inflammatory drugs, two infiltrations and an intensive rehabilitation program. Should this fail or the diagnosis be uncertain, arthroscopic examination is proposed to assess the lesions accurately and perform a debridement. The results of the debridement are difficult to appreciate because many factors are involved, including the sport itself and the level of performance, the age of the patient, the severity of the tendinous lesions and the damage to the posterosuperior labrum and glenoid.

Andrews et al,[9] who first emphasized the partial tears of the undersurface of the rotator cuff in the throwing athlete, reported that 76% of the patients returned to their preinjury level of athletic performance after a simple articular debridement, 9% returned to the same sport but at a lower level of competition, and 15% did not return at all. These results are consistent with our experience: of 104 arthroscopic debridements performed between 1990 and 1995; 20 patients were unable to return to their sport.[10]

Surgical principles

Arthroscopy has three goals.

(1) Diagnosis: to determine the contact between the tendinous and labral lesions with the arm in abduction–external rotation and retropulsion, and confirm the absence of an isolated superior labrum anterior to posterior (SLAP) lesion or an anterior instability with a Bankart lesion;

(2) Prognosis: assess the tendinous lesions of the undersurface of the supra- and infraspinatus and classify them according to Snyder et al[11] to evaluate the posterosuperior labrum: meniscal-shaped or non-meniscal-shaped labrum, proper insertion, physiologic or pathologic detachment;

(3) Treatment: to perform articular debridement.

The major risk of arthroscopy is to over- or underestimate the importance of the impingement and lesions observed. As a matter of fact, this contact is physiologic and will be found in the vast majority of individuals. Therefore, it may be difficult to correlate pain definitely with the arthroscopic appearance. This is the reason why it is important to perform a dynamic exploration with the arm in abduction–forced external rotation and retropulsion to avoid the risk of misinterpreting degeneration or fraying of the anteroinferior labrum as an anterior instability or misinterpreting lesions of the superior labrum as an isolated SLAP lesion.

We have never had any complications other than those usually associated with any regional anesthesia and diagnostic and/or therapeutic arthroscopy.

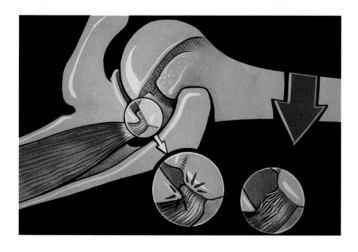

Figure 23.1

In abduction–external rotation and retropulsion there is an impingement between the articular side of the cuff and the posterosuperior part of the glenoid.

Surgical technique

The patient is positioned in the lateral decubitus position with the arm in vertical and horizontal double traction, or in a beach-chair position, according to the surgeon's preferences. Should a painful form of anterior instability still be suspected, it is advisable to position the patient in the beach-chair position, which will allow the use of an anterior deltopectoral approach, if necessary. The anterior and posterior aspects of the shoulder should be draped free, and the arm should be protected by sterile drapes as the surgeon will need to move the arm during the dynamic exploration. Regional anesthesia using an interscalene block is sufficient.

The arthroscope is introduced through a posterior portal located 1.5 cm inferior and medial to the posterolateral acromion angle. A 30° arthroscope is appropriate.

Step 1

The first arthroscopic step is the exploration of lesions, which should be performed methodically, beginning at the superior aspect of the joint and continuing with the superior labrum, biceps, and superior glenohumeral ligament. This is followed by exploration of the anterior aspect of the joint continuing with middle and inferior glenohumeral ligaments, labrum subscapularis tendon, and then its inferior aspect: labrum, and axillary pouch; and posterior aspect: the humeral sulcus inferiorly, and then the attachments of the rotator cuff muscles, namely, the teres minor, infraspinatus and supraspinatus. Simple rotation of the shoulder and arthroscope will provide good visualization of their tendinous attachments onto the humerus. The posteroinferior labrum and the posterosuperior labrum are subsequently explored.

Step 2

The second arthroscopic step is the palpation of the different structures by inserting a probe through an anterior portal that is created in an inside-out direction using a Wissinger rod. When there is a partial tear of the undersurface of the rotator cuff, the Wissinger rod should be advanced along the anterosuperior wall of the joint, above the long head of the biceps tendon, to gain easy access to the posterosuperior attachment of the rotator cuff onto the greater tuberosity. In the absence of a rotator cuff tear, the Wissinger rod should be advanced inferior to the long head of biceps and superior to the subscapularis, through the angle formed by the subscapularis and the middle glenohumeral ligament. An 8-mm anterior cannula is inserted over the Wissinger rod using a retrograde technique. Exploration

is resumed step by step as previously described, using palpation to more accurately define the lesions.

The biceps tendon and the superior glenohumeral ligament are usually intact, but in three of our cases, the intra-articular portion of the biceps tendon was frayed (Figure 23.2), and this was attributed to posterosuperior impingement. In fact, incomplete tearing of the deep surface of the supraspinatus had resulted in partial denudation of the greater tuberosity; during abduction and external rotation–internal rotation movements, the long head of the biceps repeatedly rubbed against the denuded area of the greater tuberosity like a windscreen wiper, causing severe injury to the tendon (Figure 23.3).

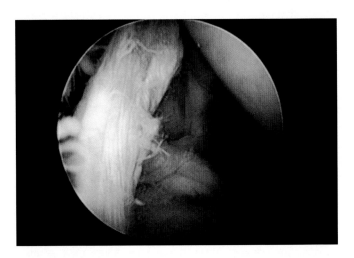

Figure 23.2

Partial tear and fraying of the deep part of the intra-articular portion of the long head of the biceps.

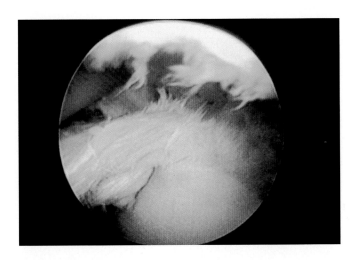

Figure 23.3

During dynamic exploration with the arm abducted, internal–external rotations produce rubbing of the long head of the biceps against the bare area of the greater tuberosity (articular side tear of the supraspinatus).

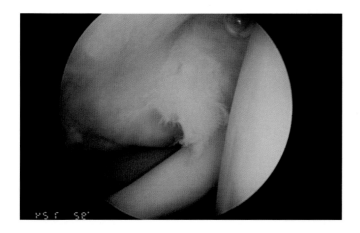

Figure 23.4

Articular side partial tear of the supraspinatus (grade II according to Snyder et al[11]).

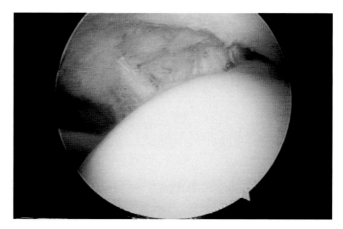

Figure 23.5

Articular side partial tear of the supraspinatus (grade III according to Snyder et al[11]).

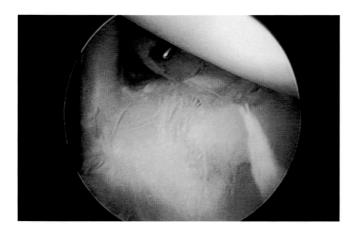

Figure 23.6

Meniscal-shaped type labrum.

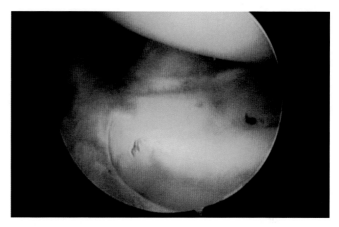

Figure 23.7

Meniscal-type labrum physiologically detached.

The insertion of the superior labrum is palpated for detection of a possible pathologic detachment that may result from superior impingement occurring when the arm is placed in more than 140° of abduction.

The anterior aspect of the joint is usually unaffected. However, it is important to carefully palpate the anteroinferior insertion of the labrum to detect a possible Bankart lesion, as in this case, the problem is a painful form of anterior instability rather than posterosuperior impingement.

The inferior aspect of the joint is usually normal. In fact, most lesions affect the posterior and posterosuperior aspects of the joint.

Lesions of the deep aspect of the rotator cuff

These mainly affect the supraspinatus, but in some cases the infraspinatus may also be involved. Patients present with partial rupture of varying severity, ranging from minor fraying of the articular capsule to a two-thirds rupture of the tendon (grade III) (Figures 23.4 and 23.5).

Lesions of the posterosuperior labrum

The lesions are different according to whether or not the labrum has a meniscal shape (Figure 23.6). With a meniscal-shaped labrum, the labrum can be normally inserted on the glenoid where it protects the supraspinatus from direct contact with the sharp edge of the cartilage, physiologically detached (Figure 23.7) or detached due to repeated contact (Figure 23.8).

It may also be torn or frayed with numerous loose flaps (Figure 23.9). During the arthroscopic maneuver, with the arm placed in the throwing position (abduction–external rotation, retropulsion), it is crucial that the superior labrum be tested to determine whether or not

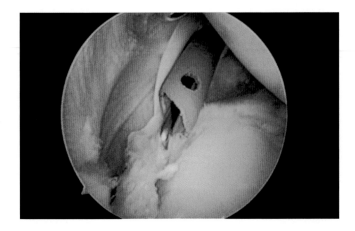

Figure 23.8
Meniscal-type labrum pathologically detached.

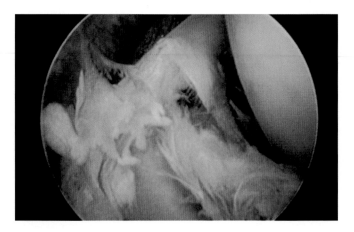

Figure 23.9
Torn posterosuperior labrum.

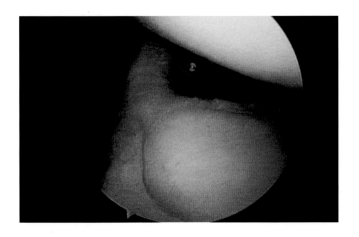

Figure 23.10
Non-meniscal-shaped labrum.

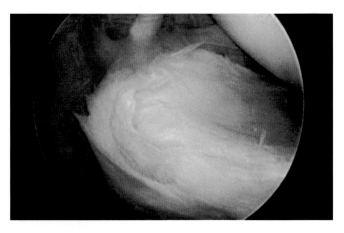

Figure 23.11
Frayed, detached non-meniscal type labrum.

it is in contact with the glenoid. The labral lesion may also extend superiorly and reach the biceps insertion that may be affected, suggesting a SLAP lesion.

In the case of a non-meniscal-shaped labrum (Figures 23.10 and 23.11), the examiner should evaluate for an avulsion or tearing at the cartilage–labrum junction, which often appears only in the cocking-phase maneuver.

Lesions of the posterior glenoid rim

Various lesions have been demonstrated using a profile view of the glenoid or a computed tomography (CT) scan but these lesions are not always easy to detect or to figure. On a plain radiograph, ossification or bone spicules, or periosteal spurs may appear as partial fractures of the posterior glenoid rim. Abrasion of the posterior rim (Figure 23.12) is mainly visible on a CT

scan, possibly comparative. On arthro-CT scans, these minor lesions are often obscured by the contrast medium. Chondromalacia of the glenoid cartilage visualized at arthroscopy may have different appearances with cartilage softening demonstrable by palpation and minor crevices parallel to the posterior rim (Figure 23.13). These posterior lesions are typically located in the upper part of the glenoid, which differs from the Bennett lesion as described in pitchers, which is located in the posteroinferior portion of the glenoid.

Lesions of the humeral head cartilage

These are rare but may be diagnosed on plain radiographs or CT scans (geodes or cysts). They lie in the posterosuperior portion, often superior to the sulcus, and appear as osteochondral fractures limited in size. Differentiation from Hill–Sachs lesions is easy. Their

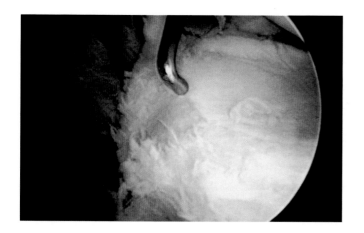

Figure 23.12

Abrasion of the posterosuperior cartilage.

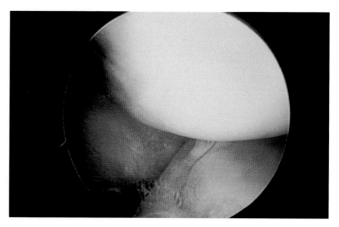

Figure 23.13

Cartilage softening and crevices of the posterosuperior glenoid.

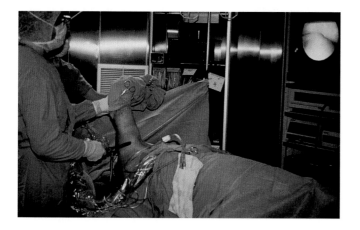

Figure 23.14

The surgeon grasps the patient's forearm and places it in abduction–external rotation and retroplusion, while observing what is occuring in the joint. (Patient is in the lateral decubitus position.)

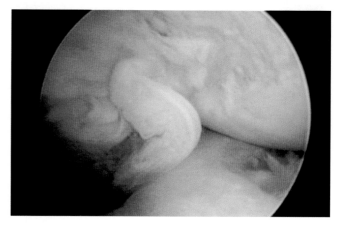

Figure 23.15

Impingement occurs at 9 o'clock between the superior part of the infraspinatus (torn and frayed) and the intact meniscal-type labrum.

pathogenicity is unknown as we have never been able to restore lesion–labrum contact while the arm is cocked. They are possibly traumatic and may occur following violent forced motions; however, they may also occur as degenerative changes (geodes) resulting from excessive stresses such as those encountered in arthritis.

Step 3

The third arthroscopic step is the dynamic exploration: the probe is removed whereas the anterior cannula can remain in situ. The arthroscope is positioned posteriorly in the midsection of the joint, and directed toward the superior aspect of the joint. The surgeon grasps the patient's forearm, which is protected by the sterile drapes, and places it carefully in abduction, external

rotation, and retropulsion, while observing what is occurring in the joint (Figure 23.14). There are different types of impingement.

Impingement in which the lesions are in contact may occur at 90° or 100° of abduction, most often between the superior portion of the infraspinatus attachment and the posterior aspect of the glenoid and labrum, in the area between 9 and 10 o'clock (Figure 23.15). The impingement may also occur between 120° and 160° of abduction between the supraspinatus and the glenoid rim between 10 and 12 o'clock (Figure 23.16).

Lesions of the rotator cuff are often emphasized and sometimes revealed by this maneuver, and they should be evaluated again. Lesions of the posterosuperior labrum and glenoid cartilage are also observed in a new light. Clear detachment of the labrum or crevices in the cartilage resulting from tendon contact can be evidenced by this maneuver. Last but not least, contact may occur

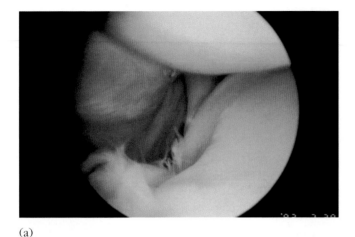

(a)

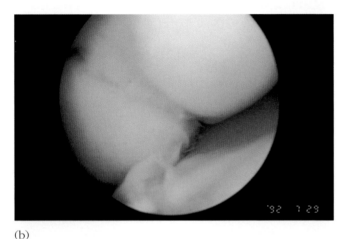

(b)

Figure 23.16

(a) and (b) impingement occurs between 10 and 12 o'clock between the supraspinatus and the posterosuperior part of the glenoid (detached non-meniscal labrum).

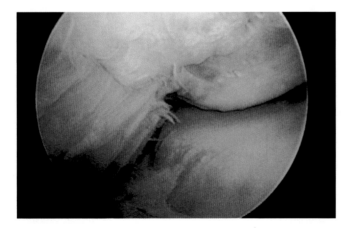

Figure 23.17

Impingement occurs between the tendon and the glenoid cartilage where the labrum retracts posteriorly during the maneuver.

either between the tendons and the attached or partially detached labrum, or between the tendons and the glenoid cartilage where the labrum is absent or retracts posteriorly during the maneuver (Figure 23.17).

This dynamic exploration is critical and allows better evaluation and understanding of the lesions. Patients can actually visualize the lesions under regional anesthesia, and thus better understand their condition and the part played by the cocking motion in their symptoms in abduction–external rotation and retropulsion. Besides, it seems essential to us to differentiate between impingements occurring between the tendon and the labrum, and those occurring between the tendon and the cartilage or bone.

Step 4

The fourth arthroscopic step is the debridement of lesions. The patient's arm is brought back to its initial position and a 6-mm full radius resector is inserted into the anterior cannula. Placing the shoulder in internal and external rotation facilitates the shaving of the rotator cuff lesions. All the tendinous frays should be resected to provide a surface as smooth and even as possible. In cases where detachment of the supraspinatus has caused partial denudation of the greater tuberosity, the denuded area is abraded down to the bleeding bone using a 6-mm diameter spherical burr.

Regarding the posterosuperior labrum and glenoid cartilage, we modulate our technique to the situation. We routinely resect the frayed or torn portion of the labrum, but we do not systematically excise a detached labrum because we do not know whether it should be considered a painful and non-indispensable structure or a non-painful structure that assists in protecting the tendon from direct contact with the posterior margin of the glenoid. If it is severely damaged with multiple tears, we remove it; if it is detached (generally in the area between 10 and 1 o'clock) and undamaged, we decorticate the posterior edge of the scapula facing the detachment site so as to promote healing. This is performed using a spherical burr down to the cancellous bone. We have never reattached the labrum with suture anchors as suggested by Burkhart and Morgan.[12]

In cases where the intra-articular portion of the long head of biceps is damaged, we release it from its glenoid attachment and address it later on, at the end of the procedure, through a short incision made under the pectoralis major tendon. We perform a tenodesis using non-absorbable sutures and reattach the tendon at the humeral insertion site of the pectoralis major. In fact, we believe that simple tenotomy of the long head of biceps in young patients results in an unsightly deformity of the arm that is not well accepted.

Step 5

The fifth step is the bursoscopy which should be performed routinely to detect a possible superficial rotator cuff lesion.

Postoperative protocol

The arm is immobilized in a sling for 8 days, after which patients are encouraged to use their arm for the normal activities of daily living, avoiding any external rotation motion until the end of the first postoperative month, and extreme or forced external rotation until the end of the second postoperative month. During these first 2 months, any sporting activities in which excessive stress is placed on the operated shoulder are strictly prohibited. Return to work is authorized in the same conditions of relative rest.

Physical therapy is begun 1 week after the operation and gentle exercises are performed for progressive recovery of full range of forward elevation, respecting the limits set for external rotation. Static and dynamic exercises involving the internal and external rotators as well as strengthening of the scapular adductors (rhomboideus major and minor), are begun at the end of the first postoperative month.

At the end of the second postoperative month, patients are allowed to return to sports. However, they are advised to modify their cocking motions and avoid any forced abduction–external rotation and retropulsion motion for some time.

The average time to return to competition varies according to the sport, the level of performance, and the athlete's schedule. As regards tennis, this generally takes place towards the fourth postoperative month.

References

1. Walch G, Liotard JP, Boileau P et al. Un autre conflit de l'épaule. 'Le conflit glénoïden postero-supérieur'. *Rev Chir Orthop* 1991; **177**:571–4.
2. Walch G, Boileau P, Noel E. Impingement of the deep surface of the supra-spinatus tendon on the postero superior glenoid rim. An arthroscopic study. *J Shoulder Elbow Surg* 1992; **1**:238–45.
3. Walch G. Perspectives in postero–superior impingement AANA Meeting 14th Annual Fall Course, December 7–10, 1995, San Antonio, Texas.
4. Jobe CM, Sidles J. Evidence for a posterior glenoid impingement upon the rotator cuff. *J Shoulder Elbow Surg* 1993; **2**:S19.
5. Davidson PA, Elattrache NS, Jobe CM et al. Rotator cuff and posterior–superior glenoid labrum injury with increased glenohumeral motion: a new site of impingement. *J Shoulder Elbow Surg* 1995; **4**:384–90.
6. Jobe CM. Posterior–superior glenoid impingement: expanded spectrum. *Arthroscopy* 1995; **11**:530–6.
7. Jobe CM. Superior glenoid impingement. *Clin Orthop* 1996; **330**:98–107.
8. Jobe FW, Tibone JE, Pink MM et al. The shoulder in sports. In: Rockwood CA, Matsen F. eds. *The Shoulder*, 2nd edn. Philadelphia: WB Saunders, 1998; 1214–37.
9. Andrews JR, Broussard TS, Carson WG. Arthroscopy of the shoulder in the management of partial tears of the rotator cuff: a preliminary report. *Arthroscopy* 1985; **1**:117–22.
10. Riand N, Levigne Ch, Renaud E, Walch G. Results of derotational humeral osteotomy in postero–superior glenoid impingement. *Am J Sports Med* 1998; **26**:453–9.
11. Snyder SJ, Pachelli AF, Del Pizzo W et al. Partial thickness rotator cuff tears: results of arthroscopic treatment. *Arthroscopy* 1991; **7**:1–7.
12. Burkhart SS, Morgan CD. The peel-back mechanism: its role in producing and extending posterior type II SLAP lesions and its effect on SLAP repair rehabilitation. *Arthroscopy* 1998; **14**:637–40.

24 Arthroscopic treatment of calcific tendinitis

Suzanne L Miller, Jonathan B Ticker and James N Gladstone

Introduction

Calcific deposits in the rotator cuff leading to tendinitis are a common cause of shoulder pain, peaking in the fourth and fifth decades of life. Codman described the calcification as being located primarily within the supraspinatus tendon adjacent to the insertion on the greater tuberosity, but it also can be found within the subscapularis, infraspinatus and teres minor.[1] Considerable controversy remains regarding the etiology of this condition. Codman proposed that degenerative changes were necessary before the tendon would calcify. Conversely, Uhthoff and Loehr do not believe degeneration plays a role in calcium deposition, and state that calcification is actively mediated by cells in a viable environment.[2] The age distribution and the self-limiting course of the disease argues against degeneration as the cause, according to Uhthoff and Loehr.

The clinical manifestations range from an incidental radiographic finding without symptoms to functional impairment with acute, debilitating pain. Most authors describe two phases: a formative (chronic) and a resorptive (acute) phase. In the formative phase, calcium crystals are deposited in matrix vesicles and the calcium appears chalk-like if removed. The resorptive phase is characterized by spontaneous resorption of calcium with an influx of macrophages and multinucleated giant cells. In this stage the calcium deposit can be grossly characterized as thick and creamy. It is during this phase that pain usually occurs and patients seek medical attention.

Physical examination and plain radiographs are essential for an accurate diagnosis. Pain is the most common complaint. Neer describes four mechanisms for the pain associated with calcific tendinitis.[3] The first is chemical irritation of the tissue by calcium. Second, the calcium imbibes water and causes swelling which increases pressure within the tendon. Third, thickening of the bursa in response to the calcium may occur causing a bursitis or impingement, and fourth, pain may occur due to adhesive capsulitis from decreased activity. Unlike other diseases of the musculoskeletal system, calcific tendinitis may be present with minimal symptoms for an indefinite period of time during the formative phase. This is usually followed by the acute onset of pain (patients can often pinpoint the time) corresponding to the resorptive phase. Ruling out other causes of shoulder pain is mandatory, as calcium deposits can be incidental findings on radiographs not related to signs detected on physical examination. Tenderness over the involved area is important in establishing the calcium deposit as the source of pain.

Plain radiographs are valuable for two reasons. The first is for diagnosis and localization of the calcific deposit. The second is to follow changes during treatment. A routine shoulder series is initially obtained, including anteroposterior (AP) in internal rotation (IR) and external rotation (ER), supraspinatus outlet, and axillary views. These can be supplemented with additional views if further localization of calcium is needed. Most of the calcium deposits are located in the supraspinatus tendon and can be seen on an AP view of the glenohumeral joint (Figure 24.1). AP views in IR

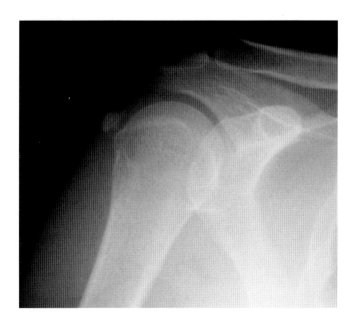

Figure 24.1

AP radiograph demonstrating calcific deposit in the supraspinatus tendon.

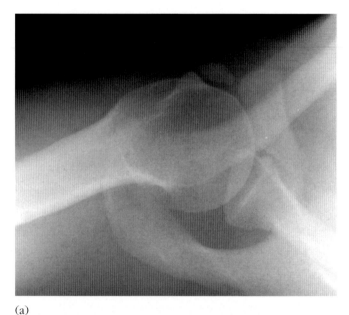

(a)

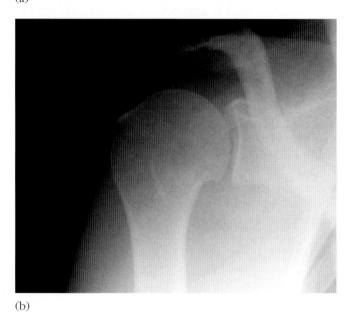

(b)

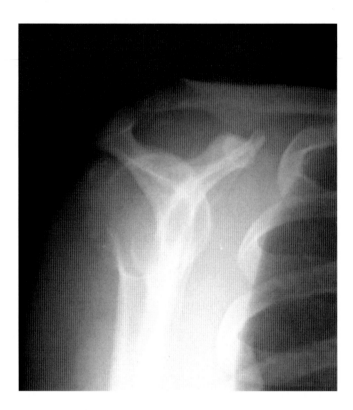

Figure 24.2

Supraspinatus outlet view demonstrating infraspinatus deposit, posteriorly.

Figure 24.3

(a) Axillary view demonstrating subscapularis deposit anteriorly. Compare with (b) AP view of the same patient (note difficulty identifying calcium deposit).

and ER are used to further localize deposits in the infraspinatus and supraspinatus, respectively. The supraspinatus outlet view helps to localize supraspinatus deposits in the anterior-to-posterior direction and to identify deposits in the infraspinatus seen posteriorly (Figure 24.2), in addition to determining the acromial morphology and the presence of any subacromial osteophytes. The axillary view is useful for identifying deposits within the subscapularis tendon (Figure 24.3). If the Zanca view for the acromioclavicular joint (10° cephalic tilt) is part of a routine shoulder series, the calcific deposit superiorly is often seen quite clearly. DePalma and Kruper describe calcifications on radiographs as dense and well defined in the formative stage, but cloudlike or irregular in the resorptive phase.[4] Calcific tendinitis must be distinguished from dystrophic calcification associated with rotator cuff disease, which occurs closer to the tendon insertion. The latter carries a worse prognosis and is not associated with the eventual resorption of calcium and a resolution of symptoms.

Non-surgical treatment consisting of initial rest, ice, anti-inflammatory medication, analgesics, home exercises and physical therapy will usually relieve the symptoms in either the formative or resorptive phase. During the formative phase, some authors recommend subacromial

injections to relieve impingement pain.[2] However, Lippmann warns that corticosteroids may inhibit the cellular activity that produces disruption of the calcium deposit.[5] Needling a calcium deposit with or without lavage during the resorptive phase is a treatment that has met with variable success.[4,6] If a patient presents with acute shoulder pain and difficulty with motion and demonstrates calcific deposits on radiography, we will attempt needling with a combination of anesthetic and steroid into the suspected area of the deposit and into

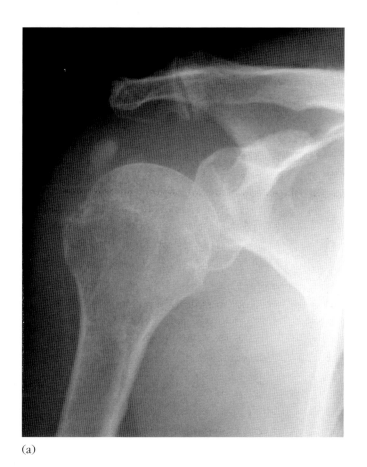
(a)

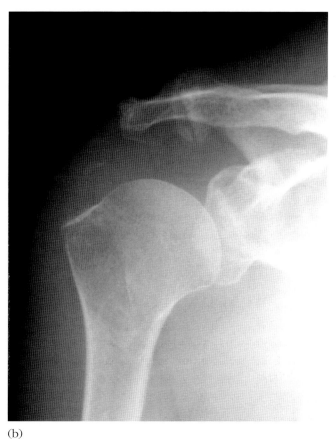
(b)

Figure 24.4

(a) Pre-needling radiograph of calcific deposit in the supraspinatus tendon. (b) Eight weeks after needling, showing dissolution of calcium deposit.

the subacromial space. This will often provide immediate and significant relief (Figure 24.4). During the needling procedure, a white aspirate may be obtained. This indicates a direct hit of the deposit. The non-surgical program is then initiated.

If non-surgical efforts to relieve pain and restore function are unsuccessful, and other diagnoses have been eliminated, a surgical approach to the problem is justified. Most often this is necessary in the chronic formative phase. Traditionally, this was done as an open procedure.[7] Bosworth, in 1941, described open surgery as being the quickest and most dependable way to eliminate pain and avoid an impending frozen shoulder.[7] More recently, arthroscopic techniques have been developed. Advantages may include a shorter rehabilitation time, a better functional result, and a better cosmetic appearance. Several studies have attempted to establish the efficacy of arthroscopic treatment for refractory cases of calcific tendinitis.[8–10]

Ark et al treated 23 patients with calcific tendinitis with an arthroscopic excision.[8] Concomitant subacromial

decompression was performed in three patients who demonstrated a 'bony acromial overhang'. Nine patients (91%) had a good or satisfactory result. In this series, complete removal of calcium was not achieved in 14 patients, but 12 of these obtained significant pain relief. The authors concluded that complete excision of the calcium deposit was not necessary, nor was an acromioplasty, with the exception of those exhibiting signs and symptoms of impingement.

Jerosch et al evaluated 48 out of 57 patients treated arthroscopically for calcific tendinitis.[9] Constant scores improved from 38 before surgery to 86 after surgery. In their series acromioplasty was not associated with a significant improvement in the results. High success rates have been reported by Mole et al in a multicenter study conducted by the French Society of Arthroscopy.[10] Eighty-eight per cent of the patients had complete disappearance of the calcific deposit and 82% were satisfied with their result. In this series acromioplasty did not influence the outcome.

Surgical principles

To ensure optimal results, complete removal of the calcium deposit should be attempted. Therefore, pinpoint accuracy in localizing the deposit prior to surgery is essential. As described previously, this can be achieved with the use of specific radiographs to highlight different planes. Other studies, such as magnetic resonance imaging and ultrasonography, may provide additional useful information as to calcium location (Figure 24.5). When the location of the deposit is clearly understood, the surgical procedure may be undertaken.

Equipment includes the usual arthroscopic instrumentation along with a pump, an electrocautery device, a spinal needle, an arthroscopic knife and a small, non-aggressive shaver. The arm should be draped free to allow easy rotation in order to bring the affected area of the cuff into position. When a rotated and/or abducted position is required to expose the deposit, a McConnell intraoperative arm positioner (McConnell Orthopedic Manufacturing Co., Greenville, TX, USA) can be helpful to maintain this position. Viewing the tendon surface from all portals (posterior, lateral, and anterior) may help to identify the calcium deposit and assist with its release. Judicious use of the spinal needle will decrease the number of holes made in the tendon. A marking suture, as outlined below, can help localize the calcium deposit. If exposing the deposit results in a large or deep defect in the tendon, a repair of the tendon should be considered and the equipment for a tendon repair should be available.

In addition to the usual arthroscopic complications that can occur, complications from a calcium release include incomplete excision of calcium, causing residual pain;

rotator cuff tendon disruption or damage; deltoid damage; and postoperative capsulitis. All can be avoided or managed with meticulous attention to detail in the surgical technique and appropriate rehabilitation.

Surgical technique

The procedure may be performed under interscalene regional block or general endotracheal tube anesthesia. The patient may be placed in either the beach-chair or the lateral decubitus position. We perform the procedure with an interscalene regional block in the beach-chair position with the back elevated approximately 70°. All bony prominences are carefully padded. A shoulder hydraulic table (Tenet Medical, Calgary, AB, Canada) specifically designed for the beach-chair position greatly simplifies this set-up. An antibiotic, usually a cephalosporin unless contraindicated, is administered preoperatively. An examination under anesthesia is documented prior to the usual preparation and draping of the extremity. The bony landmarks of the shoulder, including the acromion, acromioclavicular joint, and coracoid, as well as the planned portal sites, are marked on the skin with a marking pen. An injection of 20 ml of local anesthetic solution with epinephrine (adrenaline) is given into the portal sites and subacromial space to aid with hemostasis. In addition, 2 ml of epinephrine in a 1:1000 solution is injected into each 3-liter bag of arthroscopic saline solution. An arthroscopic pump, usually set at 40 mmHg, is preferred. This pressure and the flow can be adjusted for visualization and distension. Attention should be paid to avoid excessive extravasation of fluid.

The posterior soft spot of the shoulder is palpated. This is approximately 2 cm inferior and 1 cm medial to the posterolateral corner of the acromion. The exact position is then localized with an 18-gauge spinal needle directed anteriorly into the joint toward the coracoid tip; 50 ml of saline is injected into the joint, and brisk backflow of fluid through the spinal needle confirms placement within the joint and suggests an intact cuff. Fluid distension of the glenohumeral joint allows for an easier entry with less chance of damaging articular surfaces. Since the majority of the work is to be carried out in the subacromial space, the posterior portal can be placed slightly superiorly if desired to facilitate placement of the arthroscope into this space. This allows easier maneuvering above the humeral head. After the skin incision is made, the blunt trocar and sheath are inserted into the top third of the glenohumeral joint, which is confirmed with backflow of fluid through the sheath.

A careful inspection of the glenohumeral joint is carried out and any intra-articular pathology is identified and treated appropriately. In order to ensure good visualization, even if just for diagnostic purposes, an

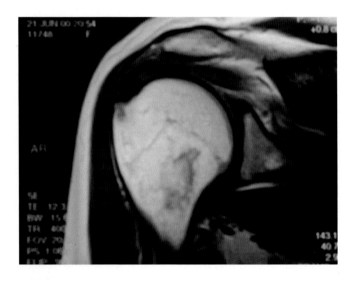

Figure 24.5

Calcific deposit in the supraspinatus tendon appears black on magnetic resonance imaging.

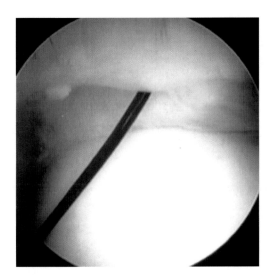

Figure 24.6

Intra-articular view of marking suture placed through the rotator cuff localizing the deposit.

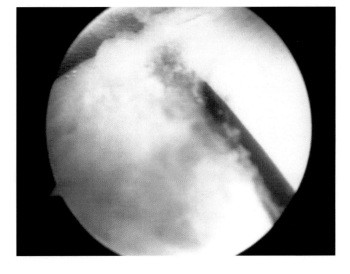

Figure 24.7

The same marking suture shown in Figure 24.6, seen subacromially after bursa has been resected.

outflow is beneficial. If an anterior portal is required, the outflow can be through a cannula placed anteriorly. If no anterior portal is used, an 18-gauge spinal needle can be placed via an anterior approach and connected to the outflow tubing of the arthroscopic pump. The needle can be used to gently probe any suspicious areas. However, an anterior portal is recommended.

The undersurface of the rotator cuff, particularly in the area of the suspected calcium deposit, should be carefully inspected for any suspicious bulge, area of hyperemia, or signs of damage. If a suspicious area is identified, an 18-gauge spinal needle is inserted directly through this portion of the rotator cuff from a lateral entry and a #1 colored monofilament suture is placed as a marking stitch (Figure 24.6). Through the anterior portal, a grasper is used to retrieve the intra-articular limb of the suture. If an anterior portal is not used, the suture is pushed well into the joint so that it remains across the tendon when the needle is removed. Careful planning is used to keep the lateral entry of the suture away from the site of the lateral portal that will be created to perform the subacromial portion of the procedure. We also take into account the confines of the bursa when placing the marking suture, as the posterior margin of the bursa is usually located at the midportion of the acromion. If the suture is placed outside of the bursa, usually posteriorly, it will be more difficult to identify. If the calcific deposit is located more posteriorly, this may be unavoidable.

After work in the glenohumeral joint is completed, the arthroscopic cannula with blunt trocar is redirected into the subacromial space from the posterior portal. Wide, sweeping motions are made to clear the bursa, particularly in the lateral subacromial and subdeltoid area, to facilitate visualization for creation of the lateral portal. It is useful at this point for the anesthesiologist to keep the patient's blood pressure as low as is medically safe in order to minimize bleeding.

The subacromial space needs to be cleared of most of the bursa to ensure complete visualization. We routinely use a radiofrequency ablation probe that allows clearing of thick subacromial bursa and provides concomitant hemostasis. This can also be started through the anterior portal and completed after the lateral portal is established. A lateral portal is established under direct visualization with the aid of an 18-gauge spinal needle. This is usually placed at the junction of the anterior and middle thirds of the lateral acromion (often in line with the posterior aspect of the acromioclavicular joint), and distally enough (1–2 cm with the arm at the side) from the lateral edge of the acromion so that instruments can enter the subacromial space easily.

Although its necessity is not supported by the literature, one author (JNG) always performs an acromioplasty. If preoperative imaging demonstrates a subacromial spur, it is removed to create a flat acromion. If on the other hand no spur is present, a minimal acromioplasty is performed to create slightly more space for the supraspinatus, which may thicken slightly after the procedure from scarring. If a patient demonstrated preoperative acromioclavicular tenderness and arthritic changes on radiography, a distal clavicle resection can be performed at this time.

At this point, attention is turned toward the rotator cuff. There is usually a thin veil of bursa remaining overlying the tendon. It can usually be removed with a full-radius resector with little or no bleeding. A supraspinatus calcium deposit is usually located in this

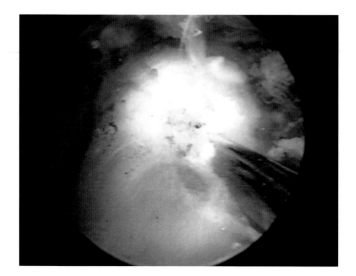

Figure 24.8
Spinal needle used to locate the calcific deposit.

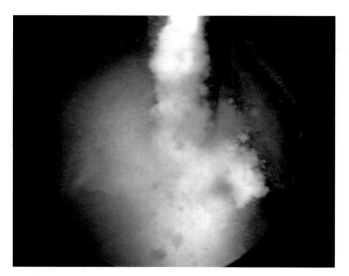

Figure 24.9
The 'snowstorm' effect after needling the deposit.

area. The blue color of the polypropylene marking suture can normally be identified at this point (Figure 24.7). With internal or external rotation of the shoulder and abduction as needed, the involved area of the tendon can usually be brought into clear view within easy access from the lateral portal. If the calcium deposit is not easily identified, an 18-gauge spinal needle is used to penetrate the rotator cuff in the region of the marking stitch until the calcium deposits become apparent. If a marking suture has not been placed, the bursal surface of the tendon is inspected for a suspicious bulge, an area of hyperemia, or any signs of damage. It is then needled to identify the calcium deposit (Figure 24.8). If a particular area is suspected, further bursa can be removed to expose more tendon. In addition, the preoperative radiographs should be available in the operating room for further review.

As the deposit is needled, calcium is liberated and will often be seen as a 'snowstorm' (Figure 24.9). With the precise location of the calcium identified, an attempt is made to remove the entire deposit. If the calcium is readily seen, it can be removed using either a small curette or a small, straight or curved, full-radius resector (Figure 24.10). If the location has been identified but the calcium is not readily seen, a knife can be used to open the tendon longitudinally, directly over the deposit. An attempt is made to incise the tendon in line with its fibers. We pay particular attention to trying to remove all of the calcium. If there is any question as to whether an incomplete removal has been performed, or the location cannot be identified, an intraoperative radiograph can be taken. Fluoroscopy can also be used.[11] In the event that insufficient calcium is excised or the deposit cannot be found, a 'mini-open' approach can be

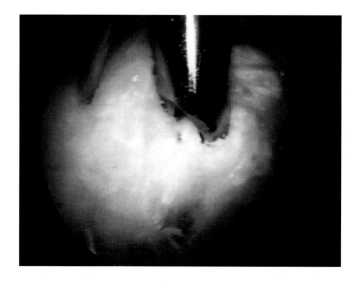

Figure 24.10
A shaver is used to debride any remaining calcium in the tendon or any loose debris.

performed and the cuff palpated manually to find the calcium deposits.

The resulting damage to the tendon must now be assessed. If the tendon involvement is superficial or if there is a small longitudinal split, no further treatment is necessary. If the split appears more involved or if the tendon is damaged to the point of concern, sutures can be placed arthroscopically to close the defect. We prefer using long-acting, braided, absorbable sutures. If the tendon insertion to the greater tuberosity is found

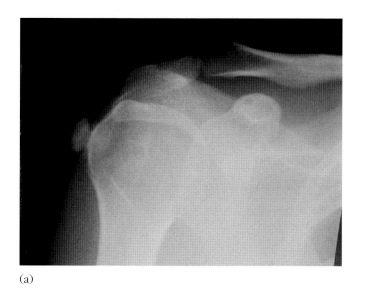

(a)

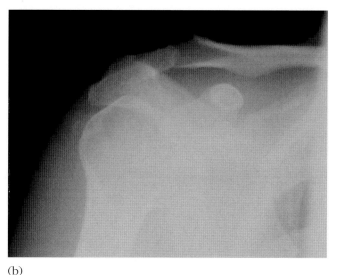

(b)

Figure 24.11

(a) Preoperative radiograph showing calcific deposit in the supraspinatus tendon. (b) Postoperative radiograph after arthroscopic removal of calcific deposit.

to be disrupted, it must be repaired either arthroscopically with a suture anchor, or with a 'mini-open' technique.

As a final step, the subacromial space is irrigated to flush out any remaining calcium crystals that could potentially cause inflammation. A catheter placed in the subacromial space and connected to a pump that delivers continuous local anesthetic solution may be useful to provide postoperative pain relief (Zimmer, Warsaw, IN, USA). If this technique is chosen, a separate posterolateral approach is used for insertion of the catheter. The tip of the catheter is placed in the region of calcium release, and the catheter is carefully secured where it exits the skin to avoid unintentional removal. The arthroscopic instruments are removed, and the portals are closed with nylon sutures. Sterile dressings are applied, and the arm is placed in a sling. Cryotherapy may be used to provide cold compression in the postoperative period.

Postoperative protocol

Appropriate analgesia is important to diminish pain during the early postoperative period as well as during rehabilitation. If used, an anesthetic pump should also be able to provide bolus doses for breakthrough pain in the period immediately following surgery. These devices are usually removed by the patient after approximately 48 hours. A series of radiographs (Figure 24.11) are

obtained at the first postoperative visit to demonstrate the removal of the calcium. Unless a rotator cuff tear has been repaired, rehabilitation is much the same as that following an arthroscopic acromioplasty. Passive range-of-motion exercises as well as pendulum and active-assisted range-of-motion exercises with a stick are begun immediately. Pulley exercises are added when the patient demonstrates sufficient rotator cuff control. These exercises are progressively increased as tolerated in order to restore full range of motion as promptly and as comfortably as possible. Premedicating with analgesics will help to control pain during the exercise regimen. Application of heat as a warm-up prior to stretching exercises and application of cold following rehabilitation and home exercises are beneficial. In general, patients are encouraged to use the arm as normally as possible, within the range of comfort.

When full range of motion has been restored and pain is controlled, active exercises are initiated with progression to a resistance exercise program. The goal is to have the patient using the arm for light activities of daily living by 2–3 weeks, and involved in normal activities by 2–3 months. Return to upper-extremity sports or activities may require additional time for specific strengthening and functional rehabilitation. Careful follow-up should be performed and the physician-directed rehabilitation adjusted appropriately for any flare-ups. Occasionally, postoperative inflammation limits a patient's progress. When this occurs, non-steroidal anti-inflammatory medications and/or, in certain cases, a subacromial injection with a steroid may be beneficial.

References

1. Codman EA. Calcified deposits in the supraspinatus. In: *The Shoulder: Rupture of the Supraspinatus Tendon and Other Lesions in or about the Subacromial Bursa*, Boston: Thomas Todd, 1934; 178–215.

2. Uhthoff HK, Loehr JW. Calcific tendinopathy of the rotator cuff: pathogenesis, diagnosis, and management. *J Am Acad Orthop Surg* 1997; **5**:183–91.

3. Neer CS. Less frequent procedures. In: Neer CS, ed. *Shoulder Reconstruction*. Philadelphia: WB Saunders, 1990; 427–8.

4. DePalma AF, Kruper JS. Long term study of shoulder joints afflicted with and treated for calcific tendinitis. *Clin Orthop* 1961; **20**:61–72.

5. Lippmann RK. Observations concerning the calcific cuff deposit. *Clin Orthop* 1961; **20**:49–60.

6. Rokito AS, Loebenberg MI. Frozen shoulder and calcific tendinitis. *Curr Opin Orthop* 1999; **10**:294–304.

7. Bosworth BM. Examination of the shoulder for calcium deposits. *J Bone Joint Surg* 1941; **23**:567–77.

8. Ark JW, Flock TJ, Flatow EL, Bigliani LU. Arthroscopic treatment of calcific tendinitis of the shoulder. *Arthroscopy* 1992; **8**:183–8.

9. Jerosch J, Strauss JM, Schmiel S. Arthroscopic treatment of calcific tendinitis of the shoulder. *J Shoulder Elbow Surg* 1998; **7**:30–7.

10. Mole D, Kempf J, Gleyse P et al. Results of arthroscopic treatment of tendinitis of the rotator cuff of the shoulder. Second part: calcified lesions of the rotator cuff. *Rev Chir Orthop* 1993; **79**:532–41.

11. Imhoff AB. Arthroscopic decompression of calcium deposits. In: Fu FH, Imhoff AB, Ticker JB, eds. *An Atlas of Shoulder Surgery*. London: Martin Dunitz, 1998; 159–65.

25 Calcific tendinitis: The role of arthroscopic treatment

Mark S Falworth and Roger J Emery

Introduction

Pain from calcific tendinitis can occur following the deposition of calcium within periarticular tissues. The tendons of the rotator cuff are commonly affected although calcific deposits are not infrequently seen in other regions of the body.[1-3] Duplay identified the subacromial bursa as a source of shoulder pain in 1872;[4] however, the radiological appearance of calcific tendinitis was not documented until 1907.[5] At the time the calcific deposit was believed to be located within the bursa, although Codman later demonstrated its intra-tendinous location.[6]

Incidence

The incidence of calcific tendinitis of the shoulder is reported to be between 2.7% and 23.6%.[7-9] Bosworth's clinical and fluoroscopic review of 6061 company employees (12 122 asymptomatic shoulders) revealed that 165 (2.7%) patients had calcific deposits in one or both shoulders over a 3-year period.[7] When symptomatic shoulders are considered, Harmon reported a series of 2580 painful shoulders in which 609 (23.6%) were attributed to calcific tendinitis,[8] although Molé has reported a lower incidence of 7%.[10]

Calcific tendinitis occurs most commonly in women, with incidences of 60–64% being reported in those affected.[11,12] The average age at presentation is 30–50 years.[7,11,13] Geographic variations are reported: a series from Taiwan demonstrated a male predominance (74%) and an older age at presentation – 69% were older than 60 years, 24% were aged 40–59 years and only 7% were less than 40 years old.[14]

The calcific deposit is commonly confined to a single tendon, with the supraspinatus having the highest incidence (63–80%).[14-16] However, analysis of either plain radiographs or magnetic resonance images has verified the presence of multiple calcific deposits affecting more than one tendon,[10,12,15,17] with the supraspinatus and subscapularis tendons being jointly affected in 20% of cases.[15] Bilateral symptomatic shoulder involvement is reported in 6–11%;[13,18,19] however, this incidence can rise to 47% when both shoulders are examined radiographically, even in the absence of symptoms.[7,17]

Pathogenesis

The aetiology of calcific tendinitis is unclear. Initial theories suggested that degenerative changes in the collagen fibres were the cause.[6] The deposits were believed to arise in a hypovascular area of the tendon where a fibrinoid mass develops and subsequently becomes calcified.[20] Codman identified this area as being just proximal to the insertion of the supraspinatus tendon, and termed it the 'critical portion'.[6]

The vascular supply to this area has been extensively investigated.[21-23] This critical portion, or zone, corresponds to the anastomosis between the osseous and tendinous vessels within the supraspinatus tendon. Rothman and Parke suggested that this hypovascularity was age-related and was not itself a pathological state.[22] This was challenged by Rathbun and Macnab who found this zone of relative avascularity in specimens of all ages, with a degree of perfusion that was related to shoulder position.[23] Indeed, calcific tendinitis has been reported in a patient as young as 3 years old,[24] suggesting that metabolic causes may be involved. This could also explain how calcific periarthritis affects multiple sites, sometimes simultaneously.[2] In addition, we have also seen occurrences in family groups and a case has been reported in 23-year-old monozygotic twins,[25] suggesting a genetic predisposition.

Uhthoff et al suggest that the calcific formation is due to a multifocal, active, cell-mediated process rather than degeneration.[26] Indeed, their series of 46 patients demonstrated no histological evidence of inflammatory infiltrate or scarring which would be expected in a degenerative process. They postulate that calcific tendinitis is a self-healing tendinopathy which is a dynamic process of four phases. In the precalcific phase, a combination of mechanical factors and a decrease in the vascular perfusion within the critical zone lowers the tissue oxygen tension, resulting in the asymptomatic transformation of tendinous tissue into fibrocartilage. This stimulus is the initial stage prior to mineralization. There follows the formative or calcific phase, during which chondrocyte-mediated calcification occurs within the tendon and calcific deposits are formed. This phase may be asymptomatic or may result in various degrees of pain. The subsequent resorptive phase is characterized by a period of vascular proliferation. Normal tissue perfusion and oxygen tensions are restored, enabling resorption of the calcific foci through phagocytosis.

Histological examination confirms that the resorptive phase coincides with symptoms of pain.[2,19,26,27] In the final post-calcific or reparative phase, new tendon matrix is synthesized to restore the normal tendon architecture. This phase may last several months.

This typical sequence of formation and resorption is not always followed. The periods between formation and resorption are variable, and separate foci may be in different stages of formation and resorption at any one time. Furthermore, symptomatic deposits may persist, and post-calcific tendinitis and its biomechanical consequences may develop to the extent that intervention is warranted.

Composition

The precise composition of the calcific deposit is not fully known. Infrared spectroscopy has revealed variable concentrations of water, carbonate and phosphate, but there are no significant differences in composition in either the acute or chronic stages of the disease. Studies using X-ray diffraction revealed poorly crystallized hydroxyapatites lattice in both. With no apparent differences in either the crystal lattice or chemical composition, it has been suggested that the initiating factor for phagocytosis – and hence the resorptive phase – is a change in the bonding capacity between the organic molecules.[28]

Clinical presentation

The clinical presentation is dependent on the phase of the disease process. In the formative phase the process is hypovascular and thus lacks the cellular component of the disease. The intratendinous pressure will therefore not be significantly raised. In these individuals there may be no pain; indeed, Bosworth reported that 65.4% of 202 calcific deposits were symptom-free.[7] If present, symptoms are usually mild and consist of a painful arc syndrome of varying intensity. Pain is often poorly localized and may be referred down the arm or into the neck. Night pain is also reported.

The acute onset of pain is believed to occur during the resorptive phase of the disease. An increase in the vascular and cellular components of the lesion results in a raised intratendinous pressure such that the condition may be comparable to a sterile abscess. As resorption continues the resultant oedema gives rise to pain,[2,26,27] which is often so severe and incapacitating that no shoulder movement is tolerated and the arm is held in a position of adduction and internal rotation. The pain is usually localized to a specific site of the shoulder and is of shorter duration than the chronic form, with symptoms often settling after 2–3 weeks. Systemic symptoms including malaise and fever have been reported,[29,30] and there may be an elevated erythrocyte sedimentation rate and neutrophilia.[30] Residual pain after this period has been termed the subacute stage, and may persist for 1–6 months.[11]

The clinical course of this disease demonstrates a cycle rather than two separate entities. Recognition of this, and accurate determination as to where the patient is in the cycle, is imperative in establishing the correct treatment protocol.

Investigations

Radiography

The identification and localization of calcific deposits using radiographs was first reported in 1907 and remains the main mode of investigation.[5] The radiological appearances of the deposits vary during their clinical course (Figure 25.1) and can be linked to changes in

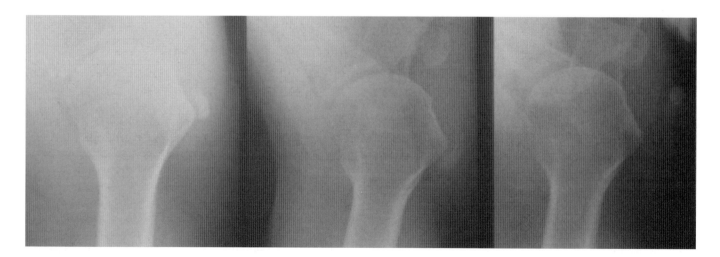

Figure 25.1

Serial radiographs demonstrating resorption of a calcific deposit.

the clinical presentation of the disease process. The size of a calcific deposit may also vary, but this appears to have little bearing on the symptoms associated with calcific tendinitis unless the size of the lesion causes secondary impingement.

Anteroposterior films are required, with the arm in neutral, internal rotation and external rotation.[7,31] An axillary view, taken perpendicular to these films, can also prove helpful in locating the deposit. A lateral view in the scapular plane[32] and outlet views[33,34] have also been recommended. Failure to take a full series of films may result in deposits being missed at both the diagnostic and therapeutic stages of management.

Calcific lesions in the supraspinatus tendon are most easily seen on the neutral or internal rotation films (Figure 25.2). Infraspinatus and teres minor lesions require radiographs taken with the arm in internal rotation, and subscapularis deposits with the arm in external rotation.

Ultrasound

Ultrasonography has a role in both the diagnosis and localization of a calcific deposit prior to needling, or excision.[35] Deposits can be identified as a hypoechogenic signal. This is helpful in determining the presence of all forms of calcific deposit but may be of particular benefit when investigating lesions in their acute phase, as these may be unclear on plain radiographs.

Magnetic resonance imaging

Deposits can be identified on T_1-weighted images as areas of decreased signal intensity with 95% accuracy (Figure 25.3).[15] Their location can be verified by analysing images taken in two perpendicular planes. In contrast, T_2-weighted images may reveal a perifocal band of increased signal intensity around the calcific deposit. This is suggestive of oedema, and if there is additional evidence of a partial or full-thickness rotator cuff tear subacromial impingement may also be present.

Differential diagnosis

Periarticular calcifications are not necessarily specific for calcific tendinitis. Dystrophic calcifications, characterized by small flecks of calcific material just above the greater tuberosity, may be associated with degenerative processes including cuff tear arthropathy and the neuropathic shoulder. Partial or full-thickness tears of the rotator cuff can further complicate the diagnostic process.

In chronic cases the diagnosis of calcific tendinitis may be complicated by the development of a subacromial spur or enthesophyte. This may further compound the clinical symptoms and signs of the condition owing to the presence of secondary impingement.

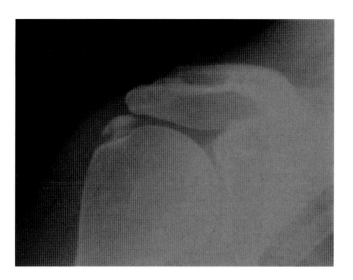

Figure 25.2
Anteroposterior view demonstrating a supraspinatus deposit.

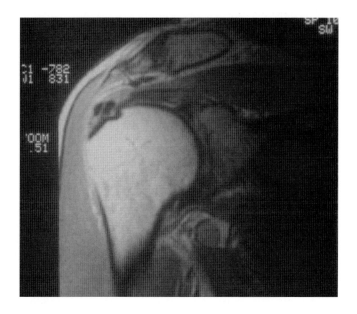

Figure 25.3
Magnetic resonance T_1-weighted image.

Classification

Several classifications have been proposed based on both the clinical and radiographic features of the disease.

Clinical

Clinically the condition is often divided into two groups, acute and chronic.[6] In practice these groups may be so distinct that it questions Uhthoff's concept that these are different stages of the same pathological cycle.

During the chronic initial phase, a calcific deposit is gradually formed within the tendon. This phase may result in minimal but prolonged clinical symptoms. As the calcific deposit undergoes resorption, the acute painful phase develops, due to the raised intratendinous pressure which follows the oedema and proliferative phase of the disease process.[26,27] A subacute type has also been reported.[6,11]

Radiographic

Bosworth based the earliest radiological classification system on size.[7] However, the radiological appearances of the calcific lesions were later categorized into two groups: type I (amorphous), and type II (homogenous).[11] It was the observation that these structural characteristics could be linked to the clinical presentation of the disease[1,27] that led to the more modern classification systems.

Gärtner proposed a radiographic classification in which the calcific lesions are graded into three types.[36] Type I lesions are clearly circumscribed and have a dense appearance; pain is an inconsistent feature. Type III deposits have a translucent or cloudy appearance and are usually associated with resorption and pain that can persist for 2–3 weeks. When the deposit does not clearly fall into one of these categories and demonstrates features of both type I and type III lesions, it is classified as type II. The percentage distribution of these lesions is type I 18%, type II 42% and type III 40%.

The French Arthroscopic Society[37] has also introduced a classification system that has been widely used, particularly in Europe (Table 25.1). Types A and C are similar to the type I and III lesions as proposed by Gärtner; however, the type B deposit is more precisely defined as multilobular. A type D has also been introduced for dystrophic calcifications. It is still unclear whether these morphologies are distinct or transitional phases, hence limiting their value in assessing outcome. We have adopted this classification because its definition of the type B deposit is more precise than the corresponding

Gärtner type II deposit. This is important as this subgroup of deposits accounts for 42–60% of all lesions.[36,38,39]

Non-operative treatment

Once a diagnosis has been established the need for treatment must be clarified. Treatment options are based on the presenting clinical features and on the understanding of the pathological process.

Conservative

Longitudinal studies have reported that chronic calcific tendinitis may last for years but is often self-limiting and may resolve spontaneously without any intervention.[7,27,40] However, pain associated with the acute form of the disease may be so severe that shoulder immobilization is necessary. Once the pain has subsided shoulder mobility should be encouraged. Pain in all phases of the disease may require the use of non-steroidal anti-inflammatory drugs.

Physiotherapy and pulsed ultrasound treatment can be used to maintain and improve function. Ultrasound has been shown to be a viable method of treatment in chronic calcific tendinitis where clearly circumscribed calcium deposits were seen.[41] In a prospective randomized trial, Ebenbichler et al reported that after 24 treatment sessions, each lasting 15 minutes, early improvements in both shoulder function and in the radiological resolution of the deposit were possible.[41] However, little difference was seen between those managed with or without pulsed ultrasound at 9 months following treatment. This approach may be impractical for some patients because of the lengthy period of treatment required.

Temporary relief of shoulder pain may be achieved with local anaesthetic injections into the subacromial

Table 25.1 French Arthroscopic Society radiographic classification

	Radiographic appearance		
	Shape	Texture	Borders
Type A	Unilobular	Dense	Clearly circumscribed
Type B	Multilobular	Dense	Clearly circumscribed
Type C	Irregular	Translucent or cloudy	Ill-defined

bursa. The addition of corticosteroids is commonly advocated to decrease the secondary inflammatory response of the bursa.

Extracorporeal shock-wave therapy

Single-impulse acoustic waves can be used to achieve disintegration of the calcareous deposit. In a controlled, prospective trial of 100 patients Rompe et al[42] used either low- or high-energy shock waves to achieve complete disintegration of the deposits in 50% and 64% of the patients respectively. Clinically, this translated as 52% of the low-energy group and 68% of the high-energy group reporting results of 'good' or 'excellent' after 24 weeks' follow-up. However, no improvement was reported in 24% of the low-energy group and 10% of the high-energy group. Similar results have been reported by others,[43] with the conclusion that this treatment may have a role in the management of chronic pain due to calcific tendinitis in those who are resistant to conservative measures.

Semi-invasive puncture techniques

Needle irrigation has been advocated as a means of facilitating the natural resorption of the calcific deposit. Various techniques involving needle irrigation[29] and multiple needle punctures[8,11] of the calcific deposits have been advocated. More recently, needle irrigation with the aid of fluoroscopic guidance has been suggested,[12,17,44] and its use with ultrasound guidance is currently being evaluated (Figure 25.4).

Once the calcific deposit has been located local anaesthetic solution is administered to the subcutaneous tissue, muscle and bursa immediately over the point of maximal tenderness. Needle irrigation is performed by inserting an 18-gauge needle into the centre of the calcific deposit and injecting small amounts of saline. Subsequent aspiration may result in plumes of the calcific deposit appearing in the aspirate, confirming accurate needle placement. The ruptured deposit is then repeatedly distended and aspirated until as much calcific material is removed as possible.[17] The use of more than one syringe has also been advocated.[44]

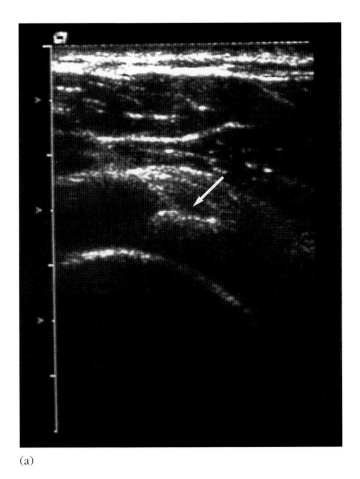

(a)

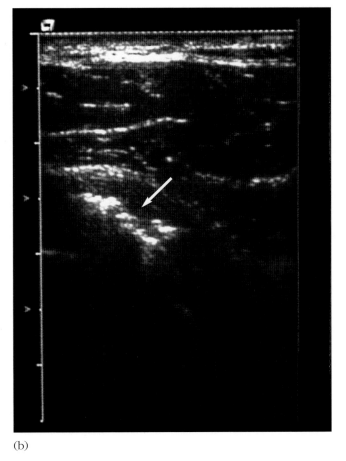

(b)

Figure 25.4

(a) Ultrasonographic localization of calcific deposit; (b) calcium liberated from deposit after needling.

Using a single syringe technique, Pfister and Gerbar reported that they were able to aspirate calcareous material in 47 of 62 cases (76%) of chronic calcifying tendinitis.[17] There was a clear reduction in the size of the deposit 2 months after the procedure and a 50% reduction in the pain after 6 months. Failure of this procedure was postulated as an indication for surgical intervention.

Gärtner compared the outcome of needling procedures with the radiological classification of the deposit.[36] Type II deposits responded most favourably, with resolution of the symptoms and resorption of the deposit occurring in 50% of cases. Type III lesions underwent complete resorption in 85% of cases, although these were already in their resorptive phase. Complete resorption was only seen in 33% of type I lesions. Needling was therefore only advocated for type II lesions.

Following needling procedures it is thought that the resulting hyperaemia enhances dissolution and absorption of any of the remaining calcific material.[11] The additional use of corticosteroid injections has been suggested,[12,17] but others claim the outcome was not affected by its inclusion.[8,13] Indeed, intratendinous injection of corticosteroid may weaken the rotator cuff[45] and its anti-inflammatory properties may prevent the resorption of the calcareous material.

Surgical principles

Arthroscopic treatment

The most common indication for operative treatment is chronicity. If pain has persisted for more than 1 year and non-operative management has failed, intervention should be considered. Indeed, non-operative treatment is reported to be satisfactory in only 50% of cases.[46] In the acute form of calcific tendinitis, attention must be given to the phase of the disease, as Uhthoff has shown that intervention during the resorptive phase of the disease is rarely indicated.[47] However, if the resorptive phase produces excessive pain immediate intervention is indicated and can be gratifying to both patient and surgeon alike. Intervention may also be necessary in patients presenting with subacromial impingement due to distortion of the supraspinatus tendon.

Arthroscopic technique

Arthroscopic techniques provide the best means with which to remove the calcific deposit, but they can be technically demanding. A full clinical and radiological evaluation of the shoulder is therefore necessary to determine the nature of the deposit, its location and any other associated pathologic changes such as secondary spur formation.

We advocate the use of an interscalene block in all cases of shoulder arthroscopy. Intravenous sedation or general anaesthesia can be added as necessary, but is rarely indicated. A beach-chair position is favoured, permitting easy internal and external rotation of the shoulder during the procedure. A standard posterior portal for glenohumeral arthroscopy is used. The glenohumeral joint is assessed for any associated, or unsuspected, pathological condition, and the undersurface of the rotator cuff is then examined.

The arthroscope is then reinserted into the subacromial bursa through the same posterior portal. Clean entry into the bursa is essential to facilitate clear visualization of the bursal and acromial surfaces. Subacromial bursoscopy is performed without a bursectomy, although some clinicians advocate its use.[32,34] In the presence of hypertrophic bursitis, visualization of a calcific deposit can be improved by minimal debridement of the subacromial bursa, using a power shaver through a lateral portal positioned 1 cm posterior and 4 cm lateral to the anterior lateral edge of the acromion. When inserting the instrument, aim towards the surface of the lateral acromion to facilitate entry into the bursa. An arthroscopic pump is used with the pressure and flow set at a level that permits adequate visualization but does not encourage excessive postoperative swelling and tissue oedema.

A thorough examination should be made of the bursal surface of the rotator cuff and the undersurface of the acromion for the presence of an impingement lesion. Next, the bursal surface of the rotator cuff can be more closely examined for the presence of a calcific deposit. Rotation and forward flexion of the arm during the examination is helpful, particularly for lesions located on the anterior aspect of the cuff.

Calcific deposits vary in appearance. Superficial deposits appear as a single, or multilocular, yellowish-white mass just deep to the bursal layer of the rotator cuff (Figure 25.5). There may be an area of hyperaemia with associated vascular proliferation, but widespread bursitis is uncommon. In many cases there may only be a few whitish spots, or a slight alteration in the colour of the tendon, making localization more difficult. These calcifications are sometimes more easily located by lightly probing the cuff. Chalky deposits can be felt in this manner, although their presence may only be located with the aid of extra preoperative planning.

Occasionally a calcific deposit located deep within the supraspinatus tendon may only be identifiable from the articular surface of the rotator cuff. Large calcific deposits can cause chondral erosions of the humeral head (Figure 25.6); alternatively, there may be an area of localized synovitis on the articular side of the involved tendon. Snyder referred to this as the 'strawberry lesion'.[48] To locate the lesion from the bursal side, a spinal needle can be passed from the lateral edge of the acromion into the rotator cuff such that the needle passes through the calcific deposit. Once the needle has been accurately placed a suture can be passed down the needle lumen (Figure 25.7). When this is seen entering the articular side

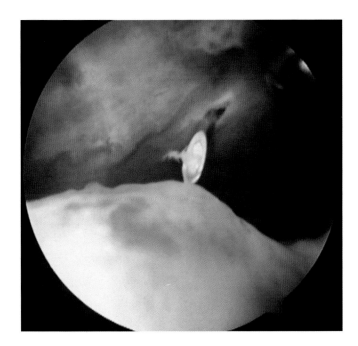

Figure 25.5
Superficial calcific deposit.

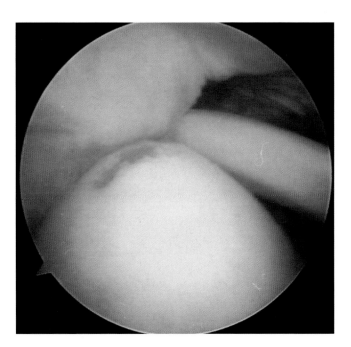

Figure 25.6
Chondral erosion of humeral head.

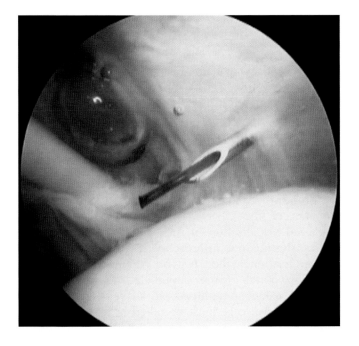

Figure 25.7
Placement of marker suture.

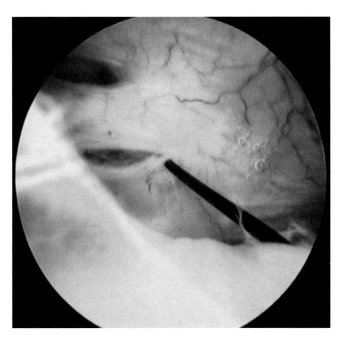

Figure 25.8
Marker suture traversing the subacromial bursa and entering the cuff.

of the joint the needle can be removed, leaving the suture within the tendon. Subsequent bursoscopy, and identification of the marking suture, will help reveal the deposit deep within the supraspinatus tendon (Figure 25.8).

Care must be taken to locate all the deposits as more than one may be present. Deposits within the supraspinatus tendon are most easily seen by placing the arm in external rotation. A secondary lesion can be present in the infraspinatus tendon in 15–20% of cases.[38] These lesions are most easily located with the arm in internal rotation. Subscapularis lesions are rare. The arthroscopic instrumentation of these deposits is difficult and may be more easily achieved using anterolateral and anteromedial portals.[16]

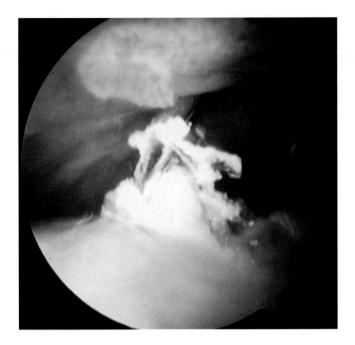

Figure 25.9

Needle liberation: the 'snowstorm' effect.

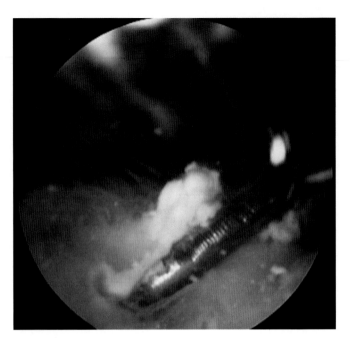

Figure 25.10

Paste-like calcium release.

Needling and lavage

Superficial deposits can be released by needling the lesion. An 18-gauge spinal needle is passed from the lateral end of the acromion under the direct view of the arthroscopist. Single or multiple passes of the needle can release the calcareous material into the subacromial bursa. Jerosch et al reported that as few as 17.5% of cases may demonstrate visual evidence of the calcific deposit on bursoscopy alone.[34] Needling suspected areas, as predicted by preoperative radiographic evaluation, may therefore be the only way of determining the location of these deposits. The periphery of calcific deposits can also be needled. This is believed to create new vascular channels that facilitate the resorption of any remaining material,[33] and also help the reparative process.

The appearance of the calcific material is dependent on the phase of the resorptive process. Chronic lesions appear as a granular conglomerate when seen as a dry specimen. Under arthroscopic conditions needling may result in plumes of liberated calcium that float freely into the subacromial space creating a 'snowstorm' effect (Figure 25.9). A more creamy or toothpaste-like consistency is indicative of an acute (resorptive) state (Figure 25.10). This type of deposit is often more difficult to release and may require encouragement by 'milking' the material out, pressing the angle of an arthroscopic probe, or indeed the convexity of a small curette, around the site of the collection. A mixed picture is also possible during cases of active resorption and is reported in 10–15% of cases.[38]

Curettage

Calcific deposits that are resistant to simple needling may require further debridement by means of curettage. These are often chronic deposits with a chalk-like consistency. An arthroscopic probe is introduced into the cavity containing the deposit and then longitudinal sweeps of the probe can be used to split the tendon in the line of its fibres, giving greater access to the deposit. This causes minimal damage to the cuff, and the probe (or curette) can then be used to remove the contents of the cavity (Figure 25.11). To aid this, improved visualization of the 'crater' can be achieved by transferring the arthroscope to the lateral portal. Further instrumentation can be continued through the posterior portal. Large superficial deposits can be debrided using an arthroscopic shaver (Figures 25.12 and 25.13), but care must be taken to avoid damaging sound cuff tissue.

Incision

Deeper deposits may be inaccessible by this technique and may only be reached by incising the overlying cuff.[16,32] A double-sided Beaver™ blade (Beaver, Becton, Dickinson & Co., Franklin Lakes, NJ, USA) can be used to create small longitudinal incisions in the tendon directly over the calcific deposit. Curettage of the underlying cavity can be performed to evacuate any remaining calcareous material. Horizontal and full-thickness incisions of the tendon should be avoided to preserve the integrity of the rotator cuff.

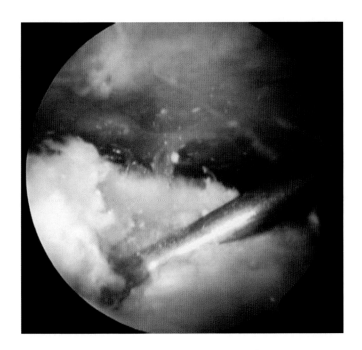

Figure 25.11

Arthroscopic probe liberation of calcium.

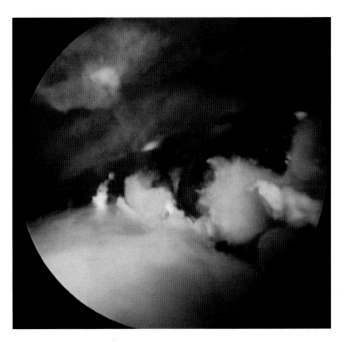

Figure 25.12

Arthroscopic shaver debridement.

Deposits observed during glenohumeral arthroscopy, and identified with a marking suture, can be excised from the acromial side of the cuff. A small incision in the line of the tendon fibres is made and deepened as the marker suture is followed down into the tendon. Once identified, the deposit should be completely excised by curettage. In the case of multilocular deposits a spinal needle can be used to locate other deposits. Despite adequate preoperative investigation, and diligent exploration at the time of the procedure, some deeper deposits may prove difficult to locate. For these lesions intraoperative fluoroscopy may be useful.

Thorough irrigation is believed to be an important factor in the management of this condition, as the calcific material is believed to have an irritant effect on the bursa. Irrigation can be aided by suction lavage. Failure to remove the calcific material from the subacromial space is believed to inflame the bursa and result in a hyperalgesic crisis, which is observed in 10–15% of cases.[38]

Subacromial decompression

There has been a long-standing question as to whether subacromial decompression should be performed at the same stage as arthroscopic excision of the calcific deposit. A multicentre study reported a series of 295 cases of calcific tendinitis treated by calcific excision and acromioplasty, isolated calcific excision, or isolated acromioplasty.[40] It was concluded that acromioplasty did not improve functional results. These findings are supported by other studies.[34,40] However, a prospective

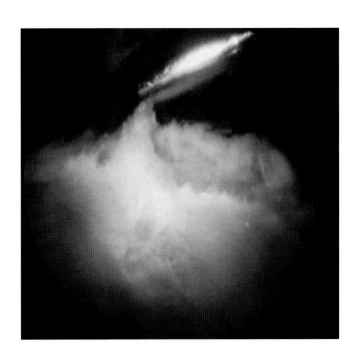

Figure 25.13

Crater formation during debridement.

randomized trial involving 99 shoulders has demonstrated a greater improvement in postoperative function when acromioplasty was undertaken in patients who demonstrated a type C lesion radiographically.[40]

It is our feeling that the primary objective in managing calcific tendinitis is to remove the deposit.

However, release of the coroacromial ligament is sometimes indicated. Presence of the calcific deposit causes oedema within the tendon; with large calcific deposits there may also be a degree of mechanical impingement on the overlying coracoacromial arch. Resection of the coracoacromial ligament encourages the free excursion of the humeral head during the postoperative recovery phase. Detachment of the coracoacromial ligament may also facilitate localization of deposits within the anterior aspect of the supraspinatus and subscapularis tendons.

Subacromial decompression may be indicated in patients who demonstrate an alteration in acromial morphology, such as spur formation and a type III acromion.[49] Usually these cases demonstrate clear evidence of impingement. Furthermore, if a partial-thickness rotator cuff tear is identified in association with an impingement lesion, functional outcome has been shown to improve following an arthroscopic subacromial decompression.[50] We also advocate the use of subacromial decompression in patients in whom a calcific lesion has been confirmed radiographically, but no deposit can be found at arthroscopy. Other authors support this view.[33]

Rotator cuff tears

Calcific tendinitis and rotator cuff tears are two separate clinical entities but they may coexist. The incidence of this is variable. In a series of 295 shoulders undergoing arthroscopy for calcific tendinitis, 4% were reported to have either a complete or an intratendinous tear at the time of arthroscopy.[40] Similar incidences have also been reported.[15] However, using arthroscopy Hsu et al investigated a series of 82 patients from Taiwan with calcific tendinitis and reported a surprisingly high incidence of 28%.[14] Although ethnic factors may account for some of this difference, the study concluded that the presence of a cuff tear was linked to the radiographic nature of the deposit, with 77.9% of patients in the non-tear group demonstrating deposits that had an ill-defined and 'moth-eaten' appearance.

Postoperative protocol

Although the use of regional anaesthesia necessitates the use of a sling immediately postoperatively, an interscalene block does allow passive exercises to be initiated early in the postoperative course. Active, and active assisted, exercises in forward flexion and external rotation are encouraged thereafter. Isometric exercises are deferred for 6 weeks, or until the pain has settled.

This postoperative physiotherapy regimen is aimed at restoring shoulder mobility and preventing postoperative complications such as adhesive capsulitis. In patients suffering calcific tendinitis, adhesive capsulitis has been reported in 6–20% of shoulders following glenohumeral arthroscopy.[10] We feel that this incidence could be reduced during needling procedures by avoiding the introduction of the needle into the articular side of the joint. This can inadvertently introduce calcific material into the glenohumeral joint, which may result in irritation, pain and eventually a frozen shoulder.

Open surgery

We believe that open techniques are rarely, if ever, indicated. Open surgery is associated with longer postoperative recovery times, longer periods of hospitalization and worse cosmesis. However, open procedures may have a role in the surgical management of calcific tendinitis if the expertise for arthroscopic excision is not available. Furthermore, inaccessible deposits located within the subscapularis tendon may require an open approach using a deltopectoral incision.

It has been postulated that calcific deposits should be excised with a cuff of tendinous tissue.[18] This is technically difficult to perform arthroscopically, and there is little evidence to support tendon debridement and suture repair of the cuff either arthroscopically or using open techniques.

Conclusion

When calcific tendinitis does not display its normal self-limiting course, the use of arthroscopic excision can be a relatively non-invasive technique in dealing with this enigmatic condition. The risk of causing adhesive capsulitis, with its associated morbidity, must be balanced against the technical satisfaction and therapeutic benefits of locating and dispersing the calcific material. Management of this condition can therefore be both frustrating and challenging.

Although technical tips to achieve the therapeutic aims are provided here, the role of acromioplasty remains controversial. Its use is advocated where distortion of the supraspinatus tendon has led to secondary effects in the coracoacromial arch, in particular the formation of an impingement lesion or bony spur.

Acknowledgements

The authors thank Dr S Burnett, MRCP FRCR, consultant radiologist at St Mary's Hospital, London, for the ultrasound images reproduced here.

References

1. Sandstrom C. Peritendinitis calcarea: a common disease of middle life: its diagnosis, pathology and treatment. *Am J Roentgenol* 1938; **40**:1–21.
2. Pinals RS, Short CL. Calcific periarthritis involving multiple sites. *Arthr Rheum* 1966; **9**:566–74.
3. Holt PD, Keats TE. Calcific tendinitis: a review of the usual and unusual. *Skeletal Radiol* 1993; **22**:1–9.
4. Duplay S. De la periarthrite scapulo–humerale et des raideurs de l'epaule qui en sont la consequence. *Arch Gen Med* 1872; **2**:513–42.
5. Painter CF. Subdeltoid bursitis. *Boston Med Surg J* 1907; **156**:345–9.
6. Codman EA. *The Shoulder*. Boston: Thomas Todd, 1934.
7. Bosworth BM. Calcium deposits in the shoulder and subacromial bursitis: a survey of 12 122 shoulders. *JAMA* 1941; **116**:2477–82.
8. Harmon PH. Methods and results in the treatment of 2580 painful shoulders with special reference to calcific tendinitis and the frozen shoulder. *Am J Surg* 1958; **95**:527–44.
9. Reifor HJ, Krodel A, Melzer C. Examinations of the pathology of the rotator cuff. *Arch Orthop Trauma Surg* 1987; **106**:301–8.
10. Molé D. Calcifying tendinopathies. Proceedings of the European Symposium of the Shoulder (SECEC), St Etienne, France 1996; 200–1.
11. DePalma AF, Kruper JS. Long term study of shoulder joints afflicted with and treated for calcific tendinitis. *Clin Orthop* 1961; **20**:61–72.
12. Lippmann RK. Observations concerning the calcific cuff deposits. *Clin Orthop* 1961; **20**:49–60.
13. Friedman MS. Calcified tendinitis of the shoulder. *Am J Surg* 1957; **94**:56–61.
14. Hsu H, Wu J, Jim Y et al. Calcific tendinitis and rotator cuff tearing: a clinical and radiographic study. *J Shoulder Elbow Surg* 1994; **3**:159–64.
15. Loew M, Sabo D, Wehrle M, Mau H. Relationship between calcifying tendinitis and subacromial impingement: a prospective radiography and magnetic resonance imaging study. *J Shoulder Elbow Surg* 1996; **5**:314–19.
16. Molé D, Roche O, Sirveaux F. Removal techniques for calcific deposits. Proceedings of the Second Advanced Course on Shoulder Arthroscopy (SECEC), Val d'Isère, France, 1998; 90–8.
17. Pfister J, Gerber H. Chronic calcifying tendinitis of the shoulder. Therapy by percutaneous needle aspiration and lavage: a prospective open study of 62 shoulders. *Clin Rheumatol* 1997; **16**:269–74.
18. Litchman HM, Silver CM, Siman SD, Eshragi A. The surgical management of calcific tendinitis of the shoulder. An analysis of 100 consecutive cases. *Int Surg* 1968; **50**:474–9.
19. McKendry RJR, Uhthoff HK, Sarkar K, George-Hyslop P. Calcifying tendinitis of the shoulder: prognostic value of clinical, histologic and radiologic features in 57 surgically treated cases. *J Rheumatol* 1982;**9**:75–80.
20. Steinbrocker O. The painful shoulder. In: Hollander JE, ed. *Arthritis and Allied Conditions*, 8th edn. Philidelphia: Lea & Febiger, 1972. 1461–510.
21. Moseley HF, Goldie I. The arterial pattern of the rotator cuff of the shoulder. *J Bone Joint Surg* 1963; **45B**:780–9.
22. Rothman RH, Parke WW. The vascular anatomy of the rotator cuff. *Clin Orthop* 1965; **41**:176–86.
23. Rathbun JB, Macnab J. The microvascular pattern of the rotator cuff. *J Bone Joint Surg* 1970; **52B**:540–53.
24. Nutton RW, Stothard J. Acute calcific tendinitis in a three year old child. *J Bone Joint Surg* 1987; **69B**:148.
25. Cannon RB, Schmid FR. Calcific periarthritis involving multiple sites in identical twins. *Arthr Rheum* 1973; **16**:393–6.
26. Uhtoff HK, Sarkar K, Maynard J. Calcifying tendinitis. A new concept of its pathogenesis. *Clin Orthop* 1976; **118**:164–8.
27. McLaughlin HL. Lesions of the musculotendinous cuff of the shoulder: III. Observations of the pathology, course and treatment of calcific deposits. *Ann Surg* 1946; **124**:354–62.
28. Gärtner J, Simons B. Analysis of calcific deposits in calcifying tendinitis. *Clin Orthop* 1990; **254**:111–20.
29. Patterson RL, Darrach W. Treatment of acute bursitis by needle irrigation. *J Bone Joint Surg* 1937; **19**:993–1002.
30. Speed CA, Hazleman BL. Calcific tendinitis of the shoulder. *N Engl J Med* 1999; **340**:1582–4.
31. ViGario GD, Keats TE. Localization of calcific deposits in the shoulder. *Am J Roentgenol* 1970; **108**:806–11.
32. Ark JW, Flock TJ, Flatow EL, Bigliani LU. Arthroscopic treatment of calcific tendinitis of the shoulder. *Arthroscopy* 1992; **8**:183–8.
33. Ellman H, Gartsman GM. *Arthroscopic Shoulder Surgery and Related Procedures*. Philadelphia: Lea & Febiger, 1993. 219–32.
34. Jerosch J, Strauss JM, Schmiel S. Arthroscopic treatment of calcific tendinitis of the shoulder. *J Shoulder Elbow Surg* 1998; **7**:30–7.
35. Rupp S, Seil R, Kohn D. Preoperative ultrasonographic mapping of calcium deposits facilitates localization during arthroscopic surgery for calcifying tendinitis of the rotator cuff. *Arthroscopy* 1998; **14**:540–2.
36. Gärtner J. Tendinosis calcarea – Behandlungsergebnisse mit dem Needling. *Z Orthop* 1993; **131**:461–9.
37. Molé D, Kempf JF, Gleyze P et al. Résultats du traitement arthroscopique des tendinopathies non rompues de la coiffe des rotateurs. 2: les calcifications de la coiffe des rotateurs. *Rev Chir Orth Rep* 1993; **79**:532–41.
38. Kempf JF. Arthroscopic treatment of rotator cuff calcifications by isolated excision. Proceedings of the European Symposium of the Shoulder (SECEC), St Etienne, France, 1996; 206–8.
39. Porcellini G, Campi F, Paladini P. Arthroscopic treatment of calcifying tendinitis of the shoulder: clinical and ultrsonographic findings. Proceedings of the European Society for Surgery of the Shoulder and the Elbow, Windsor, UK, 2001. Paper no. 25, 77.
40. Kempf JF, Molé D. Arthroscopic isolated excision of rotator cuff calcium deposits. Proceedings of the Second Advanced Course on Shoulder Arthroscopy (SECEC), Val d'Isère, France, 1998; 93–8.
41. Ebenbichler GB, Erdogmus CB, Resch KL et al. Ultrasound therapy for calcific tendinitis of the shoulder. *N Engl J Med* 1999; **340**:1533–8.
42. Rompe JD, Burger R, Hopf C, Eysel P. Shoulder function after extracorporeal shock wave therapy for calcific tendinitis. *J Shoulder Elbow Surg* 1998; **7**:505–9.
43. Loew M, Daecke W, Kusnierczak D et al. Shock-wave therapy is effective for chronic calcifying tendinitis of the shoulder. *J Bone Joint Surg* 1999; **81B**:863–7.
44. Comfort TH, Arafiles RP. Barbotage of the shoulder with image intensified fluoroscopic control of needle placement for calcific tendinitis. *Clin Orthop* 1978; **135**:171–8.
45. Kennedy JC, Willis RB. The effects of local steroid injections on tendons: a biomechanical and microscopic correlative study. *Am J Sports Med* 1976; **4**:11–21.
46. Noel E, Brantus JF. Les tendinopathies calcifantes de la coiffe des rotateurs: treatment médical a propos de 124 épaules. *J Lyonn Epaule* 1993; **547**:199–213.
47. Uhtoff HK. Calcifying tendinitis. *Ann Chir Gynaecol* 1996; **85**:111–15.
48. Snyder SJ. Arthroscopic evaluation and treatment of calcifications around the shoulder. In: Snyder SJ, ed. *Shoulder Arthroscopy*. New York: McGraw-Hill, 1994. 215–27.
49. Bigliani LU, Morrisson DS, April EW. Morphology of the acromion and its relationship to rotator cuff tears. *Orthop Trans* 1986; **10**:459–61.
50. Falworth MS, Sforza G, Shariff S et al. Arthroscopic subacromial decompression in the treatment of partial thickness tears; clinical outcome in 120 patients. Proceedings of the 68th Annual Meeting of the AAOS, San Francisco, 2001; 619.

26 Acromioclavicular joint: Distal clavicle resection

Ariane Gerber and Christian Gerber

Introduction

Development of the procedure

Described independently by Mumford[1] and Gurd,[2] the open resection of the lateral clavicle is a well defined and widely used procedure to treat painful acromioclavicular (AC) arthropathies. Reliable pain relief has been reported after open lateral clavicle resection for AC joint osteoarthritis,[3] AC joint separation[4] and osteolysis of the lateral clavicle,[1,2,5] but long-lasting postoperative weakness has been described, especially in weight-lifting athletes.[4]

As a logical step in the successful development of therapeutic arthroscopy of the shoulder, the feasibility and the clinical potiential of arthroscopic AC joint resection has been evaluated. Ellman[6] and Esch et al[7] described approaching the AC joint from the subacromial space to remove inferior AC osteophytes after acromioplasty. However, recent studies[8,9] have shown that partial resection of the inferior capsule and inferior osteophytes or violation of an asymptomatic AC joint during acromioplasty can lead to substantial symptoms. Therefore the integrity of the joint capsule of asymptomatic AC joints should be preserved. On the other hand, if inferior osteophytes have to be removed for adequate acromioplasty, the AC joint should be resected completely.

Gartsman et al[10] showed in a cadaveric study that complete AC joint resection can be performed effectively and predictably by arthroscopy from a subacromial approach. Flatow et al[11] compared arthroscopic resection of the lateral clavicle through a superior approach with open resection. Although sastisfactory results have been presented by the same group,[12] the subacromial approach remains the standard approach for AC joint resection.

Clinical presentation and indication

The AC joint is a common site of shoulder pain related to idiopathic osteoarthritis, to secondary osteoarthritis after intra-articular fracture of the distal clavicle or AC joint separation or to osteolysis of the lateral clavicle after repetitive microtrauma as in heavy lifting and gymnastics.

Because painful AC arthropathy is very often associated with other disorders of the shoulder/neck region, the diagnosis can be difficult. As a matter of fact, failure to diagnose concomitant AC arthropathy is a common source of poor surgical results of shoulder surgery performed for other conditions. Pain over the AC joint, which radiates proximally in the anterolateral neck, in the trapezius–supraspinatus region, and in the anterolateral deltoid, associated with a significant or complete relief after injection of local anesthesia in the joint helps to confirm the diagnosis.[13] Symptoms at the AC joint do not correlate with its radiologic appearance.[14]

In patients with a chronic isolated painful AC joint we perform an X-ray-controlled AC joint infiltration with steroids and local anesthesia in a diagnostic and therapeutic attempt, and we can confirm that a good response to intra-articular injection predicts a good outcome (C Spormann and C Gerber, personal communication). In many patients such a procedure leads to definitive managment of the pain. In some cases pain relief is present for a limited period of time. Recurrence of pain to the same level within 2–4 weeks after infiltration is an indication for arthroscopic AC joint resection. In cases of recurrence of symptoms after 6 weeks or longer, we advise repetition of the injection. In patients in whom another (arthroscopic or open) procedure is planned and a concomitant AC arthropathy is present, the AC joint is resected.

Reported results

Many reports have demonstrated that symptomatic AC arthropathies can be treated effectively and safely with arthroscopic techniques. Bigliani et al[12] showed 90% excellent results after resection of stable painful AC joints through a superior approach. However, in patients with a painful AC joint after grade II AC joint separation, only 37% satisfactory results were obtained. Snyder et al[15] reported 94% excellent and good results after resection of the lateral clavicle through a subacromial approach. In a small series,[16] subacromial AC joint resection led to excellent subjective and functional results in all patients. Our own results are somewhat less favorable. The key information derived from our own study is that lateral clavicle resection of a painful AC joint with radiologic osteoarthritis has a significantly better outcome than excision of the lateral clavicle in a painful joint without radiological signs of osteoarthritis (C Spormann and C Gerber, personal communication).

Surgical principles

General considerations

The two important goals of AC joint resection are the removal of the pathologic clavicular articular surface and the articular disc, with the creation of enough space between the resected distal clavicle and the medial acromion to avoid painful contact between these bones for any movement of the shoulder. Whereas these goals are achieved by resection of the distal clavicle in an open procedure, a resection of the lateral clavicle is often associated with some shaving of the medial acromion. Doing so, the AC ligaments and the anterosupero-posterior joint capsule are preserved. As they are known to restrain the motion of the distal clavicle,[17,18] abutment between the acromion and the clavicle will not occur even if a smaller amount of bone has been resected.

Materials

The standard 4-mm arthroscopic equipment including a 30°-angled lens and an arthroscopic pump system (Linvatec Corp, Largo, FL, USA) are used. A 5.5-mm soft-tissue suction shaver (Linvatec 5.5-mm full radius resector; Figure 26.1), a 5.5-mm burr (Linvatec 5.5-mm spherical burr, Figure 26.1) and an electrosurgical pencil (Valleylab, Boulder, CO, USA or Mitek Surgical Products Inc, Westwood, MA, USA; Figure 26.2) are also intruments required for AC joint resection. Additionally, one or two 20-gauge puncture needles are used as marker pins. A normal saline solution with 1:3000 ephedrine added is employed.

Anesthesia and positioning

Regional anesthesia consisting of an interscalene brachial plexus block and maintained for up to 1–3 days postoperatively with a catheter is used whenever possible. This technique allows intraoperative analgesia and relaxation of the operated arm and is an efficient method for postoperative pain control.[19,20] AC joint resection can principally be achieved in a sitting (beach-chair) or lateral position. As we routinely perform shoulder arthroscopy in a lateral decubitus position and AC joint resection through a subacromial approach, the following description will deal exclusively with these modalities.

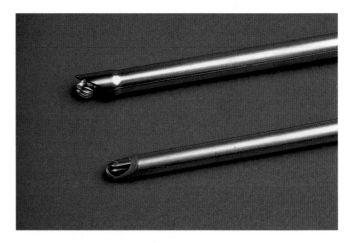

Figure 26.1
Linvatec 5.5 mm full radius resector and 5.5 mm spherical burr.

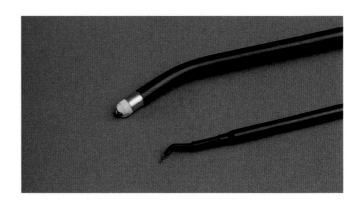

Figure 26.2
Valleylab and Mitek VAPR electrosurgical pencils.

Complications and technical problems

Intraoperative and postoperative complications are rare for shoulder arthroscopy generally. The most frequently encountered problem after AC joint resection is an inappropriate area and amount of bone resected leading to persisting pain. The key point for adequate resection is an optimal visualization of the anatomical landmarks given by:

1. Correct positioning of the portals;
2. Sufficient subacromial and intra-articular soft tissue debridement;
3. Systematic bone resection;
4. Meticulous hemostasis.

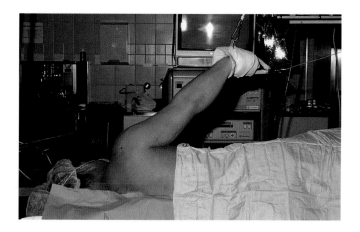

Figure 26.3

The patient is placed in a lateral position. The arm is placed in traction with 3–5 kg weight at 30° abduction.

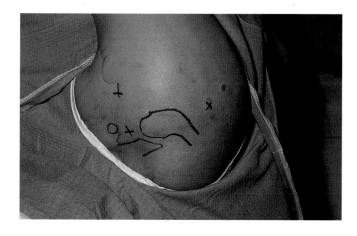

Figure 26.4

Glenohumeral arthroscopy, subacromial endoscopy and AC joint resection can be performed through three portals: the posterior arthroscope portal, with the anterolateral and anterior working portals.

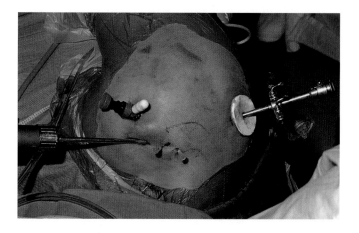

Figure 26.5

Note the two puncture needles to define the orientation of the AC joint.

Surgical technique

After the interscalene brachial plexus block has been set, the patient is placed in a lateral position on an inflatable bean bag covered with a silicon gel sheet allowing for stable and comfortable positioning. The arm is placed in traction with 3–5 kg weight at 30° abduction (Figure 26.3). Disinfection and draping are performed after definitive positioning of the patient.

Portals

A complete subacromial AC joint resection can be performed through three portals (Figure 26.4).

Posterior portal

This is the standard portal for the arthroscope in glenohumeral arthroscopy and is situated 2 cm below and 2 cm medial to the lateral scapular spine. For AC joint resection a too-medial position of this portal leads to a tangential view of the joint space and increased torque on the instrument is required to keep the joint in view.

Anterolateral portal

This portal lies 3–4 cm distally to the anterolateral corner of the acromion and is used mainly for subacromial bursectomy and landmark identification. Placing the portal too far distally can lead to a lesion of the axillary nerve.

Anterior portal

The AC joint resection is performed through this portal. For an even resection of the medial acromion and the distal clavicle the instrument must approach the joint space in line. If the portal is chosen too far laterally the intruments will approach the joint obliquely leading to excessive resection anteriorly and poor resection posteriorly. As the AC joint can show important individual variation of inclination, it is worthwhile to define the position of the joint with puncture needles and set the anterior portal just in front of and in line with the AC joint space (Figure 26.5).

Technique

Glenohumeral arthroscopy

A diagnostic glenohumeral arthroscopy and appropriate treatment of intra-articular lesions are performed in all patients.

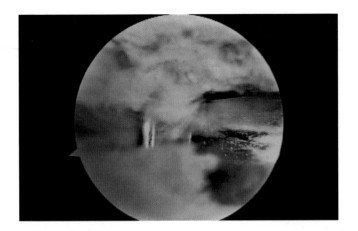

Figure 26.6

The puncture needles help in the identification of the AC joint.

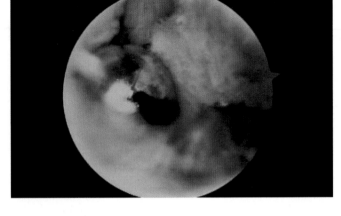

Figure 26.7

Resection of the inferior capsule with the shaver.

Subacromial endoscopy and debridement

After glenohumeral arthroscopy the arthroscope is withdrawn leaving the scope sheath in place. A blunt obturator is introduced. The instrument is then withdrawn from the joint while still remaining under the deltoid muscle. The sheath is aimed superiorly and advanced in the subacromial space. Shifting the instrument mediolaterally will open the subacromial space and facilitate initial identification for the shaver. The blunt obturator is removed and the arthroscope is inserted again. Fluid inflow is achieved through this sheath and the arthroscope, fluid outflow through the shaver.

A plastic canula with a round-tipped obturator is introduced through the anterolateral portal (Figure 26.5). The tip of the canula is directed upward to reach the subacromial space sliding over the rotator cuff. The next step consists in a systematic shaving of the subacromial bursa and allows identification of the anatomical landmarks. First the bursa is resected in the most posterior aspect of the subacromial space. As the shaving process progresses in the anterior direction, the inferior portion of the AC joint capsule appears and the anteromedial and anterolateral borders of the acromion become exposed. The puncture needles help in identification of the AC joint (Figure 26.6).

The subacromial bursa is a well-vascularized tissue and bleeding due to shaving may impair visualization. Other sources of hemorrhage are the AC branch of the thoracoacromial artery, which can be cut while identifying the anterior margin of the acromion, as well as muscular branches of the supraspinatus and infraspinatus. The most efficient way to control bleeding is the immediate identification of the bleeding vessels and coagulation with an electrosurgical pencil. The use of epinephrine (adrenaline) in the irrigation fluid, hypotensive anesthesia, the increase of pump pressure up to 100–120 mmHg or the interruption of the procedure for a few minutes

are other possibilities for controlling bleeding. Therapeutic procedures such as acromioplasty, cuff repair or removal of calcifications are performed if indicated.

AC joint resection

The shaver is introduced directly through the anterior portal (Figure 26.5). Before bony resection can be performed systematically, the medial border of the acromion and the lateral end of the clavicle have to be visualized. To do so, all soft tissues, including the inferior AC joint capsule and the intra-articular disc are removed, ensuring complete exposure of the most posterior, superior and anterior aspect of the joint while preserving the joint capsule and the ligaments there (Figures 26.7–26.9). Here too, bleeding vessels have to be coagulated immediately.

The burr is inserted anteriorly with the cutting area oriented to the lateral clavicle. A burr width (5.5 mm) of bone is resected from the inferior cortex of the clavicle. A constant amount of bone is removed taking care to preserve the posterior, superior and anterior part of the capsule (Figure 26.10).

The instrument is then oriented to the medial acromion and 2–3 mm of bone are resected (Figure 26.11). Finally an 8–10-mm wide space is created between the remaining lateral clavicle and the acromion so that the burr can be driven through the joint easily.

Prominent inferior and superior osteophytes from the lateral clavicle as well as the medial acromion are trimmed to avoid subacromial impingement and to restore a normal shoulder contour (Figure 26.12). The visualization and palpation of the posterior, superior and anterior capsule is the confirmation of a complete resection (Figure 26.13). Before the intruments are withdrawn irrigation is performed to clean the subacromial space of bony debris. The portals are closed with simple non-resorbable sutures.

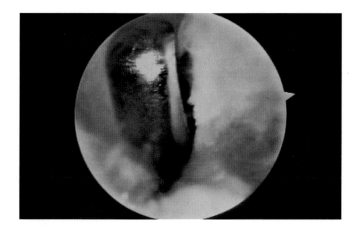

Figure 26.8

Resection of the intra-articular disc with the shaver.

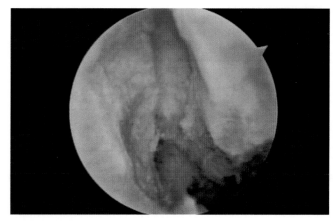

Figure 26.9

After soft tissue resection, exposure of the superior, anterior and posterior portions of the capsule is ensured.

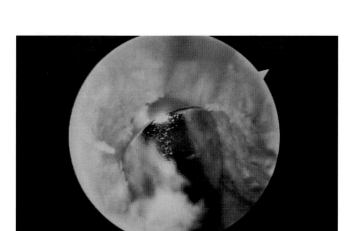

Figure 26.10

The burr is inserted anteriorly with the cutting area oriented to the lateral clavicle and a burr width (5.5 mm) of bone is resected.

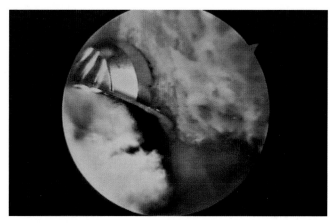

Figure 26.11

The instrument is then oriented to the medial acromion and 2-3 mm of bone are resected.

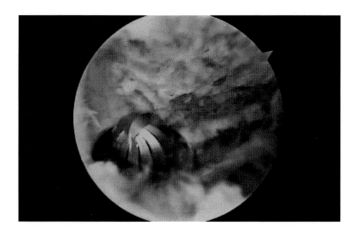

Figure 26.12

Prominent inferior osteophytes are trimmed.

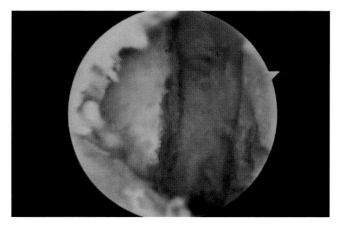

Figure 26.13

Visualization of the intact posterior, superior and anterior capsule is then confirmation of a complete resection.

Postoperative protocol

Arthroscopic AC joint resection is known to be less painful than open resection and can be performed principally as an ambulatory procedure. As long as a continuous regional anesthesia is used, the patients can take advantage of an almost complete analgesia for 1–2 days after the operation and will be instructed on a home exercice program during this time. Passive exerscises are started immediately after the operation and active movements as soon as the continous interscalene block has resolved. Strenghtening is started at 3 weeks and return to manual work, contact and upper extremity sports at 6–8 weeks.

References

1. Mumford E. Acromioclavicular dislocation. A new operative treatment. *J Bone Joint Surg* 1941; **23**:799–802.
2. Gurd F. The treatment of complete dislocation of the outer end of the clavicle. An hitherto undescribed operation. *Ann Surg* 1941; **113**:1094–8.
3. Worcester J, Green D. Osteoarthritis of the acromioclavicular joint. *Clin Orthop* 1968; **58**:69–73.
4. Cook F, Tibone J. The Mumford procedure in athletes. An objective analysis of function. *Am J Sports Med* 1988; **16**:97–100.
5. Cahill B. Osteolysis of the distal part of the clavicle in male athletes. *J Bone Joint Surg* 1982; **64A**:1053–8.
6. Ellman H. Arthroscopic subacromial decompression: analysis of 1–3 year results. *Arthroscopy* 1987; **3**:173–81.
7. Esch J, Ozerkis LR, Meigager JA et al. Arthroscopic subacromial decompression: results according to the degree of cuff tear. *Arthroscopy* 1988; **4**:241–9.
8. Fischer BW, Gross RM, McCarthy JA, Arroyo JS. Incidence of acromioclavicular joint complications after arthroscopic subacromial decompression. *Arthroscopy* 1999; **15**: 241–8.
9. Kuster M, Hales P, Davis S. The effects of arthroscopic acromioplasty on the acromioclavicular joint. *J Shoulder Elbow Surg* 1998; **7**:140–3.
10. Gartsman GM, Combs AH, Davis PF, Tullos HS. Arthroscopic acromioclavicular joint resection. An anatomical study. *Am J Sports Med* 1991; **19**:2–5.
11. Flatow E, Cordasco F, Bigliani L. Arthroscopic resection of the outer end of the clavicle from a superior approach: a critical, quantitative, radiographic assesment of bone removal. *Arthroscopy* 1992; **8**:55–64.
12. Bigliani L, Nicholson G, Flatow E. Arthroscopic resection of the distal clavicle. *Orthop Clin North Am* 1993; **24**:133–41.
13. Gerber C, Galantay R, Hersche O. The pattern of pain produced by irritation of the acromioclavicular joint and the subacromial space. *J Shoulder Elbow Surg* 1998; **7**:352–5.
14. Petersson C, Redlund-Johnell I. Radiographic joint space in normal acromioclavicular joints. *Acta Orthop Scand* 1983; **54**:431–3.
15. Snyder S, Banas M, Karzel R. The arthroscopic Mumford procedure: an analysis of the results. *Arthroscopy* 1995; **11**:157–64.
16. Kay S, Ellman H, Harris E. Arthroscopic distal clavicle excision. *Clin Orthop* 1994; **301**:181–4.
17. Fukuda K, Craig EV, An KN et al. Biomechanical study of the ligamentous system of the acromioclavicular joint. *J Bone Joint Surg* 1986; **68A**:434–40.
18. Branch TP, Burdette HL, Shahriari AS et al. The role of the acromioclavicular ligaments and the effect of distal clavicle resection. *Am J Sports Med* 1996; **24**:293–7.
19. Borgeat A, Schappi B, Biasca N, Gerber C. Patient-controlled analgesia after major shoulder surgery: patient-controlled interscalene analgesia versus patient-controlled analgesia. *Anesthesiology* 1997; **87**:1343–7.
20. Borgeat A, Tewes E, Biasca N, Gerber C. Patient-controlled interscalene analgesia with ropivacaine after major shoulder surgery: PCIA vs PCA. *Br J Anaesth* 1998; **81**:603–5.

Section V – Rotator cuff pathology

27 Mini-open rotator cuff repair

Vladimir Martinek and Andreas B Imhoff

Introduction

The treatment of rotator cuff lesions has improved since the 1980s as a consequence of new arthroscopic techniques, novel instruments and modern rehabilitation. Increasing knowledge about the biology of tendon healing and biomechanics of the shoulder, greater understanding of the clinical spectrum of rotator cuff pathology, and advancements in magnetic resonance imaging have led to a better understanding of rotator cuff disease and its treatment.

Rotator cuff tears present usually with impingement pain, night pain and loss of shoulder function. Since the incidence of rotator cuff tears increases from 11% in 60-year-olds to 50% in 70-year-olds and 80% in 80-year-olds, the degenerative rotator cuff lesion can be seen as the end result of an accelerated ageing process.[1] For this reason, many patients with a rotator cuff disorder can be successfully managed with conservative measures including physiotherapy to relieve pain. Operative treatment is reserved for physically active people with persistent symptoms. Although early satisfactory results are reported with debridement and subacromial decompression without rotator cuff repair in patients with full-thickness tears,[2] we do not support this management, especially in active persons. It results in recurrence of the symptoms and in progression of the tendon tear.

Since the benefits of subacromial decompression in patients with rotator cuff tears have been clearly demonstrated, this procedure should be an obligatory part of operative treatment.[3] In our management of the operative rotator cuff treatment, we combine the arthroscopic subacromial decompression with a mini-open rotator cuff repair using an anterolateral 4-cm split of the deltoid. This technique has advantages in comparison with both open and arthroscopic rotator cuff repair techniques. The arthroscopic approach allows an arthroscopic examination and treatment of associated intra-articular injuries of the labrum, articular cartilage or partial undersurface cuff tears, which is not possible with the classic open rotator cuff repair.[4] However, the most important benefit of the arthroscopic acromioplasty is preservation of the deltoid origin. Patients report reduced postoperative pain, and the intact deltoid muscle permits faster rehabilitation. Also, later catastrophic situations such as an anterosuperior glenohumeral instability or deltoid insufficiency are avoided. A completely arthroscopic rotator cuff repair is a procedure suitable for partial or minor rotator cuff tears. However, the stability of the repair is questionable, especially in cases with poor tendon quality and with retracted tendon edges requiring extended releases. In such cases an adequate mobilization of the entire rotator cuff is more important for the successful outcome than the better cosmetic result of the arthroscopic procedure. The reported results of the arthroscopically assisted mini-open rotator cuff repair are good to excellent in 84–94% of the cases.[5,6] These results are thus slightly better than the results obtained with open techniques. For large rotator cuff tendon tears requiring muscle transpositions, or in cases of isolated subscapularis tendon rupture, the classic open approach should be used for the rotator cuff reconstruction.[7,8]

Surgical principles

The four most important principles of a rotator cuff repair are (according to Neer[9]) the complete closure of the defect, the avoidance of an impingement underneath the coracoacromial arch, the preservation of the deltoid muscle insertion, and competent rehabilitation to prevent shoulder stiffness on one side and failure of the sutures on the other side. Besides these criteria, which must be fulfilled regardless of the chosen operative technique, biological considerations have to be taken into account by every surgeon who wants to be successful.

In general, degenerative rotator cuff lesions originate from a chronic lack of blood supply and insufficient nutrition at the tendon insertion site. In most cases, the tendon tissue at the area of the tear is of a poor quality. Although no vascularity is expected in this degenerative tissue, intraoperative ultrasound measurements showed blood flow reaching the edge of supraspinatus tendon tears, which macroscopically did not bleed.[10] For this reason, only the necrotic tissue from the end of a ruptured tendon should be excised, and excessive debridement of the tendon to the bleeding edge should be avoided. For the rotator cuff repair, a good mechanical quality of the tendon for secure placement of the traction sutures is far more important than a bleeding tendon end. The subdeltoid bursa should also not be removed completely, only what is necessary to ensure a good view of the rotator cuff tendons.[11]

The extra- and intra-articular mobilization of the retracted cuff is one of the key points of the procedure. Only a well-mobilized rotator cuff allows tension-free closure of the tear, which is essential for a successful repair.[12] For the mobilization, the use of traction sutures is better than holding and squeezing the tendon with a sharp clamp. The extra-articular mobilization involves the subacromial space and, if the area of the cuff is included, also the supraspinous and infraspinous fossae as well as the subcoracoid area, where the coracohumeral ligament should be separated from the base of the coracoid process. Intra-articularly, the release should be performed especially superiorly between the long biceps and the supraspinatus tendon, and posteriorly around the glenoid area.

To improve the healing of the tendon margins to the greater tuberosity, the bony surface should be prepared. We support the biological assumption that the rotator cuff tendon heals more readily to a bleeding cancellous surface providing mesenchymal pluripotential cells and a variety of growth factors than to cortical bone.[13] However, bleeding should be achieved by only roughening the bony surface with a curette or arthroscopically with a shaver. It is absolutely not required to create a deep groove in the greater tuberosity, as removal of the cortical bone impairs the mechanical strength of the cuff fixation. This is especially important in the typical elderly patient with a degenerative rotator cuff lesion and a high incidence of inactivity-induced osteoporosis. An extensive deepening of the bony surface increases also the distance between the tendon and the fixation site and results in increased tension of the repaired rotator cuff.

The tension in the supraspinatus tendon during active 30° abduction has been reported to be as high as 300 N.[14] For this reason, a rotator cuff reconstruction should withstand at least these forces to allow adequate postoperative rehabilitation. However, most transosseous fixation techniques fail at 200 N.[15] Caldwell et al demonstrated a stable transosseous rotator cuff fixation with a distal position of 20 mm from the top of the greater tuberosity and with a minimum distance between the drill holes of 10 mm.[16] The addition of a plate-like augmentation device for the transosseous suture fixation at the lateral humeral cortex can improve the failure strength of the rotator cuff repair from 140 N to 329 N.[15] Meanwhile several suture anchoring devices, such as Corkscrew (Arthrex, Naples, FL, USA), Statak (Zimmer, Warsaw, IN, USA), Harpoon (Biomet, Warsaw, IN, USA) and Superanchor (Mitek, Westwood, MA, USA), with improved designs are available for rotator cuff fixation, which show failure at ultimate loads comparable to those of transosseous fixation.[15,17] However, in elderly patients with osteoporotic humeral bone, transosseous sutures will offer a more secure fixation than the suture anchors. The Concept Rotator Cuff Repair kit (Linvatec, Largo, FL, USA) is helpful in creating tunnels and in passing the sutures through the tunnels where they can be tied over the greater tuberosity. To enhance the fixation strength we routinely use a titanium plate (Synthes, West Chester, PA, USA), which is placed over the holes on the lateral proximal humerus (see Figures 27.7 and 27.8).[18]

An ideal rotator cuff fixation includes the use of sutures with a high degree of initial strength that do not elongate with time and keep their mechanical strength until the

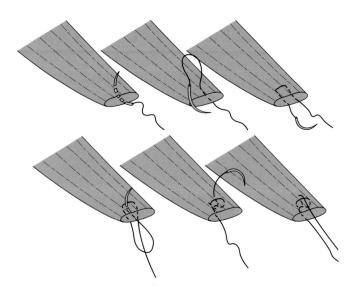

Figure 27.1

Technique of the Mason–Allen suture.

tendon-to-bone healing is completed. Although resorbable or monofilament sutures show good in vitro tensile strength, they are not suitable for the rotator cuff reconstruction. For this reason, non-absorbable braided polyester sutures (Ethibond, Ethicon, Somerville, NJ, USA) #3 or #6 are recommended for the transosseous refixation of the rotator cuff. Gerber et al evaluated different suture techniques for the rotator cuff tendon on cadavers and found that a modified Mason–Allen suture possesses the highest tensile strength (Figure 27.1).[15] Besides a good mechanical strength, this self-locking Mason–Allen suture results in less compromise of the microcirculation of the sutured tendon than with conventional sutures.

Surgical technique

Following induction of general anaesthesia and, in selected cases, additional regional anaesthesia with an interscalene block, both shoulders are examined under relaxed conditions for increased glenohumeral translation or capsular stiffness. The patient is then placed in the beach-chair position with the table at 70°, and the arm is wrapped and attached to a sterile, articulated armholder (McConnell Orthopedic Manufacturing Co., Greenville, TX, USA). This positioning allows free movements in all planes and permits traction of the shoulder without the possible neuropraxia of the brachial plexus associated with traction of the arm in the lateral decubitus position.

Prior to the start of the operative procedure, the arthroscopic portals and the anterolateral skin incision site are infiltrated with diluted epinephrine (adrenaline) to improve haemostasis and visualization. Using the standard posterior portal, an arthroscopic examination of the glenohumeral joint is performed. The entire rotator cuff and the long biceps tendon are carefully examined to judge the true extent of the tear and to choose the subsequent procedure. If it is not possible to ascertain whether the tear is partial or full-thickness, a probe through an additional standard anterior portal is used to evaluate it further. Small intra-articular tears of the rotator cuff can be treated arthroscopically with debridement of the lesion to induce healing in association with arthroscopic subacromial decompression. During the arthroscopic examination, all parts of the labrum are thoroughly visualized since anteroinferior instability may produce secondary rotator cuff tears. Young participants in throwing sports can also present with posterior labral and rotator cuff tears from traction on the rotator cuff over the posterior glenoid rim during repetitive load.[19] All concomitant capsulolabral and superior labrum anterior to posterior (SLAP) lesions are repaired arthroscopically if necessary with suture anchors (FASTak, Arthrex, Naples, Florida, USA) or just debrided if frayed.

Once glenohumeral arthroscopy is completed, the subacromial space is entered from the posterior portal by repositioning the arthroscope with a blunt trocar underneath the acromion. After distension of the subacromial space by the irrigant inflow, an additional portal is placed about 2 cm lateral to the acromion edge and 2 cm posterior to the anterolateral corner of the acromion. Next, the bursa and periosteum are debrided with a full-radius shaver and electrocautery (ArthroCare, Sunnyvale, CA, USA) in order to obtain a good view of the entire subacromial space including the undersurface of the lateral clavicle and the bursal side of the rotator cuff. Before the subacromial decompression is performed, all soft tissue should be removed and bleeding sites coagulated. It is important to visualize the acromion, especially the anterior and lateral borders. An arthroscopic burr is then introduced through the lateral portal to remove 4–8 mm of the acromial undersurface from the anterior 2 cm of the acromion. Saving the coracoacromial ligament, the anteromedial acromion is resected initially to the desired depth and the resection continues laterally to the lateral border of the acromion and proceeds dorsally, converting the underside to a flat surface. If necessary, spurs on the undersurface of the acromioclavicular joint are removed or arthroscopic resection of the acromioclavicular joint is completed.

After sufficient decompression of the subacromial space, the arthroscopic part of the procedure is finished. A 4-cm skin incision is made from the anterolateral edge of the acromion in continuation of the supraspinatus fossa along the Langer's skin lines (Figure 27.2). After incision of the fascia, the deltoid fibres are split proximally to the acromion leaving the deltoid insertion intact.

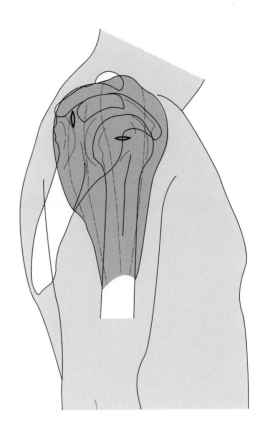

Figure 27.2

The posterior arthroscopic portal is created 2 cm posterior and 2 cm medial to the posterolateral corner of the acromion and the lateral portal is created 2–3 cm lateral to the middle portion of the acromion. The mini-open incision is made from the anterolateral edge of the acromion in continuation of the supraspinous fossa.

Distally, the deltoid split should not exceed 4 cm to avoid possible axillary nerve injury (Figure 27.3). A self-retaining retractor with smooth blades is used for the deltoid retraction (Figure 27.4). Rotation of the shoulder in 30° abduction internally and externally allows the subacromial bursa to be excised and the rotator cuff tear easily exposed. After minimal debridement of the rotator cuff edges, the tendon is tagged with two or three modified Mason–Allen sutures (Figure 27.5; see also Figure 27.8B). These self-locking sutures (Ethibond #6, Ethicon), can be also used for traction during the mobilization of the rotator cuff. The release is first performed extra-articularly in the subacromial space and in the supraspinous fossa, and, if necessary, in the infraspinous fossa and in the subcoracoid area, where concave scissors can be used to separate the coracohumeral ligament from the base of the coracoid process. Rarely, intra-articular mobilization of the supraspinatus and infraspinatus tendon in the periglenoidal area is needed for complete closure of the cuff defect. A shallow trough is then created with a rongeur or a curette adjacent to the articular margin of

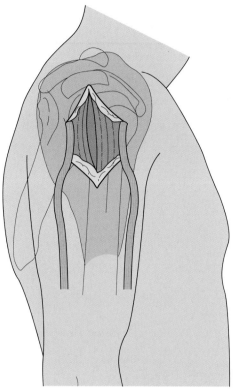

Figure 27.3

The deltoid fascia is split along the course of the fibres leaving the deltoid insertion at the acromion intact.

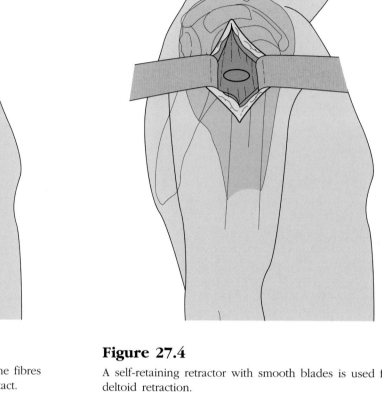

Figure 27.4

A self-retaining retractor with smooth blades is used for deltoid retraction.

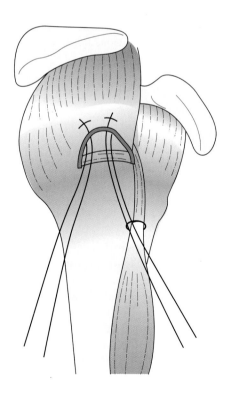

Figure 27.5

The tendon is tagged with two or three modified Mason–Allen sutures.

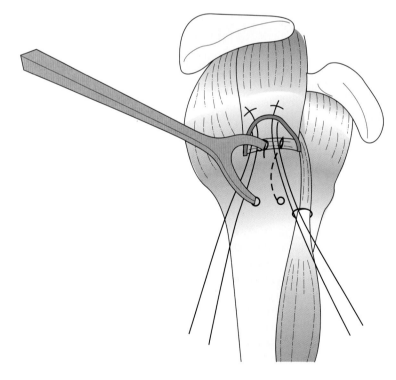

Figure 27.6

The cortical gouge punch is used to create a transosseous hole in the greater tuberosity.

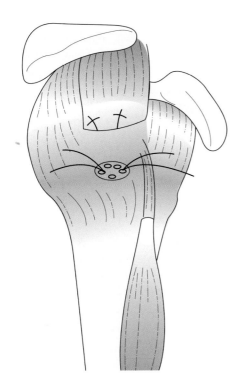

Figure 27.7

After passage of the suture using an appropriately sized suture retriever lateral to the greater tuberosity, the sutures are tied over a titanium augmenting device.

the humeral head. A cortical gouge punch and a corresponding circle rasp (Concept Rotator Cuff Repair, Linvatec) are used first to create two or three rounded osseous tunnels through the bone trough in the greater tuberosity (Figure 27.6; see also Figure 27.8C). The sutures holding the rotator cuff edge are then passed through the osseous tunnels in the tuberosity laterally (Figure 27.8D) and tied over a titanium augmenting device (Figures 27.7, 27.8E,F). Any excess material is removed and the arm is taken through a full range of motion to rule out a subacromial impingement of the reconstructed rotator cuff.

If the rotator cuff tear is larger than expected and cannot be reconstructed through this limited approach, conversion to a conventional open repair is performed easily by extending the skin incision medially and detaching 2–3 cm of the deltoid from the anterior and lateral acromion. However, this is usually not necessary if a thorough preoperative clinical examination and appropriate diagnostic imaging have been applied.

Finally, the superficial deltoid fascia is closed with #1-0 absorbable interrupted sutures. The subcutaneous tissue is closed in a routine fashion with absorbable #2-0 sutures, and a subcuticular closure with non-absorbable #3-0 sutures is effected on the skin. No drain is necessary. A dressing is attached over a thin layer of cotton

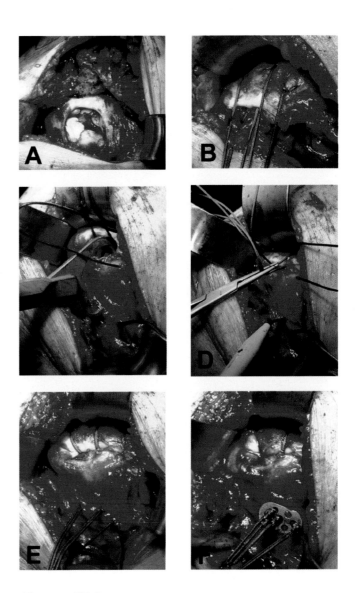

Figure 27.8

Mini-open rotator cuff repair. (A) Visualization of the supraspinatus tendon lesion by retraction of the deltoid. (B) Tagging of the tendon with modified Mason–Allen sutures. (C) Creating the transosseous holes through the bone trough with a cortical gouge punch. (D) Passing the suture laterally with a suture retriever. (E) Adapting the tendon edge. (F) Tying the sutures over a titanium augmenting device.

padding and a cold-therapy cuff (Aircast, Summit, NJ, USA) is applied for the first two postoperative days.

Postoperative protocol

To facilitate a supervised rehabilitation, the majority of patients undergoing mini-open rotator cuff repair are admitted to hospital for about a week. For the first three

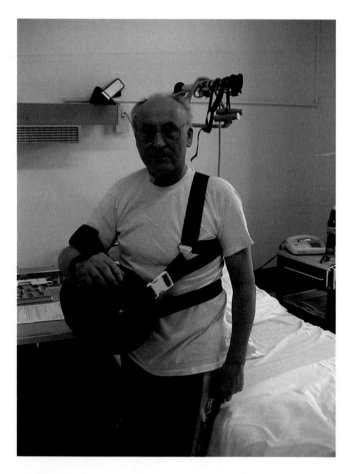

Figure 27.9

The upper extremity is placed on an abduction cushion in 45° flexion and 45° abduction for 6 weeks to diminish the tension at the repair site.

postoperative days, a scalene catheter with repeated injection of local anaesthetic solution gives good pain control. While the patient is still under anaesthesia, the treated shoulder is placed on an abduction cushion in 45° flexion and 45° abduction to diminish the tension strength at the repair site (Figure 27.9). The abduction cushion is used to maintain this position for 24 hours a day for 6 weeks postoperatively. Passive exercises with a range of motion from 45° flexion and abduction up to the horizontal plane and free rotation are initiated on the first postoperative day. The patients are encouraged to use the elbow and the hand for all activities of daily living as far as possible. The main goal of rehabilitation during the first six postoperative weeks is the maintenance of a full range of motion in the operated shoulder. Active assisted motion is started at 4 weeks, followed by active exercises at 6 weeks when the abduction cushion is removed. Rotator cuff strengthening

consists of external and internal rotation of the adducted, and later of the abducted, shoulder against a progressive resistance, e.g. with rubber bands of varying stiffness. Patients are allowed to return to unrestricted activities after 3 months, but are instructed to continue their exercises indefinitely.

References

1. Milgrom C, Schaffler M, Gilbert S, van Holsbeeck M. Rotator-cuff changes in asymptomatic adults. The effect of age, hand dominance and gender. *J Bone Joint Surg* 1995; **77B**:296–8.
2. Ogilvie-Harris DJ, Demaziere A. Arthroscopic debridement versus open repair for rotator cuff tears. A prospective cohort study. *J Bone Joint Surg* 1993; **75B**:416–20.
3. Esch JC, Ozerkis L, Helgager JA et al. Arthroscopic subacromial decompression: results according to the degree of rotator cuff tear. *Arthroscopy* 1988; **4**:241–9.
4. Payne LZ, Altchek DW. Arthroscopic assisted rotator cuff repair. In: Fu FH, Ticker JB, Imhoff AB, eds. *An Atlas of Shoulder Surgery.* London: Martin Dunitz, 175–82.
5. Liu SH. Arthroscopically-assisted rotator-cuff repair. *J Bone Joint Surg* 1994; **76B**:592–5.
6. Paulos LE, Kody MH. Arthroscopically enhanced 'miniapproach' to rotator cuff repair. *Am J Sports Med* 1994; **22**:19–25.
7. Cofield RH. Subscapular muscle transposition for repair of chronic rotator cuff tears. *Surg Gynecol Obstet* 1982; **154**:667–72.
8. Neviaser JS, Neviaser RJ, Neviaser TJ. The repair of chronic massive ruptures of the rotator cuff of the shoulder by use of a freeze-dried rotator cuff. *J Bone Joint Surg* 1978; **60A**:681–4.
9. Neer CS. Cuff tears, biceps lesions, and impingement. In: Neer CS, ed. *Shoulder Reconstruction.* Philadelphia: WB Saunders, 1900; 141–2.
10. Rathbun JB, Mcnab J. The microvascular pattern of the rotator cuff. *J Bone Joint Surg* 1970; **52B**:540–53.
11. Bigliani LU, Rodosky MW. Techniques of repair of large rotator cuff tears. *Tech Orthop* 1994; **9**:133–40.
12. Debeyre J, Patte D, Elmelik E. Repair of ruptures of the rotator cuff of the shoulder. *J Bone Joint Surg* 1965; **47B**:36–42.
13. Uhthoff HK, Sano H, Trudel G, Ishii H. Early reactions after reimplantation of the tendon of supraspinatus into bone. A study in rabbits. *J Bone Joint Surg* 2000; **82B**:1072–6.
14. Wallace WA. Evaluation of forces, the ICR and the neutral point during abduction of the shoulder. *Trans Orthop Res Soc* 1984; **9**:5.
15. Gerber C, Schneeberger AG, Beck M, Schlegel U. Mechanical strength of repairs of the rotator cuff. *J Bone Joint Surg* 1994; **76B**:371–80.
16. Caldwell GL, Warner JP, Miller MD et al. Strength of fixation with transosseous sutures in rotator cuff repair. *J Bone Joint Surg* 1997; **79A**:1064–8.
17. Craft DV, Moseley JB, Cawley PW, Noble PC. Fixation strength of rotator cuff repairs with suture anchors and the transosseous suture technique. *J Shoulder Elbow Surg* 1996; **5**:32–40.
18. Imhoff AB. Rekonstruktion von Rotatorenmanschettenläsionen. Arthroskopisch assistierte mini-open Technik. In: Imhoff AB, König U, eds. *Schulterinstabilität-Rotatorenmanschette.* Darmstadt: Steinkopff, 1999; 228–45.
19. Walch G, Liotard JP, Boileau P, Noel E. Postero–superior glenoid impingement. Another impingement of the shoulder. *J Radiol* 1993; **74**:47–50.

28 Mini-open rotator cuff repair with transosseous tunnels

Jonathan B Ticker, Evan L Flatow and William W Colman

Introduction

The mini-open rotator cuff repair technique, with splitting of the deltoid from the edge of the anterolateral acromion, was developed to offer the surgeon an alternative to an open rotator cuff repair technique while avoiding the traditional approach that required complete detachment of the deltoid from the anterior acromion.[1-5] While the deltoid detachment was necessary as part of the traditional open rotator cuff tendon repair and enabled the surgeon to perform an anterior acromioplasty, reattachment of the deltoid to the acromion was required.[6] The mini-open technique utilizes the advances made with arthroscopic techniques to complete the subacromial decompression, including the anterior acromioplasty, while preserving the deltoid attachment.[7] In addition, the glenohumeral joint can be inspected and any additional problems identified.

This arthroscopically assisted technique proved effective, particularly with small tears of the supraspinatus, and medium tears of the supraspinatus and anterior portions of the infraspinatus.[1-5,8] A shorter hospital stay, quicker rehabilitation, and an earlier return to full activity are expected, compared with a traditional open repair. Extending the indications to large and massive tears was not so successful.[1] The limited exposure provided by the deltoid split, among other things, often resulted in inadequate releases. However, it is clear that advances with arthroscopic techniques for rotator cuff repairs may change – or at least modify – this outlook. Employing arthroscopic techniques to release and mobilize a retracted two- or three-tendon tear and combining this with the mini-open repair may lead to improved results with these more challenging tears.[9]

Surgical principles

Neer described four major objectives of surgery for rotator cuff tears: closure of the cuff defect, eliminating the impingement lesions of the coracoacromial arch, preserving the origin of the deltoid muscle, and rehabilitation that prevents stiffness postoperatively without disrupting the repair.[6] In addition, the steps developed with traditional open repairs included excision of the inflamed bursa, debridement of the edges of the tear, mobilization of the tendon, preparation of the bone in the sulcus between the articular margin and the greater tuberosity, and closure of the defect with tendon-to-tendon sutures and/or fixation of tendon to bone via transosseous sutures.[6,10-15] Finally, a tension-free, water-tight repair was the goal.[16,17] All these goals can be achieved with the mini-open rotator cuff repair technique. In this chapter, one method for transosseous fixation is described.

The following technique employs the Link Rotator Cuff Repair Instrumentation (Link Orthopedics, Rockaway, NJ, USA), specifically designed instruments to facilitate rotator cuff repair. A self-retaining Kölbel retractor

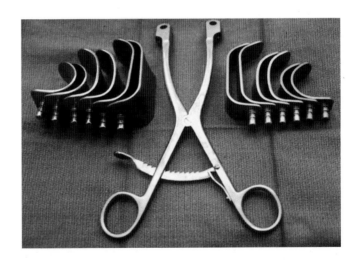

Figure 28.1

The Link Kölbel self-retaining retractor with standard and narrow blades, in lengths of 36 mm, 53 mm, and 68 mm.

handle with modified narrow blades (18-mm width rather than the standard 36 mm; Figure 28.1), bi-curved to protect the deltoid, optimizes exposure of a rotator cuff tear through the deltoid split to complete the tendon mobilization, preparation and repair. Curved awls and suture passers (Figure 28.2), with matching curvature, create uniform transosseous tunnels and pass single or multiple sutures through the tunnels to accomplish the tendon repair to bone. Two different sizes of these instruments allow tunnel placement to be varied in the proximal to distal direction along the greater tuberosity

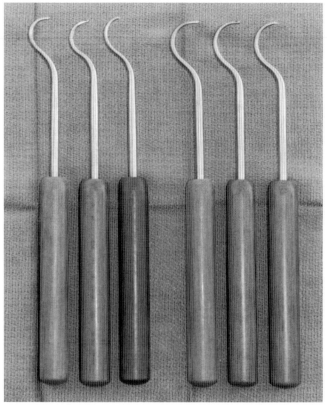

(a)

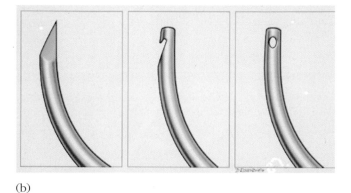

(b)

Figure 28.2

(a) The instrumentation for creating transosseous tunnels and passing sutures, with 9.5 mm or 11.5 mm radius of curvature. (b) The instrument tips.

to avoid stress risers, as well as to take advantage of the thicker cortical bone more distally.[18] Additional special instrumentation that should be available includes small Richardson retractors to enhance exposure when needed, a flat rasp to insure a smooth undersurface of the acromion, a rongeur and curettes to prepare the sulcus to bleeding bone without creating a formal trough, and chisels to remove larger bony excrescences at the greater tuberosity. For osteopenic bone, augmentation at the lateral aspect of the greater tuberosity is desirable,[18,19] and the Cuff Link (Mitek, Norwood, MA,

USA) is easily deployed into the tunnel opening created laterally on the tuberosity with the Link instrumentation.

A successful technique requires additional considerations. Resection of the bursa serves to enhance exposure of the torn edge of the rotator cuff to facilitate the repair, as well as remove potentially inflammatory tissue.[20] However, this tissue might provide blood flow and add to the healing response of the repaired tendon. Bigliani and Rodosky recommended removing only the superficial bursa for this reason,[21] and other surgeons recommend removing only the portion of the bursa that is thickened and scarred or limits exposure of the rotator cuff tear in order to preserve the gliding function of the bursa.[12,22] A limited bursectomy is recommended for these reasons.

If mobilization of the tendon is indicated, arthroscopic releases (techniques described in the arthroscopic rotator cuff repair chapters of this book) may be performed. These include developing the plane between the undersurface of the tendon and the glenoid rim anteriorly, superiorly, and posteriorly as needed. The coracohumeral ligament can be incised as part of the rotator interval release. These maneuvers can be carried out through the deltoid split. However, the larger the tear, the more difficult this endeavor will be, and it is in this regard that the arthroscopic releases are best utilized. When this is considered, it appears that the mini-open approach may serve as a transitional step in the development of the surgeon's treatment of rotator cuff tears. With each tear repaired by a mini-open technique, the surgeon has the opportunity to develop skills, step by step, which will eventually allow the performance of arthroscopic repairs. In concert with hands-on cadaveric courses teaching arthroscopic rotator cuff repair techniques and simulation models, performing arthroscopic rotator cuff repairs is a reasonable and achievable goal.

Early techniques for rotator cuff tendon mobilization included placing tenaculums or forceps on the free edge of the torn rotator cuff.[11,23] Although this may provide the surgeon with a good grip of the tissue, the tendon that is crushed beneath clamps will be considerably less viable, affecting the tissue's ability to hold a suture and to heal. Tenaculums or towel clips may create large holes in the tendon and are not forgiving when used for traction. Placement of traction sutures evenly along the torn edge of the rotator cuff tendon is a better way of applying tension on the cuff tissue during mobilization and repair.[6] In addition, taper needles rather than cutting needles should be used when passing these sutures through the tendon to minimize tissue damage and the size of the hole created in the tendon for the suture.

As part of the repair, the edge of the tendon must be prepared. Neer recommended removing only a 'thin margin' of the edge of the tear.[6] It would seem that a minimal debridement of the torn rotator cuff tendon edge is all that necessary at this stage of the procedure to remove 'degenerated tissue' and 1–2 mm has been suggested.[20,21,24–26] A bony trough into the cancellous bone at the sulcus, once thought to be essential for tendon healing, is not necessary.[21,27] Removal of soft tissue to expose bleeding bone on the surface of the sulcus is carried out with curettes or rongeurs, though occasionally a burr is used to expose bleeding bone.

Gerber et al suggested that the 'ideal repair should have high initial fixation strength, allow minimal gap formation and maintain mechanical stability until solid healing'.[28] A single or double loop of suture placed in a simple fashion has been suggested by some surgeons for the transosseous repair, and a mattress suture technique has been suggested by others.[6,12,26] Compared with a single mattress suture, two securely tied simple suture loops are more effective,[29,30] and are clearly adequate for small tears without tension.[28] For tendon repairs under some tension, a modified Mason–Allen locking suture technique is preferred.[28] It has also been recommended that sutures be tied laterally on the greater tuberosity.[6,13] Suture material that could subsequently cause impingement, such as non-absorbable suture in the subacromial space, should be avoided.[22] For this reason, Neer has also recommended that side-to-side sutures be buried.[6] While braided non-absorbable polyester was formerly felt to be the best suture for repair,[28] the introduction of longer-lasting braided absorbable material (Panacryl, Ethicon, Somerville, NJ, USA) has made this an alternative suture material for rotator cuff tendon repair. While suture anchors have been recommended for rotator cuff repairs, we prefer to use transosseous tunnels in mini-open and open procedures.[31]

The quality of the repair is dependent upon careful management of the soft tissues and strong fixation to bone during the healing process. However, the extent of preoperative motion, the quality of the tissue, the amount of muscle atrophy, a diligent rehabilitation program and patient motivation, among other factors, will affect the overall outcome, despite an optimal repair technique. Postoperative pain management is an essential component of the recovery process. Patient-controlled infusion devices that deliver an anesthetic solution to the surgical site are effective in reducing pain in the early postoperative period.[32–36] The pump used by one author (JBT) is a device (Zimmer, Warsaw, IN, USA) that allows constant infusion of a basal rate of anesthetic solution and a bolus for additional pain relief, which is especially useful during initial passive range of motion exercises.

There are limitations to this technique because of the constraints of the deltoid split. It is not advised to attempt repairs of the subscapularis with this approach, as additional exposure is required.[37] Larger tears that are not mobilized adequately will be difficult to attach to the sulcus and there is likely to be excessive tension that could compromise the repair. Furthermore, we do not recommend repair to a prepared surface medial to the sulcus, which would involve removal of a portion of the articular cartilage. Complications of this procedure, and of rotator cuff tear repairs in general, include failure of tendon healing, recurrence of the tear, infection, post-operative stiffness and persistent pain or weakness. Some reports for all rotator cuff repairs include axillary nerve

injury, hematoma, and greater tuberosity or acromial fracture, among other complications.[38] Larger tears are more likely to have a complication, particularly failure of the tendon repair.

Surgical technique

Interscalene anesthesia is preferred for its advantages of providing excellent anesthesia, avoiding a general anesthesia, and providing postoperative analgesia.[39] After anesthesia is administered, the shoulder is examined. Occasionally, mild limitations of motion are detected, and a manipulation is performed. Significant passive motion limitations should be addressed prior to undertaking surgery. The patient is then placed in the beach-chair position; this position is facilitated by using a device secured to the operating table (T-Max, Tenet Medical, Calgary, AB, Canada), ensuring surgeon and patient comfort. Care is taken to pad down all surfaces. Arm position during the procedure is maintained with the McConnell sterile articulated arm holder (McConnell Orthopedics, Greenville, TX, USA) or the Spyder hydraulic arm positioner (Tenet Medical). The arm is then prepared and draped in the usual sterile fashion. Landmarks are outlined and lidocaine (lignocaine) 1% with epinephrine (adrenaline) is injected into the planned portal sites, the planned mini-open incision, and the subacromial space. The incision is usually placed in such a way as to extend the lateral portal in a transverse fashion along Langer's lines. A vertical incision can be used, although it is less cosmetically pleasing.

The shoulder arthroscopy proceeds in the usual fashion beginning with the glenohumeral joint. Prior to making the posterior portal incision, a spinal needle is inserted from a posterior direction towards the coracoid tip to enter the glenohumeral joint, which is then insufflated with 45–60 ml of normal saline. This serves to separate the articular surfaces to allow for easier entry of the arthroscopic sheath. Brisk backflow of fluid into the syringe or through the end of the spinal needle suggests that the rotator cuff is at least partially intact. After withdrawing the needle, a posterior incision is made and the blunt trocar and sheath are inserted into the joint. Again, backflow through the sheath is assessed. The arthroscope is then introduced and the glenohumeral joint is visualized.

An anterior portal is placed lateral and superior to the coracoid tip, in such a way as to allow the insertion of a disposable cannula into the triangle formed by the biceps tendon, the subscapularis tendon and the glenoid labrum. A needle is used to localize this portal prior to incision and its precise placement can be varied, depending upon the planned surgical procedure. In particular, if a distal clavicle resection is planned, a more medial placement closer to the acromioclavicular joint is desirable to allow greater access to the acromioclavicular joint. The anterior portal is used as a working portal, as well as to view the posterior aspect of the glenohumeral joint. Any lesion of the biceps is addressed first, as well as any other treatable intra-articular problem. If the supraspinatus insertion is not fully identified, slight traction or abduction of the arm with rotation is helpful. If a partial-thickness tear is suspected, a marking suture is placed through the area of tendon concerned. This helps to identify the suspected area on the bursal side of the tendon when the arthroscope is in the subacromial space. A spinal needle is introduced through the lateral aspect of the shoulder (not in the position planned for the lateral portal) and passed through the region of the suspected partial tear. If the needle is introduced from a point too far anteriorly, posteriorly or distally, identifying the suture may be more difficult unless additional bursa is removed. The stylet of the spinal needle is removed and a colored #1 monofilament suture is placed into the joint through the needle and retrieved through the anterior portal. Both ends are then clamped together and placed aside until the subacromial portion of the procedure.

If there is damage to the biceps, a tenotomy can be performed at this time. An arthroscopic approach is preferred for its clear visualization and access, and because it is not always as easy to do this step through the deltoid split, particularly if the tear is small. Prior to the tenotomy, a suture is passed through the tendon as a tag suture. A narrow basket forceps releases the biceps tendon at its insertion at the superior glenoid tubercle. The suture is then brought out through the anterior portal and clamped in the event a biceps tenodesis is planned. While this can be performed arthroscopically, the tenodesis is easily accomplished through the deltoid split. On rare occasions, when tearing of the biceps is minimal, a debridement can be carried out.

The arthroscope is now withdrawn at the completion of the glenohumeral portion of the surgery and the joint is suctioned, unless plans include returning into the glenohumeral joint. The blunt trocar and sheath are then introduced from the posterior portal into the subacromial space and swept medially and laterally to lyse any scarred tissue and to clear bursa. The arthroscope is inserted and evaluation of the subacromial space is completed, including assessment of wear under the acromion, involvement of the tendon and the position of the marking suture. A lateral portal is established with a spinal needle to localize the optimal position, usually in line with the posterior aspect of the acromioclavicular joint and 2 cm lateral to the edge of the acromion. The skin incision is made, taking care not to cut across the fibers of the deltoid muscle. A disposable cannula with a blunt trocar is inserted into the subacromial space and the bursectomy is completed with a full-radius resector.

The subacromial decompression is then performed viewing from posteriorly and working laterally. The undersurface of the acromion is prepared by removing the soft tissue with a shaver and electrocautery, with ablation. This includes releasing a sufficient amount of the coracoacromial ligament to expose the anterior tip of the acromion. Care is taken to respect the margins of the acromioclavicular joint, if it is not involved. An oval burr (about 4.0 mm) is used to begin the acromioplasty, resecting bone from lateral to medial from the undersurface of the anterior third of the acromion. An anterior to posterior motion is used as the burr progresses medially. We prefer to complete the finishing touches of the acromioplasty with the cutting-block technique, using switching sticks to place the burr posteriorly and the arthroscope laterally.[40] The size of the burr and outer sheath are used to determine the thickness of bone removed, using the preoperative supraspinatus outlet radiograph as a guide. At times, using the burr in the reverse mode permits less aggressive bone resection.

After the subacromial decompression is completed, the rotator cuff tear pattern is fully assessed by viewing from both the posterior and lateral portals, as needed. The edge of the tear is debrided minimally to healthy tissue. If the tear is found to be greater 1 cm or so (a small tear), the mobility of the retracted tendon should be assessed. A monofilament suture is placed along the lateral edge, using a Caspari suture punch (Linvatec, Largo, FL, USA), Spectrum Suture Hook (Linvatec) or similar device. Lateral traction is applied to evaluate mobility of the tendon edge onto or over the sulcus. In addition, longitudinal components of a tear must be appreciated to determine if margin convergence with side-to-side repair will be an element of the tendon repair.[29,30] If the tear is larger than 3–4 cm, involving two tendons and retracted more than 2 cm medially approaching the glenoid rim, the surgeon must decide whether or not to proceed with a mini-open repair. This type of tear will require more advanced releases, arthroscopically and through the deltoid split, to complete the repair. In addition, massive rotator cuff tears, particularly those including the subscapularis, might be better repaired through other surgical approaches. If mobilization is not necessary, a burr may be used to prepare the sulcus at this time. Alternatively, the sulcus can be prepared after the mini-open incision and deltoid split are performed, using a burr or rongeur.

After all the arthroscopic techniques are completed, the lateral portal is extended 3–4 cm. Skin flaps are developed and the deltoid is split 4 cm from the lateral edge of the acromion, in line with the defect in the deltoid created when the lateral portal was established. A suture is placed at the distal aspect of the split to protect the deltoid from extending further and potentially damaging the axillary nerve. The Kölbel self-retaining retractor with narrow blades is placed for exposure (Figure 28.3). If placed, the monofilament suture is used as a landmark to approach the tear. Additional bursectomy may be required at this time for visualization, particularly laterally. The undersurface of the acromion is palpated and a flat rasp is applied, as needed, to achieve a smooth, flat acromioplasty. The wound is irrigated at this point and at various times throughout the remainder of the procedure.

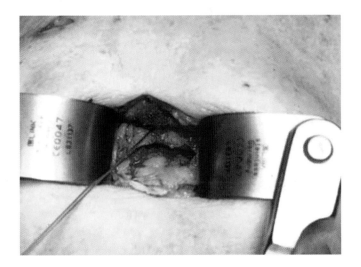

Figure 28.3
With the retractor in place, the rotator cuff tear with traction suture is viewed through the deltoid split.

Additional, braided #0 non-absorbable traction sutures are spaced along the tendon edge, using a taper needle, to assist with mobilization and traction of the tendon during suture tying. Mobilization of the tendon is assessed and finished at this point. A Cobb elevator or similar instrument is placed along the bursal surface of the rotator cuff and advanced medial to the glenoid from anterior to posterior beyond the margin of the tear to ensure no adhesions are present. This is then done on the intra-articular side of the tear between the tendon and the glenoid rim to ensure the tear is mobile in a lateral direction. The larger the tear and the greater the medial retraction of the tendon edge, the more effort and attention to mobilization are needed. More advanced steps include releasing the rotator interval and coracohumeral ligament from the base of the coracoid,[24] as well as a posterior interval slide, as required.[21,41,42] Preparation of the sulcus is now completed. If a large excrescence is present on the greater tuberosity, an osteotome can be used to remove it, which will also serve to expose bone for tendon-to-bone healing.

If the biceps tendon is involved in the pathologic process, it is now addressed. If a tenotomy is planned, it can be performed during the arthroscopic portion of the procedure or at this time. Otherwise a tenodesis is performed. In medium to large tears, the rotator cuff defect is used to view the biceps insertion. Anatomic landmarks are identified to help recreate the appropriate amount of tension on the biceps during the tenodesis. Place a traction suture through the biceps tendon lateral to the insertion, and release the biceps from its insertion on the superior glenoid tubercle. These steps can be performed arthroscopically if desired, as noted above, particularly in small tears. By externally rotating and elevating the arm in the scapular plane, the intertubercular groove is exposed. We prefer an interference screw technique using an absorbable

screw of 20–23 mm in length and 8–9 mm in diameter, usually the same size as the drilled hole.[43] The socket is drilled at the superior aspect of the intertubercular groove and the groove is roughened with a curette or lightly with a burr. This drill hole is oriented medial to the location of the planned tunnels for the rotator cuff repair. With the tendon inserted into the socket at the desired tension, the absorbable screw is fully inserted for firm interference fixation.

In rotator cuff tears that have a longitudinal component, simple sutures that will be buried are now placed for the side-to-side repair, but not tied. For the tendon-to-bone repair, transosseous tunnels are created laterally on the greater tuberosity. The positioning for the tunnels depends upon the size of the repair. Small tears usually have one or two tunnels, medium tears often require two or three tunnels, large tears can typically be repaired with three or four tunnels, and massive tears (which are not typically repaired through a mini-open approach and could only be performed through this approach if the retracted tendon were released appropriately) usually require five or even more tunnels. In addition, an acute tear that requires little mobilization and has minimal tension can be expected to be more easily repaired with slightly fewer sutures compared with a chronic tear of the same size that requires extensive releases and exhibits more tension. Two braided sutures, either non-absorbable or long-acting absorbable, as desired, will occupy each tunnel. Tunnel position is varied in a proximal to distal direction laterally to avoid a 'postage stamp' appearance along the greater tuberosity, which is not optimal. This is achieved by alternating the two different curvatures of awls and/or by changing the angle of entry so that the awl tip exits the sulcus in a more medial or lateral placement, as desired. Preparation of the sulcus should be completed prior to tunnel placement.

The tunnels are placed along the greater tuberosity from one edge of the tear to the other, starting either posteriorly or anteriorly. The Penetrating Awl is placed against the cortex of the greater tuberosity at the desired level (Figure 28.4a). While the awl is held by one hand, pressure is applied with the contralateral thumb to assist in perforating the cortex (Figure 28.4b). The tip of the Penetrating Awl is advanced into the metaphyseal bone with continued pressure, guiding the sharp tip along its arc of curvature into the sulcus, lateral to the articular margin at the humeral head (Figure 28.4c). The handle of the awl is now inferior to the incision. The awl is gently removed as the handle is brought up to follow its arc of curvature, resulting in a uniform transosseous tunnel with walls of impacted bone (Figure 28.4d). The corresponding size of Crochet Hook suture passer is passed through the transosseous tunnel in the same motion used to create the tunnel, and its tip exits in the sulcus. As the tip of the Crochet Hook is deeper within the surgical site, a clamp is used to place a free braided non-absorbable suture securely in the tip of the hook

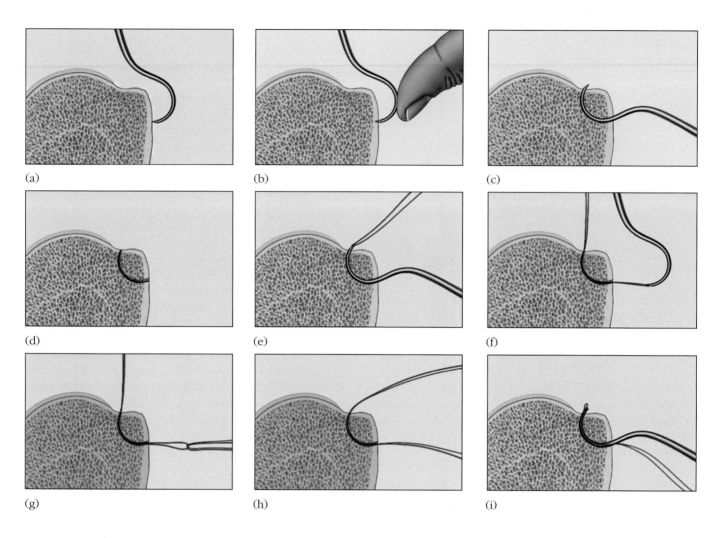

Figure 28.4

(a) The Penetrating Awl is placed on the cortex. (b) Pressure is applied for the awl tip to enter the bone. (c) The handle of the awl is brought inferiorly as the tip is advanced through bone medially and superiorly, along its arc of curvature, into the sulcus. (d) The transosseous tunnel is created. A passing suture is placed in the tip of the Crochet Hook (e), and maintained, as a loop (f) is brought through the tunnel. (g) The sutures that will be used for the tendon-to-bone repair are placed inside the loop of the passing suture. (h) The sutures for the repair are now in position through the transosseous tunnel. (i) The Hollow Lumen Suture Passer can be used, alternatively, to pass a suture from lateral to medial, as desired.

(Figure 28.4e). The Crochet Hook with suture is then removed from the tunnel using the same motion as previously described along its arc of curvature. This delivers a loop of the suture through the tunnel (Figure 28.4f). Alternatively, the tip of the hook can be used to pass one or both limbs of a previously placed suture through the tunnel.

The suture is kept within the tunnel and used as a passing suture by placing the ends of two free braided (non-absorbable or absorbable) sutures inside the loop (Figure 28.4g). The loop is then pulled back through the transosseous tunnel out of the sulcus, delivering the two free sutures for the tendon-to-bone repair (Figure 28.4h). Each pair of suture limbs is clamped together. If only one transosseous suture is desired, then the loop is broken by bringing one end of the suture out laterally.

An alternative is to use the Hollow Lumen Suture Passer to pass a loop of suture from laterally through the transosseous tunnel into the sulcus (Figure 28.4i). This loop can be used to pass additional sutures or be retrieved as a single suture. Each subsequent transosseous tunnel is prepared with sutures in a similar fashion. The sutures are kept in sequential order with an Alice clamp, if necessary, for subsequent placement in the tendon edge. A gentian violet marker can be used, if desired, to help differentiate and identify individual sutures if the same type is used within each tunnel. Alternatively, the use of differently sized or colored sutures will simplify suture identification.

Sutures are placed within healthy tendon, using a tapered needle, approximately 5 mm from the tendon edge and spaced according to the number of sutures available and to the size of the tear. The previously placed traction sutures are used to bring the torn edge of the tendon laterally over the sulcus to approximate the position of the tendon after the repair. This assists with the planning and the placement of the sutures. We have been alternating simple suture placement with modified Mason–Allen sutures for a more secure repair: in other words, one suture within each tunnel is placed in a sliding fashion and the second suture is placed in a locking fashion. At this point, it is worthwhile reassessing the sutures that might have been placed along the longitudinal component of the tear. If these sutures are positioned as desired, they can be securely tied at this time, starting with the most medial. The most lateral suture is often tied after the tendon-to-bone sutures are securely tied, especially if the tear pattern is Y-shaped.

Prior to tying the tendon-to-bone sutures, the surgeon must determine if the bone laterally requires augmentation. Recognizing the need for supplemental augmentation of the bone laterally on the greater tuberosity is essential to avoid the sutures cutting out of the transosseous tunnel. Creating the transosseous tunnel may suggest whether augmentation is necessary, depending upon how easy it is to penetrate the lateral cortex and the bone of the sulcus with the tip of the Penetrating Awl. In these cases we prefer to use the Cuff Link, which allows the lateral limbs of both sutures within each tunnel to be passed through its lumen. Once the sutures are passed through the Cuff Link, this plastic device is slid along the sutures and into place at the greater tuberosity, filling the tunnel entrance laterally. The opening created by the Penetrating Awl accommodates the device and no further instrumentation is required.

The sutures are now tied securely. For L-shaped tears, the sutures are tied starting with the side of the tear with the least amount of tension and progressing from there. We try to avoid clamping the suture after the first throw as it can damage the suture material and compromise the repair. If the first throw is slipping prior to placing the second throw and locking the knot, the side of a curved clamp is placed across the first throw to stabilize it as the second throw is pulled tight. Occasionally, a smooth needle-holder is used. Care is taken to place the knots laterally, and preferably distally, along the greater tuberosity to avoid any knots occupying a position within the subacromial space. This is particularly important when tying the sutures passed in the Mason–Allen fashion as these cannot slide after being tied. The simple knots can be moved more laterally after being tied, but this is less desirable because of potential friction of the suture on the bone edge and the possibility of loosening the knot. For Y-shaped tears, the sutures on one side of the tendon-to-bone repair and then the other side are tied, working toward the center. The last transosseous suture can be passed through both sides of the tear with the Y pattern, if desired. A final side-to-side suture can then be tied. The wound is irrigated with saline after the rotator cuff repair has been completed.

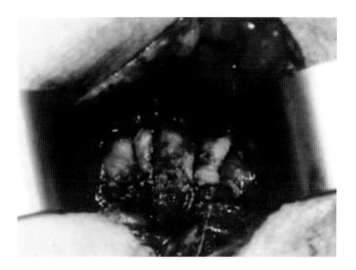

Figure 28.5

The final tendon repair, in this case using braided non-absorbable sutures.

The arm is taken through a range of motion, and the stability of the repair is assessed and noted for reference during the postoperative rehabilitation (Figure 28.5). If an anesthetic infusion pump is to be used it is introduced at this stage. The angiocatheter provided is introduced into the subacromial space from a separate posterolateral approach under direct visualization. The needle is removed and the sheath is maintained in position. An epidural-type catheter is passed through the sheath into the subacromial place and maintained in this position as the angiocatheter sheath is removed. The catheter is placed at the desired position, typically over the repair and under the acromioplasty site. The catheter can be flushed during the closure to avoid blood backing up into it and clotting. (The pump will be started after the wound is completely closed and the dressing applied.) Next, the Link self-retaining retractor is removed and the stay stitch in the deltoid is removed. The deltoid and superficial tissues are irrigated and the deltoid is approximated with #2 braided long-lasting absorbable suture. Particular attention is paid to securely tying the first stitch placed at the deltoid insertion on the lateral edge of the acromion. After the deltoid closure is completed, the subcutaneous tissues are closed with #2-0 short-lasting braided absorbable sutures. A #3-0 absorbable monofilament suture is used to close the skin in a subcuticular fashion and adhesive strips are applied. With the arm protected, the catheter is secured to the skin and a sterile dressing is applied. Cryotherapy, such as a Cryocuff (Aircast, Summit, NJ, USA), is helpful to relieve pain and swelling and is applied at this time. If the repair is large or exhibits tension, a sling with an abduction pillow can be used, though use of these devices is not routine.

Postoperative protocol

An understanding of a tissue's response to injury and its mechanisms of repair is helpful when designing a rehabilitation program.[44] The healing process proceeds in much the same manner for all soft tissues, with a surgical repair creating a more controlled healing environment. The initial inflammatory phase is followed by a reparative phase. The healing tissue is weaker and at risk of the tear recurring early on, so a careful regimen to avoid overstressing the repaired tissue is essential. This phase may last 3–6 weeks. The remodeling phase then progresses for many months and will influence decisions regarding return to activities.

The rehabilitation process actually begins preoperatively when the surgeon explains to the patient the planned operative procedure, the perioperative course and the demands of the postoperative rehabilitation. In this manner, the patient's and the surgeon's expectations are understood by both parties. The primary goals of the rehabilitation program are to control pain, protect repaired tissue during the healing process, restore function and avoid recurrence of symptoms. The size of the tear, as well as the quality of the tissue and the quality of the repair, are taken into account by the surgeon as the rehabilitation program progresses. The sling is maintained for 4–6 weeks, with the longer period needed for larger tears. Passive range of motion exercises usually begin immediately, based on patient ability and comfort, primarily as pendulum exercises. Analgesics are given to diminish pain and encourage earlier progression of motion. Avoiding arm extension initially following a rotator cuff repair is helpful to limit tension on the repair and decrease pain.

A physician-supervised physical therapy rehabilitation program is an important component of the recovery process. The surgeon must communicate with the physical therapist to set initial limits and to advance the rehabilitation. During the initial stages of healing following a repair, gaining motion is the focus of the rehabilitation. Phase I, the acute or protective stage, is generally designed to manage postoperative pain and inflammation, protect the repair, initiate passive and then active-assisted range of motion exercises for the involved joint, initiate isometric exercise for the unaffected muscles, and resume motion to the uninvolved joints, especially the elbow, wrist, and hand. Initial motion limits, increased as tissue healing progresses, are based on the surgeon's intraoperative assessment of the safe zone for motion following the repair. This phase generally lasts 4–6 weeks following surgical repair. Pulley exercises are initiated toward the end of this phase; inflammation can occur if these are started too early.

Phase II, the subacute or recovery stage, begins when sufficient tissue healing is achieved, after 4 to 6 weeks, again depending upon the size of the tear and the quality of the tissue and its repair. The phase clearly begins much sooner following repair of a small rotator cuff tear than following repair of a large tear. This phase includes active range of motion exercises, advanced stretching to restore full motion, and light then more advanced strengthening of the affected muscles and the entire shoulder girdle.

Phase III, the functional stage beginning at 8–10 weeks, maximizes the strengthening and stretching, with the addition of sports or activity-related exercises and a maintenance program. Judicious application of heat promotes soft tissue flexibility and facilitates stretching. Stretching of the posterior capsule should not be overlooked. Slow, gradual stretching exercises are preferred over rapid, ballistic-type movements. Activities are resumed in stages, based on the demands such activities will place on the repair.

References

1. Levy HJ, Gardner RD, Lemak LJ. Arthroscopic assisted rotator cuff repair: preliminary results. *Arthroscopy* 1990; **6**:55–60.
2. Liu SH. Arthroscopic-assisted rotator cuff repair. *J Bone Joint Surg* 1994; **76B**:592–5.
3. Liu SH, Baker CL. Arthroscopically assisted rotator cuff repair: correlation of functional results with the integrity of the cuff. *Arthroscopy* 1994; **10**:54–60.
4. Paulos LE, Cody MH. Arthroscopically enhanced 'mini-approach' to rotator cuff repair. *Am J Sports Med* 1994; **22**:19–25.
5. Pollock RG, Flatow EL. Full-thickness tears: mini-open repair. *Orthop Clin North Am* 1997; **28**:169–78.
6. Neer CS. Cuff tears, biceps lesions, and impingement. In: *Shoulder Reconstruction*. Philadelphia: WB Saunders, 1990; 141–2.
7. Ellman H. Arthroscopic subacromial decompression: analysis of one to three year results. *Arthroscopy* 1987; **3**:173–81.
8. Warner JJ, Goitz RJ, Irrgang JJ, Groff YJ. Arthroscopic-assisted rotator cuff repair: patient selection and treatment outcome. *J Shoulder Elbow Surg* 1997; **6**:463–72.
9. Yamaguchi K. Mini-open rotator cuff repair: an updated perspective. *J Bone Joint Surg* 2001; **83A**:764–72.
10. Bosworth DM. An analysis of twenty-eight consecutive cases of incapacitating shoulder lesions, radically explored and repaired. *J Bone Joint Surg* 1940; **22**:369–92.
11. Codman EA. Complete rupture of the supraspinatus tendon. Operative treatment with report of two successful cases. *Boston Med Surg J* 1911; **164**:708–10.
12. DePalma AF. Disorders associated with biologic aging of the shoulder: painful arc syndrome (impingement syndrome). In: DePalma AF, ed. *Surgery of the Shoulder*, 3rd edn. Philadelphia: Lippincott, 1983; 245–65.
13. McLaughlin HL. Lesions of the musculotendinous cuff of the shoulder: I. The exposure and treatment of tears with retraction. *J Bone Joint Surg* 1944; **26**:31–51.
14. Post M. Injuries to the rotator cuff. In: Post M, ed. *The Shoulder: Surgical and Nonsurgical Management*. Philadelphia: Lea & Febiger, 1978; 304–28.
15. Ticker JB, Warner JJP. Rotator cuff tears: principles of tendon repair. In: Iannotti JP, ed. *The Rotator Cuff: Current Concepts and Complex Problems*. Rosemont: AAOS, 1998; 17–24.
16. McLaughlin HL. Rupture of the rotator cuff. *J Bone Joint Surg* 1962; **44A**:979–83.
17. McLaughlin HL. Repair of major cuff ruptures. *Surg Clin North Am* 1963; **43**:1535–40.
18. Caldwell GL, Warner JJP, Miller MD et al. Strength of fixation with transosseous sutures in rotator cuff repair. *J Bone Joint Surg* 1997; **79A**:1064–8.

19. France EP, Paulos LE, Harner CD, Straight CB. Biomechanical evaluation of rotator cuff fixation methods. *Am J Sports Med* 1989; **17**:176–81.

20. Post M, Silver R, Singh M. Rotator cuff tear: diagnosis and treatment. *Clin Orthop* 1983; **173**:78–91.

21. Bigliani LU, Rodosky MW. Techniques of repair of large rotator cuff tears. *Tech Orthop* 1994; **9**:133–40.

22. Iannotti JP, ed. *Rotator Cuff Disorders: Evaluation and Treatment*. Park Ridge: AAOS, 1991; 1–74.

23. Wilson PD. Complete rupture of the supraspinatus tendon. *JAMA* 1931; **96**:433–9.

24. Bigliani LU, Cordasco FA, McIlveen SJ, Musso ES. Operative repair of massive rotator cuff tears: long-term results. *J Shoulder Elbow Surg* 1992; **1**:120–30.

25. Ellman H, Hanker G, Bayer M. Repair of the rotator cuff. *J Bone Joint Surg* 1986; **68A**:1136–44.

26. Poppen NK. Soft-tissue lesions of the shoulder. In: Chapman MW, ed. *Operative Orthopaedics*, 2nd edn. Philadelphia: Lippincott, 1988; 1651–71.

27. St Pierre P, Olson EJ, Elliott JJ et al. Tendon-healing to cortical bone compared with healing to a cancellous trough. *J Bone Joint Surg* 1995; **77A**:1858–66.

28. Gerber C, Schneeberger AG, Beck M, Schlegel U. Mechanical strength of repairs of the rotator cuff. *J Bone Joint Surg* 1994; **76B**:371–80.

29. Burkhart SS, Athanasiou KA, Wirth MA. Margin convergence: a method of reducing strain in massive rotator cuff tears (technical note). *Arthroscopy* 1996; **12**:335–8.

30. Burkhart SS, Fischer SP, Nottage WM et al. Tissue fixation security in transosseous rotator cuff repairs: a mechanical comparison of simple versus mattress sutures. *Arthroscopy* 1996; **12**:704–8.

31. Burkhart SS, Diaz Pagan JL, Wirth MA, Athanasiou KA. Cyclic loading of anchor-based rotator cuff repairs: Confirmation of the tension overload phenomenon and comparison of suture anchor fixation with transosseous tunnels. *Arthroscopy* 1997; **13**:720–4.

32. Mallon WJ, Thomas CW. Patient-controlled lidocaine analgesia for acromioplasty surgery. *J Shoulder Elbow Surg* 2000; **9**:85–8.

33. Savoie FH, Field LD, Jenkins N et al. The pain control infusion pump for postoperative pain control in shoulder surgery. *Arthroscopy* 2000; **16**:339–42.

34. Duralde SA, McCollam S, Scherger A. Postoperative pain management following outpatient open rotator cuff repair: a comparison of interscalene block analgesia vs. Marcaine pump. American Academy of Orthopaedic Surgeons, San Francisco, March 2001.

35. Sallay P. A comparison of pain following outpatient rotator cuff repair with and without subacromial bupivacaine infusion. American Academy of Orthopaedic Surgeons, San Francisco, March 2001.

36. Barber FA, Herbert MA. The effectiveness of an anesthetic continuous-infusion device on postoperative pain control. *Arthroscopy* 2002; 18: 76–81.

37. Ticker JB, Warner JJP. Single-tendon tears of the rotator cuff: evaluation and treatment of subscapularis tears and principles of treatment for supraspinatus tears. *Orthop Clin North Am* 1997; **28**:99–116.

38. Mansat P, Cofield RH, Kersten TE, Rowland CM. Complications of rotator cuff repair. *Orthop Clin North Am* 1997; **28**:205–13.

39. Brown AR, Weiss R, Greenberg C et al. Interscalene block for shoulder arthroscopy: comparison with general anesthesia. *Arthroscopy* 1993; **9**:295–300.

40. Caspari RB, Thal R. A technique for arthroscopic subacromial decompression. *Arthroscopy* 1992; **8**:23–30.

41. Codd TP, Flatow EL. Anterior acromioplasty, tendon mobilization, and direct repair of massive rotator cuff tears. In: Burkhead WZ, ed. *Rotator Cuff Disorders*. Baltimore: Williams & Wilkins, 1996; 323–34.

42. Hill JM, Norris TR. Open rotator cuff repair. In: Fu FH, Ticker JB, Imhoff AB, eds. *An Atlas of Shoulder Surgery*. London: Martin Dunitz, 1998; 133–44.

43. Molé D, Sirveaux F. Principes de technique chirurgicale. *Rev Chir Orthop* 1999; **85**:100–4.

44. Johnson DL, Ticker JB. Soft-tissue physiology and repair. In: Beaty JR, ed. *Orthopaedic Knowledge Update 6*. Rosemont: AAOS Press, 1999; 1–18.

29 Arthroscopic repair of rotator cuff tears: Principles and techniques

Stephen S Burkhart

Introduction

The major prerequisite for biologic healing of surgically repaired tissues is structural strength of the repaired construct. This is as true for rotator cuff repairs as it is for fracture fixation or vascular anastamoses. Security and biomechanical integrity are paramount.

I have previously described a number of principles that I have found valuable in achieving secure arthroscopic rotator cuff repairs.[1-11] I firmly believe that application of these principles to a stepwise technique of arthroscopic rotator cuff repair is essential to maximizing the strength of our repair constructs, thereby optimizing our clinical results.

Surgical principles

Arthroscopic evaluation allows a much more accurate assessment of cuff tear configuration than open inspection. Tears can be viewed through various arthroscopic portals to afford three-dimensional views of tear patterns that generally are superior to the views obtained by open means, particularly for large tears.

Rotator cuff tears can broadly be classified into two patterns:

1. Crescent-shaped tears; or
2. U-shaped tears.

Crescent-shaped tears, even large ones, typically pull away from bone but do not retract far. Therefore, they can be repaired to bone with minimal tension (Figure 29.1). U-shaped tears generally extend much farther medially than crescent-shaped tears, usually extending to the glenoid or even medial to the glenoid (Figure 29.2a–c). It is important to realize that this medial extension of the tear does not represent retraction, but rather represents the shape that an L-shaped tear assumes under physiologic load from its muscle–tendon components.[12] Closing such a tear is much like closing a tent-

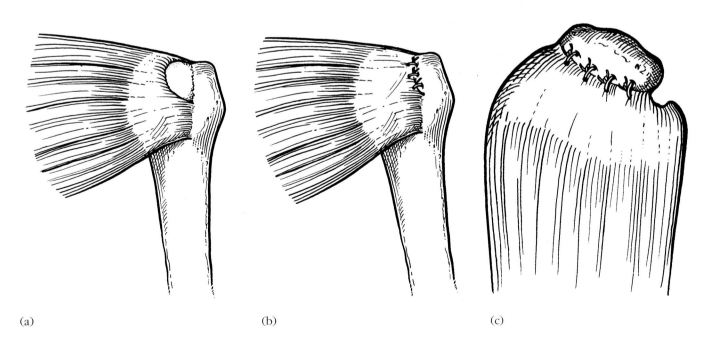

(a) (b) (c)

Figure 29.1

(a) Crescent-shaped rotator cuff tear without much retraction can be repaired directly to bone with minimal tension. (b) Repair of crescent-shaped rotator cuff tear (posterior view). (c) Repair of crescent-shaped rotator cuff tear (superior view).

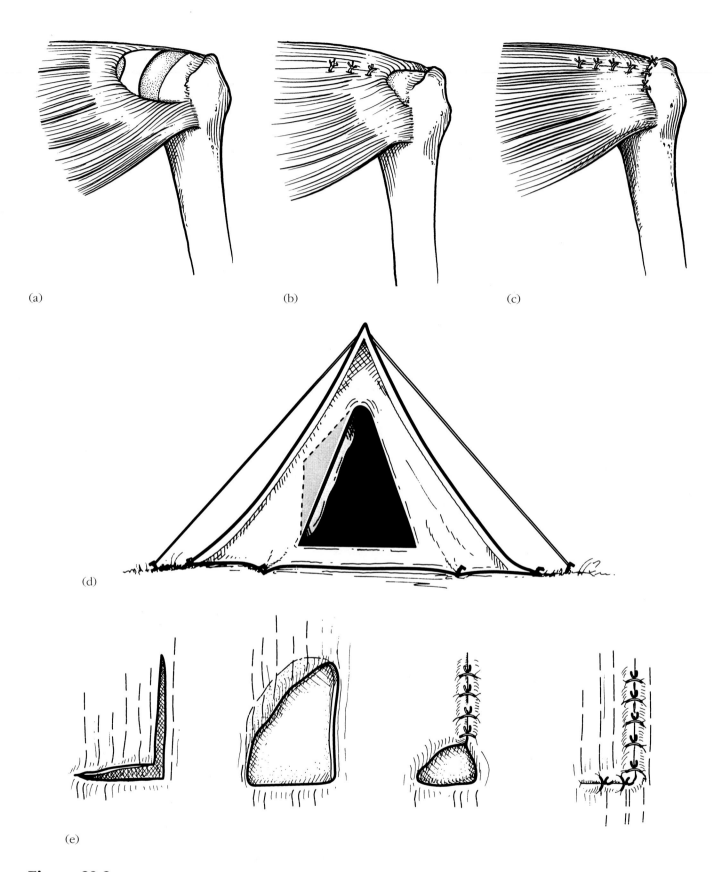

(a)   (b)   (c)

(d)

(e)

Figure 29.2

(a) Large U-shaped cuff tear extending to glenoid. (b) Repair of U-shaped cuff tears begins with side-to-side sutures that converge the free margin of the cuff toward the bone bed (margin convergence). (c) After placing side-to-side sutures, the free margin of the cuff is repaired to bone with suture anchors. (d) Closing an L-shaped or U-shaped tear is much like closing a tent flap. (e) Closure of a U-shaped tear involves first side-to-side closure of the vertical limb of the tear, then tendon-to-bone closure of the transverse limb.

flap; one must reconstitute the two limbs of the L (Figure 29.2d, e). One must not make the mistake of trying to mobilize the medial margin of the tear from the glenoid and scapular neck enough to pull it over to the humeral bone bed. The large tensile stresses in the middle of such a repaired cuff margin would doom the repair to failure.[7,8,13]

The crescent-shaped tear

This type of tear can be easily repaired to bone (Figure 29.1). The surgeon must decide whether to do a transosseous bone tunnel repair or a suture anchor repair. We have previously shown that, under conditions of physiologic cyclic loading, bone fixation by suture anchors is stronger than bone fixation by transosseous bone tunnels.[8] Therefore, I now use suture anchors for rotator cuff repairs instead of bone tunnels. I prepare a bone bed on the humeral neck, just off the articular margin, by means of a power shaver, so as not to decorticate the bone. Decorticating the bone would weaken the anchor fixation in bone and so should be avoided. A bleeding bone surface rather than a bone trough is all that is necessary for satisfactory healing of tendon to bone.[14]

The suture anchor should be inserted at an angle of approximately 45° (deadman angle) to increase the anchor's resistance to pull-out (Figure 29.3).[4] Most of the permanent suture anchors today have adequate pull-out strengths to resist physiologic loads.[15,16]

The crescent-shaped margin of the tear must be respected in the repair and therefore the suture anchors should be placed in a crescent array just 4 or 5 mm off the articular surface to avoid tension overload at any of the fixation points (Figure 29.4). Tension overload has

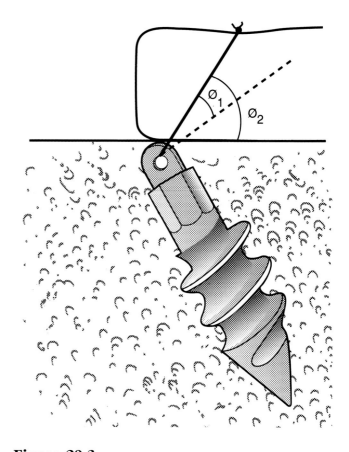

Figure 29.3

Suture anchor should be inserted at a 45° deadman angle.

been shown experimentally to cause failure of cuff repairs subjected to physiologic cyclic loads.[7,8]

Suture capture of the tendon can be done arthroscopically by either simple sutures or mattress sutures.

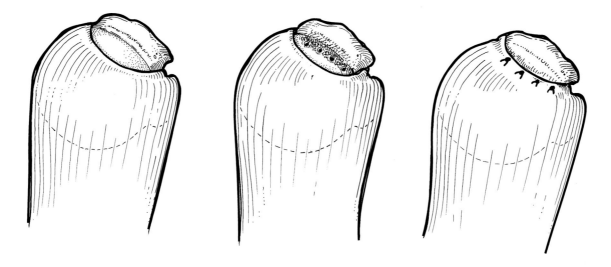

Figure 29.4

Respecting the crescent-shaped margin of a crescent-shaped tear will help avoid tension overload of the repair.

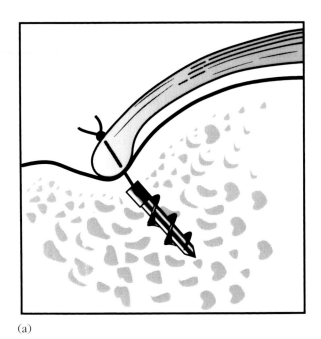

(a)

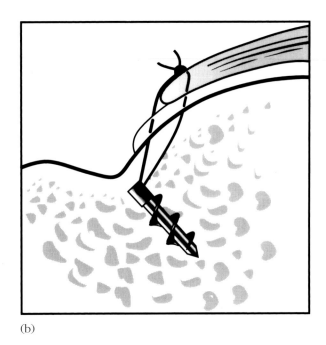

(b)

Figure 29.5

(a) A tight, secure loop maintains apposition of tendon to bone (loop security). (b) A loose loop will allow the tendon to pull away from bone no matter how secure the knot may be.

The strength of simple sutures of #2 Ethibond (Ethicon, Somerville, NJ, USA) has been shown in the laboratory to be adequate for maximal loading conditions of the rotator cuff.[5,11]

Loop security is defined as the ability to maintain a tight suture loop as a knot is tied. Knot security is defined as the effectiveness of a given knot at resisting slippage or breakage when load is applied. Little has been written about loop security, but it is at least as important as knot security, since a loose loop will allow loss of soft tissue fixation even though its associated knot may be very strong (Figure 29.5).[10] Loop security has been shown to be better achieved with an arthroscopic double-diameter knot pusher than with a standard knot pusher.[10] Although some complex sliding knots (Duncan loop, Roeder knot, Nicky's knot, buntline hitch) may also maintain adequate loop security, these complex knots were not investigated in our study.[10]

The literature pertaining to knot security is vast and confusing.[17–30] Unfortunately, virtually all of these studies deal only with the issue of how to tie the strongest knots, whereas all the surgeon really needs to know is the minimal strength that the knot must possess to avoid failure under maximal physiologic load. That is, which knots are strong enough to hold the repair? Beyond that, all discussion about knot security is academic. We would never need to tie a complex knot that is several times stronger than it would ever have to be to resist physiologic loads.

As we consider knot security, there are a couple of important points to keep in mind. First of all, #2

Ethibond breaks at approximately 30 lbs. (133.5 N).[11] However, we have shown in the lab that the common four-throw configurations of half hitches (s=s=s=s, sxsxsxs, s//s//s//s, s//xs//xs//xs) (Figure 29.6) fail by suture slippage rather than breakage, so load to knot slippage becomes the important parameter. The s=s=s=s knot, in which the half-hitches are all in the same direction, fails at a much lower load than the other three configurations, which all fail in the 35–50-N range.[11]

One must keep in mind that knot security is dependent on three factors: friction, internal interference, and slack between throws.[11] Friction will obviously be greater for braided multifilament suture than for slick monofilament suture. Internal interference refers to the 'weave' of the two sutures relative to each other, and it can be increased by changing posts between throws of the knot and/or reversing the direction of consecutive half-hitches. Slack is effectively removed by two maneuvers: removing any twists between the two suture limbs before each half-hitch is tightened, and past-pointing (Figure 29.7) to tighten each half-hitch. Therefore one can maximize knot security by using a braided suture, reversing post suture limbs and/or loop direction, removing all twists between suture limbs, and past-pointing to tighten each half-hitch.

Now that we have maximized the strength of our knot and the tightness of our loop, we can analyse the knot to see whether it is strong enough to resist maximal loading conditions of rotator cuff repair. We have previously shown in the laboratory that rotator cuff repair

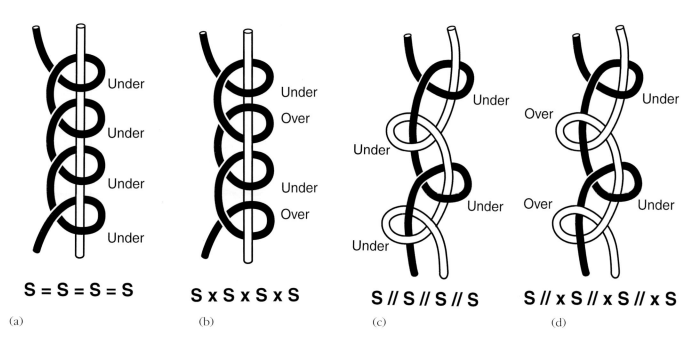

Figure 29.6

(a) Same post, same loop knot configuration (s=s=s=s). (b) Same post, reverse loop knot configuration (sxsxsxs). (c) Reverse post, same loop knot configuration (s//s//s//s). (d) Reverse post, reverse loop knot configuration (s//xs//xs//xs).

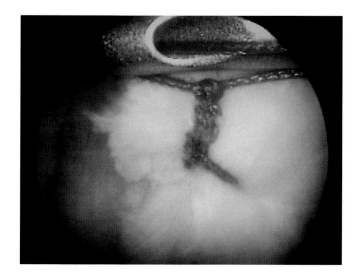

Figure 29.7

Past-pointing, in which the arthroscopic knot pusher is 'run past' the knot, is a useful technique for removing slack between throws.

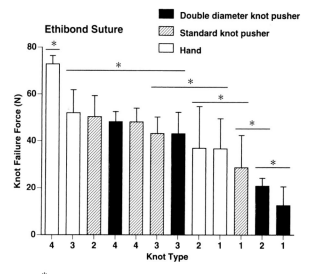

*Groups under same line are not significantly different (p<0.05).

Figure 29.8

Ultimate strength of various knot types tied with #2 Ethibond suture (#1: s=s=s=s; #2: sxsxsxs; #3: s//s//s//s; #4: s//xs//xs//xs).

constructs subjected to large single-pull loads experience suture failure, whereas rotator cuff repair constructs subjected to cyclic loading undergo biologic failure (bone failure or suture pull-out from tendon) rather than suture failure.[5,7,8] Therefore, suture failure would be most likely to occur with a sudden single-pull load caused by

a maximal contraction of the repaired cuff, as in a fall or sudden reflexive arm movement.

To estimate the likelihood of suture failure, one must be able to calculate the load across each suture that might be caused by a sudden forceful contraction and see if the load exceeds the ultimate strength (failure

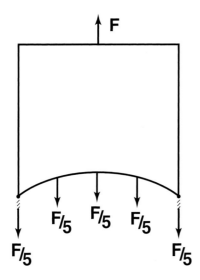

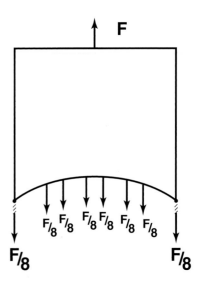

Figure 29.9

If there is one suture per anchor, there will be five fixation points for three anchors.

Figure 29.10

If there are two sutures per anchor, there will be eight fixation points for three anchors.

strength) for the various knot configurations. Failure strength for four stacked half-hitches of #2 Ethibond in an s=s=s=s configuration was determined to be less than 30 N, whereas the ultimate strength for the other common configurations (sxsxsxs, s//s//s//s, and s//xs//xs//xs) was generally in the 35–50-N range (Figure 29.8).[11] Assuming a cuff tear of 4 cm anterior-to-posterior length in the rotator crescent, the maximum muscle force that could be generated across the tear would be 302 N (see Appendix). This tear can be fixed with three suture anchors located 1 cm apart. If each anchor has one suture, then there would be five fixation points (three sutures, two tendon attachments; Figure 29.9) that could be assumed to equally share the load of 302 N. The load per suture during a maximal muscle contraction would be 302 N ÷ 5 = 60.4 N, a load that would cause failure of all the commonly used half-hitch configurations. Assuming two sutures per anchor, there would be eight fixation points (six sutures and two tendon attachments; Figure 29.10). Therefore, the load per suture during a maximal muscle contraction would be 302 N ÷ 8 = 37.75 N, which is a load that all but one of the knot configurations in this study could withstand without failure. One should note that, to simplify the model, we assume that the sutures resist in a direction directly opposite the rotator cuff pull; in the clinical situation, there will be a small angle between the cuff force and the suture, causing a slightly higher tension to develop in the suture. This model allows us to predict the adequacy of a given knot configuration under maximum physiologic loading conditions.

We have recently completed a study to examine optimization of stacked half-hitch knots.[31] By definition,

optimization of knot-holding capacity or knot security would be an enhancement of that knot, which converts its mode of failure from slippage to breakage. The above-referenced study determined that any knot, including complex sliding knots such as the Duncan loop and buntline hitch, can be optimized (i.e. converted to failure by breakage rather than slippage) by adding three half hitches in which the post is consecutively reversed for each half hitch. In addition, Chan and Burkhart[32] have described an easy way to reverse the post without having to rethread the knot pusher, simply by tensioning the wrapping limb in order to 'flip' the post.

The U-shaped tear (so-called 'retracted' tear)

It is critical to recognize that the so-called 'retracted' massive tears are not retracted at all. These large U-shaped tears are actually L-shaped tears with a vertical split from lateral to medial; they have assumed a U-shape by virtue of the elasticity of the involved muscle–tendon units. McLaughlin recognized this pattern and advocated an anatomic L-shaped repair.[12] I have also advocated this type of repair, advising initial side-to-side closure of the anterior and posterior leaves of the tear in order to accomplish margin convergence.[6] Margin convergence refers to the phenomenon that occurs with side-to-side closure of large cuff tears, in which the free margin of the tear converges toward the greater tuberosity as side-to-side repair progresses (Figure 29.11). The creation of

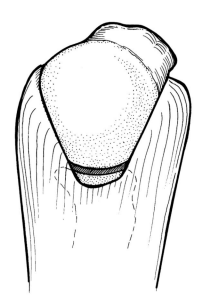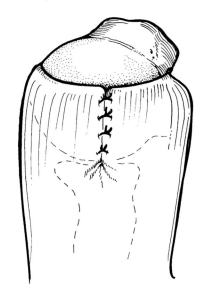

Figure 29.11

Margin convergence occurs with side-to-side closure of a U-shaped tear as the free margin of the cuff converges toward the greater tuberosity. This margin convergence is accompanied by decreased strain in the cuff margin.

this 'converged' cuff margin has the very useful accompaniment of decreased strain in the cuff margin. This gives an added safety factor to the repair to bone, since decreased strain means that there will be a lower likelihood of failure of fixation to bone (for either suture anchors or bone tunnels).

In performing the side-to-side repair, I prefer #2 Ethibond sutures with the knots placed over the posterior leaf of the tear to avoid 'knot impingement'. As with crescent-shaped tears, loop security and knot security are extremely important and demand attention to detail.

In repairing large U-shaped tears, there are two biomechanical principles that must be sequentially followed in order to produce a functional rotator cuff. These principles are:

1. Margin convergence;[6] and
2. Balance of force couples.[2]

As shown above, margin convergence is accomplished by side-to-side closure of anterior and posterior leaves of the cuff. Next, the surgeon must shift the deficient leaf (usually the posterior leaf of the cuff) proximally in order to maximize the moment produced by the repaired cuff, thereby creating a balanced force couple between the anterior and posterior cuff forces. This balance allows the shoulder to establish a stable fulcrum of glenohumeral motion. Suture anchors are very useful in accomplishing this proximal shift. Loop security and knot security are vital to maintaining the shift and the balanced anterior–posterior force couple. If complete closure of cuff to bone cannot be accomplished, the force couple can still be effective even though a hole is left in the superior portion of the cuff. Such partial cuff repairs have been shown to be very effective if at least half of the infraspinatus can be repaired to bone.[9] Partial

repairs are recommended whenever complete closure of the defect is not possible. We advise against rotator cuff tendon transfers (e.g. subscapularis transfer), which change the mechanics of the shoulder and can significantly weaken the transferred muscle–tendon units. For tears that have very rigid margins that cannot be shifted proximally on the bone bed to a mechanically more favorable insertion site, I recommend consideration of the interval slide technique (see Chapter 30).

For large U-shaped tears, loop security and knot security are vitally important, and can be achieved as discussed earlier. Multiple sutures per anchor will reduce the load per suture below the failure point.

Summary of repair

Tear recognition
(A) Crescent-shaped tear
    (1) Repair to bone
    (2) Respect crescent shape during repair (anchor placement 4 or 5 mm off the articular surface)
    (3) Suture anchors at 45° 'deadman angle'
    (4) Loop security
    (5) Knot security
    (6) Multiple sutures per anchor
(B) U-shaped tear
    (1) Side-to-side repair (margin convergence)
    (2) Shift posterior leaf proximally to achieve balanced force couple
    (3) Loop security
    (4) Knot security
    (5) Multiple sutures per anchor
    (6) Partial repair if defect not fully reparable
    (7) Consider interval slide

The sum of its parts

Much of the history of rotator cuff repair has been checkered by ill-advised attempts to simply cover the hole in the cuff. By ignoring shoulder mechanics, many of these methods can actually make the shoulder worse. This chapter is an attempt to relate biomechanical principles to a stepwise approach to arthroscopic rotator cuff repair that will maximize the strength of the repair. Meticulous attention to detail at every step is critical. A loose suture or a poorly placed anchor can mean loss of integrity of the entire construct. In orthopedic surgery, as in structural engineering, structural integrity is built one step at a time. The finished product is never more than the sum of its parts. Therefore, as surgeons, we must strive to maximize the quality of each part. The natural laws that govern biomechanical relationships are not new, but they are sometimes obscure. By clarifying these relationships, we can, to some degree, harness the forces of nature to work in our favor. Natural laws never change. Nature will not conform to humans; we must conform to nature.

Surgical technique

Repair of crescent-shaped tear

The tear pattern is assesssed by testing the mobility of the tear margin with an atraumatic tendon grasper (Arthrex, Naples, FL, USA). Prior to initiating the repair, the surgeon must have a clear view into the lateral gutter, which necessitates removing the lateral shelf of the subacromial bursa (Figure 29.12) so that the entire greater tuberosity can be visualized (Figure 29.13). If the tear can be easily brought directly to the bone bed with minimal tension (Figure 29.14), then it can be repaired directly to bone with suture anchors. I prefer screw-type anchors (Corkscrew; Arthrex). With a screw-type anchor, the suture must be passed through the tendon after the anchor has been placed in bone. After preparation of the bone bed with a shaver, the anchors are placed at a 30–45° deadman angle approximately 5–10 mm from the articular margin (Figure 29.15). The eyelet of the anchor is directed toward the cuff margin so the suture will slide easily (Figure 29.16). Anchors are placed 1 cm apart (Figure 29.17).

Suture passage is done by passing a suture retriever such as a Penetrator (Arthrex) through the superior aspect of the cuff in line with the sutures, which can then be easily retrieved and pulled back out through the cuff. The correct angle of approach through the cuff is obtained by backing the scope out enough to obtain a panoramic view of the suture passer and sutures (Figures 29.18 and 29.19), then 'lining up the putt' so that the suture retriever ends up close enough to the suture to easily capture it (Figure 29.20). For the anterior portion of the cuff, the angle of approach through the cuff and to the suture is often more easily accomplished with an angled suture retriever (BirdBeak; Arthrex; Figures 29.21 and 29.22). I prefer separate soft tissue fixation points for each suture and I utilize posterior, anterior, and modified Neviaser portals for suture passage.

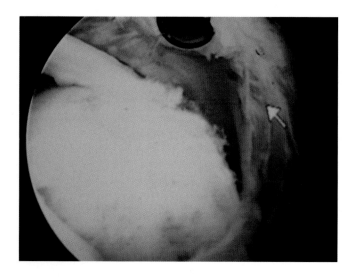

Figure 29.12

In this right shoulder, the lateral bursal shelf (arrow) partially obscures the bone bed. It must be resected to provide a good view of the bone bed on the greater tuberosity.

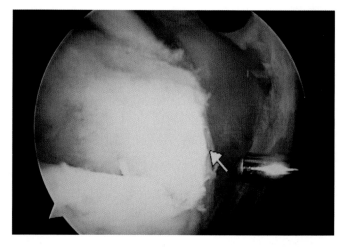

Figure 29.13

After the lateral bursal shelf has been partially resected, the surgeon can easily see the superolateral 'corner' of the greater tuberosity (arrow). The posterior leaf of the rotator cuff tear can also be seen and there is a good view down into the lateral gutter.

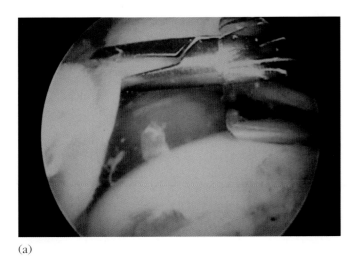

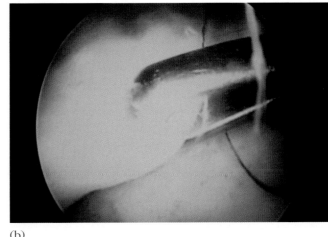

(a)

(b)

Figure 29.14

(a) An atraumatic tendon grasper is used to grasp the apex of this crescent-shaped tear. (b) The tendon grasper is able to easily position the margin of the rotator cuff tear over the bone bed with minimal tension.

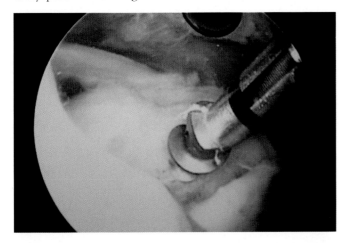

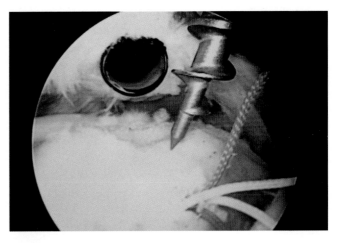

Figure 29.15

Suture anchors are placed 5–10 mm from the articular margin, at a 30–45° deadman angle.

Figure 29.17

Suture anchors are placed approximately 1 cm apart on the prepared bone bed, at the previously described deadman angle.

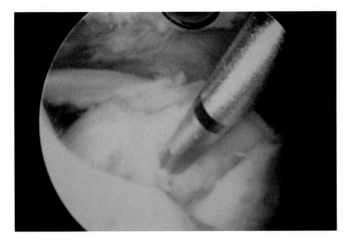

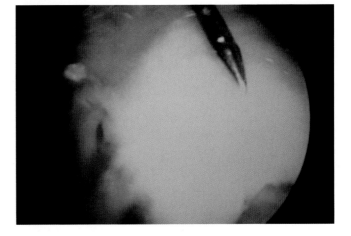

Figure 29.16

The vertical hash marks on the corkscrew inserter indicates the orientation of the eyelet of the anchor. The eyelet is positioned toward the free margin of the cuff so that the suture will slide easily.

Figure 29.18

A panoramic view is obtained to visualize the angle of approach of the suture passer toward the sutures of the suture anchor. The suture passer should penetrate the tendon approximately 1.5–2 cm from the free margin of the rotator cuff tear.

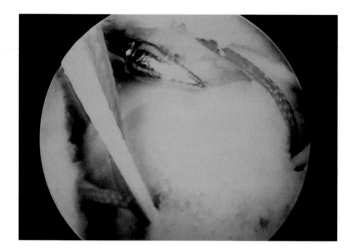

Figure 29.19

After the Penetrator suture passer has gone through the cuff, it is visually lined up with the suture in order to grasp it for passage back through the cuff.

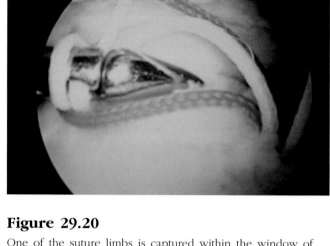

Figure 29.20

One of the suture limbs is captured within the window of the Penetrator, and the suture is wrapped once around the passer to decrease the possibility of suture slippage through the opening of the window of the passer.

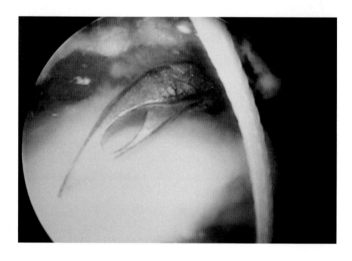

Figure 29.21

The BirdBeak with its angled tip, is frequently the most versatile suture passer for penetrating the anterior portion of the rotator cuff at the proper angle.

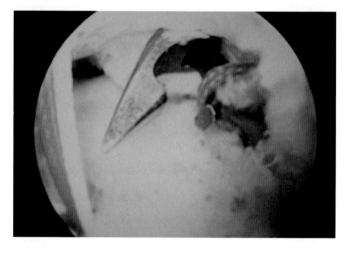

Figure 29.22

After passage through the cuff, the jaws are opened to capture the suture and pull it back through the anterior portion of the rotator cuff.

I prefer to pass all the anchor sutures prior to tying any knots. After suture passage, I tie knots starting with the sutures nearest to the intact cuff insertions and then proceed to those that pass through the central part of the tear. In this way I sequentially decrease the amount of tension that the central suture will have to withstand. By passing all the sutures prior to tying, it is easier to manipulate the suture retriever under the cuff margin, as the cuff is not bound down by sutures that have already been tied.

Suture management is important. Obviously, if one passes all the sutures from multiple anchors before tying

any knots, a tangled mess may result (Figure 29.23). However, the tangling is easily remedied as the suture pairs are retrieved for knot-tying. By grasping suture pairs proximal to the entanglement (Figure 29.24) and pulling the pairs to be tied, one pair at a time, through a dedicated cannula (usually lateral) for knot-tying, the entanglement is never an issue for suture pairs as they are being tied (Figure 29.25).

The knots are tied with a double-diameter knot pusher (Surgeon's Sixth Finger; Arthrex). The knot is delivered to the top of the cuff margin (Figure 29.26),

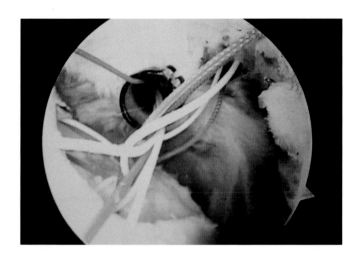

Figure 29.23

After passage of all sutures in a large crescent-shaped rotator cuff tear, there can be tangling of sutures that can initially look to be an irretrievable mess.

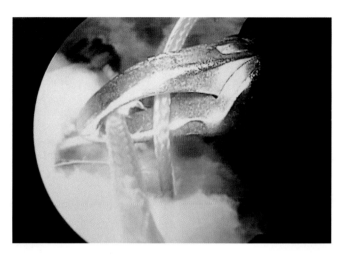

Figure 29.24

If the surgeon grasps the two limbs of a given suture pair proximal to the entanglement, and pulls them through a dedicated lateral cannula for knot tying, the tangling as noted in Figure 29.23 is of no consequence.

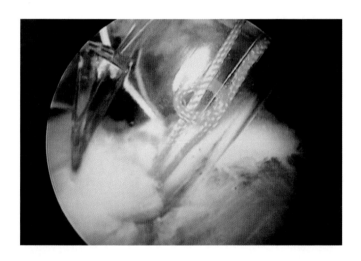

Figure 29.25

With knot tying, the surgeon must be careful to have only the two suture limbs involved in the knot going through the cannula when tying. A clear cannula enhances visualization.

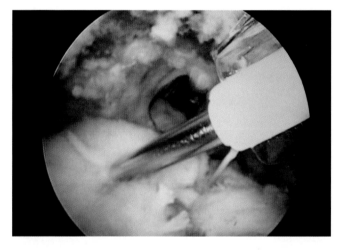

Figure 29.26

A Surgeon's Sixth Finger knot pusher is used to deliver the knot to the top of the rotator-cuff tissue. This placement of the knot allows for a more secure suture loop than if the knot is placed over the bone.

Continuous tension is maintained in the post limb to avoid loosening of the soft tissue loop. Post-switching is accomplished without rethreading the knot pusher, simply by tensioning the wrapping suture limb (Figure 29.27). This maneuver provides additional knot security. An angled basket cutter facilitates suture cutting after the knot has been tied (Figure 29.28). The completed repair should demonstrate a crescent shape to the repaired cuff margin (to avoid tension overload centrally) with separate fixation points for each suture pair (Figure 29.29).

Repair of U-shaped tear

The U-shaped tear is generally easy to recognize. The apex of the tear is located at or medial to the glenoid margin (Figure 29.30). The posterior leaf of the tear has typically been pulled inferomedially in the direction by the infraspinatus force vector, but usually is quite mobile and easily approximated to the anterior leaf (Figure 29.31). Once the U-shaped tear pattern has been recognized, the bone bed on the humeral neck and greater tuberosity is prepared to a bleeding surface with a power

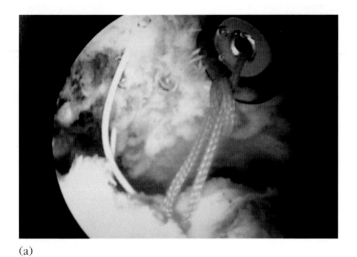

(a)

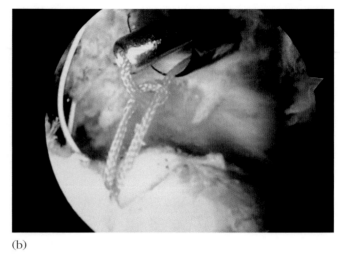

(b)

Figure 29.27

(a) Once the first two throws of half hitches (or the initial sliding knot) have been placed, and the knot has enough friction so that it will not back off, the post should be sequentially switched three times to maximally enhance knot security. In this figure, the post suture is the one that is threaded through the knot pusher, and the wrapping limb circles around the post suture. (b) By tensioning the wrapping limb, it straightens out and becomes the post limb, while the suture that is threaded through the knot pusher has become the wrapping limb. This has, in effect, flipped (or reversed) the post.

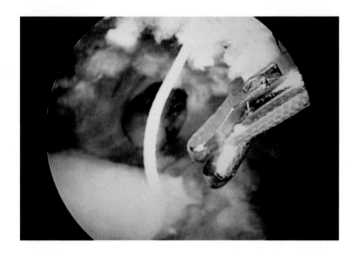

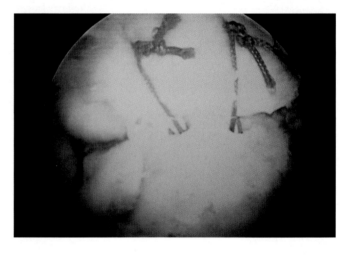

Figure 29.28

An angled basket cutter provides a more natural angle for cutting the suture than a straight basket cutter.

Figure 29.29

Completed repair. Note that the repaired margin of the rotator cuff has been maintained in a crescent shape in order to avoid tension overload of the central portion of the repair. In addition, each suture has a separate fixation point through the tendon. Since each anchor has two sutures, there are six fixation points in this repair.

shaver. Braided #2 Ethibond sutures are passed through the posterior and anterior leaves of the repair for side-to-side closure, using a 'hand-off' technique between suture passers (e.g. Penetrator or BirdBeak) that have been separately passed through the leaves of the cuff (Figure 29.32). Knots are tied through a posterior cannula, with the knot positioned over the posterior leaf, to avoid knot impingement under the acromion (Figure 29.33). As the side-to-side sutures are tied, the free margin of the cuff converges over the previously prepared bone bed (Figure 29.34).

Suture anchors are placed approximately 1 cm from the posterior and anterior leaves of the cuff in order to shift the leaves to the anchors as the knots are tied (Figure 29.35). Sutures from the posterior anchor are passed through the posterior leaf by 'lining up the putt' with a

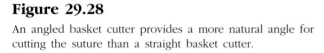

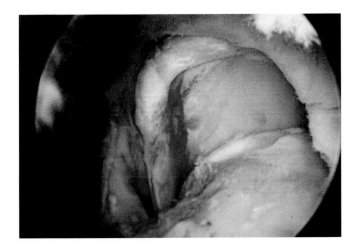

Figure 29.30

This is a massive U-shaped tear in a right shoulder, as viewed through a lateral portal. Note that the posterior leaf is drawn inferiorly because that is the direction of the infraspinatus force vector.

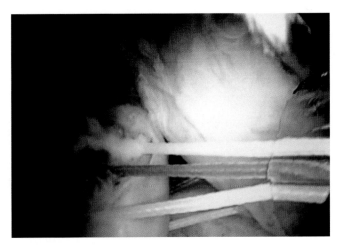

Figure 29.31

After three side-to-side sutures have been placed, the suture limbs have been drawn through an anterior portal in order to determine the mobility of the posterior leaf. With a minimal amount of tension on the sutures, the posterior leaf can be approximated to the anterior leaf.

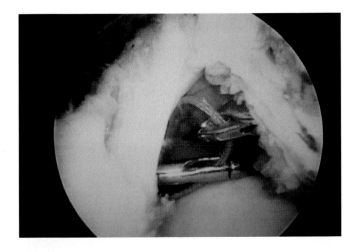

Figure 29.32

A Penetrator suture passer has carried a #2 Ethibond suture through the posterior leaf of the rotator cuff, and this has been 'handed off' to a BirdBeak suture passer which has been passed through the anterior leaf of the rotator cuff.

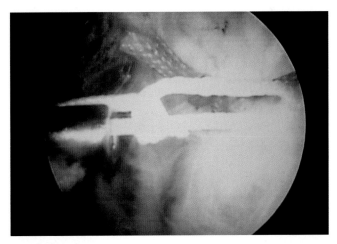

Figure 29.33

The side-to-side sutures are tied sequentially through a posterior cannula so that the knots will be positioned in a posterior location that will avoid the knot impinging under the acromion.

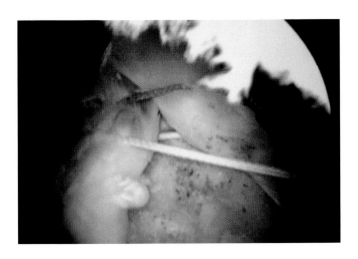

Figure 29.34

Side-to-side repair of the posterior leaf to the anterior leaf has resulted in 'margin convergence', so that the free margin of the cuff now lies over the prepared bone bed.

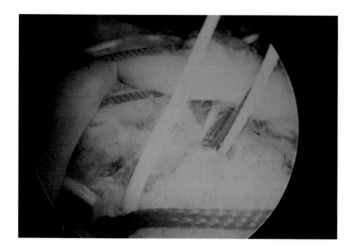

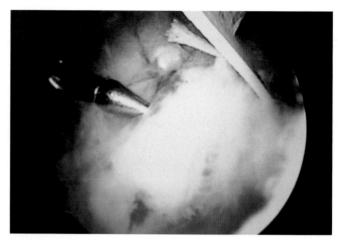

Figure 29.35

Suture anchors have been placed approximately 1 cm from the edges of the anterior and posterior leaves of the rotator cuff in order to obtain an additional 'shift' of each leaf toward the anchor as the sutures are tied. This will optimize the force couple created by the anterior and posterior leaves of the repair.

Figure 29.36

A Penetrator suture passer is used to pass the sutures from the suture anchor through the posterior leaf for fixation to bone. This photograph illustrates how the surgeon 'lines up the putt' in order to pass the suture retriever at the correct angle.

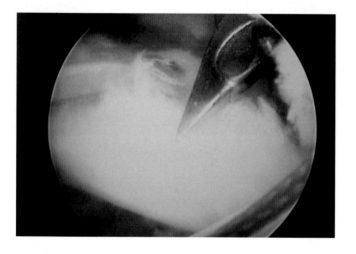

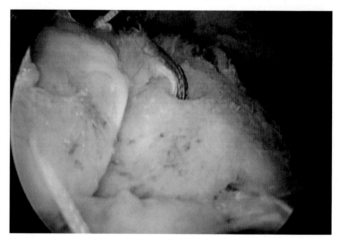

Figure 29.37

The angled BirdBeak suture passer is useful for passing the sutures from the anchor through the anterior leaf.

Figure 29.38

Completed repair. The 'converged margin' of the repair is held snugly to bone by the sutures that have been passed from the suture anchors.

Penetrator suture passer (Figure 29.36). The angled BirdBeak suture passer is used to pass sutures through the anterior leaf (Figure 29.37). The completed repair shows the 'converged margin' repaired snugly to bone by means of suture anchors (Figure 29.38).

Visualization can be enhanced in a tight subacromial space by means of a Muscle Jack (Arthrex). This device has a pointed tip and deployable 'wings' (Figure 29.39). The tip is placed onto the greater tuberosity through an accessory lateral portal (Figure 29.40). Then the wings are deployed, lifting up the deltoid and

providing an additional 1–2 cm space in which to work (Figure 29.41).

Appendix

Average cross-sectional area[33] of supraspinatus–infraspinatus muscle combination that subtends the rotator crescent is 8.8 cm². Maximal contraction of muscle per unit area is 3.5 kg/cm².[34] Assume that homogeneous loading

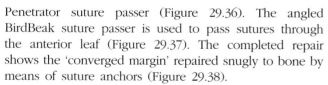

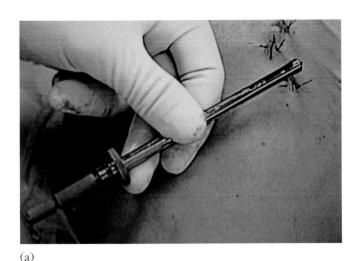

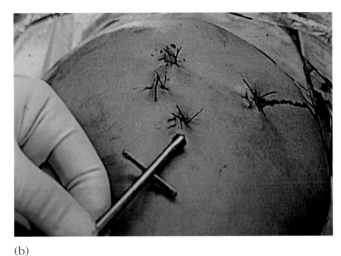

(a)   (b)

Figure 29.39

(a) The Muscle Jack is a useful device that can retract the deltoid muscle in a tight subacromial space. This photograph shows the cylindrical Muscle Jack with its straight profile so that it can be easily inserted through a standard portal. (b) When the wings of the Muscle Jack are deployed, one can see how they would retract the deltoid if the tip of the Muscle Jack were fixed against the greater tuberosity.

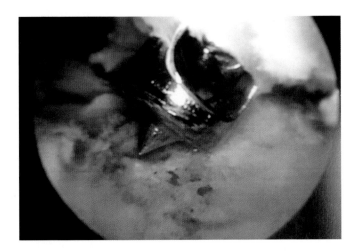

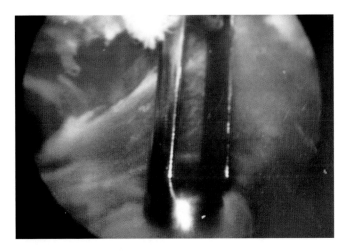

Figure 29.40

Arthroscopic subacromial view of a right shoulder in which the tip of the Muscle Jack has been set against the bone bed on the greater tuberosity.

Figure 29.41

The wings of the Muscle Jack have now been deployed and elevate the deltoid away from the greater tuberosity in order to provide more space in which to operate in cases in which deltoid swelling has compromised the subacromial space.

exists across the cross-section, resulting in uniform loading. Therefore, maximal muscle contraction force across the rotator crescent is $8.8 \, cm^2 \times 3.5 \, kg/cm^2 = 30.8 \, kg = 302 \, N$.

References

1. Burkhart SS, Esch JC, Jolson RS. The rotator crescent and rotator cable: an anatomic description of the shoulder's 'suspension bridge'. *Arthroscopy* 1993; **9**:611–16.

2. Burkhart SS. Current concepts: reconciling the paradox of rotator cuff repair versus debridement: a unified biomechanical rationale for the treatment of rotator cuff tears. *Arthroscopy* 1994; **10**:4–19.

3. Burkhart SS, Nottage WM, Ogilvie-Harris DJ et al. Partial repair of irreparable rotator cuff tears. *Arthroscopy* 1994; **10**:363–70.

4. Burkhart SS. Technical note: The deadman theory of suture anchors: observations along a South Texas fence line. *Arthroscopy* 1995; **11**:119–23.

5. Burkhart SS, Fischer SP, Nottage WM et al. Tissue fixation security in transosseous rotator cuff repairs: a mechanical comparison of simple versus mattress sutures. *Arthroscopy* 1996; **12**:704–8.

6. Burkhart SS, Athanasiou KA, Wirth MA. Technical note: margin convergence: a method of reducing strain in massive rotator cuff tears. *Arthroscopy* 1996; **12**:335–8.

7. Burkhart SS, Johnson TC, Wirth MA et al. Cyclic loading of transosseous rotator cuff repairs: 'tension overload' as a possible cause of failure. *Arthroscopy* 1997; **13**:172–6.

8. Burkhart SS, Diaz-Pagàn JL, Wirth MA et al. Cyclic loading of anchor-based rotator cuff repairs: confirmation of the tension overload phenomenon and comparison of suture anchor fixation with transosseous fixation. *Arthroscopy* 1997; **13**:720–4.

9. Burkhart SS. Partial repair of massive rotator cuff tears: the evolution of a concept. *Orthop Clin North Am* 1997; **28**:125–32.

10. Burkhart SS, Wirth MA, Simonich M et al. Technical note: loop security as a determinant of tissue fixation security. *Arthroscopy* 1998; **14**:773–6.

11. Burkhart SS, Wirth MA, Simonich M et al. Knot security in simple sliding knots and its relationship to rotator cuff repair: how secure must a knot be? *Arthroscopy* 2000; **16**:202–7.

12. McLaughlin HL. Lesions of the musculotendinous cuff of the shoulder: the exposure and treatment of tears with retraction. *J Bone Joint Surg* 1944; **26A**:31–51.

13. Caldwell GL, Warner JJP, Miller MD et al. Transosseous rotator cuff fixation: the weak link? a biomechanical evaluation. *Orthop Trans* 1995; **19**:368 (abstract).

14. St. Pierre P, Olson FJ, Elliott JJ et al. Tendon healing to cortical bone versus a cancellous trough: a biomechanical and histological model in the goat. Presented at the 14th Annual Meeting of The Arthroscopy Association of North America. San Francisco, CA, May 4–7, 1995.

15. Barber FA, Herbert MA, Click JN. The ultimate strength of suture anchors. *Arthroscopy* 1995; **11**:21–8.

16. Barber FA, Herbert MA, Click JN. Internal fixation strength of suture anchors: update 1997. *Arthroscopy* 1997; **13**:355–62.

17. Brouwers JE, Dosting H, deHaas D, Klopper PJ. Dynamic loading of surgical knots. *Surg Gynecol Obstet* 1991; **173**:443–8.

18. Gerber C, Schneiberger AG, Schlegel U. Mechanical strength of repairs of the rotator cuff. *J Bone Joint Surg* 1994; **76B**:371–80.

19. Gunderson PE. The half-hitch knot: a rational alternative to the square knot. *Am J Surg* 1987; **154**:538–40.

20. Herrman JB. Tensile strength and knot security of surgical suture materials. *Am J Surg* 1971; **37**:209–17.

21. Holmlund DE. Knot properties of surgical suture materials. *Acta Chir Scand* 1974; **140**:355–62.

22. Loutzenheiser TD, Harryman DT, Yung SW et al. Optimizing arthroscopic knots. *Arthroscopy* 1995; **11**:199–206.

23. Loutzenheiser TD, Harryman DT II, Ziegler DW et al. Optimizing arthroscopic knots using braided or monofilament suture. *Arthroscopy* 1998; **14**:57–65.

24. Mishra DK, Cannon WD Jr, Lucas DJ et al. Elongation of arthroscopically tied knots. *Am J Sports Med* 1997; **25**:113–17.

25. Rodeheaver GT, Thacker JG, Edlich RF. Mechanical performance of polyglycolic acid and polygalactin 91D synthetic absorbable suture. *Surg Gynecol Obstet* 1981; **153**:835–41.

26. Taylor FW. Surgical knots. *Ann Surg* 1938; **107**:458–68.

27. Tera H, Aberg C. Tensile strength of twelve types of knots employed in surgery, using different suture materials. *Acta Chir Scand* 1976; **142**:1–7.

28. Trimbos JB, Booster M, Peters AAW. Mechanical knot performance of a new generation Polydiaxanon suture (PDS-2). *Acta Obstet Gynecol Scand* 1991; **70**:157–9.

29. Trimbos JB, Van Rijssel EJC, Klopper PJ. Performance of sliding knots in monofilament and multifilament suture material. *Obstet Gynecol* 1986; **68**:425–30.

30. Van Rijssel EJ, Trimbos JB, Booster MH. Mechanical performance of square knots and sliding knots in surgery: a comparative study. *Am J Obstet Gynecol* 1990; **162**:93–7.

31. Chan KC, Burkhart SS, Thiagarajan P, Goh JCH. Optimization of stacked half-hitch knots for arthroscopic surgery. *Arthroscopy* 2001; **17**:752–9.

32. Chan KC, Burkhart SS. Technical note: how to switch posts without re-threading when tying half-hitches. *Arthroscopy* 1999; **15**:444–50.

33. Bassett RW, Browne AO, Morrey BF et al. Glenohumeral muscle force and mechanics in a position of instability. *J Biomech* 1990; **23**:405–8.

34. Ikai M, Fukunaga T. Calculation of muscle strength per unit of cross-sectional area of human muscle by means of ultrasonic measurement. *Int Z Angew Physiol* 1968; **26**:26–30.

30 Rotator cuff tear: Arthroscopic repair

Brian S Cohen and Anthony A Romeo

Introduction

Rotator cuff dysfunction is a common source of shoulder pain in patients over the age of 40 years. Disruption of the integrity of the rotator cuff forms one pathologic entity that can be potentially painful and disabling for many patients. 'Rotator cuff surgery' reliably decreases pain, and improves motion and function as well as the general health status of the patient.[1,2] The objectives of the surgical repair of a torn rotator cuff are to decrease pain, increase range of motion and improve function.[2] Complete or partial anatomic restoration of the rotator cuff accomplishes these goals by restoring 'biomechanical stability' to the shoulder complex.[3] The operative approach for rotator cuff repairs has evolved from the classic open approach to a mini-open, or deltoid-sparing, approach, then finally to an 'all-arthroscopic' repair.[4,5] The surgical evolution has been stimulated by an improvement in the understanding of rotator cuff tear patterns, as well as the availability of arthroscopic instrumentation specifically designed for soft tissue repair techniques. Furthermore, surgical concepts such as margin convergence have provided repair strategies that allow the shoulder arthroscopist to treat any rotator cuff tear, regardless of its size or retraction.[6] The ability to repair the rotator cuff without detachment or manipulation of the deltoid is a tremendous benefit to the patient. It results in decreased pain associated with the cuff repair, avoids complications that are related to deltoid reattachment, and optimizes the patient's rehabilitation process. With arthroscopic rotator cuff repairs, the rate-limiting step for recovery is biologic healing of the rotator cuff tendon to the humeral bone (estimated to be a minimum of 8–12 weeks), and the time required to strengthen the rotator cuff muscles once tendon healing is achieved.

The indications to perform a repair of a torn rotator cuff are the same, regardless of the surgical approach. Indications for repairing a torn rotator cuff are clearly defined and include pain, loss of function, and failure to improve with conservative management. The main reason that patients elect to undergo a surgical repair of their rotator cuff is the negative impact that their shoulder problem has on their 'quality of life.' The reason to perform this repair arthroscopically is solely based on the surgeon's comfort and expertise with this technically challenging approach.

A successful outcome following a rotator cuff repair is dependent on a secure, lasting repair. It is the integrity of the repair over time that has been shown to correlate with better motion and function.[7,8] The clinical results of arthroscopic rotator cuff repairs performed by advanced shoulder arthroscopists are equal to those of open rotator cuff repairs.[9–11] The ability to achieve results similar to those achieved during open repairs with reduced morbidity is appealing. We have reviewed our arthroscopic cuff repairs in a similar manner as Harryman et al,[7] and have found that cuff integrity is maintained at a similar rate as that seen with open repairs. We have also noticed better motion and function in those patients with an intact repair.[12] Therefore it is still the effectiveness and durability of the cuff repair itself, and not the surgical approach that translates into a successful patient outcome. It is the responsibility of the surgeons to select the repair technique that they are most comfortable with and affords them the opportunity to consistently repair the rotator cuff tendon securely.

Surgical principles

Arthroscopic rotator cuff surgery offers a repair technique that not only protects the deltoid origin, which is compromised during a classic open repair, but avoids aggressive deltoid retraction seen during difficult mini-open repairs. The keys to a successful arthroscopic cuff repair are first, understanding the tear configuration, and second, implementing the appropriate repair technique based on the tear configuration (Figures 30.1–30.3). By utilizing the arthroscope to view the cuff tear from all available portals, the surgeon has a better understanding of the three-dimensional nature of the cuff tear pattern and its repairability.[13,14]

Rotator cuff fixation is accomplished with arthroscopic suture anchors, which have been shown to provide better fixation than cuffs repaired through bone tunnels.[15] The ideal repair location is at the rotator cuff tendon's anatomic insertion, approximately 5–10 mm lateral to the articular surface; some medialization may be required to reduce the tension on the repair. Anchors should be inserted at an angle of approximately 45°, the so-called 'deadman's angle,' to resist the pullout forces of the rotator cuff tendon (Figure 30.4).[16] Additionally, suture anchors that allow for two sutures per anchor are

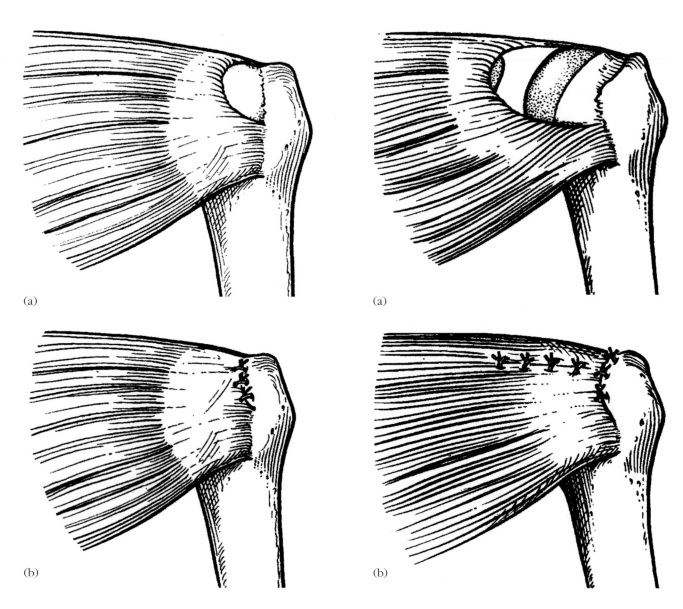

(a)

(b)

(a)

(b)

Figure 30.1

(a) Schematic representation of a crescent tear configuration repaired (b) by securing the free lateral tendon edge to bone with simple sutures from laterally placed suture anchors. (Courtesy of Stephen S Burkhart.)

Figure 30.2

(a) Schematic representation of a U-shaped tear repaired by (b) convergence of the posterior and anterior margins of the tear, followed by fixation of the lateral tendon edge to bone with simple sutures from laterally placed suture anchors. (Courtesy of Stephen S Burkhart.)

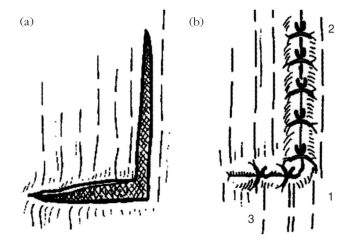

(a)   (b)

Figure 30.3

(a) Schematic representation of an L-shaped tear repaired by (b) anchor placement corresponding to the elbow of the 'L' to that point (1). Then, a side-to-side repair (2), followed by a repair of the remaining lateral margin to the bone with simple sutures from laterally placed suture anchors (3). (Courtesy of Stephen S Burkhart.)

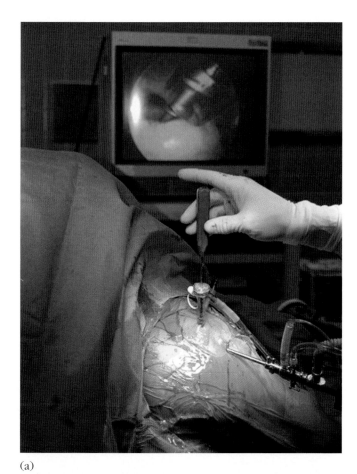

(a)

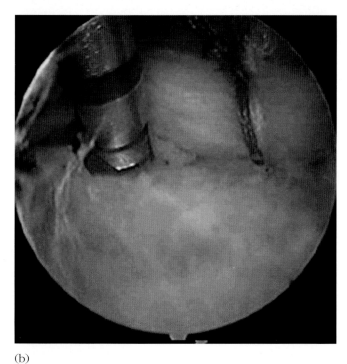

(b)

Figure 30.4

Suture anchors are inserted at a 45° angle in the lateral aspect of the area prepared on the tuberosity (a,b). This anchor may be placed through the accessory anterolateral portal, or through a small incision in the skin.

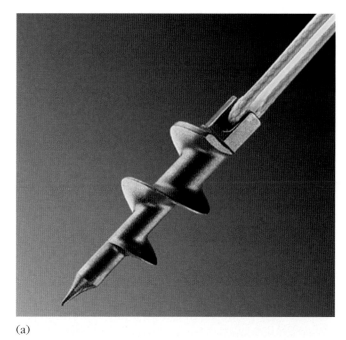

(a)

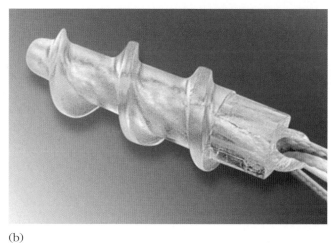

(b)

Figure 30.5

(a) 5.0 Corkscrew and (b) 5.0 Bio-Corkscrew suture anchors. (Arthrex, Naples, FL, USA)

ideally suited for a cuff repair and resistance against physiologic loads at the repair site.[15] Although, there are a number of suture anchors available, we utilize either the 5.0 Corkscrew or 5.0 Bio-Corkscrew suture anchor (Arthrex) (Figure 30.5a,b). The 5.0 mm Corkscrew suture anchor is a titanium anchor with two non-absorbable #2 Tevdek (Genzyme Biosurgery, Cambridge, MA, USA) sutures, one white and one green for easy identification. This anchor can be 'screwed' directly through the skin, does not require pre-drilling or tapping and is inserted by hand. If there is a concern with regard to the fixation of the anchor, or the anchor pulls out, there is a 6.5 mm Corkscrew anchor, which can be placed in the same insertion site for a more secure fixation. The 5.0 mm

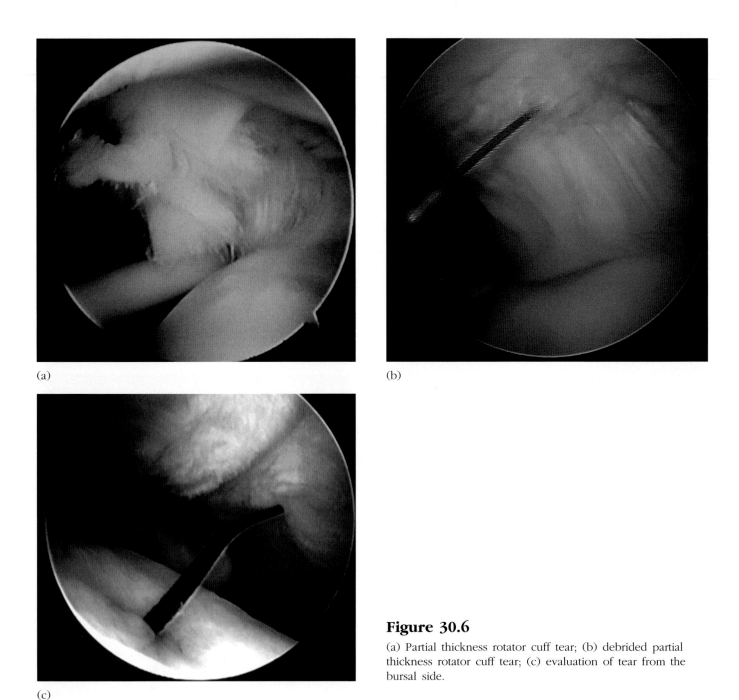

(a)

(b)

(c)

Figure 30.6

(a) Partial thickness rotator cuff tear; (b) debrided partial thickness rotator cuff tear; (c) evaluation of tear from the bursal side.

Bio-Corkscrew suture anchor requires a pilot hole to be created first by a punch. If the punch is seated easily, indicative of 'soft bone', the recommendation is to proceed with implant placement. If the bone is of appropriate 'hardness', the pilot hole is tapped prior to anchor placement. As in the situation with the 5.0 mm Corkscrew suture anchor, there is a 6.5 mm Bio-Corkscrew suture anchor available if the surgeon is concerned with the status of the anchor fixation. We utilize an anchor-first technique, which allows separation of anchor placement and tissue repair. Separating these two critical steps facilitates the goal of an anatomic cuff repair. There are a variety of suture-passing and knot-tying devices available and the surgeon needs to utilize

those instruments that allow him or her to perform a successful, reproducible anatomic reconstruction.

An arthroscopic rotator cuff repair in general follows a stepwise approach to accomplishing its goal of an anatomic reconstruction. Therefore, the surgeon must pay close attention to detail and avoid excluding or performing the basic steps of the procedure out of order since this can lead to an inadequate reconstruction. The basic steps include a thorough evaluation of the gleno-humeral joint with a close examination of the rotator cuff including the subscapularis, the supraspinatus and the infraspinatus tendons; and an inspection for additional intra-articular pathology, such as a Bankart lesion, a superior labrum anterior to posterior (SLAP) tear, or significant glenohumeral arthritis. Partial thickness rotator cuff tears need to be identified, debrided and tagged (Figure 30.6a–c) for later evaluation from the bursal side. Subacromial surgery includes a thorough bursectomy followed by an appropriate acromioplasty and a complete assessment of the rotator cuff tear pattern, mobility and repairability. Proper repair techniques based on the tear pattern are necessary to accomplish an anatomic repair; proper anchor placement at 'deadmans' angle is important for maintaining cuff integrity[16] during the 'biological healing' period; careful suture management is necessary to avoid suture entanglement and inadvertent unloading of suture anchors; and successful arthroscopic knot-tying skills are required to appropriately secure the tendon, utilizing either a sliding (Duncan loop) or non-sliding (modified Revo) knot depending on the mobility of the suture.

Treatment of partial thickness articular-sided tears with debridement versus formal repair remains controversial, but important factors for the surgeon to consider should include the depth of the partial tear, the pattern of the tear (avulsion versus degenerative) and the activity level of the patient.[2,18] At times the decision to repair a partial thickness articular-sided tear cannot be finalized from the intra-articular inspection. To further assess the area of the partial tear and its corresponding bursal-side appearance, the area is identified by passing a #0 or #1 polydioxanone (PDS; Ethicon, Somerville, NJ, USA) suture through the partial tear using an 18-gauge spinal needle (Figure 30.6). The anterior cannula and the needle are removed, and the suture is clamped together to avoid inadvertent removal.

The condition of the subacromial space is another factor in determining if a formal repair of a partial thickness rotator cuff tear is indicated. For example, if there is a paucity of inflammation or 'bursitis' in the subacromial space, the patient's shoulder pain can be attributed to the rotator cuff injury, and therefore, a formal arthroscopic repair of the partial-thickness rotator cuff tear is usually performed.

Finally, with significant partial-thickness cuff tears, the suture marker is identified in the subacromial space to evaluate the bursal integrity of the rotator cuff tendon (Figure 30.6c). In general, a non-degenerative partial-thickness tear of 50% or more of the cuff tendon in an active patient with rotator cuff symptoms is a strong indication for a surgical repair.

Complications, such as 'failure of the deltoid reattachment' seen following a classic open rotator cuff repair, or deltoid denervation following classic open and mini-open repairs, are non-existent in patient following an arthroscopic cuff repair. With proper arthroscopic portal placement, risk of neurologic injury is also avoided. The main complication seen following an arthroscopic repair is 'repair failure', which is mostly related to the patient's preoperative cuff tear size and has a similar incidence following an open or an arthroscopic cuff repair.[7,8,12]

The major disadvantage of an arthroscopic cuff repair is that it is technically more challenging, making it 'more' difficult and, therefore, 'not for everyone.' There are three theoretical concerns with the arthroscopic approach: the 'temptation to accept a marginal arthroscopic repair' rather than opening (failing); not having the tactile security of an 'adequate' open repair; and the perception of the surgery as being 'minor' places it at risk for being abused by the patient and/or the physical therapist.[18]

Surgical technique

A thorough physical examination of the injured shoulder is performed prior to patient positioning. Preoperative shoulder crepitation, range of motion, and stability are recorded and compared to that of the contralateral shoulder. Our preferred method of anesthesia is a combination of an interscalene block and general anesthesia.[19] A long-acting interscalene block reduces the amount of inhalation agents and narcotics necessary for effective general anesthesia, and provides postoperative pain relief throughout the day of surgery. More than 95% of patients using this method are discharged from our surgical facility within a few hours after completion of an arthroscopic rotator cuff repair.

Patient positioning

We prefer the beach chair position for rotator cuff repairs for several reasons (Figure 30.7). This position makes it simple for ancillary staff to set up the patient; the shoulder is oriented in a way that is familiar to the surgeon

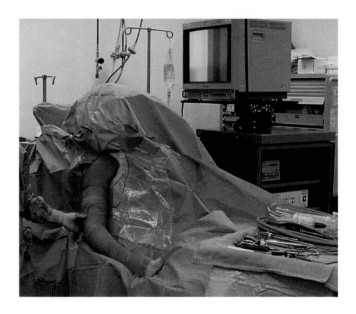

Figure 30.7
Beach chair position.

and allows the surgeon to easily move the arm and the rotator cuff during the procedure, facilitating the surgical repair. The lateral decubitus position with fixed traction on the arm is the other option and is preferred by other surgeons.[5]

Portal placement

The bony landmarks of the shoulder are outlined to identify the acromion, the clavicle, the acromioclavicular articulation, the spine of the scapula, the coracoid process and the coracoacromial ligament (Figure 30.8). In addition, the positions of the three standard portals are identified (posterior, anterior, and lateral) and infiltrated with 0.25% bupivacaine and epinephrine prior to making the incisions. The standard posterior portal is placed in the 'soft spot' of the posterior shoulder, which is approximately 2 cm inferior and 1–2 cm medial to the posterolateral corner of the acromion. The anterior portal is lateral to the coracoid process and below the coracoacromial ligament, at the level of the acromioclavicular joint externally and within the rotator interval internally. The lateral portal, which is routinely used for subacromial decompression and arthroscopic cuff repairs is positioned 2–3 cm distal to the lateral edge of the acromion and just anterior to a line that would bisect the anterior-to-posterior distance of the acromion. In addition, an accessory anterolateral portal is created after the acromioplasty and bursectomy to facilitate anchor placement, suture passage through the cuff tendon, suture management, and – most importantly – arthroscopic knot tying. The portal is located at the anterolateral corner of the acromion. Occasionally, posteriorly located tears are repaired through an accessory portal located at the posterolateral corner of the acromion.

The arthroscope is introduced into the glenohumeral joint via blunt trocar to avoid damage to the articular cartilage. The standard anterior portal is established using an inside-out technique. This is executed by advancing the arthroscope inferior to the biceps tendon and into the rotator interval. The arthroscope is then withdrawn from its sheath, and a Wissinger rod is advanced through the cannula. The rod is passed through the anterior capsule of the rotator interval, below the coracoacromial ligament and into the subcutaneous tissue lateral to the coracoid process. The skin is infiltrated with the bupivacaine and epinephrine, and a skin incision is made over the Wissinger rod. An anterior cannula (5.7 mm, Arthrex) is then advanced over the rod and into the glenohumeral joint. The outflow tubing is switched to the anterior cannula to establish directional flow of fluid. The Wissinger rod is removed, and the arthroscope is reintroduced into the shoulder through the posterior cannula. A systematic evaluation of the glenohumeral joint is then performed. Evaluation of the articular surfaces and documentation of associated

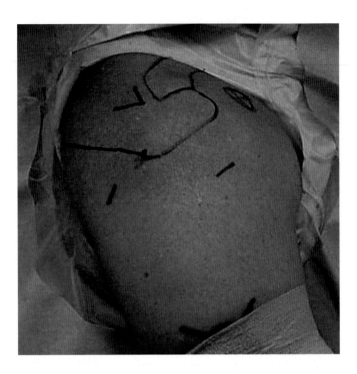

Figure 30.8

Outline of acromion, clavicle, acromioclavicular articulation, coracoid process, spine of scapula, and arthroscopic portals.

pathologies are important. Arthroscopic evidence of abnormalities related to the glenoid labrum, the biceps tendon or the subscapularis tendon might alter the preoperative plan in 10–15% of patients undergoing rotator cuff repair surgery.[20] Arthroscopic treatment of intra-articular pathology may require the placement of additional portals, such as an anterosuperior portal for repair of superior labral tears.

An arthroscopic pump is used throughout the procedure to provide fluid control and hemostasis. The inflow tubing is connected to the arthroscope sheath, while the outflow is connected to the cannula away from the arthroscope (most commonly, the anterior portal) to establish a directional flow of fluid away from the camera. The pump pressure is set at 35–40 mmHg during glenohumeral arthroscopy, and it is increased to 40–60 mmHg during arthroscopic acromioplasty and bursectomy, and then reduced to 40 mmHg during the rotator cuff repair.

Intra-articular evaluation of the rotator cuff

A meticulous evaluation of the articular side of the rotator cuff is essential prior to removing the arthroscope from the glenohumeral joint. Examination of the insertions of the subscapularis, supraspinatus, and infraspinatus can all be performed when viewing from the posterior portal. For partial thickness rotator cuff tears, tear thickness should be documented and the quality of the remaining cuff tissue should be assessed.

Before the procedure advances into the subacromial space, the arthroscope is placed through the anterior portal to re-evaluate the glenohumeral joint structures, including the posterior labrum. Evaluation of full-thickness rotator cuff tears requires documentation of the size of the tear, the number of tendons involved, and the degree of medial retraction. A final assessment of tear size and configuration is completed when the tear is viewed from the bursal surface, which provides a panoramic view of the cuff tendon.

Subacromial surgery

Direct entry from the posterior portal into the subacromial space allows for minimal bleeding and avoids causing trauma to the posterior rotator cuff tendon and muscle fibers. Improper placement of the arthroscope can lead to 'wrong-plane' dissection and inadvertent rotator cuff injury. The correct placement of the arthroscope into the subacromial space begins with a redirection of the arthroscope superiorly toward the anterior portal entry site into the space, with palpation of the undersurface of the acromion with the tip of the blunt trocar while it is still within its sheath. The blunt trocar is then removed, and a smooth Wissinger rod is passed through the cannula, below the coracoacromial ligament and outside the anterior portal incision. The anterior cannula is passed into the subacromial space over the metal rod, and the coupled cannulas are gently withdrawn and separated with in the space, creating a 'room with a view'.[5] The lateral portal is established by localizing the proper position with an 18-gauge spinal needle while viewing from the posterior portal. The lateral portal should be below the level of the lateral acromion, so that there is a direct approach to the subacromial space without interference of the acromion. In general, more superiorly positioned cannulas are favored because they allow the surgeon to 'look down' at the rotator cuff tear, and because they improve the working distance between the instruments and the rotator cuff.

Establishing and maintaining visualization is paramount to successfully completing the procedure. Hemostasis is achieved by maintaining a low systolic blood pressure (≤ 110 mmHg), using an arthroscopic pump system that maintains subacromial pressure, and an electrothermal device (i.e. Ablation probe, Oratec Interventions, Menlo Park, CA, USA) for coagulation and ablation of soft tissues. A complete bursectomy allows a comprehensive evaluation of the cuff tear size and configuration, and provides a space for an unencumbered arthroscopic repair. The initial bursectomy is performed when viewing the anterior subacromial space from the posterior portal and using a shaver or electrothermal device from the lateral portal.

In our practice, an arthroscopic acromioplasty is performed principally to increase the working space and provide a smooth surface to minimize abrasion of the repaired rotator cuff. The coracoacromial ligament is released, beginning at the anterolateral edge of the acromion and continuing medially along the anteroinferior margin of the acromion. Occasionally, the ligament is completely resected to allow for better visualization and subsequent repair of anterosuperior cuff tears. The soft tissue is removed from the anterior half of the inferior surface of the acromion. The acromioplasty is initiated at the anterolateral margin of the acromion, typically removing about 4 mm of bone using a barrel-shaped or flat-sided high-speed burr. After removing the anteroinferior section of the acromion, the arthroscope is placed in the lateral portal to visualize the slope of the acromion. The high-speed burr is then advanced through the posterior portal to the midpoint of the acromion. A 'cutting-block' technique is used to complete the acromioplasty.[21] The burr is advanced from posterior to anterior to flatten and smooth the undersurface of the acromion (Figure 30.9a,b).

Following the acromioplasty, an extensive bursectomy is performed from the posterior portal using an arthroscopic shaver to allow full visualization of the rotator cuff. However, debridement of bursal tissue in the lateral gutter should not proceed beyond the bursal reflection (3–5 cm distal) to avoid causing injury to the axillary nerve on the undersurface of the deltoid, which lies directly inferior to the bursal reflection.

Evaluation of the rotator cuff tear pattern

The evaluation of a cuff tear typically includes the size (area in cm²) of the tear based on the length of the detachment and the amount of retraction from the greater tuberosity. Similarly, tendon mobility and quality are assessed. Proper recognition of the cuff tear configuration will help determine the most effective strategy for an arthroscopic cuff repair. Crescent-shaped tears can be repaired to the tuberosity using suture anchors and simple suture patterns (Figure 30.1). For U-shaped tears, the first step in the repair is to reduce or eliminate the medial-to-lateral component of the tear configuration by converging the posterior and anterior margins with a side-to-side repair (Figure 30.2). Margin convergence is a critical step to a successful cuff repair because it facilitates an anatomic repair of the tendon and reduces the strain at the tendon–bone repair site.[6] For L-shaped tears, the elbow of the 'L' is secured to its anatomic site with simple suture from a laterally placed suture anchor, and margin convergence proceeds with passage of sutures

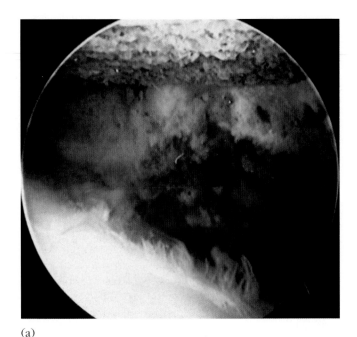

(a)

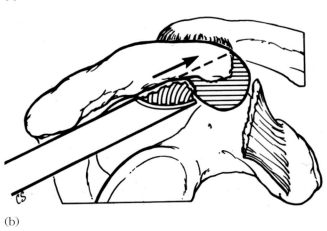

(b)

Figure 30.9

(a) Completed acromioplasty; (b) utilizing the cutting block technique.

from the posterior-to-anterior margin, followed by the securing of the lateral tendon edge to bone with simple sutures from additional suture anchors (Figure 30.3).

Preparation for the rotator cuff tendon repair

For most cuff repairs, the arthroscope will remain in the lateral portal, providing a panoramic view of the tear and the repair site. The mobility of the tendon is evaluated by grasping the tendon and gently pulling laterally. The arm is kept at 10–20° of abduction. The excursion of the tendon edge determines the position of the repair site

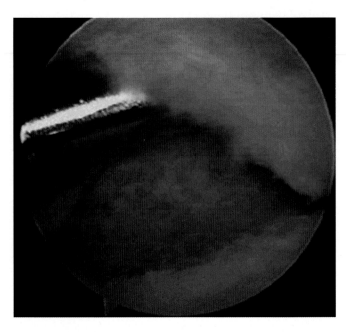

Figure 30.10

Example of a crescent-shaped tear with the normal footprint of the rotator cuff tendon insertion debrided in preparation for the rotator cuff repair.

on the tuberosity. The normal soft tissue footprint of the rotator cuff is debrided to create a bleeding bony surface just lateral to the articular cartilage for a width of 7–10 mm (Figure 30.10). Avascular and frayed edges of the tendon may also be conservatively debrided at this time, but the structural fibers of the tendon are completely preserved. An accessory anterolateral portal is then established for anchor placement, suture management and knot tying.

With chronic tears, and recurrent tears after previous surgery, tendon excursion may be increased by an intra-articular capsular release and excision of the fibrous adhesion on the bursal side. The capsular release is performed 1 cm from the edge of the glenoid to avoid injury to the labrum and the rotator cuff tendon (Figure 30.11). Release of the coracohumeral ligament may also be necessary to mobilize a retracted anterior portion of the supraspinatus tendon.[22]

Arthroscopic repair

Special instruments are required for an arthroscopic repair of the rotator cuff. For our technique, we use a crochet hook, a single-hole knot pusher, a suture cutting device and a suture passing–retrieval hand instrument. The tear configuration dictates the steps needed for the cuff repair. For tears requiring margin convergence, a side-to-side repair is performed using a

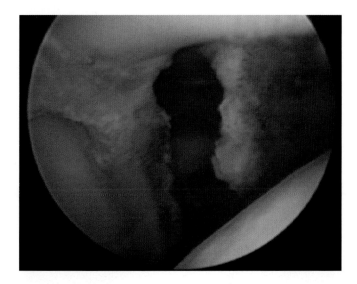

Figure 30.11

Arthroscopic capsular release performed adjacent to the glenoid may be indicated to mobilize chronic, retracted rotator cuff tears.

suture passing–retrieval instrument (i.e. Penetrator; Arthrex) with a prolonged-absorbable braided suture (Panacryl, Ethicon) passed through the posterior tendon, across the tear, and through the anterior tendon

(Figure 30.12). Occasionally, portal placement does not allow a single antegrade pass of the passing–retrieval instrument. In this case, suture passage may need to be performed in two steps, with passage first through the posterior edge, and subsequent retrieval through the anterior edge through the anterior cannula. Alternatively, a suture hook (i.e. Spectrum, Linvatec, Largo, FL, USA) helps to pass a #0 or #1 PDS suture, which is subsequently used as a shuttle to draw a prolonged-absorbable suture through the tendons (Figure 30.13).

Following suture passage, both limbs of the suture are retrieved through the accessory cannula with a crochet hook. The side-to-side repair begins medially. The suture is tied with the knot placed on the posterior side of the cuff to avoid irritation from the knot. Knot tying is prepared with multiple alternating half hitches (Revo knot), or a sliding knot followed by three alternating multiple half hitches (Duncan Loop).[23,24] The goal of the side-to-side repair is to converge the anterior and posterior tendon margins, enabling the lateral edge of the repair to rest close to the tuberosity, allowing the final repair to be made with minimal tension (Figure 30.14a,b).

Proper anchor placement is facilitated by rotating the arm while applying gentle traction to identify the site of anchor insertion. Suture anchors can be placed through

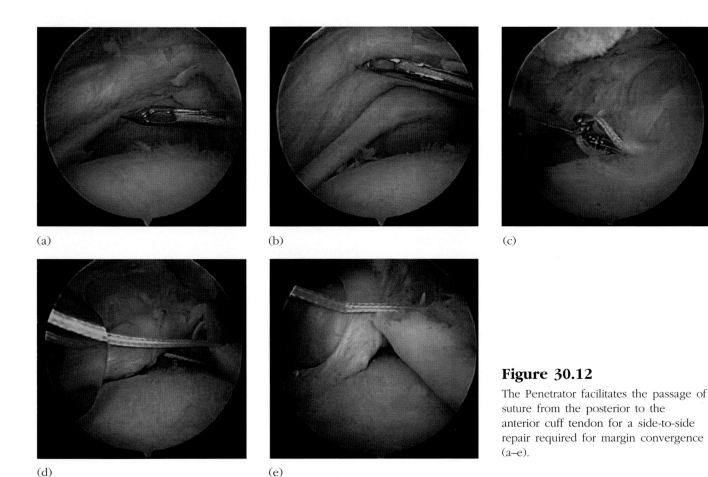

(a)

(b)

(c)

(d)

(e)

Figure 30.12

The Penetrator facilitates the passage of suture from the posterior to the anterior cuff tendon for a side-to-side repair required for margin convergence (a–e).

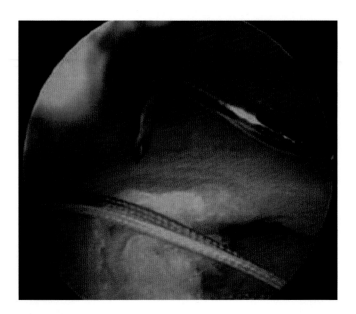

Figure 30.13

A Spectrum suture hook is helpful to pass #0 or #1 PDS suture at various angle due to the variety of left and right curve configurations. The PDS is then used to 'shuttle' a prolonged-absorbable suture through the tendon.

the accessory portal or through additional small incisions. The number of anchors used is based on the tear size. Separating each suture anchor by approximately 5–8 mm will distribute fixation proportionately over the entire insertion site and minimize excessive tension at any single fixation point.[13]

After placing the suture anchor, the next step is to pass the suture through the rotator cuff tendon edge. Typically, suture passage is most easily accomplished by passing the suture retriever to perforate the anterior supraspinatus or upper subscapularis (anterior portal), or posterior supraspinatus and infraspinatus (posterior portal), in an effort to retrieve the most medial limb of one of the two sutures loaded through the suture eyelet (Figure 30.15). The correct alignment and position of the suture is determined by visualizing the cuff, the sutures, and the tuberosity through the panoramic lateral view.

Passing a suture through the anterior half of the supraspinatus usually requires a sharp-angled suture retriever advanced through the anterior portal. Once the suture limb is passed through the tissue, visualization of the anchor is important to avoid inadvertent 'unloading' or removal of the suture from the suture anchor. Identifying the suture limbs that pass through the anchor, and pulling only the suture that leads to withdrawal from within the cannula (rather than sliding of the suture within the anchor) will avoid this frustrating event.

After the first suture limb is passed through the cuff tissue, the two limbs of the same suture (one through the tissue and one outside the tissue) are brought out through the same portal using a crochet hook or the

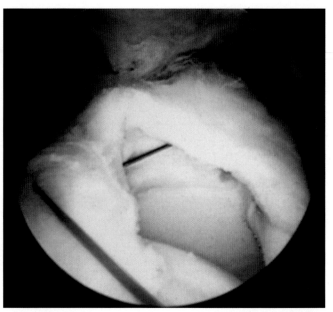

(a)

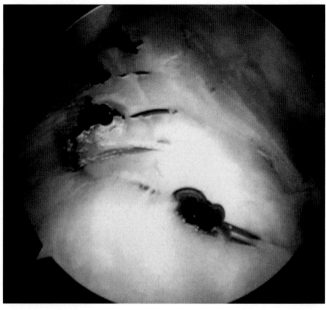

(b)

Figure 30.14

(a) A side-to-side repair is initiated at the medial aspect of the tear. The sutures are tied for a gradual progression towards the lateral aspect of the tear. The sutures are tied with the knot placed on the posterior rotator cuff. (b) The goal of margin convergence is to place the lateral edge of the tendon in close proximity to the greater tuberosity, while minimizing the strain at the repair site.

suture retrieval device to avoid suture entanglement (Figure 30.16). The second suture is passed through the cuff tissue with a similar technique, approximately 5–10 mm away from the first suture. Each suture should have independent soft tissue fixation points through the

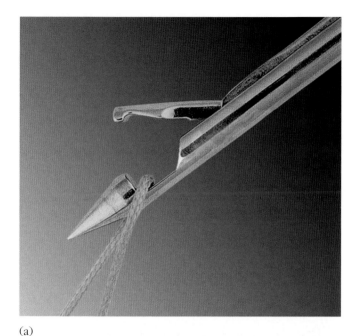

(a)

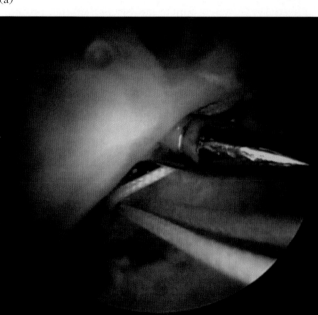

(b)

Figure 30.15

The sutures are retrieved through either the anterior or posterior portals using the suture retriever (a) after it has penetrated the rotator cuff tendon (b). Care is taken to avoid inadvertent unloading of the suture anchor.

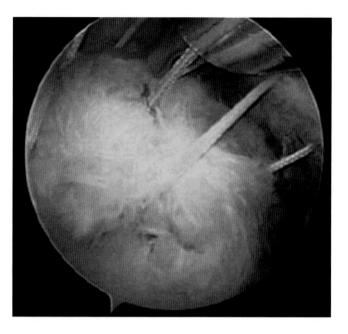

Figure 30.16

It is helpful to maintain the suture that is not being passed or manipulated through one portal (i.e. the posterior portal in this figure) and tie through a different portal (i.e. the accessory anterolateral portal).

rotator cuff tendon. The ability to pass the suture through the ideal position in the cuff is improved by rotating the arm to deliver the anterior or posterior cuff into the appropriate alignment.

Optimal suture management is accomplished by placing one anchor at a time, and securing the tendon to the bone with both sutures before placing the next anchor. Using the accessory anterolateral portal as the dedicated knot-tying portal greatly improves suture management and reliability of knot tying. The arm is rotated so that the suture, anchor, and cannula are in alignment before tying the knot. If tension is then placed on the soft-tissue limb while holding the other limb steady, the tendon is reduced to the tuberosity repair site. Multiple half-hitches with alternating posts are used to secure the suture knot (Revo knot). Alternatively, a sliding knot is tied over the soft tissue suture limb (Duncan Loop). It is important that the surgeon has the ability to tie both a sliding and non-sliding knot. As the knot slides into place, the tissue is reduced to the tuberosity. Ideally, the knots should be placed over the tendon, and not laterally over the tuberosity (Figure 30.17). Finally, a simple suture pattern is routinely used because this technique is adequate for maximal loading conditions of the rotator cuff tendon.[23]

All knots are tied with a single-hole knot pusher. Each throw includes past-pointing the suture limbs to maximize loop security. A minimum of three alternating half-hitches with alternating post limbs are included with every knot after a sliding knot or after two serial half-hitches.[23,24] At the completion of the knot tying, sutures are cut 3–4 mm from the end of the knot with a suture-cutting tool. The arm is then rotated to dynamically assess the security of the repair.

At the completion of the procedure, the four portal incisions are closed with interrupted monofilament sutures. The portal sites and subacromial space are

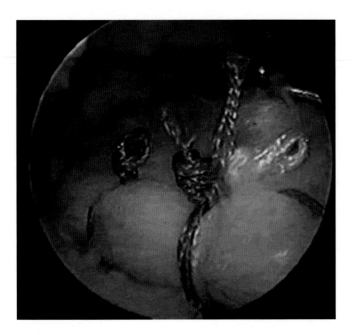

Figure 30.17

The completed arthroscopic rotator cuff repair. Knots are tied over the rotator cuff tendon and away from the greater tuberosity to minimize suture irritation.

injected with 0.25% bupivacaine and epinephrine. The arm is protected in a padded sling that has an immobilization strap.

Postoperative protocol

An arthroscopic repair of a torn rotator cuff tendon does not shorten the time required for biologic healing; therefore, protection of the repair follows the same time frame as open rotator cuff tears. The decreased surgical trauma compared to open or mini-open repairs results in decreased pain and decreased narcotic usage. The rehabilitation protocol is guided by several factors including the size of the tendon tear, the chronicity of the tear, the quality of the repair, the surgeon's assessment of repair tension, the tear location, and patient-specific factors such as chronic medical conditions.

Overall there are four phases to the rehabilitation protocol. Phase I is from 0 to 6 weeks and the repair is protected by immobilizing the patient in a sling when they are not doing their motion exercises, especially at night. During this period we allow the patient to begin active elbow motion and grip strengthening. We also allow for passive range of motion exercises of the shoulder within specific guidelines based on the nature of the tear and the stability of the repair. These passive motion exercises include forward elevation of the shoulder in the plane of the scapula, and external rotation with the

arm at the side. For patients with small tears/good quality repairs we allow 120° of forward elevation and 20° of external rotation. We also allow for light strengthening of the portion of the rotator cuff that was intact and did not require a repair.

Phase II is from 6 to 12 weeks and is the period during which we advance patients to full passive motion. The sling is no longer required, and we begin active-assisted and advance to active range of motion exercises. The patients can advance the strengthening of the intact rotator cuff, and begin light strengthening of small/good quality cuff repairs. During this phase light strengthening of the scapular stabilizers is also started. Phase III is from weeks 12 to 16 when patients undergo passive stretching at the end ranges of motion to achieve motion similar to the contralateral side. Rotator cuff strengthening of the repaired cuff is begun, and strengthening exercises of the intact cuff, small/good quality repairs, and scapular stabilizers is advanced (theraband to light weights).

Phase IV is when functional strengthening, proprioception re-education and sports-specific exercises are implemented. This is also the period of time that after a thorough rehabilitation including restoration of motion and strength patients can return to labor-intensive occupations and sporting activities.

References

1. McKee MD, Yoo, DJ. The effect of surgery for rotator cuff disease on general health status: results of a prospective trial. *J Bone Joint Surg* 2000; **82A**:970–9.
2. Matsen FA, Arntz CT. Rotator cuff tendon failure. In: Rockwood CA, Matsen FA, eds. *The Shoulder*. Philadelphia: WB Saunders, 1990: 647–73.
3. Burkhart SS. Reconciling the paradox of rotator cuff repair versus debridement: a unified biomechanical rationale for the treatment of rotator cuff tears. *Arthroscopy* 1994; **10**:4–19.
4. Gartsman GM, Hammerman SM. Full-thickness tears: arthroscopic repair. *Orthop Clin North Am* 1997; **28**:83–98.
5. Snyder SJ. Technique of arthroscopic rotator cuff repair using implantable 4-mm Revo suture anchors, suture shuttle relays, and No. 2 nonabsorbable mattress sutures. *Orthop Clin North Am* 1997; **28**:267–75.
6. Burkhart SS, Athansiou KA, Wirth MA. Margin convergence: a method of reducing strain in massive rotator cuff tears. *Arthroscopy* 1996; **12**:335–8.
7. Harryman DT, Mack LA, Wang KY et al. Repair of the rotator cuff: correlation of functional results with integrity of the cuff. *J Bone Joint Surg* 1991; **73A**:982–9.
8. Gazielly DF, Gleyze P, Montagnon C. Functional and anatomical results after rotator cuff repair. *Clin Orthop* 1994; **304**:43–53.
9. Norberg FB, Field LD, Savoie FH III. Repair of the rotator cuff: mini-open and arthroscopic repairs. *Clin Sports Med* 2000; **19**:77–99.
10. Tauro JC. Arthroscopic rotator cuff repair: analysis of technique and results at 2- and 3-year follow-up. *Arthroscopy* 1998; **14**:45–51.
11. Gartsman GM, Khan M, Hammerman SM. Arthroscopic repair of full-thickness tears of the rotator cuff. *J Bone Joint Surg* 1998; **80A**:832–40.

12. Romeo AA, Cohen BS, Primack S et al. Arthroscopic rotator cuff repair: an evaluation of integrity, strength and functional outcome. Presented at *The 8th International Congress on Surgery of the Shoulder*, Cape Town, South Africa, April 2001.

13. Burkhart SS. A stepwise approach to arthroscopic rotator cuff repair based on biomechanical principles. *Arthroscopy* 2000; **16**:82–90.

14. Gartsman GM. Arthroscopic assessment of rotator cuff tear reparability. *Arthroscopy* 1996; **12**:546–9.

15. Burkhart SS, Pagan JLD, Wirth MA et al. Cyclic loading of anchor-based rotator cuff repairs: confirmation of the tension overload phenomenon and comparison of suture anchor fixation with transosseous fixation. *Arthroscopy* 1997; **13**:720–4.

16. Burkhart SS. The dead man theory of suture anchors: observations along a South Texas fence line. *Arthroscopy* 1995; **11**:119–23.

17. Weber SC. Arthroscopic versus mini-open rotator cuff repair. Presented at the *18th Annual AANA Meeting*, Anaheim, California, 1999.

18. Brown AR, Weiss R, Greenberg C et al. Interscalene block for shoulder arthroscopy: comparison with general anesthesia. *Arthroscopy* 1993; **9**:295–300.

19. Miller C, Savoie FH. Glenohumeral abnormalities associated with full-thickness tears of the rotator cuff. *Orthop Rev* 1994, **21**:116–20.

20. McConville OR, Iannotti JP. Partial-thickness tears of the rotator cuff: evaluation and management. *J Am Acad Orthop Surg* 1999; **7**:32–43.

21. Caspari RB, Thal R. A technique for arthroscopic subacromial decompression. *Arthroscopy* 1992; **8**:23–30.

22. Tauro JC. Arthroscopic 'Interval Slide' in the repair of large rotator cuff tears. *Arthroscopy* 1999; **15**:527–30.

23. Burkhart SS, Wirth MA, Simonich M et al. Knot security in simple sliding knots and its relationship to rotator cuff repair: how secure must the knot be? *Arthroscopy* 2000; **16**:202–7.

24. Nottage WM, Lieurance RK. Arthroscopic knot tying techniques. *Arthroscopy* 1999; **15**:515–21.

25. Wilk KE, Crockett HC, Andrews JR. Rehabilitation after rotator cuff surgery. *Techn Shoulder Elbow Surg* 2000; **1**:128–44.

31 Rotator cuff tear: Arthroscopic technique with suture anchors

Dominique F Gazielly, Rami El Abiad and Luis A Garcia

Introduction

Historical perspective

The surgical treatment of full thickness tears of the rotator cuff has evolved considerably during the last 10 years with the introduction of arthroscopic technology. Arthroscopy has several well-known advantages: negligible scar; minor morbidity; less pain; easier postoperative rehabilitation due to absence of muscle detachment or incision; and shorter hospital stay. Initially, arthroscopic acromioplasty coupled with coracoacromial ligament detachment, bursectomy, and adherence release was shown to be effective in the treatment of subacromial impingement[1] and partial cuff tears.[2] However, limited success was reported in cases of full thickness cuff rupture.[3,4] Nevertheless this early period brought many advances to arthroscopic techniques within the subacromial space and a better understanding of the nature of rotator cuff tears (anteroposterior extension, degree of retraction, mobility and quality of the torn tendon stump, appearance, and coverage of the biceps).

Thus it became obvious that the association of cuff repair to the arthroscopic acromioplasty is necessary to obtain better functional results.[5] The mini-open technique, combining an arthroscopic glenohumeral exploration plus acromioplasty with an open cuff repair through a short anterior deltoid incision[6] might appear a good solution; however, it is limited to small and not retracted distal ruptures[7] and implies the loss of certain advantages of the arthroscopic technique because of the muscle incision. Thus it seems natural that orthopedic surgeons with experience in both open rotator cuff repair and arthroscopic shoulder surgery would incline toward the development of an exclusively arthroscopic repair technique. This evolution toward 'full arthroscopy' has been facilitated by technical progress in materials such as bone anchors, suture passers and arthroscopic knots.[8]

We have studied and compared the functional results, at a minimum follow-up of 2 years, of different therapeutic methods,[9] using the Constant functional score.[10] The group of isolated acromioplasty patients obtained a mean absolute Constant score of 73.5 points while the arthroscopic repair group had 87.6 points; this justifies the actual evolution and development of arthroscopic techniques for cuff repair in association with acromioplasty. We also compared the functional results after open and arthroscopic repair of the cuff: the arthroscopic technique gives, in the hands of an experienced surgeon, as good results (87.6 points) as the open technique without (84.1 points) or with RCR® Reinforcement (86.2 points) (Bionet Merck, Valence, France). These comparative results may lead the surgeon to consider this 'full arthroscopic' technique in rotator cuff tears.

Indications and contraindications

Several authors[11,12] exclusively use the arthroscopic technique for the repair of full thickness ruptures of the cuff. We believe that these indications must be tempered with regard to the patient's age and to the quality and mobility of the tendon stump. We continue to perform open repairs in patients younger than 60 years old that submit their shoulder to professional overuse with repetitive activity above the shoulder level whatever the size of the rupture. In fact, we have shown that the rate of rerupture after open repair could reach up to 25%, and is directly related to age, degree of solicitation and the size of the rupture.[13] For this reason, we use a prosthetic polypropylene reinforcement of the cuff (RCR®) in order to diminish the iterative rupture risk.[14] We reserve the 'full arthroscopic' technique for active but not manually working patients younger than 60 years, whether athletic or not. In patients older than 60 years, given their poor tolerance to morbidity resulting from deltoid splitting, it is our procedure of choice.

Preoperative clinical examination and imaging (mostly computed tomography (CT)-arthrography) are of utmost importance in all cases. In fact, shoulder stiffness or proximal migration of the humeral head suggesting massive cuff rupture with posterior extension to the infraspinatus, or advanced fatty degeneration of the cuff muscles[15] are contraindications to both the totally arthroscopic rotator cuff repair technique and the open repair. As well, anterior tear extension toward the subscapularis, either associated or not with a bicipital tendon dislocation may contraindicate this procedure and indicates an open repair technique. Within the age limits previously mentioned, our indications for an arthroscopic repair encompass full thickness supraspinatus ruptures, eventually extending backward to the infraspinatus or forward into the rotator interval, conditional to the intraoperative finding of a mobile, not retracted tendon stump, without thinning or horizontal cleavage that will weaken the tendon. If the biceps tendon is found to be dislocated or degenerated, a tenodesis or tenotomy will be performed.

Results

High rates of good and excellent results have been reported in the international literature after arthroscopic repair of the cuff: 87% by Snyder et al;[16] 84% by Gartsman et al;[17] and 92% by Tauro.[18] Yet, these studies may be criticized for their lack of confirmation, by postoperative imaging techniques, of iterative rupture, given that it is known to reach rates of 25% after an open repair. Wolf[12] has found the arthroscopically repaired cuff to be intact in 70% of cases during a second look office arthroscopy. The authors' experience stands on a series of 27 consecutive cases of arthroscopic cuff repair, limited to supraspinatus tears.[19] In this series the mean absolute Constant score improved from 58.3 to 86.6 points after a mean follow-up of 32 months. One patient suffered from postsurgical stiffness requiring manipulation under general anesthesia. No anchor migration has been found. The continuity of the repaired tendon has been studied in all cases, either by CT-arthrography (20 cases), magnetic resonance imaging (three cases), ultrasonography (two cases) or arthroscopy (two cases). Tendon healing was obtained in 20 cases (74%), a small distal leak signaling a scarring defect was found in six cases (22%). A true rerupture with tendon stump retraction was identified in one case (4%) corresponding to a poor functional result with a Constant score of 65 points.

Surgical principles

Arthroscopic cuff repair must always be performed in a shoulder that has a full range of motion. Stiffness in the shoulder is contraindicated as the result of surgery would be poor. It is better to reduce any stiffness with a program of stretching exercises before surgery. As a general rule we always prescribe a rehabilitation program of 3 months before proposing surgery to the patient. This rehabilitation allows us to test the eventual efficacy of conservative treatment, permits recovery of mobility in a stiff shoulder and shows the degree of the patient's motivation for rehabilitation.

The surgical procedure may be performed with the patient either in the 'beach-chair' position or in lateral decubitus. We prefer the latter because the patient's installation is easier and the traction to the arm is more efficiently managed. Beach-chair positioning may be the

preference of surgeons who perform the mini-open technique, which we no longer perform. In general we never carry out open surgery immediately after arthroscopy because in our opinion the tissues are swollen and the risk of infection increases. The procedure is performed under regional anesthesia (interscalenic block with double stimulation), associated with a light general anesthesia for security and comfort. The use of a pump, allowing control of flow and pressure within the joint, is essential for an optimal field of vision. The mean pressure during a standard arthroscopy is 50 mmHg. In case of bleeding, pressure is momentarily raised to 70 mmHg and lavage is performed, allowing the re-establishment of excellent vision in less than 30 seconds. We use only saline solution without glycine. In the hands of an experienced surgeon the procedure should not take more than 90 minutes, conditional on the availability of an efficient assistant with a thorough knowledge of the successive steps and the correct utilization of the different instruments necessary for the surgery.

The first step of the procedure consists of a glenohumeral diagnostic arthroscopy allowing a thorough intra-articular exploration and appreciation of the deep surface of the ruptured tendon. The second step is the subacromial partial bursectomy and treatment of the impingement by coracoacromial ligament detachment from the acromion followed by anterior acromioplasty; we accomplish this procedure with an osteotome introduced through the anterolateral portal, and we have called it the arthroscopic conventional acromioplasty or ACA.[20] Then, we explore the rupture and assess stump mobility, possibility of reattachment to the greater tuberosity without excessive tension, anteroposterior extension of the tear, tissue quality and possible horizontal cleavage tears that might weaken the repair. At this time, the decision is made whether to go on with the repair or to perform a simple debridement if a safe repair does not seem feasible.

The third step is therefore reattachment of the tendon to the greater tuberosity using braided non-absorbable sutures. Abrasion of the tuberosity permits efficient resection of all tendon remnants and cortical bone down to bleeding spongiosa with the aim of favoring a solid tendon to bone healing. In general, two or three suture anchors are necessary.

A surgeon doing arthroscopic cuff repair must master the basic shoulder arthroscopic techniques, in particular the portals, and must have the necessary equipment available. Yet, this is a demanding technique, for which the learning curve may reach around 10 cases, which does imply a number of possible pitfalls for inexperienced surgeons. The acromioplasty step must be efficient and swift in order to minimize tissue infiltration and avoid problems in the subsequent steps. Bursectomy should be as thorough as possible to allow perfect view and avoid its interposition within the different suture threads. The exploration should be meticulous and objective, the surgeon must be able to decline the repair if the tendon is too retracted and has lost mobility.

Greater tuberosity abrasion must not be too aggressive, especially in older patients because soft bone may be too weak to hold anchors. Their pull-out strength must be tested and one must not hesitate to withdraw a doubtful anchor in order to avoid material migration. Stitches must be passed through the tendon under direct, clear vision, without interposition of bursal remnants, and purchase must be solid and at a safe distance from the tendon's free edge. Four to six strands of suture may be present in the arthroscopic field at a certain moment, and the use of different coloured sutures may be extremely useful. It is fundamental to verify that the sutures are not twisting around one another and that they glide through the tendon in order to tie adequate knots that will bring back the tendon to bone contact. Arthroscopic knots should not pose a problem for the beginner surgeon, given that this technique is easily learned with in vitro models.

Complications of arthroscopic cuff repair may be per- and postoperative. The most usual peroperative complication relates to suture strands that get twisted or break down at the time of knot tying. In both cases, the anchor must be withdrawn and then replaced in the same hole after changing the suture strand. The possibility of unscrewing and rescrewing the anchor while keeping the same purchase is an advantage to this type of system compared to systems that use non-screwing anchors. This complication is not dramatic, but it takes time, demands meticulousness and patience from both surgeons and their assistants. Postoperative complications mainly involve screw migration, which can be avoided by an adequate technique.

Surgical technique

Anesthesia

We perform the procedure under regional anesthesia with an interscalene block associated with general anesthesia. The regional anesthesia permits a reduction of the dose of anesthetic drugs, facilitates fast awakening without side-effects and has a prominent analgesic role during the postoperative period allowing an immediate start of physical therapy. General anesthesia increases the patient comfort on the operating table and prevents any undesired patient movements during the procedure.

Positioning

The patient is placed in lateral decubitus (Figure 31.1) over a 'bean bag' (Olympic Vac Pac, size 31, Olympic Medical, Seattle, WA, USA) that permits a quick and accurate positioning with a posterior body inclination

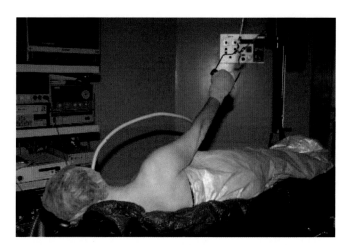

Figure 31.1

Positioning of the patient.

angle around 25°, with full safety and with no metallic supports. Particular attention is given to head and neck position; giving a slight lateral inclination and elevation of the former avoids excessive pull of the neck. Traction is delivered to the arm through a traction-positioning device (S-TRAC, Karl Storz Endoscopy, Tuttlingen, Germany) that provides accurate and adaptable position to each case. The initial traction weight is 6 kg with the shoulder at 45° of abduction and 20° of forward flexion.

Portals

The bony prominences of the shoulder, such as the acromion, clavicle, coracoid and the coracoacromial ligament are drawn on the skin with a sterile pen. Five portals are used (Figure 31.2). The posterior portal (A) placed at the 'soft point', for the arthroscope and saline

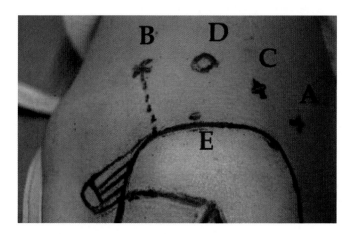

Figure 31.2

Five portals are used: (A) posterior, (B) anterolateral, (C) posterolateral, (D) lateral, (E) acromiolateral.

solution entry, is necessary for the standard gleno-humeral exploration. The subacromial step of the procedure, comprising the acromioplasty and bursectomy requires two more portals: anterolateral and posterolateral. The anterolateral portal (B) lies over a line along the anterior edge of clavicle and acromion, 4 cm distal to the acromial lateral border. A screwable 6-mm cannula, metallic or plastic and disposable (BASK, Karl Storz Endoscopy) is inserted and the outflow hose is connected to the pump (DUO, Future Medical Systems, Nice, France); this portal is established at the same time as the posterior portal for the glenohumeral step. Saline evacuation will occur through the defect in the cuff into the cannula and, if needed, can be used as an instrument portal for intra-articular procedures.

For the subacromial step we use a posterolateral portal (C), different from the posterior (A) (Figure 31.2), because vision through it is not disturbed by the natural posteroanterior arching of the acromion's inferior surface and permits a good view of the cuff and greater tuberosity from above. Placed 2 cm lateral to the posterolateral angle of the acromion, it allows one to comfortably work in triangulation with the anterolateral portal over the supraspinatus axis. A fourth lateral portal (D) is necessary for the introduction of cuff repair instrumentation. It is placed 4 cm distal to the lateral acromial edge at the midpoint between portals B and C and a 9-mm screwable cannula, either metallic and reusable or plastic and disposable (BASK, Karl Storz Endoscopy) will be screwed in. Finally, and after aiming confirmation with a long spinal needle, a small portal, just lateral to the acromion (E) will permit the introduction of specific instruments for the Revo (Linvatec, Largo, FL, USA) suture anchor positioning. However, it is important to note that specific use of portals may vary for the subacromial and cuff repair steps. We use different arrangements according to the case: the scope is posterolateral (C) and the two instrumental portals are anterolateral (B) and lateral (D), or, the scope is lateral (D) and the instrumental portals are anterolateral (B) and posterolateral (C).

General arthroscopic instruments

A technological environment and certain non-specific instruments are necessary for this kind of procedure: optical 30° wide-angle and camera, either mono CCD or better, tri CCD (Karl Storz Endoscopy), pump (Future Medical Systems), power shaving device (Karl Storz Endoscopy), monopolar electrocoagulator (Karl Storz Endoscopy) with hooked and protected electrode, allowing its use in both coagulation and cutting mode in saline solution without addition of glycine. Bipolar electrode systems like VAPR (Mitek, Westwood, MA, USA) are, in our opinion, very useful, enabling the surgeon to perform a fast and efficient bursectomy without bleeding. Finally, nowadays, it is important to record images of the proce-dure, either photographic for the patient or surgeon (DKR, Sony), or video (Sony CCD TRV 900 E camera). Specific instruments, needed for the repair itself, will be precisely described step by step.

Glenohumeral step

After verifying the articular range of motion under anesthesia, glenohumeral inspection is systematically performed. The sheath and blunt trocar are inserted through the posterior portal (A). The humeral head and posterior glenoid rim are identified by palpation with the tip of the trocar that is then pushed through the posterior capsule at the 'soft point' between the infraspinatus and teres minor. A thorough inspection of the joint is carried out after introduction of optical and camera, initially without joint distention and then after saline instillation. Outflow is established by an instrumental anterolateral cannula (B), and then a probe is inserted through the cannula and tendon defect to complete the joint examination. The size of the rupture and aspect of the articular side of the tendon will be appreciated from this approach. Several procedures may be performed if needed such as synovectomy or biceps tenotomy in cases of its instability, degenerative or prerupture changes. For these, the electrocautery, full radius resector or VAPR may be used.

Cuff tear examination in subacromial space

The scope is switched from the (A) portal to the posterolateral (C) portal. The cannula stays in place (B). The

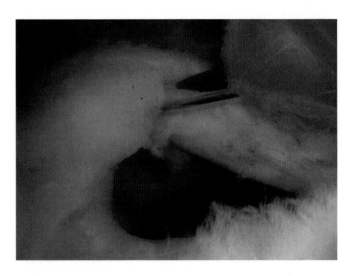

Figure 31.3
Bursal view of a repairable full thickness cuff tear after bursectomy.

first goal is to enhance visibility within the subacromial space by performing the most complete bursectomy as possible in the area of cuff tear. For this, either a full radius resector on the power shaver, the VAPR, or both are used. This subacromial debridement may be a lengthy process but is necessary in order to adequately address a subacromial impingement, analyse the rupture's features (Figure 31.3), and later repair the tendon in the best possible conditions of visibility. The next step is to assess the repairability of the cuff by arthroscopic technique. First, the tendon's free edge, usually thin, fragile and not amenable to suture holding, is resected with a shaver or basket forceps. The degree of the tendon's retraction and, most importantly, its mobility and whether it can be displaced all the way to its original insertion is evaluated by grasping it with forceps introduced through the anterolateral cannula. The anteroposterior size of the rupture is evaluated, especially its extension into the rotator interval where the biceps tendon may be uncovered at the joint entry. The defect size is measured using the cannula's diameter as reference, as proposed by Gartsman and Hammerman.[11] The cuff's quality is best appreciated from its articular side, by seeking for cleavage dissection lines. The next step is to determine the type of rupture: simple longitudinal tear – exceptional in our experience – or more often, transversal, V- or L-shaped tears. The rupture may look different according to the viewpoint, notably when a deep side partial rupture has evolved to a full thickness one. Rarely, the tear is defined intraoperatively as irreparable: usually good clinical examination and imaging studies allow the preoperative identification of a massive, irreparable cuff tear.

Coracoacromial ligament detachment

Initially, the subacromial bursa and periosteum are debrided allowing full vision of the inferior acromion and the coracoacromial ligament insertion. This is performed either with a power shaver and an aggressive full radius resector or with a bipolar electrode like VAPR, the latter having the advantages of efficacy and time-saving that compensate its price. The coracoacromial ligament is detached from its acromial insertion with an electrocautary or VAPR system, carefully keeping the instruments in bone contact to avoid injury and bleeding from the acromial artery (Figure 31.4). The cut is stopped when vertical deep deltoid fibers appear in the field. We do not resect the ligament because we believe that impingement originated in bone and that ligament resection or detachment is necessary only for allowing adequate acromioplasty. The coracoacromial ligament will reconstitute itself in its superior portion and recover its role of an anterosuperior restraint.

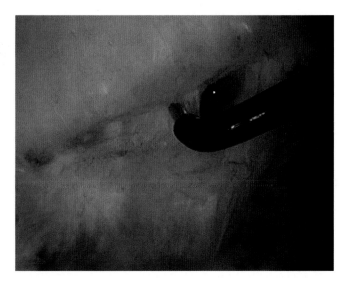

Figure 31.4

Detachment without resection of the coracoacromial ligament using an electrocautery introduced through the 6-mm anterolateral cannula.

Acromioplasty

Visualization or good exposure of the acromial spur to be resected in type 2 or 3 acromions must be perfect in order to achieve a flat, type 1 acromion. Therefore, the acromion must be cleared of all bursal, periosteal and coracoacromial ligament debris from over the inferior surface and anterior and lateral edges with a view of the deep deltoid fibers anteriorly and laterally and the acromioclavicular joint capsule medially. Since 1992 we have performed the acromioplasty with a 5.5- or 8-mm wide osteotome (Acromioplasty Set, Karl Storz Endoscopy) introduced through a 6- or 8.5-mm screwable anterolateral cannula. However, the osteotome can be introduced directly through the anterolateral portal with no cannula (Figure 31.5a). This ACA is performed starting at the anterolateral corner of the acromion and reaching as far as the acromioclavicular joint (Figure 31.5b). The first bone slice comes out of the anterior-inferior corner of the acromion and is withdrawn en bloc with a grasping forceps through the anterolateral cannula (Figure 31.6a). The anterior acromion is successively slimmed and flattened by resecting two or three bone slices. At the end, a small step may still exist between the anterior and posterior part of the inferior surface of the acromion that will be smoothened with an oval burr (Figure 31.6b) and finished with an ancillary rasp (BASK, Karl Storz Endoscopy). The ACA has the advantage of a quick, adequate subacromial decompression in contrast to an acromioplasty performed with only the motorized burr, given that the hooked anterior acromion constitutes

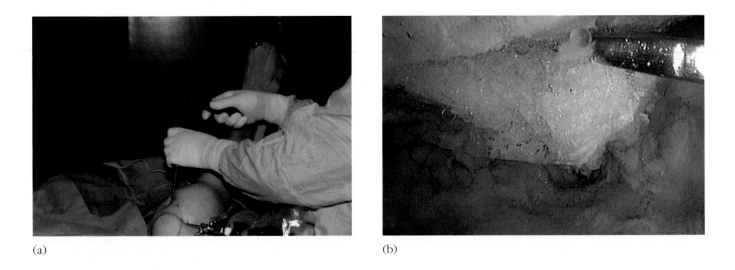

(a)   (b)

Figure 31.5

(a) Acromioplasty is performed with an osteotome introduced directly in the anterolateral portal: arthroscopic conventional acromioplasty (ACA). (b) Arthroscopic view.

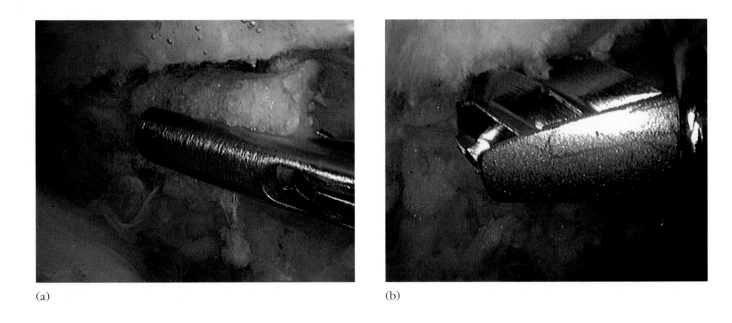

(a)   (b)

Figure 31.6

(a) The bone slices are withdrawn en bloc with a grasping forceps. (b) Regularization of the inferior surface of the acromion using an oval motorized burr introduced through the anterolateral cannula.

hard osteophytic bone that may render the procedure difficult and time consuming. An insufficient acromioplasty may be responsible for persistent cuff impingement and possible rerupture. If the preoperative X-rays show the presence of inferior osteophytes on the distal clavicle, they must be resected with a motorized burr.

Greater tuberosity preparation

After the acromioplasty has been performed, the cuff mobilized and freed of adhesions, and a bursectomy has been accomplished allowing a perfect view of the subacromial space, the next step is preparation of the greater tuberosity by clearing it of all tendinous debris

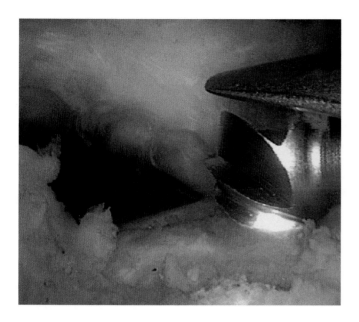

Figure 31.7

A superficial slot is located on the greater tuberosity to promote tendon healing.

either with the full radius resector or with the VAPR system. At the same time, we complete the subdeltoid bursectomy in the space between the lateral greater tuberosity and deltoid muscle in order to avoid interference with the bursa during manipulation of instruments and sutures. A 4-mm round burr, introduced through the anterolateral cannula (B), is used to prepare a cancellous bed for the tendon after removing 2 mm of cortical bone. The slot is made not to insert the tendon's edge but to promote healing of the deep surface of the reattached tendon (Figure 31.7).

Anchor and suture selection

For us, the ideal anchor must be easily inserted without the need for complex ancillary material and must allow a solid, stable fixation to the greater tuberosity avoiding all risk of material migration. We prefer a screwing system because it permits anchor withdrawal by unscrewing it if a problem such as suture rupture or twisting should arise. Its design should ensure the possibility of rescrewing an anchor in the initial hole with the same purchase. Finally its design must permit the surgeon to choose the suture type, resorbable or not, and even to pass one or two threads in one anchor. Currently, we use the rotator cuff large-eyed Revo (Linvatec) in our surgical practice. As to the suture type, resorbable monofilaments present the advantage of an

easy passage through the tendon with the different specific instruments but without the need of a suture-passer such as the shuttle-relay (Linvatec). The drawback comes from their elasticity, which makes the arthroscopic knot technique more difficult. We prefer to use #2 braided, non-absorbable, polyester sutures (Ethibond, Somerville, NJ, USA), with which we already have a 15-year experience in open surgery and which allow a reliable easy tying technique even though their use implies the utilization of a passer.

Cuff repair

In the case of an L-shaped cuff rupture, a side-to-side repair technique is used for the longitudinal arm of the tear with a Blitz suture retriever (Linvatec) or a Crescent suture hook plus a Shuttle-relay suture passer (Linvatec). Three or four stitches may be necessary. In this case the arthroscope is introduced through the lateral portal (D) while the sutures and instruments are passed through the anterolateral (B) and posterolateral (C) portals. At this time, the transverse arm of the tear is reinserted by non-absorbable sutures passed through anchors spaced 10 mm apart. In general, two or three anchors are necessary, and the technique is similar for each anchor insertion and tendon passage. The procedure is usually started at the most anterior anchor.

A spinal needle is inserted just lateral to the acromion to determine the best approach (portal E) for the Revo entry point, keeping in mind a 45° lateral inclination of the anchor in relation to the humeral axis. The Revo bone punch is then introduced through the (E) portal and aimed medially and distally following a 45° angle. Two or three holes are drilled in the most lateral border of the abraded bone area, with a mean separation of 10 mm. The 4-mm large-eyed Revo anchor, carrying one #2 non-absorbable braided suture is introduced through the acromiolateral portal (E) without any cannula and screwed in the corresponding hole down to the black ring marked on the Revo screwdriver. The anchor's eyelet is best aligned with the opening perpendicular to the cuff to avoid having a twist in the sutures after passing trough the cuff. The two strands are retrieved with a crochet hook (Linvatec) introduced through the lateral cannula (D) and the holding strength of the anchor is verified by pulling simultaneously on the suture strands (Figure 31.8). Suture twisting is avoided by the use of a suture retrieval forceps.

A modified Caspari suture punch (Linvatec) is introduced through the same lateral cannula (D); it pierces the tendon 3–4 mm away from the free edge and a shuttle relay is passed through it. The tendon purchase must be strong and placed facing the corresponding anchor. The shuttle relay is rolled in and retrieved through the anterolateral (B) cannula with the grasping

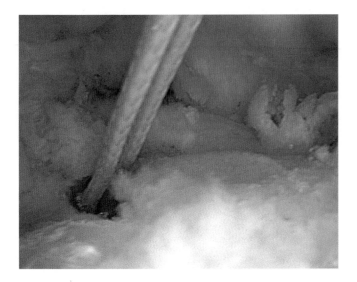

Figure 31.8

The most anterior Revo screw is put in its corresponding hole, which is located at the lateral side of the bone slot.

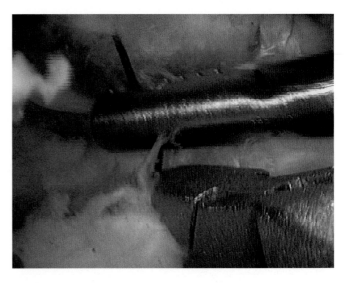

Figure 31.9

The modified Caspari punch holding the cuff tendon; the shuttle relay is retrieved using a grasping forceps introduced through the anterolateral cannula.

forceps (Figure 31.9). The eyelet of the shuttle relay suture passer is loaded with the first suture outside the lateral cannula and carried through the cuff from the bottom to the top by pulling on the opposite end. The strand already passed through the tendon is placed outside the anterolateral cannula. The same procedure is followed for the second suture strand (Figure 31.10). Now that the two suture strands have been passed through the tendon, 5–6 mm apart and 3–4 mm from the tendon's free edge, they exit through the antero-lateral portal. They are then kept outside the cannula in order to avoid mixing and twisting with the suture that will then be passed through the posterior anchor. A 'U' mattress stitch will be feasible on the tendon if the two strands are passed from the bottom to the top; this is most suitable in the intermediate suture when three stitches are needed. For the other two anchors, anterior and posterior, it is possible to perform a simple stitch by passing only one of the strands through the tendon.

When all sutures have been passed through the tendon it is time to make the arthroscopically controlled knots starting anterior, intermediate or posterior accord-ing to the surgeon's preference and tear geometry. The sutures are transferred from the anterolateral cannula to the lateral cannula. We use the Revo-knot technique described by Snyder (Knot Tying Techniques, Linvatec). In all cases, one of the strands of each suture is passed through the knot pusher to verify the absence of twist-ing. Two underhand and one overhand half hitches are performed and tightened down. After securing the knot, the remaining suture limbs are cut before tying the following stitch. At the end of the procedure the tendon

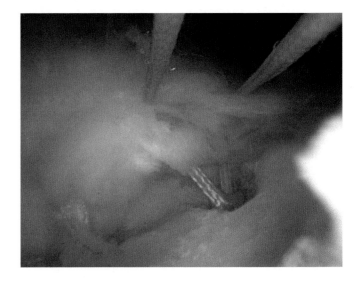

Figure 31.10

The two suture strands are passed through the tendon in front of the corresponding anchor before knot tying.

should be perfectly reattached to the tuberosity (Figure 31.11). The bone abrasion affords tendon healing to bleeding bone (Figure 31.12).

In case of suture twisting or rupture at the time of tying, it is possible to unscrew the Revo anchor with the Revo remover and then rescrew it after loading new suture into the same hole; then the above mentioned steps are repeated.

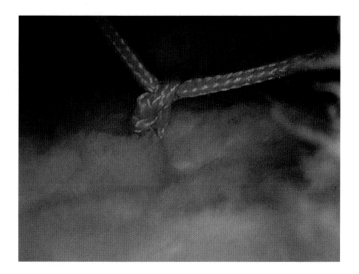

Figure 31.11
A final arthroscopic view of the arthroscopic cuff repair.

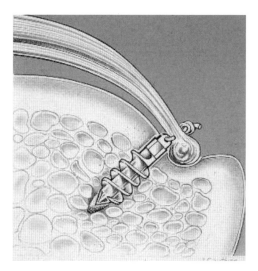

Figure 31.12
The bone slot affords the healing of the deep surface of the reinserted cuff.

Postoperative protocol

The involved arm is rested in a simple, removable sling. Rehabilitation is started the day after the surgery with passive mobilization: pendulum exercises, elevation in supine position, extension, internal and external rotation with the patient in the standing position. This passive rehabilitation lasts for 6 weeks until joint motion has been fully restored. Assisted active motion is started at the sixth week so that full active shoulder motion can be recovered by the end of the third month. At this stage, proprioception and depressor muscle strengthening exercises are introduced until the sixth postoperative month.

Return to labor and sports depends on the age and level of activities and is usually possible between the third and the sixth postoperative months.

References

1. Ellman H. Arthroscopic subacromial decompression, analysis of one to three year results. *Arthroscopy* 1987; **3**:173–81.
2. Snyder SJ, Pachelli AF, Delpizzo W et al. Partial thickness rotator cuff tears: results of arthroscopic treatment. *Arthroscopy* 1991; **7**:1–7.
3. Gartsman GM. Arthroscopic acromioplasty for lesions of the rotator cuff. *J Bone Joint Surg* 1990; **72A**:169–80.
4. Ellman H, Kay SP, Wirth M. Arthroscopic treatment of full-thickness rotator cuff tears: 2–7 years follow-up study. *Arthroscopy* 1991; **9**:195–200.
5. Montgomery TJ, Yerger B, Savoie FM. Management of rotator cuff tears: a comparison of arthroscopic debridement and surgical repair. *J Shoulder Elbow Surg* 1994; **3**:70–8.
6. Paulos LE, Kody MH. Arthroscopically enhanced 'mini-approach' to rotator cuff repair. *Am J Sports Med* 1994; **22**:19–25.
7. Gartsman GM. Combined arthroscopic and open treatment of tears of the rotator cuff. *J Bone Joint Surg* 1997; **79A**:776–83.
8. Snyder SJ. Arthroscopic evaluation and treatment of the rotator cuff. In: *Shoulder Arthroscopy.* New York: McGraw-Hill, 133–78.
9. Gazielly DF, Gleyze P, Thomas T (eds). *The Cuff.* Paris: Elsevier.
10. Constant CR, Murley AMG. A clinical method of functional assessment of the shoulder. *Clin Orthop* 1987; **214**:160–4.
11. Gartsman GM, Hammerman SM. Arthroscopic repair of full-thickness rotator cuff tears: operative technique. *Tech Shoulder Elbow Surg* 2000; **1**:2–8.
12. Wolf EM. Arthroscopic rotator cuff repair. In: Fu FH, Ticker JB, Imhoff AB, eds. *Atlas of Shoulder Surgery.* London: Martin Dunitz, 1998, 167–73.
13. Gazielly DF, Gleyze P, Montagnon C. Functional and anatomical results after rotator cuff repair. *Clin Orthop* 1994; **304**:43–53.
14. Gazielly DF. Repair and RCR® reinforcement of reparable rotator cuff tears. *Annual Meeting of the American Shoulder and Elbow Surgeons,* Newport, Rhode Island, USA, 1996.
15. Goutallier D, Postel JM, Bernageau J et al. Fatty infiltration of disrupted rotator cuff muscles. *Rev Rhum Engl Ed* 1995; **62**:415–22.
16. Snyder SJ, Mileski RA, Karzel RP. Results of arthroscopic rotator cuff repair. *Annual Meeting of the American Shoulder and Elbow Surgeons,* Amelia Island, Florida, USA, 1997.
17. Gartsman GM, Khan M, Hammerman SM. Arthroscopic repair of full-thickness tears of the rotator cuff. *J Bone Joint Surg* 1988; **80A**:832–40.
18. Tauro JC. Arthroscopic rotator cuff repair: analysis of technique and results at 2 and 3 years follow-up. *Arthroscopy* 1998; **14**:45–51.
19. Gazielly DF, Gleyze P, Pasquier B et al. Functional and anatomical results of 27 arthroscopic repair of complete rotator cuff tears. *The 7th International Congress on Surgery of the Shoulder.* Sydney, Australia, 1998.
20. Gazielly DF. Arthroscopic conventional acromioplasty (ACA). *Annual Meeting of the American Shoulder and Elbow Surgeons.* La Quinta, California, USA, 1995.

32 Arthroscopic repair of rotator cuff tears: Absorbable Panolok RC anchors with Panacryl sutures

Laurent Lafosse

Introduction

In ruptures of the rotator cuff, the only way to achieve satisfactory muscle recovery to restore the painless and functional state of the shoulder is by means of tendon repair combined with acromioplasty.[1]

The advent of arthroscopy first made it possible to resolve the subacromial conflict by means of isolated acromioplasty without reinserting the tendons of the cuff.[2] Satisfactory results in terms of pain and function can be obtained, but the shoulder never recovers anything approaching normal muscular strength, which constitutes a definite disability.[3]

In order to combine arthroscopic acromioplasty with cuff repair surgery, mini-open techniques have been used. This mixed surgery still has some of the drawbacks of open surgery in reinserting the tendons, and notably requires detachment and splitting between the bundles of the deltoid muscle.[4] Various arthroscopic techniques for cuff repair are now available; some of them involve intra-osseous implants combined with transtendinous suture.[5,6]

Surgical principles

The results of athroscopic repair of the cuff using titanium 'Super Anchors' (Mitek, Westwood, MA, USA) and Ethibon dec. 6 non-absorbable sutures (Mitek) show that this technique is reliable.[7] Secure anchorage and suturing are essential during tendon healing, but afterwards these devices no longer serve any useful purpose.

The use of a combination of slowly absorbed devices should make it possible to combine sufficient initial mechanical strength during tendon cicatrization with subsequent gradual disappearance of the retention without excessive inflammatory reactions. This can be achieved using Panalok RC anchors (Mitek) and Panacryl suture (Mitek), both of which are composed of absorbable polylactic acid (PLA), which is absorbed within 2 years. The short follow-up time for the small number of cases having undergone surgery with those implants makes it impossible to draw any conclusions,

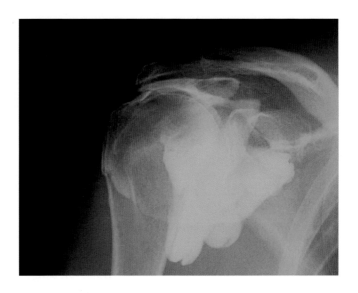

Figure 32.1
AP arthrography, right shoulder. Tear of superspinatus/infraspinatus with intermediate retraction.

even of a preliminary nature, from the results. Here we will simply describe the surgical technique, which is now clearly defined, based on the method for non-absorbable anchors and braided sutures.

Surgical technique

The patient selected has a tear of supra- and infra-spinatus tendon (Figure 32.1). Local/regional anesthesia using inter-scalene C6 bloc is administered; a catheter may be inserted for post-operative analgesic purposes. The patient is placed in a beach chair position (Figure 32.2), the elbow in extension and the arms and forearms under horizontal traction, using jersey attached to the skin to apply 3 kg traction. Before surgery begins, 20 cc of xylocaine with epinephrine is injected into the gleno-humeral joint (Figure 32.3) and subacromial space. This potentiates the local/regional anesthesia and reduces peroperative bleeding.

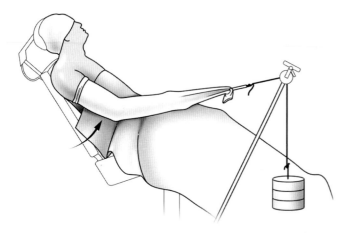

Figure 32.2

Beach chair position for arthroscopy.

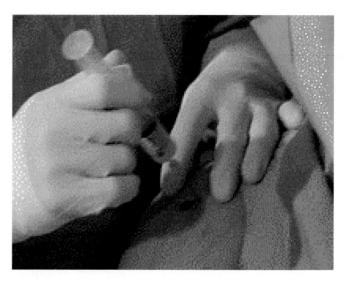

Figure 32.3

Infiltration of the glenohumeral joint and the subacromial space with xylocaine and epinephrine.

Four portals are required for this operation (Figure 32.4):

- the conventional posterior portal
- the posteroexternal subacromial portal (adjacent to the posteroexternal angle of the acromion, level with its external margin) used for subacromial viewing
- the anteroexternal subacromial portal, an accessory working portal
- and the anterior subacromial portal, for placement of the instruments used to repair the cuff and carry out the acromioplasty.

The glenohumeral joint is injected with 60 cc of air from posterior, the treocar and arthroscopic sheath are inserted into the joint, and the arthroscopy begins in order to carry out a thorough assessment of the cartilage, ligaments, rim, biceps and cuff. The cuff is explored from front to back, beginning with the subscapularis tendon, the intra-articular upper third of which is visible. Intratendon ruptures or upper disinsertions of the deep surface are only relieved by relaxing the tendon with internal rotation of the arm. The biceps, which has already been explored from its insertion on the superior glenoid, is now explored thoroughly from the intra-articular portion to where it enters its groove by passing above and below it and by adjusting the eyepiece as required. The walls of the bicipital groove are constituted to the front by the terminal part of the external coracohumeral ligament, above by the interval rotator and behind by the anterior foot of the supraspinatus tendon. The stability of the biceps tendon is tested during internal rotation and, above all, during external rotation to check for anterior subluxation. This exploratory stage is very important, because it is possi-

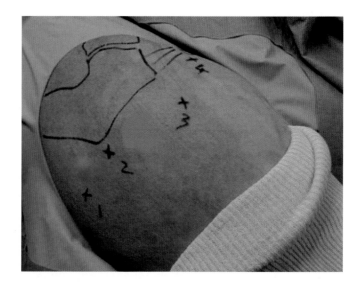

Figure 32.4

Portals for arthroscopy: portals 1 and 2 for the scope, portals 3 and 4 for instruments.

ble, although difficult, to repair subscapular lesions and/or subluxations of the biceps using arthroscopy.

We will consider here only the situation of single lesions of the supra- and infraspinatus tendons. These tendons are explored from front to back, with the scope directed superiorly in order to assess the degree of vascularization of the deep surface, to determine the location and extent of disinsertion in the sagittal and frontal plane and to evaluate intratendinous cleavage, which is often posterior or a non-transfixing rupture of

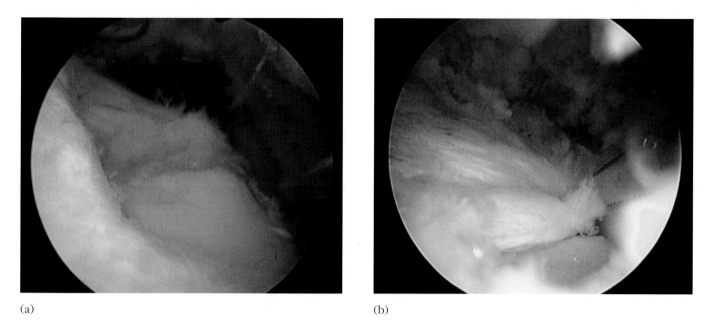

(a)

(b)

Figure 32.5

Testing the reducibility of the tear. The medium-sized tear (a) is reducible with a medial to lateral traction (b).

the deep surface. We will use the classification for distal, intermediate or retracted ruptures in the sagittal plane and anterior, superior or posterosuperior rupture in frontal plane. A needle, followed by a graduated probe, is introduced via the subacromial anteroexternal portals to measure the size of the rupture. In small ruptures, it is sometimes necessary to fill the joint with fluid to provide distension before it is possible to see the disinsertion zone, towards which the scope is pushed before being inserted as far as the subacromial space.

After determining the site, type and size of the rupture by comparison with the preoperative imaging studies, the possibility of reducing the rupture by introducing forceps through the subacromial anteroexternal portal is determined (Figure 32.5). This portal position may have to be slightly modified depending on the position of the tear. The reducibility of the rupture is more important than its size in deciding whether to continue with the arthroscopic tendon repair. Abduction and internal or external rotation movements are used to help to assess the facility and site of tendon reinsertion.

If it is only possible to achieve partial reduction, arthroscopy is continued because we know that anatomical re-insertion can be achieved by means of periglenoid capsulotomy and peritendinous release. If arthroscopic repair is considered to be impossible or risky, the operation can be continued after opening, without being hampered by infiltrated fluid, because the arthroscopy will have been carried out using ambient air which causes no problem. If the decision to continue with the arthroscopic repair is taken, the joint is distended with

saline, using a pump fitted with an input and output pressure regulating system.

After washing the joint, the arthroscope is removed from the joint and then reinserted via a subacromial posteroexternal portal in order to carry out a bursoscopy. The usual method is slightly modified in that the scope is inserted right beside the posterior angle of the acromion along its external margin in order to avoid subsequently being hindered by fat and by the deep aponeurosis of the deltoid. The rupture of the cuff is reduced again, but this time it is assessed by subacromial viewing, which makes it easier to determine the best rotation position as well as the number and site of the future attachment points. Abrasion of the greater tuberosity of humerus with no tendon insertion is done using a shaver or milling cotter via the anteroexternal approach. This step is essential for the subsequent reinsertion of the tendon edge onto the bone and should not go beyond simple removal of the cortex. A 7-mm cannula is then inserted via the same incision and attached to the skin (using the same method as for the attachments of thoracic drains for instance) to keep it in place while the instruments are being moved through it.

The repair of the supraspinatous processes is then carried out by introducing a 45° right or left Wolf (Linvatek) hook with a doubled monofilament PDS #2 (Ethicon, Mitek), leaving the loop formed at its distal end (Figure 32.6). The hook chosen is the opposite of the shoulder being repaired (left hook for a right shoulder and vice versa). The anterior subacromial portal through which the hook is introduced is located flush with the

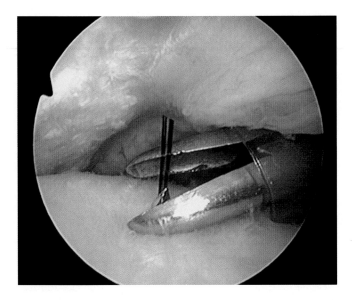

Figure 32.6

Suture hook loaded with a doubled monofilament PD2#2 used as a shuttle relay.

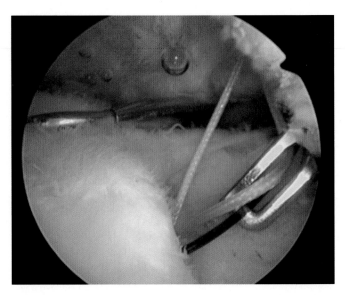

Figure 32.7

Passage of the Panacryl strand through the cuff by means of the PDS shuttle.

coracoacromial ligament. The portal is localized from outside inwards with a needle that approaches the cuff tangentially at the level of the tear. The hook is introduced from front to back, perpendicular to the direction of the cuff, and manipulated to perforate the tendon from top to bottom and then from bottom to top to create a mattress or U-suture. Using this anterior portal to pass the suture through the cuff rather than using the antero-external subacromial portal makes it possible to choose a more or less proximal site relative to the end of the tendon rupture, which is essential for the suture to hold well.

The loop of PDS (Ethicon, Mitek) is now advanced by turning the small wheel and recovered using an ordinary hook slipped into the cannula in the antero-external subacromial portal (Figure 32.6). The PDS loop is pulled through the cannula sufficiently to make it possible to insert the Panacryl (Mitek) braided suture. The step of passing the PDS through first is necessary because a braided suture cannot be fed through a Wolf hook. The Wolf hook is then removed, with the two ends of the PDS suture exiting the anterior subacromial portal. The Panalok RC anchor, with the Panacryl suture attached, is mounted on an inserter. For this arthroscopic technique, the needles on the suture are removed. One of the two strands of Panacryl is passed through the loop of PDS (Figure 32.7). The two ends of the PDS suture are pulled so that the Panacryl passes through the cuff from the antero-external subacromial portal to the anterior subacromial portal (Figure 32.7). In this way, the anterior suture is passed through the cuff and emerges through the anterior portal. The posterior strand remains initially in the antero-external portal via the external cannula and remains attached to the anchor mounted on its inserter (Figure 32.8).

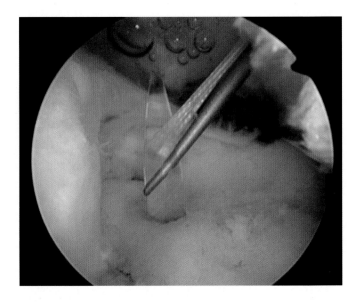

Figure 32.8

Insertion of the Panalok RC anchor.

The hole into which the anchor is inserted is made using a #3.2 bit introduced via the cannula, in the external cortical bone of the greater tuberosity of humerus, flush with the external margin (Figure 32.8). The anchor is then brought down into the cannula while pulling gently on the thread emerging from the anterior portal and then pushed deep into the bone of the greater tuberosity, taking care not to make a loop with the Panacryl suture (Mitek). The inserter is then removed,

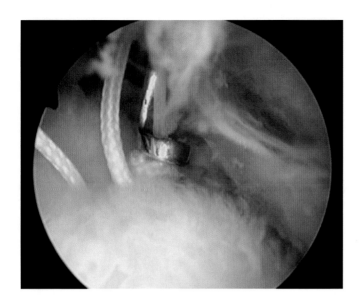

Figure 32.9

Easy Knot to fix the tendon to the bone.

and the posterior suture is pulled in order to check that the suture slides freely through the anchor.

A hook is then used to grasp the anterior suture through the cannula. Both sutures are therefore brought out through the antero-external subacromial portal cannula. A knot is then tied, either an Easy Knot if the sutures glide freely, or alternatively by a descending series of half-hitches if they glide with difficulty (Figure 32.9). The tear in the cuff is then reduced with the assistance of an arm position in abduction and slight internal rotation. The rupture of the cuff is thus repaired with a single anchor or several if the size of the rupture makes this necessary, beginning at the front and working towards the posterior margin. After all subsequent anchors and sutures are placed and securely tied, the acromioplasty is then carried out in the usual fashion. The repair is then checked by the subacromial approach, and then by the intra-articular approach.

Postoperative protocol

The postoperative instructions are usually straightforward. The repair is relieved by using a small abduction cushion for 45 days making it possible to carry out immediate passive rehabilitation. The patient is then permitted to resume activity cautiously over a further 45 days.

References

1. Ellman H, Hanker G, Bayer M. Repair of the rotator cuff. End result study of factor influencing reconstruction. *J Bone Joint Surg Am* 1986; **68**:1136–41.
2. Rockwood CA, Burkead WZ. Management of patients with massive rotator cuff defects by acromioplasty and rotator cuff debridment. *Orthop Trans* 1988; **12**:190–3.
3. Walch G, Marechal E, Maupas J, Liotard JP. Traitement chirurgical des ruptures de la coiffe des rotateurs. Facteurs pronostiques. *Rev Chir Orthop* 1994; **80**:369–78.
4. Paulos LE, Kody M. Arthroscopically enhanced 'mini approach' to the rotator cuff. *Am J Sports Med* 1994; **22**:19–26.
5. Palette GA, Warner JJP, Altcheck DW. Arthroscopic rotator cuff repair; evaluation of results and a comparison of techniques. Presented at the 60th annual meeting of the Arthroscopc Surgeons, San Francisco, CA, USA. February 18–23, 1993.
6. Gazielly DG. Arthroscopic fixation of distal supraspinatus tears with Revoscrew anchors and permanent matress sutures; a preliminary report. In Gazielly DF, Gleyze P, Thomas T, eds. *The Cuff.* Paris: Elsevier, 1997; 282–6.
7. Lafosse L. Arthroscopic repair of rotator cuff tears with Mitek anchors. In Gazielly DF, Gleyze P, Thomas T, eds. *The Cuff.* Paris: Elsevier, 1997.

33 Arthroscopic repair of large and retracted rotator cuff tears

Joseph C Tauro

Introduction

As experience has been gained in the arthroscopic repair of small and moderate rotator cuff tears, there has been a natural progression toward the repair of larger injuries. The techniques and results of the open treatment of large rotator cuff tears are well documented, but there is limited experience with their arthroscopic repair. In an arthroscopic approach, many of the same problems found in open treatment of these tears (poor tissue quality, retraction, etc.) will be encountered and many of the principles from open repairs can be applied.[1-13]

The most significant advantage of arthroscopic repair is the elimination of deltoid morbidity, which often occurs after open surgery. Many of these patients will not recover full function of the cuff despite attempts at repair, making the loss of deltoid function an even more significant complication. The larger the cuff tear (and the more extensive the surgical exposure), the greater the potential benefit of an arthroscopic repair.

Surgical principles

Arthroscopic repair of large rotator cuff tears is technically challenging but possible using a systematic and stepwise approach. Experience in repairing smaller tears is mandatory before taking on this greater challenge. Loss of rotational stability (not only superior, but anterior and posterior as well) is one of the major causes of pain and loss of function in these patients. The repair is performed to correct this problem by closing as much of the cuff as possible. However, it is better to perform a partial repair of the cuff that will function well than to perform an unrealistic, high-tension repair of the cuff that will fail postoperatively. All of the principles of arthroscopic cuff repair discussed in Chapter 29 need to be observed. Especially critical to success is complete exposure of the tear and the identification of its configuration.

Smaller tears of the supraspinatus are usually contained within the bursa so that exposure is not difficult. Large tears will usually extend more posteriorly and therefore outside the bursa. This necessitates a more difficult extrabursal debridement but one that must be performed in order to fully expose the tear. An electro-surgical ablative device is mainly used in this exposure as the extrabursal tissue is quite vascular and will bleed if debrided with a rotary shaver alone.

Pattern configurations of large tears are the same as those described for smaller tears: crescent or longitudinal. Many tears that appear to be very large are still quite mobile. In these cases, crescent-shaped tears can be repaired directly to bone and longitudinal tears can be repaired with a combination of side-to-side repair (margin convergence) and then end-to-bone repair if necessary. Some retracted tears, however, have poor mobility. Inability to close the cuff tear because of intrinsic muscle atrophy and fibrosis is not correctable with primary repair. Poor cuff mobility secondary to attachment to contracted capsular tissue is correctable with arthroscopic releases.

In large tears, we subdivide the crescent and longitudinal patterns into non-retracted and retracted categories (Figures 33.1–33.4). Note how in Figures 33.3 and 33.4

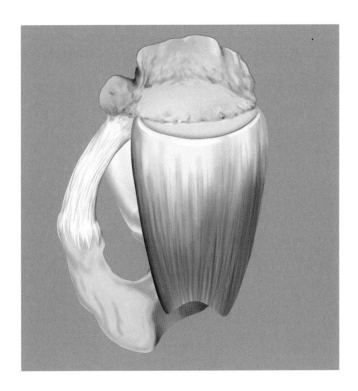

Figure 33.1

Non-retracted crescent-shaped tear.

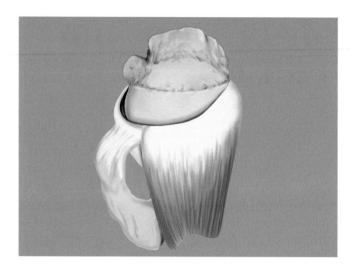

Figure 33.2

Retracted crescent-shaped tear.

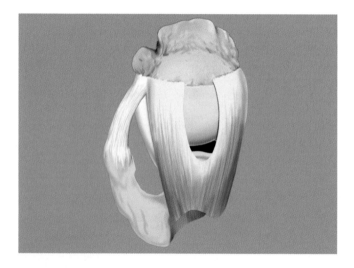

Figure 33.3

Non-retracted longitudinal tear.

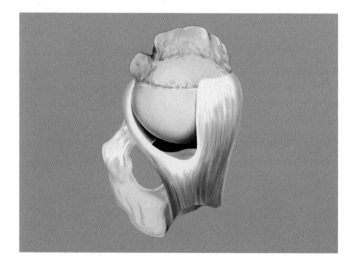

Figure 33.4

Retracted longitudinal tear.

the supraspinatus tendon is tethered by the contracted coracohumeral ligament and the attached rotator interval capsule. Retracted tears must be released from these tissues to achieve the maximum closure possible. Other special considerations when repairing large cuff tears arthroscopically are outlined below.

Surgical technique

Preparation, releases and acromioplasty

All arthroscopic cuff repairs are performed as outpatient procedures, usually under general anesthesia. Scalene block anesthesia is used if there is a patient preference or a medical contraindication to general anesthesia. The patient is placed in the lateral decubitus position with the arm in 45° of abduction and 15° of forward flexion and with 4.5 kg (10 lb) of traction. Excessive abduction should be avoided because it will block access to the greater tuberosity. Routine diagnostic arthroscopy is performed first in the glenohumeral joint to assess the size and shape of the tear. An atraumatic grasper is inserted through the lateral subacromial portal, and cuff mobility is assessed from the articular side (Figure 33.5). If supraspinatus tendon mobility is poor, a superior capsular release should be performed at this time, using an arthroscopic elevator or electrosurgical cutting device inserted through the lateral subacromial portal. The release is carried out by cutting through the capsule between the cuff tendon and the glenoid rim from the biceps anteriorly to the posterosuperior corner of the

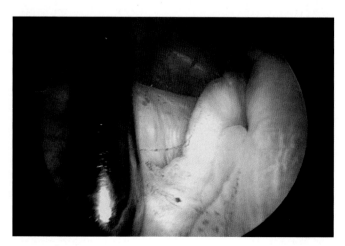

Figure 33.5

Tissue tensioner applying lateral tension to the rotator cuff.

glenoid (Figure 33.6). Now manually try to close the tear again with the tissue tensioner. At this point if a crescent-shaped tear will not reduce to bone or a longitudinal tear will not close from side to side, then an arthroscopic 'interval slide' should be performed. This soft-tissue release is simply an arthroscopic adaptation of the open interval slide.

Perform the release while viewing from the posterior intra-articular portal. Insert a narrow basket punch into the lateral subacromial portal, through the tear in the cuff and into the joint (Figures 33.7 and 33.8). The interval between the anterior border of the supraspinatus and the superior capsule (rotator interval) is divided laterally to medially. This will also release the tendon from the contracted coracohumeral ligament on the bursal side. With the biceps intact, the release is made just caudad to the tendon. If the biceps is not intact, the release is started approximately at the anterosuperior pole of the glenoid, but can be judged also by the character of the tissue being cut. It is helpful in most cases to establish a small percutaneous portal, just adjacent to the lateral subacromial portal, to help pull laterally on the tendon as it is released. Once the release is completed past the medial border of the capsule, mobility is generally greatly improved. The completed releases are illustrated in Figures 33.9 and 33.10.

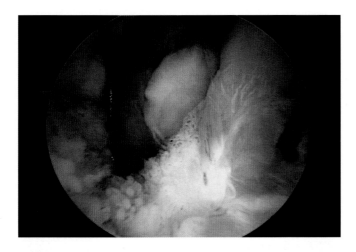

Figure 33.6
Superior capsular release.

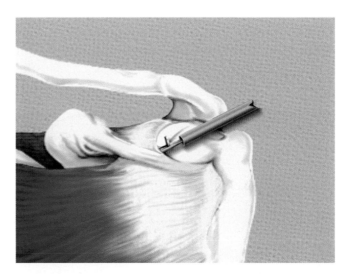

Figure 33.7
Basket punch inserted through the lateral subacromial portal to begin the interval release.

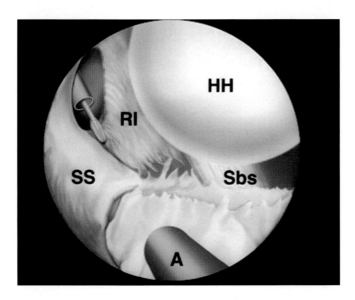

Figure 33.8
Interval slide as viewed from the posterior intra-articular portal. The basket punch is inserted through the tear to begin the release (biceps absent in this case).

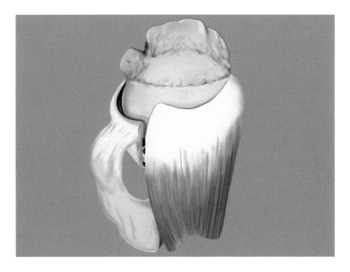

Figure 33.9
Completed interval slide release, crescent-shaped tear.

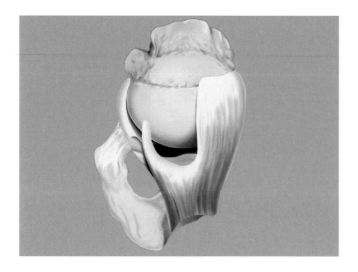

Figure 33.10

Completed interval slide release, longitudinal tear.

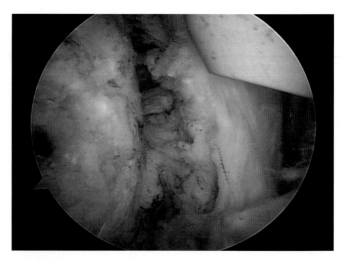

Figure 33.11

Coracoacromial ligament released from the acromion as a sleeve.

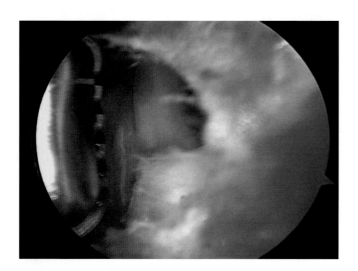

Figure 33.12

Posterior view of the bursa before debridement. The posterior extent of the cuff tear is obscured.

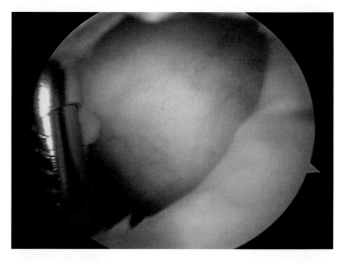

Figure 33.13

Posterior view after bursal debridement. The complete extent of the tear is exposed.

The arthroscope is now moved into the bursa. Acromioplasty is routine in these cases, based on the preoperative assessment of acromial morphology determined by magnetic resonance imaging. The handling of the coracoacromial ligament is important. It should *never* be excised, since it is an important restraint against superior migration of the humeral head if the tear cannot be repaired completely or if the cuff repair fails. The ligament should be elevated as an L-shaped sleeve from the anterior and lateral acromial edge (Figure 33.11). It will then heal back to the new acromial edge after

acromioplasty. Complete hemostasis is mandatory before proceeding to cuff repair.

After acromioplasty, the bursa must be debrided until the entire extent of the cuff tear can be seen (Figures 33.12 and 33.13). This requires viewing the cuff and bursa from the posterior, lateral and sometimes anterior portals while performing the debridement. Any bursal adhesions (more common in revision repairs) are excised at this time. It is usually necessary to use arthroscopic cautery/cutting devices at this stage to control bleeding. A bursal side assessment of the cuff tear is now made,

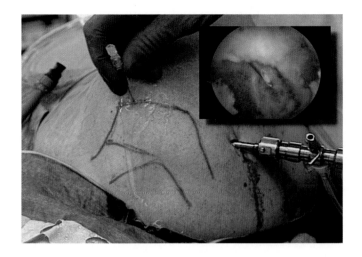

Figure 33.14

The anterolateral subacromial portal in the 'safe zone'.

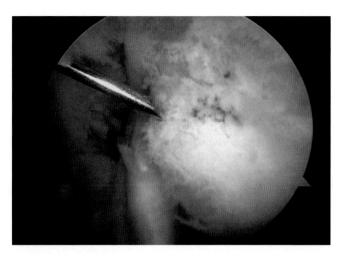

Figure 33.15

Needle localization down to the greater tuberosity, viewed from posterior portal.

once again viewing from several portals. The interval slide is checked to make sure the release is complete and, if necessary, the release can be completed from the bursal side.

Special repair considerations

There is a large 'safe zone' for portal placement in the subacromial space. Any position around the acromion from lateral to the coracoid to the posterior portal is safe as long as it is within 4 cm of the acromial margin. Needle localization for portals is very helpful. Exact portal positioning depends on the particular repair technique used and the configuration of the tear. One of the most common operative portal positions I use in supraspinatus repairs is the anterolateral subacromial portal (Figures 33.14 and 33.15).

There are two broad categories of suture and anchor insertion techniques. In 'suture first' techniques, the suture is first inserted into the tendon, followed by feeding the end of the suture that is exiting under the cuff tendon into the eyelet of a push-in anchor. The anchor is then inserted through a cannula into bone, followed by knot tying. Suture placement can be accomplished by direct insertion of #1 polydioxanone sutures (PDS) via a 7-mm open-mouthed 'Caspari' (Linvatec, Largo, FL, USA) punch, #2 braided suture with an Acufex (Smith & Nephew, Andover, MA, USA) punch (easiest), or any suture material via the use of various retrograde devices (more difficult). We employ the 'suture first' technique most often when the tear is confined to the supraspinatus. Although in theory PDS suture strength will deteriorate significantly by 8 weeks, we have been very satisfied with its performance in clinical practice.

In larger tears, and especially when repairing the infraspinatus, we often use an 'anchor first' technique. Screw-in anchors can be inserted percutaneously through small stab incisions. This is an advantage when repairing a broad cuff tear from anterior to posterior, as multiple large portals are not necessary. The preattached suture must then be pulled back through the cuff tendon using a retrograde device. The small stab incisions for percutaneous portals are all that are normally needed to insert these devices. Knot delivery, however, must always be done after transferring suture limbs to a cannula to avoid soft tissue entanglement. Non-disposable retrograde devices are recommended because they do not bend or break as easily as the disposable types.

Tears of the infraspinatus must be repaired first. This tendon is usually mobile and can be reduced fairly easily to the posterosuperior corner of the greater tuberosity. Repair of the tendon is generally performed while viewing from the lateral or posterolateral portal with instruments inserted through accessory portals as needed.

Once released, retracted supraspinatus tears that were initially crescent-shaped can be pulled down to the tuberosity and repaired directly to bone, without a side-to-side repair (Figure 33.16). To repair longitudinal tears lateral traction is applied to the released supraspinatus tendon's lateral edge with an atraumatic grasper. The posterior edge of the muscle–tendon unit is rotated adjacent to the anterior edge of the infraspinatus. The tendon is then anchored to bone, followed by a side-to-side repair to the infraspinatus. The specific techniques of end-to-bone and side-to-side repair are the same as those discussed in Chapter 29. In very large tears, this may leave an exposed area on the anterosuperior humeral head (Figure 33.17). This conforms to the

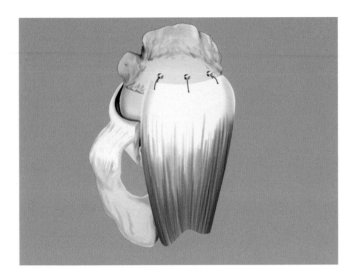

Figure 33.16

End-to-bone repair after interval slide of a crescent-shaped tear.

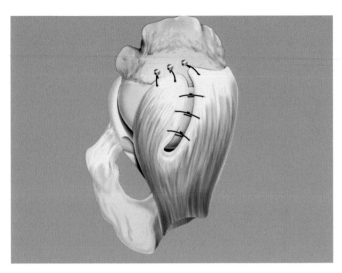

Figure 33.17

Completed repair of an oval tear. Some of the anterior-superior humeral head may still be exposed after tendon rotation in very large tears.

principle outlined above, that a partial low-tension repair is better than a complete high-tension repair that will fail. In these cases, it is important that the coracoacromial ligament should be left intact, that the interval release should be from the supraspinatus and not from the humeral head (as is done in releases for frozen shoulder), and that the subscapularis should be intact or repaired. Otherwise, anterosuperior instability of the humeral head can occur.

Postoperative care

If general anesthesia was used, 0.5% bupivacaine is injected into each of the portals and the subacromial space at the conclusion of the procedure. A 'pain pump' is usually set up, with the cannula placed in the subacromial space for 72 hours. The reservoir is filled with 0.25% bupivacaine and the pump is run at 2 ml/h with a patient-controlled bolus of 2 ml/h allowed. The patient is placed in a shoulder immobilizer and a continuous cold-therapy cuff is applied over the shoulder at the end of the procedure. Patients are prescibed rofecoxib (Vioxx) 50 mg daily for 5 days, then 25 mg daily for 5 days whether they have pain or not (pre-emptive pain control), as well as controlled-release oxycodone (Oxycontin), 20–30 mg every 12 hours as required.

Patients are instructed to remove the immobilizer, starting on the first postoperative day, when in a safe environment. They may then move the hand, wrist and elbow, but not the shoulder. Formal physical therapy begins on the third postoperative day and consists of treatment of pain and edema, passive range of movement exercises of the shoulder to full, and a parascapular mobilization and strengthening program. Depending on the size and security of the repair, progression to active range of movement exercise of the shoulder takes place 5–6 weeks postoperatively. Light resistive exercises can be added at 8–10 weeks with a very gradual increase in intensity until maximum improvement is achieved, usually by 6 months.

References

1. Bigliani LU, Cordasco FA, McIlveen SJ et al. Operative repair of massive rotator cuff tears: long term results. *J Shoulder Elbow Surg* 1994; **1**:120–30.
2. Burkhart SS, Johnson TA, Wirth MA, Athanasiou KA. Cyclic loading of transosseous rotator cuff repairs: 'tension overload' as a possible cause of failure. *Arthroscopy* 1997; **13**:172–6.
3. Cordasco FA, Bigliani FA. Large and massive tears: technique of open repair. *Orthop Clin North Am* 1997; **28**:179–93.
4. Debeyre J, Patte D, Elmelik E. Repair of the rotator cuff of the shoulder: with a note on advancement of the supraspinatus muscle. *J Bone Joint Surg* 1965; **47B**:36–42.
5. Ellman H, Hanker G, Bayer M. Repair of the rotator cuff. *J Bone Joint Surg* 1986; **68A**:1136–44.
6. Gartsman GM, Hammerman SM. Full thickness tears: arthroscopic repair. *Orthop Clin North Am* 1997; **28**: 83–98.
7. Gartsman GM, Khan M, Hammerman SM. Arthroscopic repair of full-thickness tears of the rotator cuff. *J Bone Joint Surg* 1998; **80A**:832–40.

8. Ha'eri GB, Wiley AM. Advancement of the supraspinatus in the repair of the rotator cuff. *J Bone Joint Surg* 1981; **63A**:232–8.

9. McLaughlin HL. Lesions of the musculocutaneous cuff of the shoulder. The exposure and treatment of tears with retraction. *J Bone Joint Surg* 1944; **26A**:31–51.

10. Packer NP, Calver PT, Bayley JL et al. Operative treatment of chronic ruptures of the rotator cuff of the shoulder. *J Bone Joint Surg* 1983; **65B**:171–5.

11. Rokito AS, Cuomo F, Gallagher MA, Zuckerman JD. Long term functional outcome of repair of large and massive chronic tears of the rotator cuff. *J Bone Joint Surg* 1999: **81A**:991–7.

12. Tauro JC. Arthroscopic rotator cuff repair: analysis of technique and results of 2 and 3 year follow-up. *Arthroscopy* 1998; **14**:45–51.

13. Tauro JC. Arthroscopic interval slide in the treatment of large rotator cuff tears. AANA Annual Meeting, 2001.

34 Arthroscopic subscapularis tendon repair

Stephen S Burkhart, Armin M Tehrany and Peter M Parten

Introduction

Although arthroscopic rotator cuff repair has been performed by orthopedic surgeons with increasing frequency, the torn subscapularis was generally considered not to be repairable by arthroscopic means until recently. All previous reports of subscapularis repair had involved open techniques of repair and reconstruction[1-8] until we reported our results of arthroscopic subscapularis repair.[9] In this chapter, we focus on three unique aspects of subscapularis tears:

1. Correlation of subscapularis function with a graded Napoleon test.
2. Reversal of chronic proximal humeral migration by arthroscopic repair of three-tendon tears involving the subscapularis, supraspinatus, and infraspinatus.
3. Techniques to overcome the formidable technical challenges of arthroscopic subscapularis repair.

The Napoleon test

Gerber and colleagues have described the lift-off test[1] and the belly-press test[2] as means of diagnosing subscapularis tears by physical examination. However, the lift-off test was found to be impractical in a large percentage of our patients owing to pain or loss of internal rotation which made it difficult or impossible for these patients to place a hand behind their back. The Napoleon test, described by Schwamborn and Imhoff, is a variation of the Gerber belly-press test.[10] It is named after the position in which Napoleon held his hand (over his stomach) for portraits. We graded the Napoleon test as negative (normal) if the patient could push the hand against the stomach with the wrist straight; positive if the wrist flexed 90° while pushing against the stomach; and intermediate if the wrist flexed 30–60° when the patient pushed against the stomach (Figure 34.1). In the patient with a subscapularis tear, the reason that the wrist flexes with attempts to push the hand against the stomach is that this maneuver harnesses the power of the posterior deltoid to provide a belly-press through shoulder extension. Ordinarily, one performs a belly-press by using the subscapularis to obtain near-maximal internal rotation of

the arm. In a subscapularis-deficient shoulder, the only way to perform a belly-press is to flex the wrist in order to orient the arm so that the posterior deltoid can extend the shoulder, thereby causing the hand to press against the belly. In our study, the Napoleon test could be performed by every patient, whereas the lift-off test could not be performed in the evalaution of 19 of 25 shoulders because of pain or loss of internal rotation. Consequently, the Napoleon test has been useful in predicting the extent of the tear. Tears of less than 50% of the subscapularis usually have a negative Napoleon sign; complete subscapularis tears exhibit a positive Napoleon sign; and those with tears between 50% and 100% display an intermediate Napoleon sign.[9]

Surgical principles

Tears of the subscapularis can cause a broad range of dysfunction. For tears seen arthroscopically involving the upper half of the subscapularis, the only symptoms and signs may be pain and mild weakness. Tears seen at arthroscopy involving more than 50% of the subscapularis as part of a massive tear that also involves the supraspinatus and infraspinatus are usually associated with complete loss of overhead function.

One can also encounter partial thickness, articular surface tears of the subscapularis at arthroscopy, which are analogous to the partial articular surface tear avulsion (PASTA) lesions that involve the supraspinatus. These tears cause pain and some weakness, but typically have a negative Napoleon sign. These tears are likely to be missed unless the arthroscopic surgeon views the subscapularis tendon all the way to its insertion on the lesser tuberosity. When viewing through a posterior portal, this area is best seen with the arm in approximately 45° of abduction and 30° internal rotation.

When the surgeon encounters a subscapularis tear, it is important to repair it prior to any other work in the shoulder, as the space available for instrumentation is very tight and swelling of the deltoid can compromise the space even more.

Partial thickness subscapularis tears (PASTA type) should be converted to full-thickness tears by means of electrocautery or a mechanical shaver, then repaired as full-thickness tears. The full-thickness tears may involve

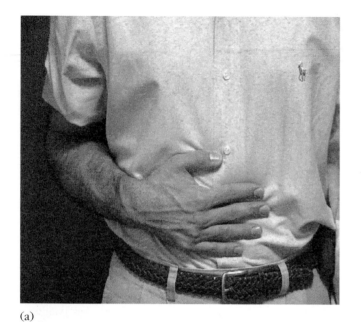

(a)

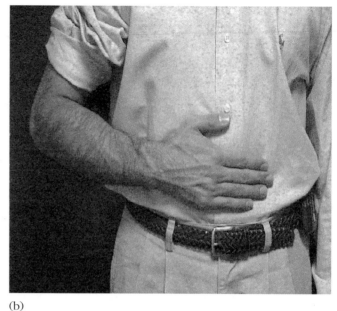

(b)

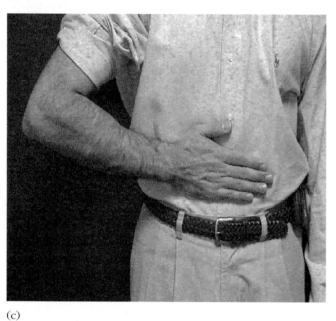

(c)

Figure 34.1

Napoleon test. (a) Positive Napoleon sign indicates a non-functional subscapularis. The patient can press on the belly only by flexing the wrist 90º, using the posterior deltoid rather than the subscapularis for this function.
(b) Intermediate Napoleon sign indicates partial function of the subscapularis. As the patient presses on the belly, the wrist flexes 30–60° owing to partial function of the subscapularis. (c) Negative Napoleon sign indicates normal subscapularis function. The patient is able to maintain the wrist extended while pressing on the belly.

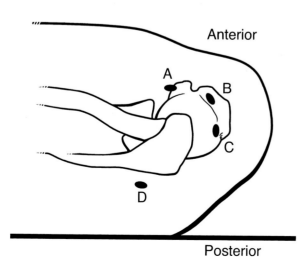

Figure 34.2

Portals for arthroscopic subscapularis repair. The anterior portal (A) is used for anchor placement and suture passage. The anterolateral portal (B) is used for subscapularis mobilization and preparation of the bone bed. The accessory anterolateral portal (C) is used for the traction sutures. The posterior portal (D) is used as the arthroscopic viewing portal.

only a portion of the subscapularis (e.g. involving the upper 50% of the tendon) or the entire tendon may be torn from its insertion on the lesser tuberosity. In addition, subscapularis tears may be isolated, or combined (e.g. associated with tears of supraspinatus and infraspinatus). Large, combined chronic tears generally require mobilization of the subscapularis tendon, whereas isolated tears involving a portion of the subscapularis generally do not. In addition, when partial-thickness tears are converted to full-thickness tears, mobilization is not needed as the intact lateral attachments have kept the tendon out to length.

In arthroscopically repairing the subscapularis tendon, four portals are used (Figure 34.2). The posterior portal is preferred for viewing, with internal rotation of the arm bringing the bone bed into view. If visualization of the insertion of the subscapularis at the lesser tuberosity is difficult, one can either change to a 70° arthroscope and remain in the posterior portal, or switch to an anterosuperolateral viewing portal. There are two anterolateral portals, one that enters the joint anterior to the biceps tendon (anterolateral portal) and the other that enters the joint posterior to the biceps tendon (accessory anterolateral portal). Care is taken to assess and protect the biceps tendon prior to the placement of these portals. The anterolateral portal is used for passage of instruments when mobilizing and repairing the tendon (arthroscopic elevators, shavers, and knot pushers), and the accessory anterolateral portal is used for manipulating the traction sutures. If the rotator interval and supraspinatus are intact, the accessory anterolateral portal is inserted above the biceps tendon at the junction of the supraspinatus tendon and the rotator interval to prevent damaging the supraspinatus tendon by the portal placement. The fourth portal is a straight anterior portal, which is used for placement of suture anchors.

Chronic, retracted subscapularis tears must be mobilized adequately to reach the lesser tuberosity bone bed. For chronic tears, the attachment is routinely medialized by preparing the bone bed 5 mm onto the articular surface. This serves both to broaden the 'footprint' of the repaired tendon and to maximize tendon-to-bone contact for healing. Indication for arthroscopic coracoplasty is judged by palpating the coracoid with a 5-mm shaver blade while the tendon is reduced over the bone bed by traction sutures. If there is less than 7 mm of clearance between the coracoid and the surface of the subscapularis, an arthroscopic coracoplasty is performed. Traction sutures in the subscapularis tendon, which are routinely placed in each case, are easily converted to 'shuttles' by tying a loop in the posterior limb of the suture and using it to pull one limb of an anchor suture through the subscapularis. Such traction shuttles are extremely useful for passing sutures from the anchors through the tendon in this confined space.

If the biceps tendon is subluxed or dislocated, or if there is a torn portion of the biceps that is not amenable to simple debridement, arthroscopic tenodesis is performed either with two suture anchors or with an absorbable interference screw. When a biceps tenodesis is planned, we first pass sutures through the biceps tendon, cut the tendon medial to the sutures, repair the subscapularis, repair any additional cuff tears, and then perform a biceps tenodesis to the anterolateral part of the greater tuberosity.

Clear cannulas are essential, as are 15° and 30° arthroscopic elevators. We prefer to use biodegradable poly-L-lactic acid screw-in anchors (Bio-Corkscrew, Arthrex, Naples, FL, USA). The Viper suture passer (Arthrex) can be useful.

Surgical technique

Burkhart technique of arthroscopic subscapularis repair

The first step is to identify the subscapularis tendon. This is easy in the case of a partial tear, but may be difficult with a chronic complete tear that may be retracted to the glenoid rim and may even be scarred to the anterior deltoid. In chronic, complete subscapularis tears, the tendon usually displays a 'comma' sign in which the superior glenohumeral ligament avulses from its humeral attachment adjacent to the subscapularis footprint and remains attached to the lateral upper margin of the subscapularis tendon, forming a comma-shaped extension above the superolateral subscapularis (Figure 34.3a, b). If the biceps is involved and a tenodesis is indicated, sutures are placed through the biceps and a biceps tenotomy is performed medial to the sutures, which are then secured until the subscapularis and remaining rotator cuff tears are repaired.

Traction sutures for the subscapularis (usually two monofilament #2 nylon sutures) are passed through the tendon by means of a spinal needle and retrieved through the accessory anterolateral portal (Figure 34.4a). In the case of a chronic retracted tear, a tendon grasper through the accessory anterolateral portal is used to pull the tendon as far lateral as possible while the traction sutures are passed. Next, while the traction sutures are pulled laterally, the retracted tendon is mobilized by means of a 15° arthroscopic elevator (Arthrex), freeing the tendon anteriorly, posteriorly and superiorly, until it can be pulled laterally to its bone bed on the lesser tuberosity (Figure 34.4b). We do not use the elevator inferiorly, and we generally do not dissect medially to the coracoid, which can be easily palpated. Dissection posterior to the tendon, in the interface between the subscapularis and the glenoid neck, is quite safe, but dissection anterior to the tendon becomes dangerous if it is carried medial to the coracoid. One must avoid any uncontrolled plunges medially or anteromedially with the elevator.

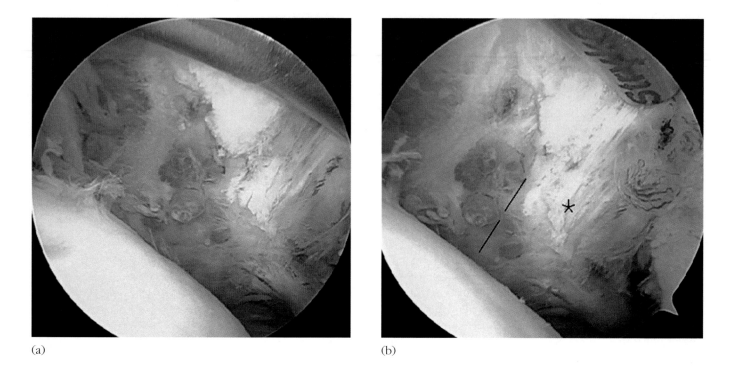

(a) (b)

Figure 34.3

(a) The retracted subscapularis tendon is difficult to identify (left shoulder as viewed through the posterior portal with patient's head toward the top of the photo, beach-chair position). (b) 'Comma' sign seen in chronic retracted subscapularis tears. The arc of the comma (asterisk) is formed by the detached superior glenohumeral ligament, which extends superior to the superolateral border of the subscapularis tendon (dotted line).

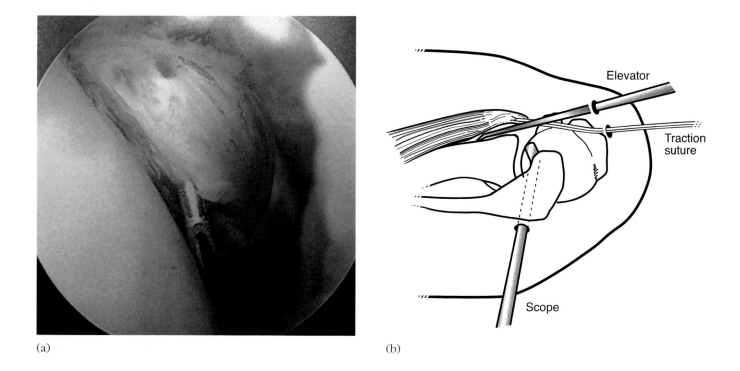

(a) (b)

Figure 34.4

(a) Traction sutures are passed through the tendon using a spinal needle to pierce the tendon and passing a nylon traction suture through the needle. (b) The traction sutures are pulled laterally while the retracted subscapularis is mobilized.

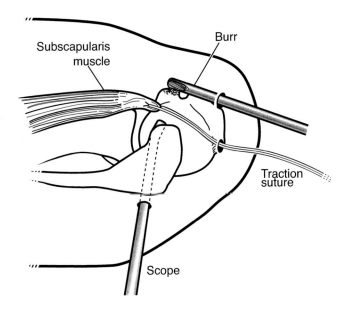

Figure 34.5

Preparation of the bone bed on the lesser tuberosity using a high-speed burr (superior view). Note: Figures 34.5–34.9 are all positioned in the beach-chair perspective.

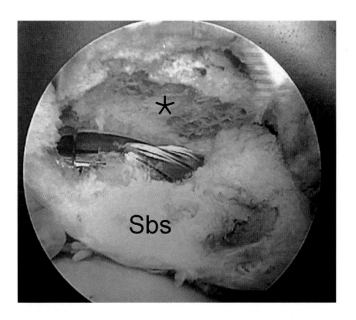

Figure 34.6

Left shoulder, posterior viewing portal. Arthroscopic coracoplasty, demonstrating more than 7 mm space between the subscapularis (Sbs) and coracoid (*) after arthroscopic coracoid decompression is completed.

Once the tendon has been released enough to reach the lesser tuberosity, the bone bed is prepared with a burr through the anterolateral portal (Figure 34.5). We usually medialize the bone bed approximately 5 mm by removing the adjacent 5 mm of articular cartilage in order to provide a broad 'footprint' for subscapularis healing to bone. At this point, we determine whether a coracoplasty will be required. We have found that in many cases of subscapularis tears, the coracoid encroaches tightly onto the bone bed to which the tendon will be repaired, especially with the arm in internal rotation. To avoid this coracoid impingement, the guideline used is that there must be at least 7 mm of space between the subscapularis tendon (when it is held reduced over its bone bed) and the coracoid. If there is less than 7 mm of space, an arthroscopic coracoplasty is performed (Figure 34.6). The palpable soft tissues on the posterolateral tip of the coracoid are made up entirely of the coracoacromial ligament. These soft tissues are removed with a combination of electrocautery and power shaver, and then bone is removed in the plane of the subscapularis tendon by means of a high-speed burr until there is a 7-mm space between the coracoid and the subscapularis. During the coracoplasty we use the posterior viewing portal and place the burr through either the anterolateral or the accessory anterolateral portal, depending on which portal gives the best angle of approach for the burr.

An anatomic study of 18 cadaver shoulders has shown that the average subscapularis tendon 'footprint' is 2.5 cm in length, from superior to inferior (Tehrany AM,

Burkhart SS, Wirth MA, unpublished data.) This information is useful in judging how much of the subscapularis is torn. If there is an exposed footprint of 1.25 cm, for example, then 50% of the tendon has been torn. To repair the tendon to bone, we use one or two suture anchors, depending on the amount of tendon that has been torn. As a general guideline, if the tear involves 50% or less of the tendon we use one anchor, and if it involves more than 50% we use two.

In placing the biodegradable screw-in anchors, we use a spinal needle to determine the angle of approach to the bone bed. We try to place the anchors at a 30–45° 'deadman's angle', approximately 5 mm from the articular margin. Each anchor is doubly loaded with two #2 polyester sutures (Ethibond, Ethicon, Somerville, NJ, USA).

Sutures can be passed in one of two ways. If the tendon is quite mobile and the space is not compromised excessively by swelling, a Penetrator or BirdBeak (Arthrex) suture passer can be brought through the tendon from an anterior portal, retrieving the suture directly. The Viper (Arthrex) suture passer allows easy antegrade suture passage through the tendon via the anterolateral portal. Alternatively, if the space is tight and visualization on both sides of the tendon is poor due to swelling, we prefer to use the 'traction shuttle' technique, in which the traction sutures are used to shuttle the sutures from the anchor through the tendon (Figure 34.7). For the lower anchor, the posterior limb of the lowermost monofilament traction stitch is retrieved through the accessory anterolateral portal along with one

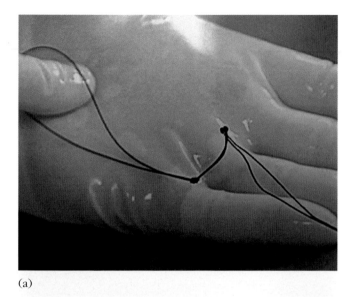

(a)

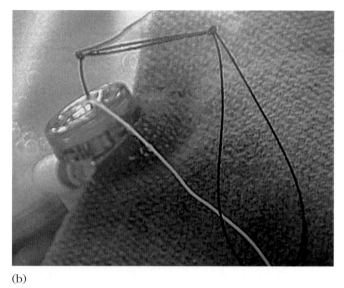

(b)

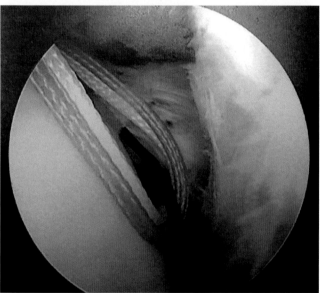

(c)

Figure 34.7

A traction shuttle technique is used to shuttle sutures from the anchor through the tendon. (a) A loop is tied in the posterior limb of the traction suture. (b) One limb of each #2 polyester suture from the suture anchor is threaded through the loop. (c) Left shoulder, posterior viewing portal. The anterior limb of the traction suture is pulled, advancing the loop and anchor sutures through the subscapularis tendon.

limb of each suture pair from the anchor. A loop is tied in the limb of the traction stitch, and the two anchor suture limbs are passed through the loop (Figure 34.7a, b). After the anterior limb of the monofilament traction stitch has been retrieved out of the anterolateral portal, it is pulled by the surgeon in order to 'shuttle' the anchor sutures through the tendon (Figure 34.7c). In this way, a suture limb from each of the two sutures in the anchor is passed through the same transtendinous hole.

At this point, the sutures are tied while the upper traction stitch is pulled firmly through the accessory anterolateral portal. Simple suture loops rather than mattress sutures are used for fixation. If the surgeon places the upper anchor prior to tying the sutures in the lower anchor, it will be difficult to visualize the lower sutures for tying. The upper screw-in anchor is implanted after tying the sutures of the lower anchor.

The sutures are then passed and tied (Figure 34.8) in the same manner as for the lower anchor.

After the subscapularis has been repaired (Figure 34.9), associated rotator cuff tears are repaired in the manner described elsewhere in this book. This is followed by a biceps tenodesis, if indicated.

Postoperative protocol

Postoperative management of subscapularis repairs differs from that of other full-thickness rotator cuff tears in one important respect: early external rotation must be limited for 6 weeks as it would stress the repair. The patients all wear a sling with a small padded bolster (Ultrasling, D-J Ortho, Vista, CA, USA) for 6 weeks. For

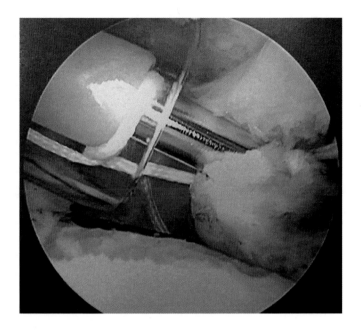

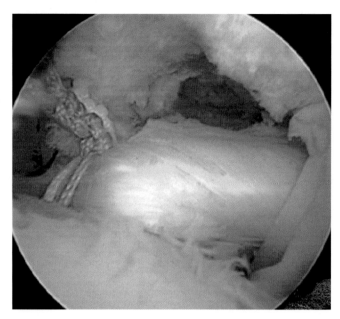

Figure 34.8

Left shoulder, posterior viewing portal. Arthroscopic knot-tying completes the subscapularis repair.

Figure 34.9

Left shoulder, posterior viewing portal. Arthroscopic view of a completed subscapularis repair.

full-thickness tears involving only a portion of the subscapularis tendon (in which there was no retraction), 20–30° of external rotation may be allowed during this period, as the tendon is supple and the repair is protected to some extent by the intact lower portion of the tendon. However, for complete full-thickness tears, particularly those that have been chronically retracted, external rotation beyond 0° is prohibited for 6 weeks. After that, the patient may progress with active and active-assisted external rotation as tolerated, in addition to overhead stretching.

Strengthening exercises are delayed until 12 weeks postoperatively as with other varieties of full-thickness tears. A primate study has shown that it takes 12 weeks for the formation of Sharpey-like fibers after rotator cuff repairs.[11] Therefore, we believe it is not safe to begin strengthening until then. Our rehabilitation protocol emphasizes strengthening of the intrinsic and extrinsic shoulder muscles, including the rotator cuff, deltoid, biceps, and scapular stabilizers.

Results

Authors' clinical series

The senior author (SSB) performed arthroscopic subscapularis repair in 32 shoulders between August 1996 and May 2000.[9] The results were evaluated in 25 patients at least 3 months after the procedure, with an average follow-up

of 10.7 months (range 3–48 months). The average time from onset of symptoms to surgery was 18.9 months (range 1–72 months), indicating often a significant delay before surgical repair. For the entire group of patients, University of California at Los Angeles (UCLA) shoulder scores increased from a preoperative average of 10.7 to a postoperative average of 30.5 ($p < 0.0001$). Forward flexion increased from an average 96.3° preoperatively to an average 146.1° postoperatively ($p = 0.0016$). By UCLA criteria, good or excellent results were obtained in 23 patients (92%), with one fair and one poor result.

Proximal humeral migration

Seventeen of the 25 shoulders had massive rotator cuff tears that involved the subscapularis, supraspinatus, and infraspinatus, with an average tear size of 5 cm × 8 cm. Ten of these 17 shoulders had proximal humeral migration as demonstrated by an acromiohumeral interval of less than 5 mm and superior translation of the inferior articular margin of the humerus relative to the inferior articular margin of the glenoid of more than 5 mm on anteroposterior radiographs. Eight of these 10 shoulders had radiographically-proven reversal of their proximal humeral migration, and also improved overhead function from a preoperative 'shoulder shrug' with attempted elevation of the arm to functional overhead use of the arm postoperatively. Specifically, forward flexion improved significantly from 50.8° before arthroscopic repair to 135.2° after repair ($p < 0.0001$). Their UCLA scores improved significantly from 8.4 preoperatively to 27.7 postoperatively ($p < 0.0001$). In one of the two patients in whom proximal migration recurred, active forward elevation was unchanged postoperatively at only 45°, and in the other patient active forward elevation improved from 90° preoperatively to 110° after the repair. By UCLA criteria, these two patients with recurrence of proximal migration had poor and fair results, respectively, with little or no change in range of motion. This is in contrast to the significant improvement in UCLA scores and range of motion demonstrated by patients with durable reversal of proximal migration. In this series, recurrence of proximal humeral migration led to a poor outcome.

References

1. Gerber C, Krushell RJ. Isolated rupture of the tendon of the subscapularis muscle. Clinical features in 16 cases. *J Bone Joint Surg* 1991; **73B**:389–94.
2. Gerber C, Hersche O, Farron A. Isolated rupture of the subscapularis tendon. *J Bone Joint Surg* 1996; **78A**:1015–23.
3. Wirth MA, Rockwood CA. Operative treatment of irreparable rupture of the subscapularis. *J Bone Joint Surg* 1997; **79A**:722–31.
4. Ticker JB, Warner JJP. Single-tendon tears of the rotator cuff. Evaluation and treatment of subscapularis tears and principles of treatment for supraspinatus tears. *Orthop Clin North Am* 1997; **28**:99–116.
5. Deutsch A, Altchek DW, Veltri DM et al. Traumatic tears of the subscapularis tendon. Clinical diagnosis, magnetic resonance imaging findings, and operative treatment. *Am J Sports Med* 1997; **25**:13–22.
6. Resch H, Povacz P, Ritter E, Matschi W. Transfer of the pectoralis major muscle for the treatment of irreparable rupture of the subscapularis tendon. *J Bone Joint Surg* 2000; **82A**:372–82.
7. Warner JJP, Allen AA, Gerber C. Diagnosis and management of subscapularis tendon tears. *Tech Orthop* 1994; **9**:116–25.
8. Nove-Josserand L, Levigne C, Noel E, Walch G. Isolated lesions of the subscapularis muscle. Apropos of 21 cases. *Rev Chir Orthop Repar Appar Mot* 1994; **80**:595–601.
9. Burkhart SS, Tehrany AM. Arthroscopic subscapularis repair: technique and preliminary results. *Arthroscopy* 2002; **18**:488–91.
10. Schwamborn T, Imhoff AB. Diagnostik und klassifikation der rotatorenmanschettenlasionen. In: Imhoff AB, Konig U, eds. *Schulterinstabilitat-Rotatorenmanschette*. Darmstadt: Steinkopff, 1999; 193–5.
11. Sonnabend DH, Jones D, Walsh WR. Rotator cuff repair in a primate model: observations and implications. Proceedings of the 14th Annual Closed Meeting, American Shoulder and Elbow Surgeons, Manchester, Vermont, September 1997: 27.

35 Arthroscopic biceps tenodesis

Jeffrey L Halbrecht

Introduction

The appropriate treatment for injuries of the proximal long head of the biceps tendon remains controversial. For complete tears of the proximal biceps, tenodesis is often recommended for young, active patients who require supination strength,[1-3] or who wish to avoid the cosmetic deformity of a bulging muscle.[4] Older patients seem to do quite well with non-operative management.[3,5,6] Treatment for partial tears of the tendon, and chronic tenosynovitis that has not responded to conservative treatment, is not as well defined. Many authors recommend tenodesis for these conditions[1,7-10] while others recommend arthroscopic debridement of the partial tear, along with a dilatation of the bicipital groove[11] or even surgical release of the tendon, especially in the elderly.[12] For tears involving more than 50% of the tendon in young patients most authors still recommend tenodesis.[12,13]

Biceps tendonitis almost always occurs as part of an impingement syndrome and an associated subacromial decompression should be performed in most cases when surgical treatment for the tendinitis is being performed.[4,13] In rare cases of isolated biceps tendinitis caused by intertubercular groove pathology[10,14] a decompression can be avoided, and an isolated tenodesis may be warranted. The surgical treatment of biceps tendon subluxation is usually a tenodesis,[15] although a reconstruction of the bicipital groove has been described as well.[16] This author believes that tenodesis is the most predictable option in the treatment of chronic tenosynovitis and partial tears of the biceps tendon, and offers the best chance at complete return of function (Figure 35.1). Failure to tenodese in the presence of biceps pathology may indeed account for some of the poor results reported in the literature following subacromial decompression performed alone.[13,17]

The results of open biceps tenodesis as reported in the literature vary. Mostly, the poor results reported after tenodesis occurred in patients who underwent isolated tenodesis, without accompanying subacromial decompression,[17,18] or resulted from stiffness caused by the open procedure and large associated soft tissue dissection.[9] Except in the rare case of isolated bicipital groove pathology, biceps tendon injury should be considered a component of impingement syndrome and tenodesis should be accompanied by a subacromial decompression. Postoperative stiffness should be avoidable with the all-arthroscopic approach advocated.

Traditional open methods of tenodesis have been well described using either a keyhole[1] or periosteal flap[7] in

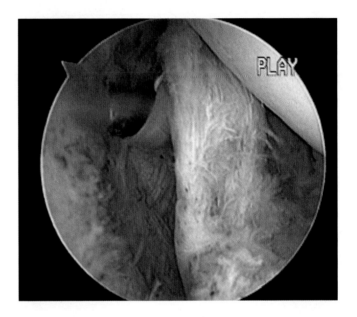

Figure 35.1

Arthroscopic appearance of a partial tear of the biceps tendon and chronic tenosynovitis.

the proximal humerus. More recent and technically easier open techniques have evolved using suture anchors to attach the tendon to a surgically roughened groove.[13,19] Snyder and Chams have described an arthroscopically assisted method of tenodesis, whereby the proximal tendon stump is debrided and tagged intra-articularly, although the tenodesis itself is still performed open.[14]

Several surgeons have begun to perform biceps tenodesis through an entirely arthroscopic approach.[20,21] There are two different approaches currently being performed: all intra-articular or subacromial, and there are various techniques for fixation using suture anchors or even an interference screw. The following will describe in detail the author's preferred arthroscopic method of tenodesis of the biceps using suture anchors through an intra-articular approach.

Surgical principles

Arthroscopic biceps tenodesis requires a familiarity with advanced shoulder arthroscopy techniques. The surgeon

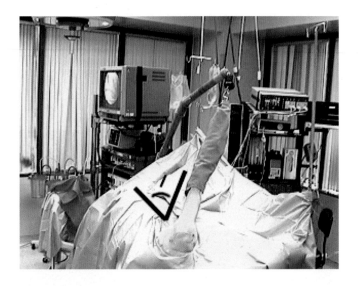

Figure 35.2

Modified lateral decubitus position of patient for arthroscopic biceps tenodesis. Arm is forward flexed to 60°.

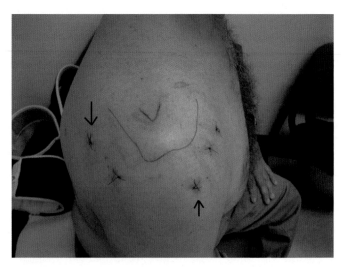

Figure 35.3

Location of portals used for arthroscopic biceps tenodesis. Note specialized 'biceps' portals (arrows).

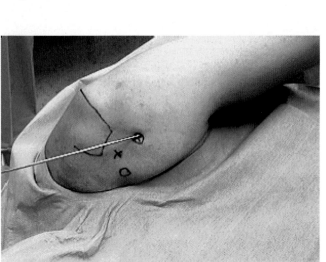

Figure 35.4

Location of anterior biceps portal, 3–4 cm distal to the antero-lateral corner of the acromion along the course of the biceps.

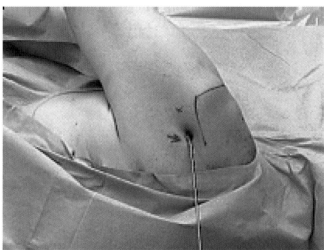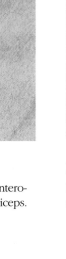

Figure 35.5

Location of posterior biceps portal, 4 cm medial and 1–2 cm distal to the posterolateral corner of the acromion.

must feel comfortable with use of multiple specialized portals and arthroscopic knot tying. The procedure is performed in a modified lateral decubitus position, with the arm in an abducted and forward elevated position. (Figure 35.2). Forward elevation facilitates access down the bicipital groove, and fixing the tendon in abduction ensures that tethering of the glenohumeral joint will not occur following tenodesis.

Two specialized portals are necessary to complete the procedure, one anterior and one posterior (Figure 35.3). The anterior 'biceps' portal is made from outside-in,

3–4 cm inferior to the anterolateral corner of the acromion (Figure 35.4). This portal is used to insert an anchor and tie sutures. This portal is lateral to the musculocutaneous nerve and cepahlic vein, but care should be taken to create this portal using blunt dissection. The posterior 'biceps' portal is made from outside-in, 4–5 cm medial and 1 cm inferior to the posterolateral corner of the acromion (Figure 35.5). The posterior portal is utilized to abrade the bicipital groove and assist in suture management. This portal is through the infraspinatus muscle and away from neurovascular

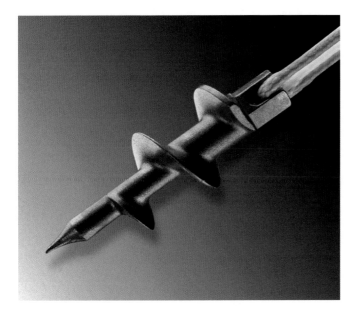

Figure 35.6

Double-armed Corkscrew anchor utilized for biceps tenodesis.

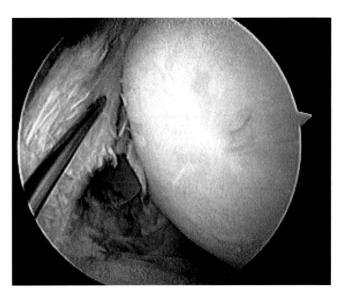

Figure 35.7

Location and direction for posterior biceps portal identified utilizing a spinal needle.

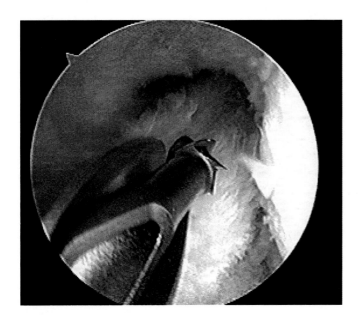

Figure 35.8

Abrade the bicipital groove using a 4.0-mm round burr from the posterior biceps portal. This portal offers direct access down the groove with the arm in forward elevation and slight abduction.

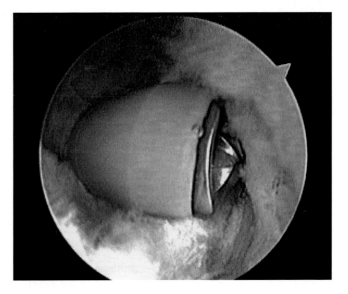

Figure 35.9

Complete the abrasion from the anterior biceps portal as necessary.

structures. For both portals, a spinal needle is used from outside-in to identify the proper location. An Arthrex 'Corkscrew' anchor (Arthrex, Naples, FL, USA) is utilized for two reasons: its small root diameter limits further damage to the tendon on insertion through the tendon; and it is preloaded with two sutures, which allows double fixation through a single anchor (Figure 35.6).

Surgical technique

The patient is placed in the standard lateral decubitus position to initiate the procedure. Once the pathology is verified, the traction device is readjusted to bring the arm into forward elevation and slight abduction. Debridement of the partially torn biceps tendon is performed.

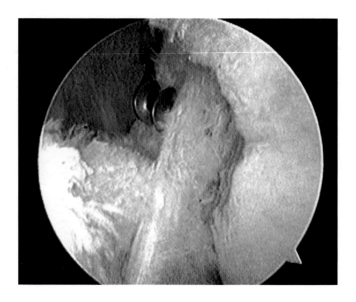

Figure 35.10

Insert a Corkscrew anchor from the anterior biceps portal directly through the biceps tendon into the abraded bony groove.

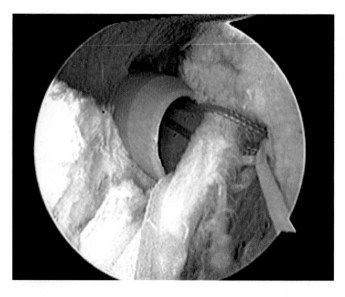

Figure 35.11

Retrieve one set of sutures out the posterior cannula, and tie the other set of sutures through the anterior cannula.

Accessory portals are now created. The posterior biceps portal is created first to gain access down the bicipital groove to debride tenosynovitis, release the transverse humeral ligament and debride the surface of the groove. A thermal ablation tool is helpful for this part of the procedure. The posterior biceps portal is made using a spinal needle from outside-in, while viewing from the standard posterior portal. The accessory posterior 'biceps' portal is made at least 4–5 cm medial to the standard posterior portal, and 1–2 cm inferior to the scapular spine, through the infraspinatus muscle. The exact location of this portal is best determined with a spinal needle (Figure 35.7). Following debridement of soft tissue around the biceps tendon in the groove, the groove is abraded to a bleeding bony bed using a 4.0-mm round burr (Figure 35.8).

At this point an accessory anterior biceps portal is created. This portal is made from outside-in using a spinal needle directly along the course of the biceps tendon so that the needle pierces the tendon and will allow a proper angle for insertion of an anchor into the groove. The location is approximately 3–4 cm inferior to the anterolateral corner of the acromion, but may vary depending on the patient's size and soft tissue bulk. This portal is utilized to complete the abrasion of the groove, and to insert the anchor (Figure 35.9).

Once abrasion is complete, the tenodesis is begun. An Arthrex Corkscrew anchor is inserted through the anterior 'biceps' portal, piercing the biceps tendon and penetrating straight through to the groove (Figure 35.10). The anchor is screwed in manually until seated in bone.

The anchor comes preloaded with two, #2 non-absorbable sutures. Upon insertion of the anchor, all four limbs of suture are through the biceps tendon and exiting the anterior cannula. One of the suture pairs is then retrieved out of the posterior 'biceps' cannula for later tying. Both limbs of the remaining suture now exit the anterior cannula but are not yet ready for tying. Since both limbs of the suture exit from the same location through the tendon, one limb of suture needs to be retrieved posterior to the tendon so that it encompasses half of the tendon when it is tied (Figure 35.11). This limb is then brought out through the anterior cannula and arthroscopic knot tying is performed (Figure 35.12). The remaining set of sutures is then retrieved posteriorly out of the anterior cannula in a similar fashion. One limb of this second suture is retrieved anterior to the biceps tendon to capture the other half of the tendon when it is securely tied. Usually a second anchor will be inserted to add additional security to the tenodesis, resulting in four separate #2 sutures providing fixation for tenodesis (Figure 35.13). Tenodesis of the tendon is in the most proximal portion of the bicipital groove, as verified by final appearance of the anchors on X-ray imaging (Figure 35.14).

The intra-articular portion of the tendon may now be resected using electrocautery and a shaver. We are not convinced that this is necessary. Leaving the tendon attached allows additional protection for the tenodesis while healing to the groove occurs, and may act as a static stabilizer to add additional stability. Neer indicated that when performing an open tenodesis he did not see

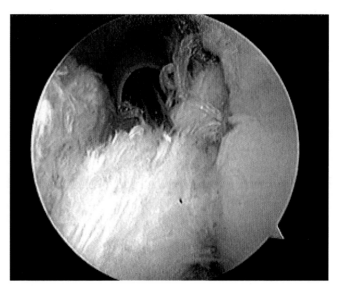

Figure 35.12

Utilize standard arthroscopic knot-tying techniques to obtain secure fixation of the tendon into the groove.

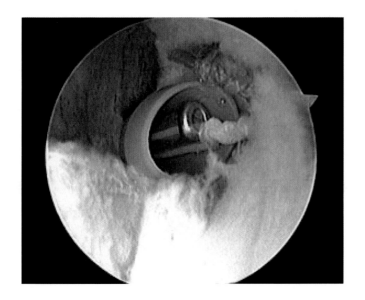

Figure 35.13

Final arthroscopic appearance of the tenodesis.

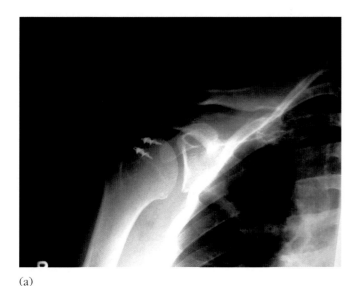

(a)

Figure 35.14

(a,b) X-ray appearance of anchors in the bicipital groove following tenodesis.

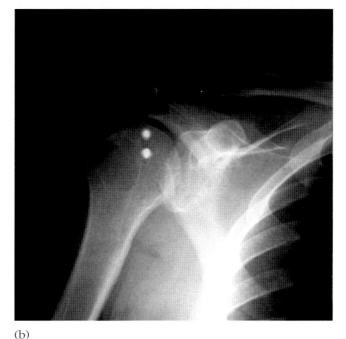

(b)

the need to resect the intra-articular portion of the tendon and often left it attached to the glenoid.[22] Some will argue that leaving the tendon attached may tether the joint. Testing the range of motion following the procedure has not supported this theory, and this has not been noticed as a problem postoperatively. As Neer

found, as long as the intra-articular portion of the tendon is left free and not sutured to the rotator cuff the joint is not tethered.

This procedure can be performed whether or not a tear of the rotator cuff is present, and an arthroscopic cuff repair can follow without compromise, if necessary.

If a rotator cuff tear is present, the tenodesis can be performed from the subacromial space as well, and this approach is preferred by some surgeons in this setting (Burkhart, personal communication).

Postoperative protocol

The patient is placed in a shoulder immobilizer for 3 weeks. Isometric exercise, avoiding the biceps, and wrist and hand motion are allowed. At 3 weeks, passive and assisted range of motion of the shoulder and elbow are begun. Active motion is initiated at 5–6 weeks. Strengthening is started at 8 weeks. Full return to activities is allowed at 12–16 weeks.

References

1. Froimson AI, Oh I. Keyhole tenodesis of biceps origin at the shoulder. *Clin Orthop* 1974; **112**:245–9.
2. Mariani EM, Cofield RH, Askew LJ et al. Rupture of the tendon of the long head of the biceps brachii: surgical versus nonsurgical treatment. *Clin Orthop* 1988; **228**:233–9.
3. Warren RF. Lesions of the long head of the biceps tendon. *Instr Course Lect* 1985; **34**:204–9.
4. Neer CS. Cuff tears, biceps lesions, and impingement. In: Neer CS, ed. *Shoulder Reconstruction*. Philadelphia: WB Saunders, 1990;135.
5. Carroll RE, Hamilton LR. Rupture of the biceps brachii—a conservative method of treatment. *J Bone Joint Surg* 1967; **49A**:1016.
6. Phillips BB, Canale ST, Sisk TD et al. Rupture of the proximal biceps tendon in middle age patients. *Orthop Rev* 1993; **22**:349–53.
7. Hitchcock HH, Bechtol CO. Painful shoulder: observations on the role of the tendon of the long head of the biceps brachii in its causation. *J Bone Joint Surg* 1948; **30A**:263–273.
8. DePalma AF, Callery GE. Bicipital tenosynovitis. *Clin Orthop* 1954; **3**:69–85.
9. Crenshaw AH, Kilgore WE. Surgical treatment of bicipital tenosynovitis. *J Bone Joint Surg* 1966; **48A**:1496–502.
10. Post M, Benca P. Primary tendinitis of the long head of the biceps. *Clin Orthop* 1989; **246**:117–25.
11. Ogilvie-Harris DJ, Wiley AM. Arthroscopic surgery of the shoulder: a general appraisal. *J Bone Joint Surg* 1986; **68B**:201–7.
12. Eakin CL, Faber KJ, Hawkins RJ, Hovis WD. Biceps tendon disorders in athletes. *J Am Acad Orthop Surg* 1999; **7**:300–10.
13. Burkhead WZ Jr. The biceps tendon. In: Rockwood CA, Matsen FA, eds. *The Shoulder*. Philadelphia: WB Saunders, 1998; 1054–7.
14. Snyder S, Chams RN. Clinical evaluation of the SCOI technique of biceps tenodesis using the C-W subpectoralis approach. Submitted for publication.
15. O'Donohue D. Subluxating biceps tendon on the athlete. *Clin Orthop* 1982; **164**:26.
16. Habermyer P, Walch G. The biceps tendon and rotator cuff disease. In: Burkhead WZ Jr, ed. *Rotator Cuff Disorders*. Media, PA: Williams & Wilkins, 1996;142.
17. Dines D, Warren RF, Ingles AE. Surgical treatment of lesions of the long head of the biceps. *Clin Orthop* 1982; **164**:165–71.
18. Becker DA, Cofield RH. Tenodesis of the long head of the biceps brachii for chronic bicipital tendinitis. *J Bone Joint Surg* 1989; **71A**:376–81.
19. Verhaven E, Huylebroek J, Van Nieuwenhuysen W, Van Overschelde J. Surgical treatment of acute biceps tendon ruptures with a suture anchor. *Acta Orthop Belg* 1993; **59**:426–9.
20. Lo KYI, Burkhart SS. Arthroscopic biceps tenodesis: Indications and technique. *Oper Tech Sports Med* 2002; **10**:105–12.
21. Boileau P, Krishnan SG, Coste JS, Walch G. Arthroscopic biceps tenodesis: A new technique using bioabsorbable interference screw fixation. *Arthroscopy* 2002; **18**:1002–12.
22. Neer CS. Cuff tears, biceps lesions, and impingement. In: Neer CS, ed. *Shoulder Reconstruction*. Philadelphia: WB Saunders 1990; 112 (Fig. 2-43I) and 136.

Section VI – Specialized arthroscopic techniques

36 Arthroscopic capsular release

Gregory P Nicholson and Jonathan B Ticker

Introduction

The diagnosis of frozen shoulder, or adhesive capsulitis, is one of exclusion. It is characterized by a limitation of both active and passive range of motion of the glenohumeral joint, which is not primarily due to some underlying condition such as arthritis, rotator cuff tear, cervical radiculopathy, or peripheral neuropathy. The etiology, diagnostic criteria, treatment methods and natural history of this condition are today still under debate and investigation.[1–6] It is felt that the pathology is a process that first involves inflammation of the synovium, resulting in subsynovial fibrosis. This leads to capsular fibrosis, thickening, and ultimately contracture of the glenohumeral capsule.[3,7] Contracture of the glenohumeral capsule can be posttraumatic and postsurgical in origin. In particular, this can result from surgical procedures designed to correct glenohumeral instability.[8–11] Whereas adhesive capsulitis is usually more global, affecting the entire glenohumeral capsule, capsulorrhaphy that is overly tightened may result in primarily anterior or posterior capsular contracture. Isolated posterior capsular contracture can also result from a traumatic traction injury.[9]

Even as our knowledge of the potential pathologic components of adhesive capsulitis has increased, it seems that there is no clear understanding of its natural history. The treatment methods have encompassed a wide variety of techniques. This demonstrates that no truly effective option has been established. Patient-performed home therapy has shown resolution of symptoms, but at a time interval of sometimes two or more years.[4,12] Physiotherapy, when performed in a more aggressive setting, has been shown to be detrimental to progress and pain relief in some reports.[4,12–14] Intra-articular steroid injections and hydraulic distention, or brisement, have also had variable results.[15–17] Operative intervention by manipulation under anesthesia has resulted in restored motion and decreased pain,[6,14,18,19] but it has been associated with complications such as fracture, tendon rupture, and neurologic injury.[5,17,19] There are reports that manipulation has not been effective and patients remained symptomatic.[6,20–23] In a few reports, some patients could not be effectively manipulated under anesthesia and required a conversion to either arthroscopic or open release.[22,24] A more invasive option, the open release through a deltopectoral approach, has been utilized to restore glenohumeral motion. This is usually reserved for treatment after previous open surgical procedures that have resulted in limitation of glenohumeral motion.[5,14,25] In the setting of isolated posterior capsular contracture following posterior capsulorrhaphy, open posterior

releases have been proposed to address the pattern of stiffness.[10]

The arthroscope has been utilized in a variety of ways in the assessment and treatment of adhesive capsulitis. It has been used to confirm the diagnosis and then to provide a hydraulic distention, or brisement, of the capsule.[16,17] The arthroscopic approach allows for documentation of the pathology, both grossly and histologically.[3,7,26,27] It has been used after manipulation to investigate the postmanipulation pathology and to address associated factors such as prominent acromion with impingement pathology, and acromioclavicular joint arthralgia.[23,27,28] Pollock et al used arthroscopy after manipulation to address these associated factors and showed satisfactory results in 83% of patients.[28]

More recent reports have utilized the arthroscope to perform the capsular release to restore motion, instead of manipulation of the shoulder for releasing or lysing the capsule. The capsular release techniques have been performed in a variety of ways. Initially manipulation would be attempted and, if not successful, then an arthroscopic capsular release would be performed with restoration of motion.[11,22,24] Other authors avoided initial manipulation and utilized an arthroscopic technique to perform an inferior capsulotomy and debridement of the synovitis. No manipulation was performed, and this technique revealed 87% good or excellent results.[29] In contrast, other authors have released only the anterior capsule and rotator cuff interval and, then, performed a gentle post-release manipulation avoiding any instrumentation to the inferior capsule. Warner et al used this technique in 23 patients with idiopathic adhesive capsulitis.[22] They reported complete pain relief and restoration of motion within 7° of the unaffected side. Most reports describe the use of an arthroscopic electrocautery device to release the capsule, though some authors have used basket forceps.[9,11,22,24,29–31] A study that utilized only a motorized shaver to release the rotator cuff interval and anterior capsule was reported by Ogilvie-Harris and Myerthall[32] in 17 diabetics. The capsular release was carried down to the inferior 6 o'clock position and the intra-articular subscapularis tendon was also debrided with the motorized shaver. Thirteen of these 17 diabetics had no pain and restoration of motion.[32] Pearsall et al[31] utilized a similar release technique dividing the capsule 1 cm lateral to the glenoid rim and releasing the same intra-articular portion of the subscapularis tendon along with the interval and anterior capsule. This was performed with an electrocautery device. Eighty-three percent of their patients felt that their shoulders were pain free and had been restored to near normal motion.[31]

Other authors have performed a more circumferential or balanced release involving the rotator cuff interval, anterior, posterior, and inferior capsular structures.[24,30] Harryman et al reported excellent restoration of motion and elimination of pain utilizing arthroscopic capsular release forceps (Smith & Nephew Endoscopy, Andover, MA, USA) to resect the capsule both anteriorly, inferiorly and posteriorly.[24] Nicholson et al reported dramatic pain relief and restoration of motion in 36 patients at an average of 3 months after release. They utilized the ArthroWand bipolar electrocautery (ArthroCare, Sunnyvale, CA, USA) and circumferentially released the capsule and rotator cuff interval off the glenoid rim preserving the labrum.[30] The capsular release technique has shown efficacy not only in idiopathic adhesive capsulitis, but also in postoperative and postinjury stiff shoulders.[9,11,22,30] A subset of patients with isolated, refractory posterior capsular contracture have similarly benefited from an arthroscopic capsular release technique addressing the involved posterior capsular structures.[9]

Indications for an arthroscopic capsular release are still evolving. The etiologic process, inciting factors, the pathophysiology, or the natural history of this condition are not fully understood. Therefore, it is difficult to classify the stage of the disease or the severity of the disease, which makes a treatment approach more difficult to define. It is important to urge the patient to be 'patient'. Conservative treatment with gentle stretching and active-assisted range of motion exercises is instituted initially. Non-steroidal anti-inflammatory medication is utilized. The synovial inflammation that is felt to be an initiator of the disease process has motivated us to use glenohumeral intra-articular steroid injections to decrease pain and, hopefully, facilitate restoration of motion. However, there are those patients who do not respond to physician-directed non-operative treatment methods. An arthroscopic capsular release is indicated if patients have had symptoms for over 3 months and have shown no progress or worsening symptoms with at least 6 weeks of home stretching and physician-directed physical therapy. With pain and shoulder dysfunction that is affecting their occupation, recreation, and/or sleep, arthroscopic capsular release is discussed.

Surgical principles

The purpose of the arthroscopic capsular release is to safely and effectively restore motion and function, relieve pain, and shorten the natural history of a painful, stiff frozen shoulder. From clinical and arthroscopic surgical experience, frozen shoulder may represent a common pathway of expression to a variety of initiating causal factors. This process could be caused by, sustained by, or be involved with any or all of the components of the glenohumeral joint capsule (anterior, inferior, posterior),

coracohumeral ligament (rotator interval) and/or the subacromial space. The arthroscope allows identification, documentation, and the ability to address all areas of pathologic involvement. It also allows the surgeon to address associated or concomitant conditions, such as a prominent acromion or acromioclavicular joint arthralgia. Arthroscopic capsular release allows for a controlled and less traumatic separation of the contracted tissue that is more complete and balanced than if done by manipulation alone. Following a release, less force is required for the final manipulation to restore full motion. If the arthroscopic capsular release is performed with an electrocautery device, there is less hemorrhage and swelling, with, possibly, less postoperative pain. If the subacromial space or the acromioclavicular joint is involved, these areas can typically be addressed arthroscopically.

To properly and safely complete the procedure, the surgeon must realize that this is a difficult arthroscopy. Initial mobility and, therefore, space within the joint is limited, and the synovium can be very friable and cause nuisance bleeding. An arthroscopic pump is vital, and it helps to be able to independently control flow and pressure. A 1:300 000 dilution of epinephrine in the arthroscopic fluid will limit bleeding. A smooth bore cannula for instruments and shavers is easier to pass into the joint than a threaded cannula. One electrocautery device that is preferable is the ArthroWand. The 3.0-mm 90° attachment is relatively stiff and small enough to access tight spots. The 90° direction of the electrodes facilitates cutting into the thickened capsule, and going around corners. The 3-mm width divides and releases a thicker 'stripe' of tissue. The bipolar mechanism arcs the electric current between the electrodes in the tip. This ablates and cuts tissue, as well as coagulates, while not penetrating into the tissue beyond the bipolar zone. This is in contrast to a monopolar hook-type device. This allows for use of a bipolar device in the inferior capsule with less risk to the axillary nerve. However, other types of electrocautery devices can be utilized to effectively release the capsule, as can manual arthroscopic basket forceps or shavers (Figure 36.1; note that all figures show views of a left shoulder).

An experienced assistant to control the arm is helpful. The joint is initially very tight and small arm movements can facilitate exposure to begin the capsular release. A sterile, articulated arm holder (McConnell Orthopedic Mfg, Greenville, TX, USA) that is attached to the operating table and secured to a sterile forearm wrap via an adapter can also assist with arm positioning throughout the procedure. An anesthesiologist who understands the problem, the surgical procedure, and the rehabilitation afterwards is an asset, in that a long-acting interscalene regional anesthetic allows for immediate therapy without pain. If an interscalene catheter is used, or if repeat blocks are planned, a good relationship with anesthesiology is essential.

Pitfalls can occur just trying to insert the arthroscopic sheath into the joint in significantly stiff shoulders. The

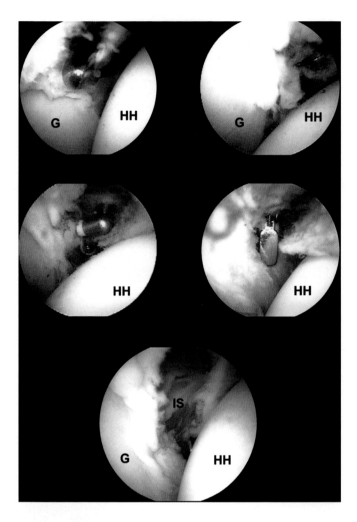

Figure 36.1

Arthroscopic view of posterior capsular release in a left shoulder. Instruments that can be utilized include a mechanical shaver, monopolar electrocautery, bipolar electrocautery, and basket forceps. Posteriorly, the release is completed when muscle fibers of the infraspinatus are visualized. HH = humeral head; G = glenoid; IS = infraspinatus.

humeral joint instability has not been a problem, even after a complete capsule release. Neurologic injury to the axillary or musculocutaneous nerves from the procedure itself or due to the increased joint excursion after the prolonged stiffness is released can occur. Another problem can arise if involvement of the subacromial space or acromioclavicular joint arthralgia is not recognized and addressed at the time of the arthroscopic capsular release. If left behind as a source of pain, these conditions can lead to treatment failure. Therefore, a preoperative clinical assessment for involvement of the subacromial space and acromioclavicular joint is routine. Radiographs, including a true AP, axillary, outlet, and Zanca projections, will assess the glenohumeral joint, acromion morphology and the acromioclavicular joint. An MRI is also obtained preoperatively to identify any associated or unrecognized pathology.

Surgical technique

We perform this procedure in the beach chair position. A long-acting interscalene block is used. A general anesthetic may also be used in combination. The arm must be mobile, as small changes in abduction, elevation, and rotation facilitate intra-articular visualization and maneuvering of the arthroscope. Once anesthesia is established, range of motion is documented for both the involved and uninvolved shoulders. It is of value to note whether the shoulder is as stiff as it was in the office. The planes of motion for measurement are glenohumeral elevation, external rotation at the side and internal rotation. Internal rotation is sometimes difficult, as patients cannot rotate behind their back, and 90° of abduction may not be possible. We try to abduct to at least 45° and assess the magnitude of rotation of the forearm as it drops into internal rotation, which allows us to assess the amount of posterior capsular involvement. Posterior capsular tightness is also evaluated by comparing cross-chest adduction in both shoulders.

Landmarks are outlined and an 18-gauge spinal needle is inserted into the glenohumeral joint from posterior and directed toward the coracoid tip, to allow for infiltration of saline. The capsule is thicker and less compliant than in other shoulder conditions and the humeral head will be tightly opposed to the glenoid. The needle is angled over the humeral head toward the superior labrum–biceps tendon origin. Only about 10–15 ml will go into the joint easily, and then significant backpressure will be felt. The arthroscopic sheath and matching trocar, with a blunt tip, are carefully introduced at the same angle and position as the needle. This will help to avoid joint surface damage. If there is a bevel on the arthroscopic cannula, the longer portion is placed superior to further decrease any chance of damaging the articular cartilage. Intra-articular placement is then confirmed by fluid backflow through the sheath.

sheath must be directed toward the origin of the long head of the biceps tendon and superior labrum. This will allow for visualization of the contracted arthroscopic triangle anteriorly and, most importantly, avoids direct injury to the articular surfaces. Care must be taken to release the capsule and not the labrum or the rotator cuff tendons. The subscapularis is at particular risk as it is covered by thickened capsular tissue. We have not felt it necessary to release any portion of its tendon. Inferiorly, the axillary nerve has the potential for injury if overzealous release or debridement is performed.[33]

Additional potential complications include inadequate restoration of motion, as well as a slow 'refreezing' of the shoulder. This has been shown to be more likely in the diabetic population.[20] On the other hand, gleno-

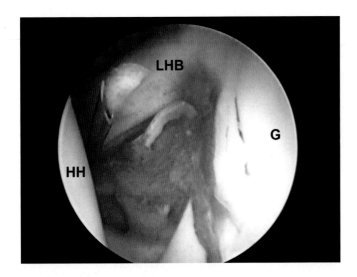

Figure 36.2

Initial view of rotator interval. Typical proliferative synovitis is seen in the contracted arthroscopic triangle. HH = humeral head; G = glenoid; LHB = long head biceps tendon.

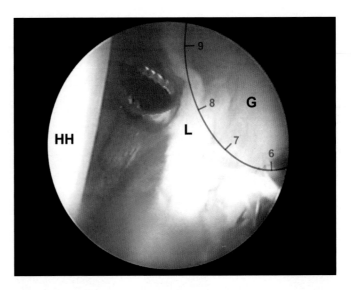

Figure 36.3

Shaver at midglenoid position. Gelatinous synovium of adhesive capsulitis covers the anterior and inferior capsule. G = glenoid; L = labrum; HH = humeral head.

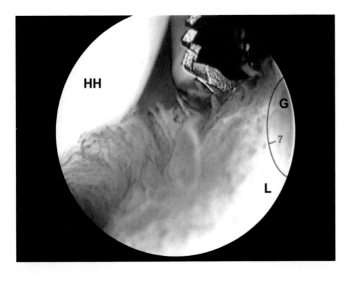

Figure 36.4

Proliferative gelatinous synovium in a contracted axillary pouch. G = glenoid; L = labrum; HH = humeral head.

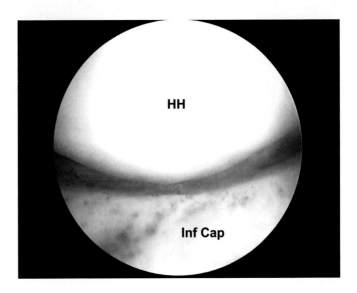

Figure 36.5

After synovial debridement, the thickened, contracted capsule in the axillary pouch is seen. Note the lack of space in the pouch. HH = humeral head; Inf Cap = inferior capsule.

The pump is typically set at a flow of 200 ml per minute and pressure of 20 mmHg. The contracted, inflamed synovium in the arthroscopic triangle between the long head of the biceps, the upper surface of the subscapularis and the glenoid rim will be visualized. Alternating irrigating and suctioning a few times can improve the view. To establish an anterior portal in an 'outside-in' method, a spinal needle is placed through the skin from just lateral to the coracoid tip into the

arthroscopic triangle under direct observation. After a skin incision in this position, a smooth 7-mm cannula (Linvatec, Largo, FL, USA) is inserted into the joint.

Gelatinous synovial material, at the root of the biceps, over the rotator cuff interval and typically down the anterior capsule into the axillary pouch, will be encountered in the majority of cases (Figure 36.2). This material is debrided with a motorized shaver, usually a 4.0- or 4.5-mm size (Figures 36.3 and 36.4). It is interesting to

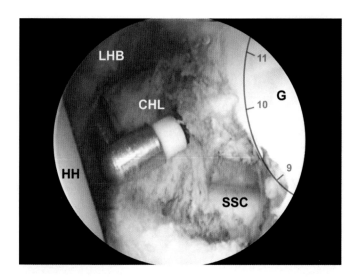

Figure 36.6

Electrocautery device is releasing thickened interval tissue. The pristine rolled upper border of the subscapularis is seen through the released capsule. CHL = coracohumeral ligament; SSC = subscapularis; LHB = long head biceps tendon; G = glenoid; HH = humeral head.

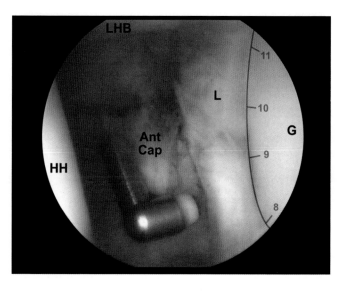

Figure 36.7

Release of base of arthroscopic triangle and continuing inferiorly. Note prominent, rolled labrum in this patient. Ant Cap = anterior capsule; L = labrum; G = glenoid; HH = humeral head; LHB = long head biceps tendon.

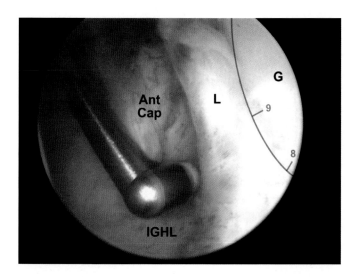

Figure 36.8

Capsular release off the glenoid, preserving the labrum. Note the position and direction of the electrocautery tip. Ant Cap = anterior capsule; L = labrum; G = glenoid; IGHL = inferior glenohumeral ligament.

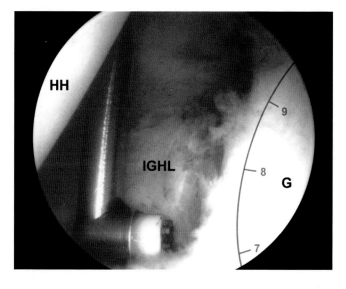

Figure 36.9

The thickened anterior portion of the inferior glenohumeral ligament (IGHL) has been released. Now at the 7 o'clock position in the left shoulder, note the increased space available between the humerus and glenoid. HH = humeral head; G = glenoid.

note that as this material is debrided it does not bleed. As much synovial hyperplasia as can easily be debrided is removed at this time (Figure 36.5). The capsular release begins with the rotator cuff interval. The release of the interval and anterosuperior capsule creates space to work in and allows us to proceed with the release inferiorly under direct visualization. At this point, the cannula is removed anteriorly and a 3.0-mm 90° AthroWand is introduced down the track of the cannula

into the joint. A 90° tip allows the surgeon to rotate the instrument and cut in 360°, including back towards the entry point of the instrument. This is especially helpful in the rotator cuff interval, where the coracohumeral ligament and interval tissues are usually quite thick and shortened (Figure 36.6). The interval is released along the 'base' of the arthroscopic triangle medially, from just anterior to the biceps down to the upper subscapularis, paralleling the glenoid rim. Electrocautery is used to

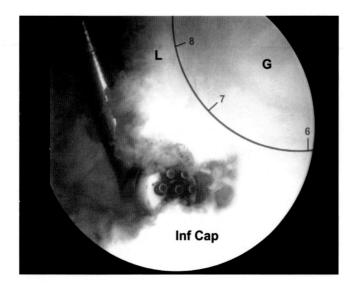

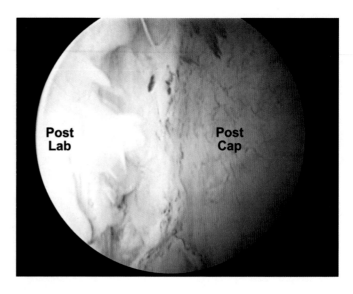

Figure 36.10

Capsular release adjacent to the inferior glenoid. The stiff bipolar electrocautery device allows the surgeon to 'turn the corner'. The tip is kept up and pointed away from the axillary nerve. Inf Cap = inferior capsule; L = labrum; G = glenoid.

Figure 36.11

View of thickened, inflamed posterior capsule from the anterior portal. Post Lab = posterior labrum; Post Cap = posterior capsule.

release the tissue parallel to the thickened upper border of the subscapularis. The capsule is released just off the glenoid rim, preserving the labrum (Figure 36.7). As the thickened capsule is released from superior to inferior, the superior glenohumeral ligament, middle glenohumeral ligament, and the very thickened anterior (superior) band of the inferior glenohumeral ligament are divided (Figure 36.8). In the normal shoulder, this region of the inferior glenohumeral ligament is approximately 3-mm thick.[34] However, it typically is very difficult to identify differences in the capsule as it is more like a 'wall of collagen'. At times, thickened tissue above the biceps can be released with a shaver or basket forceps.

By lowering the arthroscope into the joint parallel to the glenoid surface, the joint can be gently distracted, facilitating exposure as the release moves into the anteroinferior area. The electrocautery tip is oriented parallel to the anterior glenoid surface and placed between the labrum and capsular attachment (Figure 36.9). The goal is an extralabral capsular release off the glenoid, creating a sleeve of capsule. The subscapularis tendon is not routinely released or violated, and we have not found it necessary to involve this structure in the release. Exposure can be maintained with mild abduction of approximately 30–40° and alternating between 20° and 30° of internal and external rotation. With the release down to the 7 o'clock position in a left shoulder, the electrocautery is now used to release the inferior capsule. The ArthroWand tip, being bipolar, can now be oriented up, away from the axillary nerve, and placed in the 'axilla' of the capsular release (Figure 36.10). The capsule is released off the inferior glenoid rim around

to the 6 o'clock position, as the pathology allows. If the inferior capsule is dramatically thickened, the electrocautery will debulk this tissue and allow for an easier dehiscence of this tissue during the final manipulation. Alternatively, a basket forceps can be used carefully, under direct visualization, to release tissue adjacent to the glenoid rim in this region.

The posterior capsule is now assessed for involvement, which is found in the majority of patients. In the setting of an isolated posterior capsular contracture, the procedure has essentially been a diagnostic arthroscopy until this point. If additional pathology has been encountered, such as a partial tear requiring debridement, it should be addressed prior to proceeding with the posterior capsular release. The arthroscope is now placed in the anterior portal (Figure 36.11). The electrocautery is placed through the posterior portal. The posterior capsular release begins over the posterosuperior recess where the disease can obliterate this recess and tether the supraspinatus tendon to the glenoid rim. A good landmark is to start the release just posterior to the biceps tendon insertion. The release is carried down posteriorly to meet the previous anterior release. Division of the posterior capsule is performed adjacent to the glenoid rim, because the muscle of the posterior cuff tendons is superficial to the capsule at this level. Therefore, the depth of the capsular division is completed when one visualizes the muscle fibers (Figure 36.12). An arthroscopic shaver can be inserted to remove the edges of the capsule to clearly identify the release and rotator cuff muscle. If the capsule is divided more laterally, there is risk of injuring the rotator cuff tendons,

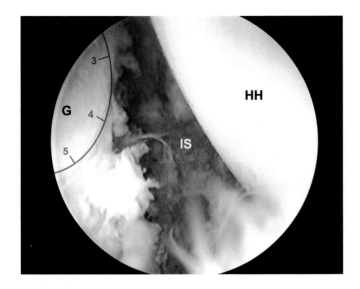

Figure 36.12

After complete posterior capsular release, reddish muscle fibers of the infraspinatus are seen. IS = infraspinatus; G = glenoid; HH = humeral head.

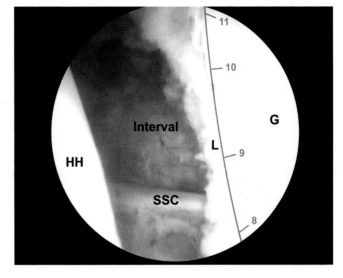

Figure 36.13

Arthroscopy after final manipulation reveals complete capsular release. Note the size of the interval and free mobility of the subscapularis. SSC = upper border subscapularis; L = labrum; G = glenoid; HH = humeral head.

which become conjoined with the capsule in this location.

Once the circumferential release is completed, the instruments are removed and the shoulder is put through a gentle range of motion with proximal humeral pressure. The manipulation proceeds in the following sequence: scapular elevation, abduction, external rotation at the side, external rotation in abduction, and internal rotation in abduction. Typically, there is a small sensation of giving way as opposed to the sudden snap felt in a traditional manipulation. The arthroscope is reintroduced into the glenohumeral joint. Typically, there is minimal bleeding. The subscapularis tendon is now seen to be freely mobile and visible anteriorly (Figure 36.13). The arthroscope can now navigate more easily through the joint, allowing for complete visualization of the cartilage surfaces and the rotator cuff superiorly.

Attention is now turned to the subacromial space. Standard bursal portals are utilized and the subacromial space is evaluated. In only approximately 20% of idiopathic frozen shoulder cases will there be significant involvement. In patients with a history of impingement syndrome, trauma such as non-displaced greater tuberosity fractures, or postsurgery, the subacromial space may require debridement and acromioplasty, particularly if a prominent acromion or osteophyte is detected on the preoperative outlet radiograph. If the subacromial space is just mildly involved and the clinical preoperative symptoms were felt to be due to the altered mechanics of frozen shoulder, then the subacromial space does not require further intervention. This is to minimize the surgical trauma, reduce bleeding, and avoid further postoperative pain and swelling. If acromioclavicular joint arthralgia is identified preoperatively, an arthroscopic acromioclavicular joint resection is performed. Our experience with indwelling catheters for anesthetic infusion following capsular release is evolving, and we have appreciated its benefits for pain relief after this procedure as well as other shoulder procedures, such as subacromial decompression or distal clavicle resection.

The portals are closed in a routine fashion. A sling and swathe are applied to protect the arm for the duration of the interscalene regional block. The arm is kept in an abducted position and neutral rotation, and not internal rotation, using an attachment to the sling, such as the Apex derotation wedge (Biomet, Warsaw, IN, USA) (Figure 36.14). A passive cold compressive device, such as the Cryocuff (Aircast, Summit, NJ, USA), is applied to the shoulder. If general anesthesia has not been utilized, the patient with the long-acting interscalene block in place goes immediately to the ward for bedside physiotherapy.

Postoperative protocol

We have used a 23-hour observation stay, and always attempt to do the capsular release procedures as the first case of the day. This allows for physical therapy to be performed twice on the operative day and once the following morning. If permitted, an additional hospital

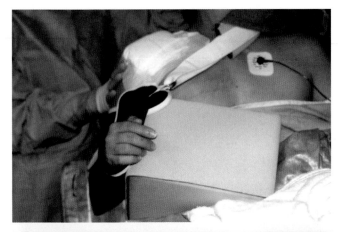

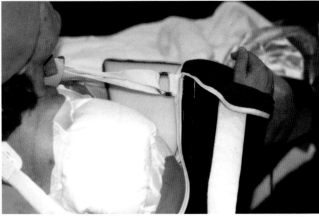

Figure 36.14

Apex derotation wedges after capsular release places patient forearm, and thus shoulder, in neutral position and slight abduction.

day may be considered. Some studies have reported protocols with repeat interscalene blocks in the morning on postoperative days 1 and 2 to allow for additional in-patient passive range-of-motion exercises with the physical therapist.[9,22] The interscalene block allows the patient and the therapist to begin immediately. This vividly demonstrates to the patient that their shoulder can be moved in a more normal range without pain, which is positive reinforcement in two ways. First, patients are pain free and see their shoulder move, especially when it is placed overhead. Second, mentally it is a tremendous experience for these patients who have suffered through time and effort and have not been able to restore motion. Clearly, a good relationship with the physical therapists is beneficial. Intramuscular and oral narcotics are utilized, as is intramuscular ketorolac, in the hospital. Oral ketorolac is continued for 4 more days. After the block has resolved, patients are encouraged to use the shoulder out of the sling and wedge device for dressing, eating, and activities of daily living. Pendulums, pulley exercises, passive external rotation with a stick,

and internal rotation both cross-body and behind the back are emphasized. A home exercise kit, with a pulley and stick, should be available. Patients are instructed to do their exercises at home three to four times a day with each session lasting only 15–20 minutes. Warm moist heat prior to, and ice after, the sessions are utilized. Premedicating with analgesics is helpful prior to home exercises and physical therapy.

Outpatient rehabilitation, with a physical therapist that appreciates the underlying problem and treatment goals, is initiated immediately upon discharge at three times per week for the first 3 weeks, then two or three times a week for the next 3 weeks. A more frequent therapy program may be considered, if permitted. Motion only is emphasized. No machines, no therabands for resistive exercises and no weights are allowed until pain-free motion has been restored. Patients will only irritate their shoulder and lose motion if strengthening is started too soon. Usually at 6–8 weeks, light theraband exercises can begin. The average time to restore pain-free final motion was 3 months, with a range from 3 weeks to 5 months, in a prospective study on arthroscopic capsular release.[30] Insulin-dependent diabetics had a somewhat longer average time to achieve pain-free motion. Strengthening exercises tended to irritate the diabetic shoulders even at 3 months following capsular release. We have reserved the use of home shoulder CPM for those patients that we feel are higher risk, such as insulin-dependent diabetic patients, and those who have a failed previous intervention, such as a manipulation. Return to normal activities of daily living, sporting activities, and full duty employment has averaged approximately 3 months. However, patients are able to return to modified duty or lighter activity around 3 weeks, but the emphasis is always upon the rehabilitation task first.

References

1. Bulgen DY, Binder AI, Hazelman BL, Roberts S. Frozen shoulder: prospective clinical study with an evaluation of three treatment regimens. *Ann Rheum Dis* 1984; **43**:353–60.
2. Grey RG. The natural history of 'idiopathic' frozen shoulder. *J Bone Joint Surg* 1978; **60A**:564.
3. Hannafin JA, DiCarlo EF, Wickiewicz TL. Adhesive capsulitis: capsular fibroplasia of the glenohumeral joint. *J Shoulder Elbow Surg* 1994; **3**:S5.
4. Miller DO, Wirth MA, Rockwood CA. Thawing the frozen shoulder: the 'patient' patient. *Orthopedics* 1996; **19**:849–53.
5. Murnaghan JP. Frozen shoulder. In: CA Rockwood, FA Matsen, eds. *The Shoulder*, Vol. 2. Philadelphia: WB Saunders, Philadelphia, 1990; 837–61.
6. Parker RD, Froimson AI, Winsberg DD, Arsham HZ. Frozen shoulder. Part I: Chronology, pathogenesis, clinical picture, and treatment. *Orthopedics* 1989; **12**:869–73.
7. Rodeo SA, Hannafin JA, Tom J et al. Immunolocalization of cytokines in adhesive capsulitis of the shoulder. *J Orthop Res* 1997; **15**:427–36.
8. Lusardi DA, Wirth MA, Wurtz D, Rockwood CA. Loss of external rotation following anterior capsulorrhaphy of the shoulder. *J Bone Joint Surg* 1993; **75A**:1185–92.

9. Ticker JB, Beim GM, Warner JJP. Recognition and treatment of refractory posterior capsular contracture of the shoulder. *Arthroscopy* 2000; **16**:27–34.

10. Warner JJP, Iannotti JP. Treatment of a stiff shoulder after posterior capsulorraphy. A report of three cases. *J Bone Joint Surg* 1996; **78A**:1419–21.

11. Warner JJP, Allen A, Marks PH, Wong P. Arthroscopic release of post-operative capsular contracture of the shoulder. *J Bone Joint Surg* 1997; **79A**:1151–8.

12. Binder AI, Bulgen DY, Hazelman BL, Roberts S. Frozen shoulder: a long term prospective study. *Ann Rheum Dis* 1984; **43**:361–4.

13. Dacre JE, Beeney H, Scott DL. Injections and physiotherapy for the painful stiff shoulder. *Ann Rheum Dis* 1989; **48**:322–5.

14. Neviaser RJ, Neviaser TJ. The frozen shoulder: diagnosis and management. *Clin Orthop* 1987; **223**:59–64.

15. Ekelund AL, Rydell H. Combination treatment for adhesive capsulitis of the shoulder. *Clin Orthop* 1992; **282**:105–9.

16. Hsu SY, Chan KM. Arthroscopic distension in the management of frozen shoulder. *Int Orthop* 1991; **15**:79–83.

17. Sharma RK, Bajekal RA, Rham S. Frozen shoulder syndrome: a comparison of hydraulic distension and manipulation. *Int Orthop* 1993; **17**:275–8.

18. Hill TJ, Bogumill H. Manipulation in the treatment of frozen shoulder. *Orthopedics* 1988; **11**:1255–60.

19. Parker RD, Froimson AI, Winsberg DD, Arsham HZ. Frozen shoulder. Part II: Treatment by manipulation under anesthesia. *Orthopedics* 1989; **12**:989–94.

20. Janda DH, Hawkins RJ. Shoulder manipulation in patients with adhesive capsulitis and diabetes mellitus: a clinical note. *J Shoulder Elbow Surg* 1993; **2**:36–8.

21. Shaffer B, Tibone JE, Kerlan RK. Frozen shoulder: a long-term follow-up. *J Bone Joint Surg* 1992; **74A**:738–46.

22. Warner JJP, Allen A, Marks P, Wong P. Arthroscopic release of chronic, refractory capsular contracture of the shoulder. *J Bone Joint Surg* 1996; **78A**:1808–16.

23. Wiley AM. Arthroscopic appearance of frozen shoulder. *Arthroscopy* 1991; **7**:138–43.

24. Harryman DT, Matsen FA, Sidles JA. Arthroscopic management of refractory shoulder stiffness. *Arthroscopy* 1997; **13**:133–47.

25. Ozaki J, Nakagawa Y, Sukurai G, Tomai S. Recalcitrant chronic adhesive capsulitis of the shoulder. *J Bone Joint Surg* 1989; **71A**:1511–15.

26. Chen SK. Arthroscopic and histologic findings in idiopathic frozen shoulder. *J Shoulder Elbow Surg* 1996; **5**:S26

27. Uitvlugt G, Detrisac DA, Johnson LL et al. Arthroscopic observations before and after manipulation of frozen shoulder. *Arthroscopy* 1993; **9**:181–5.

28. Pollock RG, Duralde XA, Flatow EL, Bigliani LU. The use of arthroscopy in the treatment of resistant frozen shoulder. *Clin Orthop* 1994; **304**:30–6.

29. Segmuller HE, Taylor DE, Hogan CS et al. Arthroscopic treatment of adhesive capsulitis. *J Shoulder Elbow Surg* 1995; **4**:403–8.

30. Nicholson GP, Lintner SA, Duckworth MA. Prospective evaluation of arthroscopic capsular release for recalcitrant frozen shoulder. *Orthop Trans* 1997; **21**:136.

31. Pearsall AW, Osbahr DC, Speer KP. An arthroscopic technique for treating patients with frozen shoulder. *Arthroscopy* 1999; **15**:2–11.

32. Ogilvie-Harris DJ, Myerthall S. The diabetic frozen shoulder: arthroscopic release *Arthroscopy* 1997; **13**:1–8.

33. Zanotti RM, Kuhn JE. Arthroscopic capsular release for the stiff shoulder: description of technique and anatomic considerations. *Am J Sports Med* 1997; **25**:294–8.

34. Ticker JB, Bigliani LU, Soslowsky LJ et al. The inferior glenohumeral ligament: geometry and strain-rate dependent properties. *J Shoulder Elbow Surg* 1996; **5**:269–79.

37 Arthroscopic decompression of periglenoid ganglion cysts

Douglas S Musgrave, Freddie H Fu and Mark W Rodosky

Introduction

Ganglion cysts located about the shoulder have become an increasingly recognized source of shoulder pain and dysfunction. These cysts are frequently associated with labral pathology,[1-4] in particular superior labrum anterior to posterior (SLAP) lesions.[5] Ganglion cysts may cause clinical symptoms by compressing the suprascapular nerve.[6-11]

The upper trunk of the brachial plexus gives off the suprascapular nerve at Erb's point. The suprascapular nerve passes behind the brachial plexus, beneath the trapezius muscle, and parallel to the omohyoid muscle to the superior edge of the scapula. There, it passes through the suprascapular notch, the roof of which is the suprascapular ligament. The suprascapular artery and vein, which travel with the nerve, pass over the suprascapular ligament. The suprascapular nerve enters the supraspinatus fossa where it provides motor innervation to the supraspinatus muscle, receives sensory branches from the glenohumeral joint, acromioclavicular joint,[12] and rotator cuff, and sends sensory and symphathetic fibers to the posterior two-thirds of the shoulder capsule.[13] The suprascapular nerve then runs around the lateral edge of the scapular spine (the spinoglenoid notch), under the spinoglenoid ligament, to enter the infraspinatus fossa as the inferior branch of the supraspinatus nerve (Figure 37.1). The suprascapular nerve is a pure motor nerve in the infraspinatus fossa, providing motor innervation to the infraspinatus muscle. There is no cutaneous sensory distribution of the suprascapular nerve.

Ganglion cysts may compress the suprascapular nerve at either the suprascapular notch, denervating both the supraspinatus and intraspinatus muscles, or more frequently at the spinoglenoid notch, causing isolated denervation of the infraspinatus muscle. Posterosuperior labral pathology can lead to synovial fluid extravasation along the posterosuperior glenoid neck. The process results in fluid accumulation at the spinoglenoid notch. The resultant spinoglenoid notch ganglion may then compress the inferior branch of the suprascapular nerve (Figure 37.2). Anterosuperior labral pathology may lead to synovial fluid extravasation along the anterosuperior glenoid neck up to the suprascapular notch. The resultant suprascapular notch ganglion cyst may compress the

suprascapular nerve proximal to its motor innervation of the supraspinatus muscle (Figure 37.3). It should be recognized that the first scenario resulting in spinoglenoid notch ganglions is more common.

Suprascapular nerve compression usually presents as deep, diffuse posterolateral shoulder pain of long-standing duration, which may radiate to the neck, arm, or upper chest wall. However, because the inferior branch of the suprascapular nerve is purely motor, nerve compression at the spinoglenoid notch occasionally does not produce pain. The pain, if present, may be aggravated by adduction and flexion of the shoulder. Patients may also present with symptoms attributable to glenoid labral pathology, such as bicipital tenderness or clicking

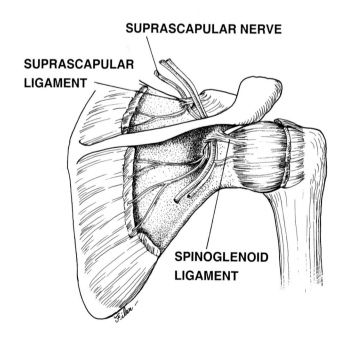

Figure 37.1

The suprascapular nerve travels through the suprascapular notch, deep to the suprascapular ligament. The suprascapular nerve exits the supraspinatus fossa by passing around the spinoglenoid notch, underneath the spinoglenoid ligament. Periglenoid ganglion cysts may cause suprascapular nerve compression at either the suprascapular notch or spinoglenoid notch.

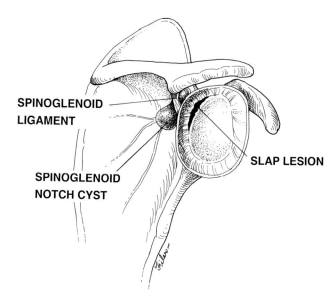

Figure 37.2

Posterosuperior labral pathology may lead to synovial fluid extravasation along the posterosuperior glenoid neck. This process may result in ganglion cyst formation at the spinoglenoid notch, possibly resulting in compression of the suprascapular nerve's inferior branch. Compression of the suprascapular nerve's inferior branch can result in infraspinatus denervation.

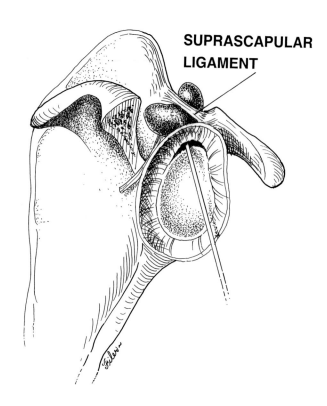

Figure 37.3

Anterosuperior labral pathology may result in synovial fluid extravasation along the anterosuperior glenoid neck. This process may result in ganglion cyst formation at the suprascapular notch with resultant suprascapular nerve compression. Suprascapular nerve compression at the suprascapular notch can result in supraspinatus and infraspinatus denervation. A blunt probe is used to identify the labral pathology and ganglion cyst.

and popping of the shoulder. Physical examination findings help suggest the diagnosis of suprascapular nerve impingement. Weakness of shoulder external rotation is the most important physical examination finding to indicate spinoglenoid notch impingement. If compression exists at the suprascapular notch, weak shoulder abduction will also be present. Infraspinatus atrophy is present with chronic nerve impingement. Tenderness to palpation over the area of nerve compression, be that either the suprascapular or spinoglenoid notch, may exist. Some authors advocate diagnostic steroid and lidocaine injections into these areas,[14–18] although accurate localization of these areas may be difficult.[19] The crossover adduction test performed with the elbow extended exacerbates the pain and tenderness by stretching the suprascapular nerve.[12,16,20] MRI can localize the ganglion cyst[21] (Figure 37.4) and nerve conduction studies can further support suprascapular nerve compression.[22]

Ganglion cysts about the shoulder should be decompressed when they are causing pain, unresponsive to conservative measures, or suprascapular nerve compression, as indicated by physical findings and nerve conduction studies. Various methods of treating ganglion cysts about the shoulder have been reported including steroid injection,[23] open surgical decompression,[6,7,9,15,20] computed tomography (CT)-directed percutaneous aspiration,[20] sonographically-directed percutaneous

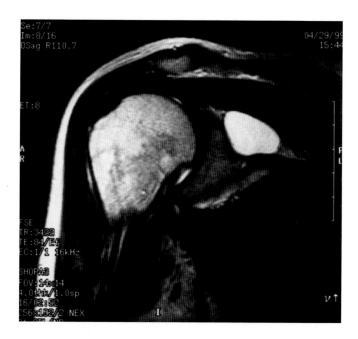

Figure 37.4

A oblique coronal T2-weighted MRI demonstrating a ganglion and an associated SLAP lesion.

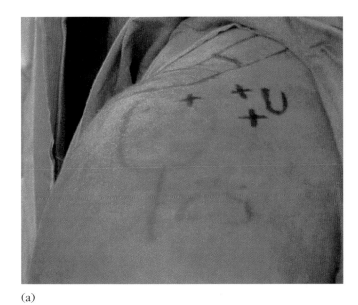

(a)

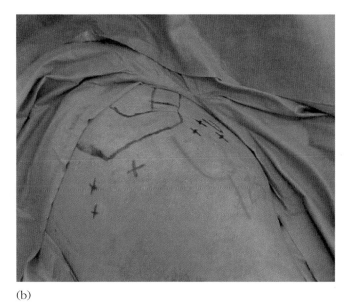

(b)

Figure 37.5

(a, b) Preoperative photograph demonstrating potential arthroscopic portals which may be used for periglenoid cyst decompression and labral repair.

aspiration,[24] and arthroscopic intra-articular cyst decompression.[1,2,4] It is hypothesized that ganglion cysts about the shoulder arise from glenohumeral joint fluid extravasation through a labral lesion, frequently a SLAP lesion. Therefore, only surgical intervention can address the etiology of the cysts, thereby minimizing recurrences. Arthroscopic intra-articular cyst decompression allows cyst decompression and labral repair without the associated morbidity of an open surgical procedure.

Five cases of arthroscopic ganglion cyst decompression have been reported in the literature.[1,2,4] The average patient age was 34.4 years, all had spinoglenoid notch cysts although in one patient the cyst extended to the suprascapular notch, four patients had infraspinatus weakness and/or atrophy, one patient presented with pain without weakness, and three patients had SLAP lesions addressed at the time of arthroscopy. One patient had two failed sonographically-directed percutaneous aspirations and one steroid injection. At a mean follow-up of 12 months (range 3–15 months), all five patients experienced resolution of their symptoms with no recurrences.

Surgical principles

Arthroscopic decompression of ganglions about the shoulder is achieved via intra-articular cyst decompression. An arthroscope is inserted via standard portals and systematic glenohumeral arthroscopy is performed. Any glenohumeral joint pathology is noted, especially labral lesions in the region of the cyst (SLAP lesions). An accessory portal is created to allow an easier approach to the

region of the cyst, and the cyst is approached through the labral lesion. If no labral lesion is present, a small capsulotomy must be performed to access the ganglion. The cyst is bluntly decompressed into the glenohumeral joint. In order to establish superior labrum/biceps anchor stability[25] and prevent ganglion cyst recurrence, it is critical to repair the pre-existing labral pathology.

Potential areas of difficulty exist in patient positioning, portal placement, capsulotomy, and labral lesion repair. Patient positioning is crucial to facilitate appropriate portal placement. The patient may be positioned either in the lateral decubitus position applying longitudinal traction or in a beach chair position. The entire upper extremity must be prepped and draped free to permit wide access to the shoulder. The standard shoulder arthroscopy portals are established slightly more lateral than normal to facilitate access to the glenoid neck. Incorrect portal placement, can preclude adequate access to a labral tear and/or the posterior glenoid neck. If a labral tear is not present, care must be taken to make a small (less than 5 mm) capsulotomy. The labrum should not be injured during capsulotomy. If the capsulotomy is larger than 5 mm, capsulotomy repair must be undertaken to prevent ganglion recurrence. If a labral tear/SLAP lesion is present, it must be surgically addressed and repaired after ganglion cyst decompression. Failure to repair the labral lesion greatly increases the likelihood of ganglion cyst recurrence.

Potential complications include infection, recurrence, labral tear, and suprascapular nerve injury. The risk of infection is likely similar to that encountered in standard glenohumeral arthroscopy and can be minimized by standard sterile technique, adequate intra-articular fluid

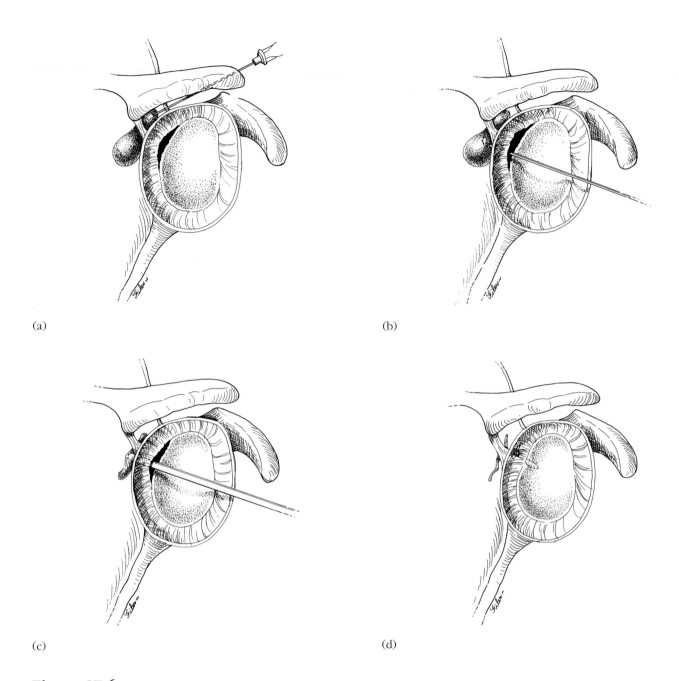

(a)

(b)

(c)

(d)

Figure 37.6

(a) A spinal needle passed from an anterior portal to probe the spinoglenoid notch cyst through the joint capsule. This technique may be used to disrupt loculations in multiloculated cysts as well as for partial cyst decompression. (b) A blunt probe is used to identify the labral tear and begin subperiosteal dissection along the posterosuperior glenoid neck. (c) A 4.2-mm resector is inserted through the labral tear and into the spinoglenoid cysts after blunt subperiosteal dissection along the posterosuperior glenoid neck. Suction is applied to facilitate cyst decompression. (d) The labral tear is repaired using a bioabsorbable suture anchor and braided suture, thereby preventing cyst recurrence.

lavage, and perioperative antibiotics. Recurrence may be minimized by thorough cyst decompression including external manual pressure over the cyst, labral tear repair, and limiting the size of the capsulotomy to less than 5 mm. Suprascapular nerve injury is possible during dissection along the posterior glenoid neck. The risk of this complication may be minimized by blunt, sub-periosteal dissection along the posterior glenoid neck.

Surgical technique

The patient is placed in the beach chair position with the head supported in a head rest and the affected shoulder freely accessible. The hand and arm may be placed in a sterile holder and attached to a McConnell arm holder or held by an assistant. Alternatively, the patient may be placed in the lateral decubitus position. A long spinal needle is used to insufflate the joint with sterile saline. The arthroscope is introduced through a posterosuperior (PS) portal located approximately 2–3 cm inferior and 1–2 cm medial to the posterolateral corner of the acromion. This portal should be slightly more lateral than usual to facilitate access to the glenoid neck. The skin is then incised and the glenohumeral joint entered using a blunt trocar followed by the arthroscope. An anterosuperior (AS) portal is then created under direct vision through the arthroscope. This AS portal should enter the joint in the region of the triangle created by the glenoid, biceps tendon, and subscapularis tendon. Systematic diagnostic arthroscopy is performed to identify any glenoid, labral, humeral head, rotator cuff, capsular, or biceps tendon pathology. Accessory portals are then created as needed to address the labral pathology. Commonly, an accessory portal is created just inferior to the AS portal to facilitate handling of suture and instruments. An accessory antero-lateral portal may be established to address certain SLAP lesions and anterior biceps tendon pathology. An accessory posterior portal directly inferior to the PS portal may be required for suture handling. Care must be taken to avoid the axillary nerve when creating this portal by not straying to far inferior. A posterolateral portal inferior to the posterolateral acromion can be created to address posterior biceps tendon pathology. Finally, an anterolateral accessory portal, just lateral to the anterolateral acromion, may be required. This portal enters the shoulder in the rotator interval, between the supraspinatus and subscapularis tendons. Figure 37.5 demonstrates the standard and potential accessory portals.

Arthroscopic decompression of a ganglion cyst usually occurs through the cyst's mouth. Occasionally, the cyst may be appreciated bulging against the joint capsule. In such cases, the cyst may be probed and partially decompressed using a spinal needle (Figure 37.6a). If a labral tear is suspected, a blunt probe should be used to confirm a detached labrum (Figure 37.6b). An arthroscopic rasp and 4.2-mm full radius resector are then used to divide any remaining fibers tethering the labrum to the glenoid. Resectors larger than 4.2 mm tend to block visualization of the cyst's mouth and are discouraged. Using the resector, rasp, and a 4.0-mm burr (if needed), the glenoid rim and labrum should be prepared for later repair. A rosette knife may be inserted through the labral detachment to facilitate blunt subperiosteal dissection along the glenoid neck. Blunt subperiosteal dissection is carried out using a probe. Once the cyst is encountered, the 4.2-mm resector may be used as a suction probe to partially decompress the cyst (Figure 37.6c). Manual pressure on the skin overlying the cyst may help decompress the ganglion into the glenohumeral joint. Following cyst decompression, the labral tear/SLAP lesion is repaired to the glenoid neck using bioabsorbable tacks or suture anchors (Figure 37.6d). The authors' preferred technique is to use bioabsorbable suture anchors and #2 braided suture. The reader is referred to Chapters 19 and 20 for further discussion of SLAP lesion repair. If a labral tear is not present,

a 5-mm capsulotomy is performed using a rosette knife near the junction of the capsule and labrum. The glenoid neck is then subperiosteally dissected using a blunt probe. The cyst is decompressed as described above. If the capsulotomy is 5 mm or smaller, no repair is performed. A larger capsulotomy should be repaired using a suture passer.

If arthroscopic cyst decompression is unsuccessful or if concerns exist regarding either the spinoglenoid ligament or suprascapular ligament contributing to suprascapular nerve compression, an open surgical approach may necessary. The open approach may be performed in conjunction with an arthroscopic approach. Spinoglenoid notch cysts are approached through a posterior, deltoid-splitting approach. The infraspinatus is retracted inferior to allow direct access to the spinoglenoid notch. Suprascapular notch cysts are approached posteriorly by first identifying and accessing the scapular spine. The trapezius is dissected off the scapular spine and reflected superiorly. Inferior retraction of the supraspinatus muscle facilitates direct access to the suprascapular notch.

Postoperative protocol

The extremity is placed in an immobilizer with the forearm across the chest and a cryotherapy dressing is applied. Patients with SLAP lesion repairs are immobilized except for gentle, gravity-assisted passive motion exercises for 3 weeks. After 3 weeks, progressive motion and then strengthening may be undertaken. The reader is again referred to Chapters 19 and 20 for further discussion regarding SLAP lesion repair and postoperative management. Patients without SLAP lesions may undergo gentle, gravity-assisted passive motion exercises when symptoms permit, followed by progressive motion and then strengthening exercises. A follow-up MRI should be obtained approximately 6–8 weeks after surgery to verify cyst decompression. If the cyst remains and adequate repair of the labral pathology was performed arthroscopically, either a CT-guided cyst aspiration or an open surgical approach may be used.

References

1. Iannotti JP, Ramsey ML. Arthroscopic decompression of a ganglion cyst causing suprascapular nerve compression. *Arthroscopy* 1996; **12**:739–45.
2. Chochole MH, Senker W, Meznik C, Breitenseher MJ. Glenoid-labral cyst entrapping the suprascapular nerve: dissolution after arthroscopic debridement of an extended SLAP lesion. *Arthroscopy* 1997; **13**:753–5.
3. Ferrick MR, Marzo JM. Suprascapular entrapment neuropathy and ganglion cysts about the shoulder. *Orthopedics* 1999; **22**:430–4.
4. Lietschuh PH, Bone CM, Bouska WM. Magnetic resonance imaging diagnosis, sonographically directed percutaneous aspira-

tion, and arthroscopic treatment of a painful shoulder ganglion cyst associated with a SLAP lesion. *Arthroscopy* 1999; **15**:85–7.

5. Snyder SJ, Karzel RP, Del Pizzo W et al. SLAP lesions of the shoulder. *Arthroscopy* 1990; **6**:274–9.

6. Hirayama T, Takemitsu Y. Compression of the suprascapular nerve by a ganglion at the suprascapular notch. *Clin Orthop* 1981; **155**:95–6.

7. Neviaser TJ, Ain BR, Neviaser RJ. Suprascapular nerve denervation secondary to attenuation by a ganglion cyst. *J Bone Joint Surg* 1986; **68A**:627–8.

8. Black KP, Lombardo JA. Suprascapular nerve injuries with isolated paralysis of the infraspinatus. *Am J Sports Med* 1990; **18**:225–8.

9. Ogino T, Minami A, Kato H et al. Entrapment neuropathy of the suprascapular nerve by a ganglion: a report of three cases. *J Bone Joint Surg* 1991; **73A**:141–7.

10. Skirving AP, Kozak TKW, Davis SJ. Infraspinatus paralysis due to spinoglenoid notch ganglion. *J Bone Joint Surg* 1994; **6B**:588–91.

11. Takagishi K, Saitoh A, Tonegawa M et al. Isolated paralysis of the infraspinatus muscle. *J Bone Joint Surg* 1994; **76B**:584–7.

12. Kopell HP, Thompson WAL. *Peripheral Entrapment Neuropathies.* Baltimore: Williams and Wilkins, 1963; 131–42.

13. Rose DL, Kelly CR. Shoulder pain. Suprascapular nerve block in shoulder pain. *J Kans Med Soc* 1969; **70**:135–6.

14. Clein LJ. Suprascapular entrapment neuropathy. *J Neurosurg* 1975; **43**:337–42.

15. Ganzhorn RW, Hocker JT, Horowitz M, Switzer HE.

16. Weaver HL. Isolated suprascapular nerve lesions. *Injury* 1983; **15**:117–26.

17. Hadley MN, Sonntag VKH, Pittman HW. Suprascapular nerve entrapment. *J Neurosurg* 1986; **64**:843–8.

18. Callahan JD, Scully TB, Shapiro SA, Worth RM. Suprascapular nerve entrapment: a series of 27 cases. *J Neurosurg* 1991; **74**:893–6.

19. Murray JWG. A surgical approach for entrapment neuropathy of the suprascapular nerve. *Orthop Rev* 1974; **3**:33–5.

20. Lauland T, Fedders O, Sogaard I, Kornum M. Suprascapular nerve compression syndrome. *Surg Neurol* 1984; **22**:308–12.

21. Fritz RC, Helms CA, Steinbach LS, Genant HK. Suprascapular nerve entrapment: evaluation with MR imaging. *Radiology* 1992; **182**:437–44.

22. Post M, Mayer J. Suprascapular nerve entrapment. *Clin Orthop* 1987; **223**:123–37.

23. Torres-Ramos FM, Biundo JJ. Suprascapular neuropathy during progressive resistive exercises in a cardiac rehabilitation program. *Arch Phys Med Rehabil* 1992; **73**:1107–11.

24. Hashimoto BE, Hayes AS, Ager JD. Sonographic diagnosis and treatment of ganglion cysts causing suprascapular nerve entrapment. *J Ultrasound Med* 1994; **13**:671–4.

25. Rodosky MW, Harner CD, Fu FH. The role of the long head of the biceps muscle and superior glenoid labrum in anterior stability of the shoulder. *Am J Sports Med* 1994; **22**:121–30.

Suprascapular nerve entrapment: a case report. *J Bone Joint Surg* 1981; **63A**:492–4.

38 Arthroscopic treatment of osteoarthritis: Debridement and microfracture arthroplasty

Steven J Klepps, Leesa M Galatz and Ken Yamaguchi

Introduction

Osteoarthritis of the shoulder in young patients is a challenging clinical problem. Non-surgical treatment options include physical therapy, therapeutic modalities (i.e. ultrasound), intra-articular corticosteroid injections, activity modification, and non-steroidal anti-inflammatory medications.[1-3] The gold standard procedure for advanced osteoarthritis in patients who have failed conservative treatment is replacement arthroplasty. However, because it is desirable to postpone joint replacement in young patients with mild to moderate osteoarthritis, several non-prosthetic options exist. These include corrective osteotomy, interpostition arthroplasty, capsular release, and arthroscopic debridement. Arthroscopy is associated with low morbidity and is helpful in terms of both diagnosis and treatment. Thus, it is an appropriate first surgical option.

Indications for arthroscopic debridement of shoulder osteoarthritis include young patients with early to moderate disease, preserved range of motion (>120° elevation, >20° external rotation at the side), concentric glenoid wear without evidence of subluxation, and minimal osteophyte formation (Table 38.1).[1,2,4] Arthroscopic debridement is also useful in patients with loose bodies or osteochondral defects who have failed conservative treatment.[5-8] Patients with more advanced osteoarthritis are not thought to gain the same benefit. Classification systems can be helpful in considering patients with osteoarthritis for arthroscopic debridement. Ahlbäck and Walch et al classify shoulder osteoarthritis by radiographic appearance (Table 38.2).[9,10] Specifically, patients beyond Ahlbäck class II or Walch class A are not considered good candidates. These classification systems are helpful in categorizing patients in order to apply a standardized approach in selecting patients for the procedure and subsequently comparing results.

Besides providing a viable treatment option for patients with shoulder osteoarthritis, arthroscopy plays an important role in diagnosis as well. In fact, it is considered the most sensitive method for diagnosing early osteoarthritis, as evidenced in several recent studies reporting the diagnosis of an osteoarthritic lesion not anticipated prior to arthroscopic evaluation.[2,6,11,12] Disorders such as rotator cuff tendinopathy, impingement syndrome, adhesive capsulitis, and biceps tendonitis often mimic osteoarthritis and are difficult to separate clinically.[11-13] By making the proper diagnosis, specific treatment may be applied maximizing the patient's opportunity for improvement.

Arthroscopic debridement has been found effective in the treatment of osteoarthritis with the majority of studies reporting success in the knee. Successful results range from 66 to 74%.[5,6,8,13-15] A few recent studies on arthroscopic treatment of osteoarthritis in the shoulder report success in patients with mild to moderate disease, ranging from 60% to 94%.[5,7,8,16] Predictably, arthroscopic debridement for severe osteoarthritis has been less effective.[8,11] Ogilvie-Harris and Wiley have reported success in 66% of patients with mild disease and 33% of patients with severe disease.[8] Although previous studies have been limited, they nevertheless provide support for the selected use of arthroscopic debridement of shoulder osteoarthritis.

Table 38.1. Indications for arthroscopic treatment of osteoarthritis

History	Examination	Radiography
Failed non-operative treatment × 3 months	Relief with glenohumeral injection	Joint space narrowing
Night pain	External rotation >20°	Concentricity maintained
Injections failed	Elevation >120°	No subluxation
Age < 60 years	Active = passive motion	Loose bodies
Joint line pain	Crepitus	Cyst formation

Table 38.2. Radiographic classification systems for osteoarthritis

Ahlbäck[9]		Walch et al[10]	
1	Joint space narrowing	A	Centralized humeral head
2	Joint space obliteration	B	Posterior subluxation of humeral head
3	Minor bone attrition		
4	Moderate bone attrition	C	Glenoid retroversion >25°
5	Severe bone attrition		
6	Subluxation		

The goals of arthroscopic treatment of shoulder osteoarthritis are primarily to relieve pain and secondarily to improve function. These goals are achieved in part by debriding loose soft tissue that causes pain and impingement during normal glenohumeral motion. Capsular release is often performed, if necessary, to restore normal range of motion. Additionally, the microfracture technique can be a useful adjunct in order to induce formation of fibrocartilage in areas of full-thickness cartilage defects. The duration of pain relief is variable and thus it is considered a temporizing procedure.[7,8,16–18] However, postponing prosthetic replacement is advantageous in young patients because of problems with premature component loosening.

The preoperative evaluation consists of patient history, examination, diagnostic injections, and imaging studies (Table 38.1). The typical history given by a patient with osteoarthritis consists of posterior joint line pain and pain that intensifies with activity. The pain may interfere with sleep. The patient may also complain of a grating sensation and may have some audible popping with motion. Physical examination in early stages reveals relatively maintained active and passive range of motion. In more advanced stages, there may be some selective loss of range of motion, especially external rotation. Crepitus may be enhanced with the 'compression rotation' test which places compression onto the glenohumeral joint during motion.[11] Coexistent disorders such as instability, rotator cuff disorders, acromioclavicular joint pain, or biceps pathology should be ruled out. Diagnostic injections are helpful in differentiating osteoarthritis from concomitant disorders. Patients with osteoarthritis should obtain relief with a glenohumeral lidocaine injection.

Radiographic studies are an important component of preoperative evaluation. X-ray views should consist of an anteroposterior (AP) view of the shoulder in internal rotation, an AP view in the scapular plane with the arm in external rotation and slight abduction, an axillary view (Figure 38.1a) and in some cases a supraspinatus outlet view. The AP view in the scapular plane and the axillary lateral are the most important views, because they are orthogonal to the plane of the joint (Figure 38.1b). To

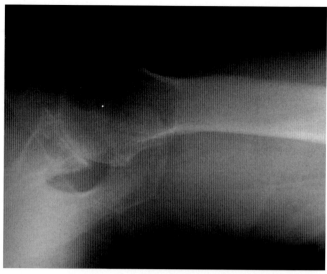

(a)

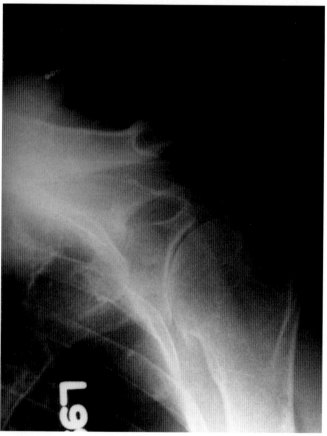

(b)

Figure 38.1

Standard radiographic evaluation of the shoulder includes (a) axillary and (b) true AP views. Note the reduced joint space, osteosclerosis, and osteophyte formation present. These findings are consistent with glenohumeral osteoarthritis. However, with no evidence of posterior glenoid wear, loss of concentricity, or bone attrition, this represents an early stage of disease (Ahlbäck-2, Walch-A). From a radiographic standpoint the patient appears to be a good candidate for arthroscopic intervention.

improve sensitivity, the AP view may be obtained with the patient in 45° of abduction to contract the deltoid and provide joint compressive force as joint space narrowing can be underrepresented in standard views.[4] Magnetic resonance imaging, computerized tomography, or ultrasonography may be helpful in evaluating concomitant disorders, however, they are not necessary in evaluating osteoarthritis.

Surgical principles

Arthroscopic treatment of osteoarthritis consists of joint lavage, labral repair or debridement, loose body removal, osteophyte resection, and synovectomy.[1,2,4,6,13,17] In addition, we have begun to employ a new technique termed microfracture arthroplasty. Originally described by Steadman, this technique has primarily been utilized in the knee. It involves creating a series of small defects in exposed subchondral bone.[17,19,20] The resultant microfracture leads to blood clot formation that undergoes metaplasia into fibrocartilage. The fibrocartilage is biomechanically less effective at reducing contact stress than hyaline cartilage, however it does provide some coverage over exposed subchondral bone. This technique is theoretically better than drilling or abrasion arthroplasty because heat necrosis does not occur.[17,18,21] The microfracture technique is indicated for full-thickness defects that are well circumscribed on the articular surface of the glenohumeral joint. The microfracture technique is contraindicated for patients with inflammatory arthritis, avascular necrosis, or significant subchondral destruction. Results using this technique in the knee have shown that it improves symptoms, reduces defect size and allows earlier return to athletic activity in patients with osteochondral defects.[17,18] Although this technique has not been reported in shoulders, the same concepts apply and our early efforts using this technique appear promising.

Complications of arthroscopic debridement include stiffness, pain, and instability. In general, complications of shoulder arthroscopy are uncommon (< 6.0%). They include infection, nerve injury, reflex sympathetic dystrophy, thromboembolic events, and hemarthrosis.[14,22]

Surgical technique

The procedure is typically performed on an outpatient basis. Anesthesia is generally at the patient's and surgeon's discretion, however, an interscalene block maximizes patient comfort and is helpful in postoperative pain control. This can be supplemented with heavy sedation or general anesthesia using a laryngeal mask airway or endotracheal tube. The patient is placed in an upright beach chair position with the head secured in a McConnell headrest (McConnell Orthopedic Mfg Co.,

Greenville, TX, USA). The patient should be placed on the operating table far enough toward the operative side such that the operative shoulder protrudes from the lateral edge of the table. This ensures access to both the posterior and anterior aspects of the shoulder in order to facilitate the arthroscopic procedure.

Examination under anesthesia is a significant part of the patient evaluation. Range of motion should be evaluated in all planes specifically forward elevation, external rotation at the side, external rotation at 90° of abduction, and internal rotation in 90° of abduction. External rotation is particularly sensitive for accessing capsular contracture, and 20° of difference between sides is considered an abnormal examination.[23] External rotation at the side evaluates the anterosuperior capsule and the rotator interval. External rotation in abduction is limited by a contracture of the anterioinferior capsule. Internal rotation in abduction allows assessment of the posterior capsule. By noting a lack of motion in any one or all of these planes, the surgeon can tell exactly which portions of the capsule are contracted. Caution should be taken in situations where there are large osteophytes as these may themselves limit rotation.

The shoulder is prepped, draped, and secured in a McConnell arm holder. Prior to insertion of the arthroscope, a preoperative injection of 0.25% Marcaine with epinephrine is placed into the glenohumeral joint in order to decrease intraoperative bleeding. Equipment necessary for arthroscopic debridement includes: (1) basic arthroscopy equipment; (2) the VAPR RF Arthroscopy System (Mitek Products, Westwood, MA, USA); and (3) the 30°, 45°, and 90° microfracture awls and arthroscopic elevator (Figure 38.2) (Linvatec Corp., Largo, FL, USA).

A posterior portal is created 2-cm inferior and 1–2-cm medial to the posterolateral corner of the acromion. The arthroscope is inserted through the skin incision aiming toward the tip of the coracoid. At this point, prior to infiltration of irrigant, assessment can be made of the amount and location of erythema and vascularity present within the synovium, biceps tendon, and anterior structures. This is a good indicator of inflammation within the joint. Next, the glenohumeral joint is expanded with irrigant, causing a reduction in erythema due to increased intracapsular pressure.

The anterior portal is placed under direct visualization. The rotator interval must be clearly visualized through the arthroscope. A large bore needle is inserted through the skin just lateral to the coracoid process aiming toward the center of the glenoid. The needle should be visualized penetrating the rotator interval. A 1-cm vertical incision is made at the base of the needle. A 7-mm shoulder arthroscopic cannula (Linvatec) is then passed through the rotator interval between the supraspinatus and the subscapularis. This anterior cannula is used for outflow and instrumentation. A diagnostic arthroscopic examination is then initiated.

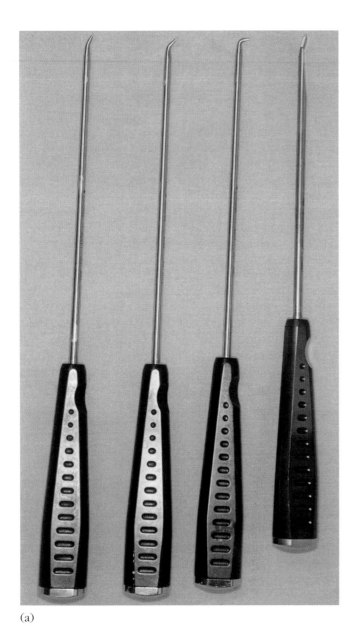

(a)

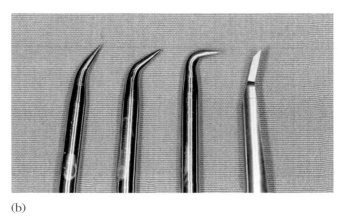

(b)

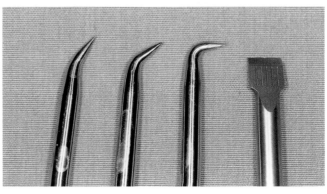

(c)

Figure 38.2

The 3–4-mm microfracture awls with 30°, 45°, and 90° angled tips, and an arthroscopic elevator, are pictured.

Diagnostic arthroscopy is performed in a systematic manner, beginning with evaluation of the humeral head and glenoid fossa for osteochondral defects. The anterior and posterior labrum are visualized and evaluated for fraying. A small probe can be used to detect any evidence of labral instability. The anterior capsule, subscapularis, and glenohumeral ligaments are assessed for tears, adhesions, and frayed tissue. The biceps tendon is evaluated for tenosynovitis, degenerative changes, or tears from its origin at the supraglenoid tubercle to the point at which it exits the joint. The portion in the biceps groove can be evaluated by inserting an Allis clamp through the anterior portal. The clamp is then placed around the biceps tendon and turned in either a clockwise or counterclockwise direction. This pulls the tendon from the groove into the joint and facilitates its examination. The rotator cuff is then evaluated for evidence of partial or full-thickness tears. It is helpful to visualize the rotator cuff by placing the arm in approximately 30° of abduction and about 10–20° of external rotation. This maneuver allows excellent visualization of the insertion of the supraspinatus and infraspinatus tendons. The arthroscope is then brought around the humeral head posteriorly in order to visualize the axillary pouch and posterior recess. It is important to visualize this area because loose bodies tend to gravitate here. Adhesions, frayed tissue, or loose bodies are debrided using a full radius motorized shaver with intermittent suction. The ability to perform diagnostic arthroscopy may be limited by joint contracture and dramatically improves following arthroscopic capsular release.

The arthroscopic capsular release is performed using VAPR RF Side-effect electrode (Mitek) placed through the anterior portal into the rotator interval. The capsule, coracohumeral ligament, and glenohumeral ligaments are

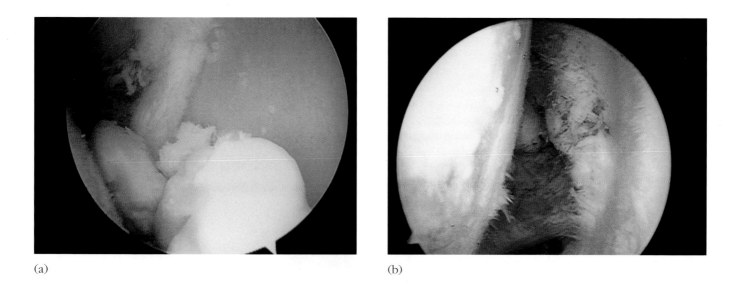

(a)   (b)

Figure 38.3

(a) Arthroscopic image of multiple loose bodies and frayed articular cartilage present in the glenohumeral joint. These undergo piecemeal removal using graspers, shavers, and suction outflow. (b) With the joint adequately debrided, the damaged articular cartilage is better visualized.

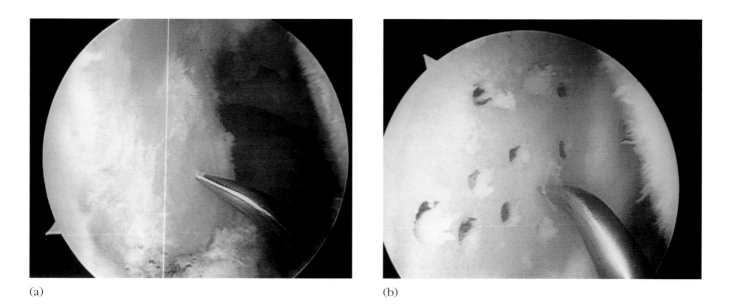

(a)   (b)

Figure 38.4

A large osteochondral defect (Outerbridge IV) is visualized on the glenoid surface. (a) The microfracture awl is positioned perpendicular to the articular surface and subsequently driven into the subchondral bone. (b) Multiple perforations are created with approximately 4–5 mm of space present between microfractures. The subchondral bone is visualized after awl placement.

released until the coracoacromial ligament is exposed and abduction–external motion is regained.[3] A posterior capsular release is rarely necessary in osteoarthritis. If this release is performed, the arthroscope should be placed through the anterior portal and the posterior lateral portal should then be used as an instrumentation portal.

Visualization is improved through arthroscopic synovectomy, which should be performed early in the evaluation. The synovectomy is performed using the VAPR RF electrode placed on the coagulation setting. This is gently applied to all accessible regions of synovium until the erythematous tissue is ablated.

Focus is now turned to the arthroscopic treatment of osteoarthritis. Initially, an attempt is made to remove loose bodies (Figure 38.3a). Loose bodies too large to fit through a standard cannula may be broken into smaller pieces for manual removal, or they can be removed through a small arthrotomy at the end of the procedure. Loose bodies in the subcoracoid region may be displaced by manual palpation of the subcoracoid region or by range of motion of the shoulder. The suction or flow may be increased during this portion of the procedure to assist in lavaging the loose bodies from the glenohumeral joint. Only large unstable tears in the glenoid labrum are removed. Smaller tears are debrided with a motorized shaver or the VAPR electrode. After adequate debridement of the soft tissues, attention is turned toward the articular surfaces (Figure 38.3b).

The glenoid and humeral head are systematically evaluated for osteochondral defects. Frayed cartilage or loose cartilaginous flaps are debrided using a motorized shaver. Several less aggressive shavers are available for this purpose. Debridement should proceed until only firm cartilage remains. If no subchondral bone is exposed, no further debridement is necessary. For defects with exposed subchondral bone (Outerbridge type III or IV lesions), microfracture pick arthroplasty is performed. A 3–4-mm microfracture awl is used to perforate the exposed surface creating subchondral defects. The awls are typically buried to the hub creating a small hole in the surface (Figure 38.4a). This should result in a small amount of blood containing fat droplets emanating from the defect. Perforations are separated by 4–5 mm of space in order to avoid overlap of the microfractures (Figure 38.4b). The glenoid is easily reached with the awl placed through the anterior portal. Treatment of the humeral head requires use of both anterior and posterior portals for instrumentation.

Fixed osseous lesions such as osteophytes may be improved by debridement (Figure 38.5). Any osteophyte that is easily accessible or appears to be causing impingement may be debrided using a motorized shaver and burr. Lesions that do not show evidence of impingement or that are exceptionally difficult to debride are left undisturbed.

Once the arthroscopic debridement is complete, the final step in the procedure is an intra-articular injection of Marcaine and corticosteroid. This is helpful for treatment of inflammation and postoperative pain control. It is easily facilitated by placing an 18-gauge needle into the joint under direct visualization from a superior direction (the Neviaser portal). The portals are closed, and the injection is performed.

Several arthroscopic techniques also exist for treating concomitant disorders such as biceps tendonitis, impingement syndrome, adhesive capsulitis, acromioclavicular arthritis, and rotator cuff pathology. The indications for bursectomy and subacromial decompression in combination with debridement for arthritis are debatable, as the clinical symptoms of rotator cuff tendinitis and osteoarthritis may overlap.[8,2,13,24]

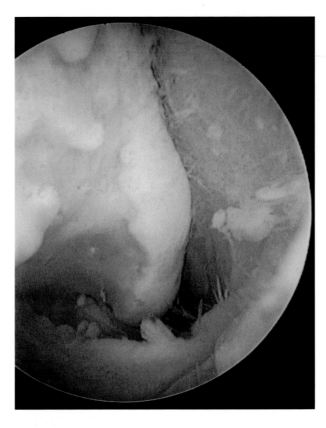

Figure 38.5

Arthroscopic view of glenohumeral joint with inferior osteophyte visible. These osteophytes undergo debridement when accessible or when the lesion shows evidence of impingement.

Postoperative protocol

The patient is placed in a sling in the immediate postoperative period, which is worn only on an as needed basis and is removed within 1 week. Physical therapy is initiated prior to discharge from the hospital. The physical therapy consists of passive and active-assisted range of motion including forward elevation, abduction, and external rotation for the first 6 weeks. Internal rotation and extension are discouraged as they may exacerbate symptoms. The patient can otherwise perform activities as tolerated. Issues such as returning to work or sporting activity are patient specific, but in general, the patient is restricted from heavy duty and overhead activity for the first 6 weeks.

Conclusion

Arthroscopic treatment of osteoarthritis is an excellent surgical option in appropriate patients. The procedure is associated with low morbidity and can potentially restore range of motion and relieve pain associated with the disease process. Early results suggest a high success rate in young patients with early to moderate disease with relatively preserved range of motion, concentric glenoid wear and minimal osteophyte formation. Microfracture arthroplasty may prove a viable and effective solution for smaller, full thickness chondral defects. Because of its low morbidity and potential for symptomatic relief arthroscopic treatment is a good first surgical option in the challenging problem of osteoarthritis of the shoulder in the young patient.

References

1. Matthews LS, Labudde JK. Arthroscopic treatment of synovial diseases of the shoulder. *Orthop Clin North Am* 1993; **24**:101–9.
2. Skedros JG, O'Rourke PJ, Zimmerman JM, Burkhead WZ. Alternatives to replacement arthroplasty for glenohumeral arthritis. In: Williams GR, Iannotti JP, eds. *Disorders of the Shoulder: Diagnosis and Management.* Philadelphia: Lippincott Williams & Wilkins, 1999; 485–99.
3. Warren CG. The use of heat and cold in treatment of common musculoskeletal disorders. In: Kessler RM, Hertling D, eds. *Management of Common Musculoskeletal Disorders.* Philadelphia: Harper & Row, 1983; 115–27.
4. Iannotti JP, Naranja RJ, Warner JJP. Surgical management of shoulder arthritis in the young and active patient. In Warner JJP, Iannotti JP, Gerber C, eds. *Complex and Revision Problems in Shoulder Surgery.* Philadelphia: Lippincott-Raven, 1997; 289–302.
5. Cofield RH. Arthroscopy of the shoulder. *Mayo Clin Proc* 1983; **58**:501–8.
6. Hayes JM. Arthroscopic treatment of steroid-induced osteonecrosis of the humeral head. *Arthroscopy* 1993; **5**:218–21.
7. Johnson L. The shoulder joint: an arthroscopist's perspective of anatomy and pathology. *Clin Orthop* 1987; **223**:113–25.
8. Ogilvie-Harris DJ, Wiley AM. Arthroscopic surgery of the shoulder. *J Bone Joint Surg* 1986; **68B**:201–7.
9. Ahlbäck S. Osteoarthrosis of the knee. A radiographic investigation (Thesis). Stockholm, Sweden. Karolinska Institute 1968; 11–15.
10. Walch G, Boulahia A, Boileau P. Primary glenohumeral osteoarthritis: clinical and radiographic classification. *Acta Orthop Belg* 1998; **64**:46–52.
11. Ellman H, Harris E, Kay S. Early degenerative joint disease simulating impingement syndrome: arthroscopic findings. *Arthroscopy* 1992; **8**:482–7.
12. Ellowitz AS, Rosas R, Rodosky MW, Buss DD. The benefit of arthroscopic decompression for impingement in patients found to have unsuspected glenohumeral osteoarthritis. Presented at the American Academy of Orthopaedic Surgeons Annual Meeting, February 1997.
13. Weinstein D, Bucchieri J, Pollock R. Arthroscopic debridement of the shoulder for osteoarthritis. *Arthroscopy* 2000; **16**:471–6.
14. Small N. Complication in arthroscopic surgery of the knee and shoulder. *Arthroscopy* 1993; **16**:985–8.
15. Jackson RW, Dieterichs C. The results of arthroscopic lavage and debridement of osteoarthritic knees based on the severity of degeneration: a 4- to 6-year symptomatic follow-up. *Arthroscopy* 2003; **19**:13–20.
16. Norris T, Green A. Arthroscopic treatment of glenohumeral osteoarthritis. Presented at Annual Meeting of American Shoulder and Elbow Surgeons, 1997.
17. Blevins F, Steadman JR, Rodrigo JJ, Silliman J. Treatment of articular cartilage defects in athletes: an analysis of functional outcome and lesion appearance. *Orthop* 1998; **21**:761–8.
18. Rodrigo JJ, Steadman JR, Silliman JF, Fulstone HA. Improvement of full-thickness chondral defect healing in human knee after debridement and microfracture using continuous passive motion. *Am J Knee Surg* 1994; **7**:109–16.
19. Frisbie DD, Trotter GW, Powers BE et al. Arthroscopic subchondral bone plate microfracture technique augments healing of large chondral defects in the radial carpal bone and medical femoral chondyle of horses. *Vet Surg* 1999; **28**:242–55.
20. Rockwood C, Williams G, Burkhead W. Debridement of degenerative, irreparable lesions of the rotator cuff. *J Bone Joint Surg* 1995; **77A**:857–66.
21. Buckwalter JA. Evaluating methods of restoring cartilaginous articular surfaces. *Clin Orthop* 1999; **367S**: S224–40.
22. Bigliani L, Flatow E, Deliz E. Complications of shoulder arthroscopy. *Orthop Rev* 1991; **20**:743–51.
23. Warner JJP, Allen A, Marks PH, Wong P. Arthroscopic release for chronic refractory adhesive capsulitis of the shoulder. *J Bone Joint Surg* 1996; **78A**:1808–16.
24. Simpson NS, Kelley IG. Extraglenohumeral joint shoulder surgery in rheumatoid arthritis: the role of bursectomy, acromioplasty, and distal clavicle excision. *J Shoulder Elbow Surg* 1994; **3**:66–9.

39 Arthroscopic treatment of inflammatory synovitis and tumors

Louis W Catalano, William N Levine and Louis U Bigliani

Introduction

The shoulder frequently becomes symptomatic in patients with inflammatory arthritis. For example, nearly 60% of patients with rheumatoid arthritis develop shoulder involvement, most commonly late in the course of the disease.[1,2] In addition, many systemic arthritides, such as psoriatic arthritis, systemic lupus erythematosus, ankylosing spondylitis, and Reiter's syndrome, can produce clinical manifestations similar to those of rheumatoid arthritis. Also, synovial osteochondromatosis and pigmented villonodular synovitis, both pathologic conditions affecting synovium, may involve the shoulder.

Arthroscopic surgery can be a useful tool in the management of these patients. An arthroscopic synovectomy has a lower morbidity than an open synovectomy, as well as a faster postoperative rehabilitation. Also, arthroscopy allows complete visualization of the diseased synovium, which is difficult with the open procedure. In addition, associated intra-articular pathology, such as rotator cuff tears and degenerative joint disease, can be evaluated and treated arthroscopically, if necessary.[3]

In rheumatoid arthritis, arthroscopic synovectomy is performed in patients whose shoulder pain is refractory to medical management with no evidence of severe degenerative changes on radiographs.[4–6] Good results following synovectomy are inversely correlated to the severity of joint destruction.[6] Ogilvie-Harris and Wiley[5] performed an arthroscopic synovectomy on 11 patients with rheumatoid arthritis. No patient had radiographic evidence of severe degenerative changes at the time of surgery. At short-term follow-up of 14 months, nine of 11 patients had significant improvement, with less pain and increased range of motion. In some patients with rheumatoid arthritis, symptomatic subacromial bursitis may require an arthroscopic subacromial decompression. Also, the acromioclavicular joint becomes painful in approximately 33% of patients with rheumatoid arthritis.[7] A symptomatic acromioclavicular joint can be resected following the arthroscopic synovectomy.

Synovial osteochondromatosis is a rare benign condition that results from synovial chondrometaplasia into hyaline cartilage nodules. The shoulder is affected in roughly 4% of cases.[2] Severe involvement can lead to multiple loose bodies and significant degenerative joint disease due to third body wear (Figure 39.1). Symptoms include pain, swelling, decreased range of motion, and crepitus. However, the diagnosis is frequently delayed as radiographs only demonstrate loose bodies in approximately 50% of cases.[3] If symptoms persist, arthroscopic synovectomy with loose body removal can produce good results.[3,8,9] However, recurrence of the disease is not uncommon.[3,10]

Pigmented villonodular synovitis (PVNS) is a proliferative disorder of synovium that presents as a monoarticular condition. Only 1% of cases involve the shoulder.[2] Hemosiderotic synovitis resulting from recurrent bleeding episodes can mimic PVNS.[11,12] Decreased range of motion and joint swelling are common presenting complaints. Pain occurs only after degenerative changes

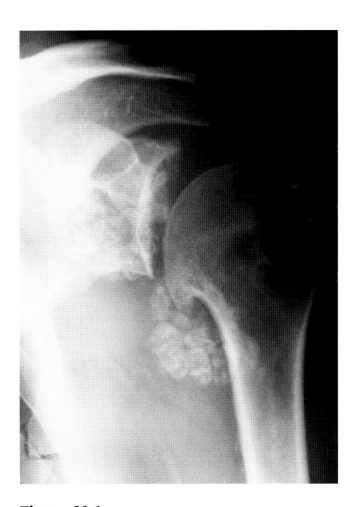

Figure 39.1

Radiograph of a patient with synovial osteochondromatosis demonstrating multiple loose bodies in the axillary recess as well as marked degenerative joint disease.

have developed. Aspiration of the involved shoulder reveals brownish-stained bloody fluid.[13] Treatment includes complete removal of the diseased synovium. An incomplete synovectomy is likely to lead to the development of a local recurrence.[12,13] The authors prefer arthroscopic treatment of PVNS due to the advantages mentioned previously.

Surgical principles

Prior to performing a synovectomy in a patient with inflammatory arthritis, the surgeon must eliminate all other possible causes of pain. Cervical spine pathology must be excluded, especially in patients with rheumatoid arthritis. Occasionally, the subacromial bursa may be the primary site of involvement in patients with inflammatory arthritis.[2] Also, the acromioclavicular and sternoclavicular joints can be symptomatic. A thorough history and physical examination, as well as responses to selective anesthetic injections, will guide the surgeon in determining the appropriate surgical procedure. When necessary, a concomitant subacromial decompression or distal clavicle excision can be performed in addition to the arthroscopic synovectomy.

The synovium of the glenohumeral joint encompasses the entire joint and then exits the joint with the biceps tendon extending beyond the transverse humeral ligament.[4] Thus, in order to expose diseased synovium distal to the superior portion of the transverse humeral ligament, the biceps tendon must be pulled into the shoulder joint. This can be performed using an arthroscopic probe. Then the diseased synovium can be carefully debrided, taking care to avoid injuring the biceps tendon.

In these patients, visualization during arthroscopy can be difficult due to marked synovial proliferation and extensive bleeding generated during the synovectomy. An infusion pump is used throughout the case to ensure adequate joint distension. Joint distension greatly enhances visualization while the hydrostatic pressure helps to control bleeding. To further minimize bleeding, the 3000-ml saline bags used for inflow during the surgery contain 1:10 000 epinephrine. If a subacromial decompression is planned, 30 ml 0.25% marcaine with epinephrine is injected into the subacromial space at the onset of the procedure. In addition, the authors use an electrocautery device (VAPR, Mitek Products, Westwood, MA, USA) to perform the synovectomy, and simultaneously maintain hemostasis. Meticulous hemostasis is critically important to avoid uncontrollable bleeding and compromised visualization. Finally, mild hypotensive anesthesia will help reduce bleeding.

Loose body removal in patients with synovial osteochondromatosis can be technically difficult. The loose bodies are generally found in the anterior and posterior portions of the axillary pouch.[4] A suction cannula can be used to rapidly remove smaller loose bodies. Larger loose bodies must be individually removed using a grasper. Depending on the size of the nodules, the portals may need to be enlarged to allow for easy extraction through the skin. A thorough inspection of the glenohumeral joint is necessary at the completion of the procedure to document thorough removal of the loose bodies. Intraoperative radiographs should be obtained as loose bodies may migrate into spaces not necessarily seen from a routine posterior portal (i.e. subscapularis bursa).

Surgical technique

The authors' preferred method of anesthesia is a regional interscalene block, which avoids the morbidity of general anesthesia and provides excellent postoperative pain relief. Standard beach chair positioning is used as it allows for unrestricted movement of the arm in all planes. Examination under anesthesia will determine the preoperative range of motion. The entire upper extremity is prepared and draped in a sterile fashion to ensure that the involved shoulder is exposed within the operative field. The acromion, clavicle, acromioclavicular joint, and coracoid process are outlined using a marking pen. Then standard posterior, lateral, and anterior portals are drawn. The portal sites are infiltrated with 2 ml 1% lidocaine with epinephrine.

If a subacromial decompression is planned, 30 ml 0.25% marcaine with epinephrine is injected into the subacromial space to minimize bleeding during the decompression. With some gentle traction applied to the arm by an assistant, the posterior portal is established for the arthroscopic camera. Joint distension is

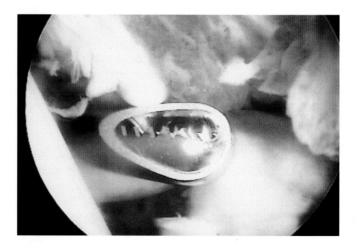

Figure 39.2

Intraoperative photograph of the glenohumeral joint in a patient with rheumatoid arthritis demonstrating diffusely hyperemic synovium.

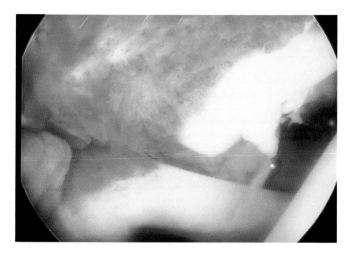

Figure 39.3

Hyperemic, hypertrophic synovium is seen partially extending down the bicipital tendon sheath of the same patient from Figure 39.2.

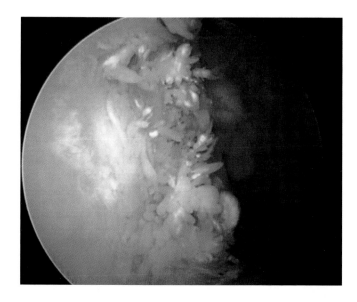

Figure 39.4

Intraoperative photograph demonstrating multiple fine rice-bodies attached to synovium in this patient with rheumatoid arthritis.

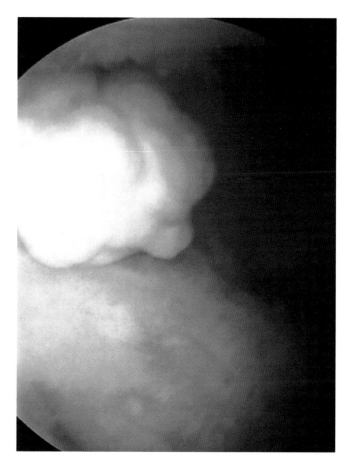

Figure 39.5

This large loose body was one of many found in the axillary recess of the patient whose radiograph is shown in Figure 39.1.

maintained using an infusion pump with inflow through the arthroscopic cannula. Upon entrance into the glenohumeral joint, the degree of synovial inflammation and/or hypertrophy is evaluated and documented with arthroscopic pictures. Again, visualization may be difficult due to synovial proliferation and bleeding. Joint distension and meticulous hemostasis will facilitate satisfactory visualization. Next, the anterior portal is created by placing a cannula in the rotator interval.

A systematic, thorough, arthroscopic examination of the glenohumeral joint is then performed. In patients with rheumatoid arthritis and other systemic arthritides, the synovium will be hyperemic causing the entire joint to appear red (Figure 39.2). Hypertrophic finger-like synovial villi may be seen, and can extend down the bicipital tendon sheath (Figure 39.3). Also, multiple fine, loose rice-bodies may be prominent (Figure 39.4).

With synovial osteochondromatosis, multiple loose bodies will be found predominantly in the axillary recess (Figure 39.5). In these patients, it is particularly important to document the degree of degenerative joint disease that exists as a result of third-body wear. In PVNS, the synovial fluid will be a bloody dark brown color mimicking a hemorrhagic effusion. In addition, the surgeon will encounter diffuse hypertrophic synovitis with long entangled synovial villi.

The diagnostic arthroscopy should also include an evaluation of the status of the rotator cuff (particularly important in patients with rheumatoid arthritis), biceps tendon, labrum, and glenohumeral ligaments. Any associated pathology identified during the glenohumeral arthroscopy is then addressed accordingly.

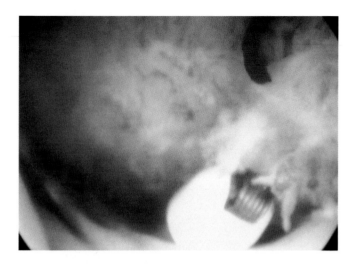

Figure 39.6

Intraoperative photograph, taken after debridement with an electrocautery, of the same patient from Figures 39.2 and 39.3.

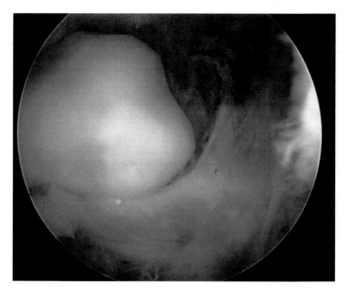

Figure 39.7

Intraoperative photograph of a loose body during extraction with a grasper via the anterior portal.

A complete arthroscopic synovectomy is then performed using anterior and posterior portals. Initially, the arthroscope is placed posteriorly and the electrocautery is brought into the joint via the anterior portal. The electrocautery is used to debride the hypertrophic, hyperemic synovium while, simultaneously, maintaining hemostasis. The majority of the synovium can be resected with the electrocautery in the anterior portal (Figure 39.6). If necessary, an arthroscopic synovial resector can be used to debride redundant synovial tissue. However, once a bleeding vessel is identified, the surgeon must stop debridement with the synovial resector and achieve hemostasis to ensure continued visualization. The biceps tendon should be brought into the joint to allow the surgeon to debride the synovium that is distal to the superior border of the transverse humeral ligament. During the synovectomy, the electrocautery should be placed on the synovium gently and quickly. The synovium must be thoroughly debrided, taking care, however, to avoid injuring the overlying rotator cuff and biceps tendon.

Access to the posterosuperior portion of the glenohumeral joint may be difficult when viewing posteriorly. To adequately debride this synovium, the arthroscope is placed through the anterior portal with the electrocautery posterior. If the axillary recess is severely involved, an accessory posterior portal is made 1.5-cm inferior and 0.5-cm lateral to the original posterior portal.[2] The axillary recess can be debrided from the accessory posterior portal while viewing from the standard posterior portal.

Arthroscopic loose body removal in synovial osteochondromatosis can be technically difficult. The majority of the loose bodies are found in the dependent axillary pouch. The smaller loose bodies can be rapidly removed with the use of a suction cannula. However, larger loose bodies must be individually removed using

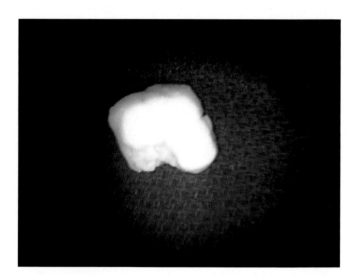

Figure 39.8

The same loose body from Figure 39.7 required the anterior portal be enlarged 1.5 cm for extraction through the skin.

a grasper (Figure 39.7). If necessary, an accessory posteroinferior portal can be created (see above) to provide easier access to the axillary pouch. In this case, the arthroscope is placed in the standard portal while the grasper is utilized though the accessory portal. In addition, depending on the size of the cartilaginous nodules, the portals may need to be enlarged to allow for simple extraction through the skin (Figure 39.8). After removal of the loose bodies, a thorough inspection of the glenohumeral joint is required to document complete removal.

A subacromial decompression is performed in patients with inflammatory synovitis whose pain is preoperatively identified to originate in the subacromial bursa. The subacromial space is visualized by redirecting the arthroscope through the posterior portal above the rotator cuff. The electrocautery is used either through the anterior or lateral portals to debride the subacromial space. The inflamed, hypertrophic bursa as well as the multiple fine rice-like bodies, if present, are removed. After debridement, the coracoacromial ligament is detached from its acromial insertion and a portion of the ligament may be excised using a grasper and electrocautery. It is critical not to detach the coracoacromial ligament in patients with large to massive rotator cuff tears as the ligament serves as a passive restraint to proximal humeral migration. Then, a standard acromioplasty can be performed if a subacromial spur exists. The authors use a 5.5-mm arthroscopic acromionizer blade (Smith & Nephew Dyonics, Andover, MA, USA) for the acromioplasty.

The acromioclavicular joint becomes painful in approximately 33% of patients with rheumatoid arthritis, and may become symptomatic in patients with other systemic arthritides.[7] An arthroscopic distal clavicle excision can be performed after the synovectomy and subacromial decompression. Accurate outlines of the osseous landmarks around the shoulder facilitate proper anterior portal placement. If a distal clavicle excision is planned, the anterior portal must be made directly in line with the acromioclavicular joint. This allows the surgeon to evenly resect the distal clavicle. With the arthroscope in the lateral or posterior portal and an arthroscopic burr in the anterior portal, the distal clavicle can be debrided. The authors use the same burr for the distal clavicle excision as for the acromioplasty. Manual downward pressure on the distal clavicle combined with a gentle upward force on the burr effectively resects the distal clavicle. If necessary, 2–4 mm of medial acromion can be debrided to facilitate visualization of the distal clavicle and acromioclavicular joint. Optimally, 6–8 mm of distal clavicle is resected. The surgeon must be sure to resect the entire distal clavicle, as it can be difficult to debride the posterior and superior aspects of the distal clavicle. Also, it is important to preserve the superior acromioclavicular joint ligaments and capsule to maintain acromioclavicular joint stability in the anteroposterior plane.

Postoperative protocol

Unless an associated rotator cuff tear is repaired, an accelerated postoperative rehabilitation program is recommended. A sling is used postoperatively for comfort only. Pendulum exercises are begun on the first postoperative day. Active-assisted and active range of motion exercises are performed without limitations. For the first 6 weeks, regaining full range of motion is emphasized. Strength and resistance exercises are added once a full range of motion is achieved. If a rotator cuff repair is performed, standard postoperative rotator cuff rehabilitation protocols are followed.

References

1. Connor PM, D'Alessandro DF. Inflammatory arthritis of the shoulder. *Orthopaedic Knowledge Update: Shoulder and Elbow* 1997; **24**:215–25.
2. Matthews LS, LaBudde JK. Arthroscopic treatment of synovial diseases of the shoulder. *Orthop Clin North Am* 1993; **24**:101–9.
3. Richman JD, Rose DJ. The role of arthroscopy in the management of synovial chondromatosis of the shoulder: a case report. *Clin Orthop* 1990; **257**:91–3.
4. Neviaser TJ. Arthroscopy of the shoulder. *Orthop Clin North Am* 1987; **18**:361–72.
5. Ogilvie-Harris DJ, Wiley AM. Arthroscopic surgery of the shoulder. *J Bone Joint Surg* 1986; **68B**:201–7.
6. Petersson CJ. Shoulder surgery in rheumatoid arthritis. *Acta Orthop Scand* 1986; **57**:222–6.
7. Petersson CJ. The acromioclavicular joint in rheumatoid arthritis. *Clin Orthop* 1987; **223**:86–93.
8. Hjelkrem M, Stanish WD. Synovial chondrometaplasia of the shoulder: a case report of a young athlete presenting with shoulder pain. *Am J Sports Med* 1988; **16**:84–6.
9. Witwity T, Uhlmann R, Nagy MH et al. Shoulder rheumatoid arthritis associated with chondromatosis, treated by arthroscopy: a case report. *Arthroscopy* 1991; **7**:233–6.
10. Satterlee CC. Osteonecrosis and other noninflammatory degenerative diseases of the glenohumeral joint including Gaucher's disease, sickle cell disease, hemochromatosis, and synovial osteochondromatosis. *Orthopaedic Knowledge Update: Shoulder and Elbow* 1997; **26**:233–40.
11. France MP, Gupta SK. Nonhemophilic hemosiderotic synovitis of the shoulder: a case report. *Clin Orthop* 1991; **262**:132–6.
12. Uhthoff HK, Sano H, Loehr JF. Calcifying tendonitis, chondrocalcinosis, heterotopic ossification, and pigmented villonodular synovitis. *Orthopaedic Knowledge Update: Shoulder and Elbow* 1997; **31**:277–87.
13. Flandry F, Hughston JC. Pigmented villonodular synovitis. *J Bone Joint Surg* 1987; **69A**:942–9.

40 Scapulothoracic bursoscopy

Michael P Staebler and Leslie S Matthews

Introduction

The normal scapulothoracic anatomy consists of the large, relatively flat scapula with its several muscular attachments, the chest wall, and the scapulothoracic bursae. Normally, the scapula glides smoothly over the congruent surface of the convex chest wall. It is cushioned from the uneven surface of the ribs by the serratus anterior and subscapularis muscles. The superior, medial, and inferior borders of the scapula are somewhat less protected by subscapular bursae at the superomedial angle between serratus anterior and the subscapularis muscles, between the serratus anterior muscle and the lateral chest wall, and at the inferior angle of the scapula.[1] The smooth motion of the scapula over the thorax may be adversely affected by a variety of pathologic processes resulting in the snapping scapula syndrome.

Etiology

First described in 1867 by Boinet,[2] snapping scapula syndrome may be defined as a palpable or audible crepi-

tus within the scapulothoracic articulation produced by movement of the scapula over the thorax. The etiology of this syndrome is multifactorial and can be divided into intrinsic and extrinsic causes as shown in the classification scheme in Table 40.1.[3] Intrinsic causes are further divided into two subsets: (1) anatomical abnormalities of the articulation, including osteochondroma,[4-8] rib or scapular fracture malunion,[4,6,7] 'rhinoceros horn-like' inferolateral border of the scapula,[9] muscle insertion avulsions causing calcifications,[10] and bone or soft tissue tumors occurring at the scapulothoracic articulation; and (2) primary idiopathic causes, either bursal inflammation/thickening or posttraumatic.

Extrinsic causes of snapping scapula are secondary to other underlying shoulder conditions and include rotator cuff disease, glenohumeral or acromioclavicular arthritis, adhesive capsulitis, instability, and fracture or posttraumatic conditions. Any of these primary conditions can lead to a compensatory overuse of the scapulothoracic motion and a resultant subscapular bursitis.

Patient evaluation

Patients presenting with snapping scapula syndrome should have a complete work-up including a proper history, physical examination and appropriate radiographs to help identify the source of the problem. Radiographic evaluation should include a lateral scapular 'Y view' of the shoulder in order to demonstrate the scapulothoracic articulation and any bony abnormalities that might be present (Figure 40.1). If the diagnosis is still unclear, computed tomography (CT) or magnetic resonance imaging (MRI) may prove helpful to rule out anatomical lesions. If no anatomical lesions are found on radiographic or clinical exam, it is important for the treating physician to look specifically for any underlying primary shoulder girdle pathology and treat this before aggressive management of a secondary scapulothoracic bursitis. Successful treatment of the primary problem will often result in resolution of the secondary snapping scapula syndrome.

It is important to recognize those patients who present with subscapular pain without associated scapulothoracic crepitus. These patients do not have snapping scapula syndrome and other sources for their pain should be carefully investigated. Other sources may include primary cardiac, intra-abdominal or intrathoracic pathology, thoracic disc herniation, or primary or metastatic neoplasm.[3]

Table 40.1 Classification of snapping scapula syndrome etiologies. Adapted from Matthews et al.[3]

Intrinsic
  Anatomic abnormalities
    Osteochondroma
    Rib or scapula fracture malunion
    Muscle insertion avulsion, calcification
    Primary bone or soft-tissue neoplasm
    Sprengel's deformity
    Luschka's tubercle exostosis
    'Rhinoceros horn' inferolateral scapular border
  Primary
    Idiopathic—inflammation
    Idiopathic—posttraumatic
Extrinsic: secondary to other forms of first-degree shoulder girdle pathology
    Acromioclavicular or glenohumeral arthritis
    Rotator cuff disease
    Adhesive capsulitis
    Fracture—posttraumatic
    Instability

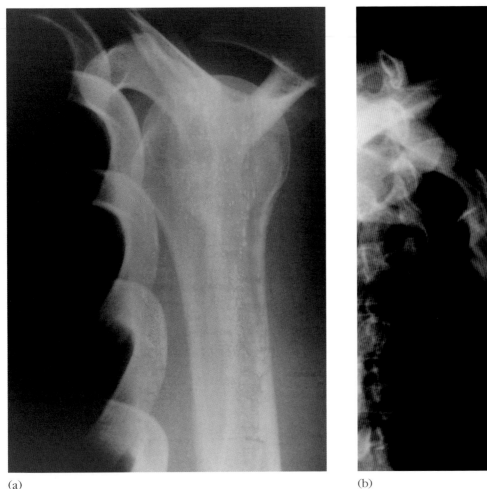

(a)

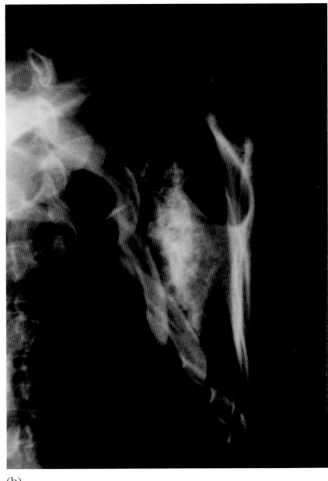

(b)

Figure 40.1

Radiographic Y views of the scapula. (a) Normal scapula and scapulothoracic articulation. (b) Large osteochondroma within the scapulothoracic articulation.

Treatment options

Proper treatment of snapping scapula syndrome depends on the etiology. Patients with extrinsic scapulothoracic bursitis should be managed by treatment of the underlying shoulder pathology. In all other patients, a trial of conservative management including rest, non-steroidal anti-inflammatory medication, activity modification, physical therapy to strengthen the scapular stabilizers, ultrasound therapy, and corticosteroid injections should be instituted as most patients will improve with these treatment modalities. Indications for surgery include failure of conservative treatment or in those patients who have a recognized anatomical lesion. Historically, surgical treatment has been performed via open techniques;[1,4,6,7] partial scapulectomy, removal of documented bony abnormalities of the scapulothoracic space, and open excision of thickened subscapular bursal tissue have all been reported as successful treatment methods for such conditions. Recently, there have

been two reports of endoscopic management of snapping scapula through resection of bursal adhesions[11] and bony resection of a prominent superomedial corner[12] with good functional outcomes.

Surgical principles

Safe and effective arthroscopic treatment of snapping scapula syndrome requires a clear understanding of the gross and arthroscopic anatomy of the scapulothoracic articulation. Improper technique can potentially lead to neurovascular injury or even penetration of the thoracic cavity.

Anatomic dissection by Ruland et al[13] has demonstrated a midline origin for the horizontal fibers of the trapezius muscle, which insert onto the superior lip of the crest of the scapular spine. The levator scapulae attaches at the superior medial border of the scapula.

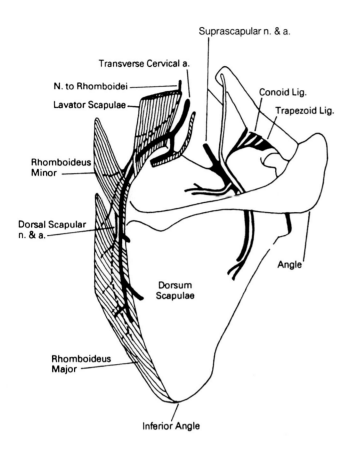

Figure 40.2

Illustration of the relationships of periscapular neurovascular structures.

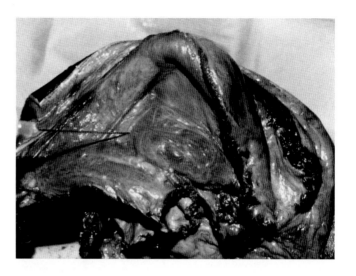

Figure 40.3

Anatomic specimen with scapula elevated from chest wall. Air insufflation demonstrates large subscapular bursa.

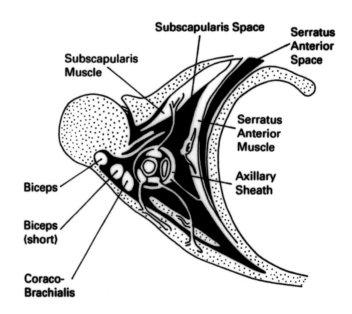

Figure 40.4

Cross-section of the axilla showing the boundaries of the serratus anterior and subscapularis spaces.

The spinal accessory nerve crosses laterally within the midsection of the muscle along the superior angle of the scapula, coursing deep to the trapezius muscle. The transverse cervical artery is divided by the levator scapulae and contains a deep branch, the dorsal scapular artery, and a superficial branch that travels with the accessory nerve (Figure 40.2). The dorsal scapular nerve and artery course along the vertebral border of the scapula deep to the rhomboid major and minor muscles, providing innervation and blood supply to both of these muscles. The rhomboid muscle fibers pass in an inferior and lateral direction to insert on the medial border of the scapula. The inferior border of the rhomboid minor lies at the level of the scapular spine. The rhomboid major inserts into the posterior surface of the medial border of the scapula from the rhomboid minor inferiorly to the inferior angle of the scapula. The serratus anterior muscle originates from the ribs of the anterior lateral wall of the thorax and inserts on the medial border of the scapula. The long thoracic nerve, which innervates the serratus anterior, lies anterolaterally on the surface of this muscle. The subscapularis muscle, which originates from the subscapularis fossa, covers most of the anterior surface of the scapular body. The axillary space, fat, and neurovascular structures lie anterior and

inferior. A large space and its bursa are located between the serratus anterior and the chest wall (Figure 40.3). This space is referred to as the serratus anterior space. The lateral extent of the serratus anterior bursa is the origin of the serratus anterior and is closely adherent to the ribs and serratus anterior muscle throughout the length of the scapula. A second, smaller subscapularis space has been identified between the scapular insertion of the serratus anterior and the subscapularis muscle extending laterally to the axilla. The axillary neurovascular contents are found within this space (Figure 40.4).[3]

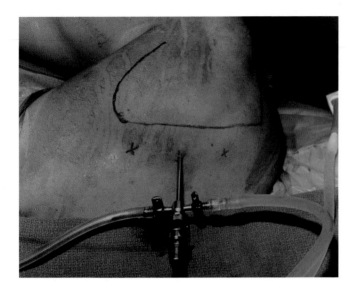

Figure 40.5

Photograph of the left shoulder in the lateral decubitus position demonstrates appropriate portal placement for subscapular bursoscopy.

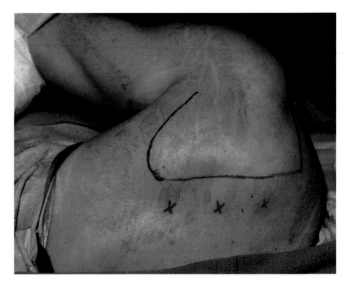

Figure 40.6

Photograph of left shoulder demonstrating optimum 'chicken wing' position to maximize scapular winging for access to the scapulothoracic bursa.

Proper portal placement in scapulothoracic bursoscopy requires that the surgeon understand the above described anatomic relationships. The superior portal is placed just below the level of the scapular spine in the interval between the rhomboid minor and major and passes though the trapezius muscle before entering the serratus anterior space. This portal provides access to the superior medial angle of the scapula. Portal placement at the superior angle should be avoided due to the close proximity of the dorsal scapular nerve and artery, the spinal accessory nerve, and the transverse cervical artery. It must be emphasized that the posterolateral boundary of the serratus anterior space is the serratus anterior muscle fibers. Penetration of these fibers with the arthroscope or operating instruments will result in penetration of the subscapularis space, placing the axillary neurovascular structures at risk for injury. Additional portals can be placed at the inferior medial border of the scapula and at a position midway between this and the first portal placement (Figure 40.5). It is important to note that all portals should be placed 2–3 cm medial to the vertebral border of the scapula to avoid injury to the dorsal scapular artery and nerve.

Surgical technique

We prefer to position our patients in the lateral decubitus position to enable complete glenohumeral and subacromial arthroscopy prior to scapulothoracic bursoscopy. The prone position has been described for scapulothoracic bursoscopy and is a reasonable alternative but it precludes the ability to perform concomitant shoulder arthroscopy.[11,12] The procedure is begun with the patient in a standard lateral decubitus position with the affected arm suspended in 5–10 lbs of skin traction. Standard glenohumeral and subacromial arthroscopic evaluation is first performed to rule out pathology in these areas. In the absence of shoulder or subacromial pathology, the surgeon can proceed with scapulothoracic bursoscopy.

After completion of the shoulder arthroscopy, the arm is removed from skin traction. The bean bag used to support the patient in the lateral decubitus position is deflated, allowing the patient to be repositioned in an anterior-oblique orientation. The shoulder is then extended and maximally internally rotated ('chicken wing position') (Figure 40.6) to maximize winging of the scapula. A spinal needle is directed into the serratus anterior space, beginning midway between the spine of the scapula and the inferior medial angle at a point 2–3 cm medial to the vertebral border. The serratus anterior space is distended with fluid to facilitate entry with the arthroscope. A stab incision is made through skin and a blunt obturator and arthroscope sleeve are introduced into the serratus anterior space. Care must be taken not to penetrate through the serratus anterior muscle into the subscapular space with its neurovascular contents as injury to these structures may occur (Figure 40.7).

Once visualization is achieved through the midscapular portal, additional superior and inferior portals can be created at the level of the scapular spine and at the

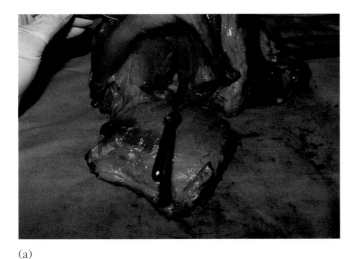

(a)

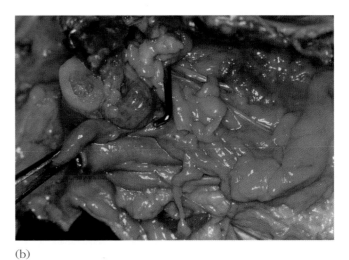

(b)

Figure 40.7

The subscapularis space. (a) Probe placed on lateral chest wall with tip in the subscapularis space. (b) Ribs of posterior and lateral chest wall elevated, showing proximity of the same probe to the axillary space fat and axillary sheath contents.

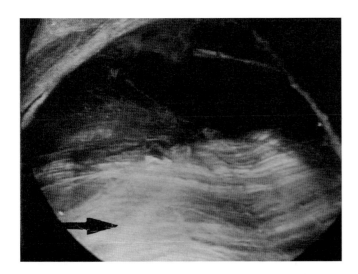

Figure 40.8

Arthroscopic view of the serratus anterior space.

inferior medial angle, respectively. Introduction of a spinal needle at accessory portal sites helps facilitate triangulation and the appropriate angle of insertion to avoid chest wall penetration.

Landmarks for orientation are few within the serratus anterior space; the undulating chest wall is the best landmark (Figure 40.8). The use of a multielectrode bipolar wand (ArthroCare, Sunnyvale, CA, USA) and motorized shaver can then be used to perform a complete bursectomy or bony debridement if necessary. As with any endoscopic procedure, bleeding control is extremely important to allow adequate visualization. This is accomplished with a combination of adequate fluid pressure within the arthroscopic field, dilute epinephrine in the irrigation fluid, and electrocautery. After surgery the portals are closed in a standard fashion and the arm is placed in a sling for comfort.

Postoperative protocol

Patients are allowed to begin range of motion immediately after surgery as symptoms allow. We routinely enroll patients in a physical therapy program to help achieve full range of motion and regain full strength of scapular stabilizers and rotator cuff musculature. Return to full activity and sports may be allowed once these parameters are met.

References

1. Sisto DJ, Jobe FW. The operative treatment of scapulothoracic bursitis in professional pitchers. *Am J Sports Med* 1986; **14**:192–4.
2. Boinet. *Bull Soc Imperiale de chir* 1867; **2**:458.
3. Matthews LS, Poehling GG, Hunter DM. Scapulothoracic endoscopy: anatomical and clinical considerations. In: McGinty JB, Caspari RB, Jackson RW, Poehling GG, eds. *Operative Arthroscopy*. 2nd edn. Philadelphia: Lippincott-Raven; 1996: 813–20.
4. Butters KP. The scapula. In: Rockwood CA, Matsen FA III, eds. *The Shoulder*. 2nd edn. Philadelphia: WB Saunders; 1998: 391–427.
5. Cooley LH, Torg JS. 'Pseudowinging' of the scapula secondary to subscapular osteochondroma. *Clin Orthop* 1982; **162**:119–24.

6. Milch H. Snapping scapula. *Clin Orthop* 1961; **20**:139–50.

7. Milch H. Partial scapulectomy for snapping of the scapula. *J Bone Joint Surg* 1950; **32A**:561–6.

8. Parsons TA. The snapping scapula and subscapular exostoses. *J Bone Joint Surg* 1973; **55B**:345–9.

9. Edelson JG. Variations in the anatomy of the scapula with reference to the snapping scapula. *Clin Orthop* 1996; **322**:111–15.

10. Strizak AM, Cowen MH. The snapping scapula syndrome: a case report. *J Bone Joint Surg* 1982; **64A**:941–2.

11. Ciullo JV. Subscapular bursitis: treatment of 'snapping scapula' or 'washboard syndrome'. *Arthroscopy* 1992; **8**:412–13.

12. Harper GD, McIlroy S, Bayley JIL, Calvert PT. Arthroscopic partial resection of the scapula for snapping scapula: a new technique. *J Shoulder Elbow Surg* 1999; **8**:53–7.

13. Ruland LJ, Ruland CM, Matthews LS. Scapulothoracic anatomy for the arthroscopist. *Arthroscopy* 1995; **11**:52–6.

Index